Diagnostic Pathology of Hematopoietic Disorders of Spleen and Liver

AF382406

Ling Zhang • Haipeng Shao • Serhan Alkan
Editors

Diagnostic Pathology of Hematopoietic Disorders of Spleen and Liver

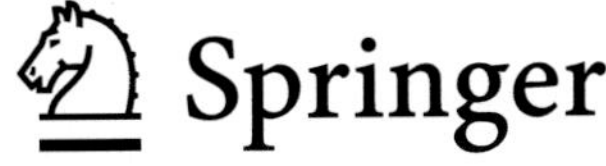

Springer

Editors
Ling Zhang
Department of Pathology
Moffitt Cancer Center
Tampa, FL
USA

Haipeng Shao
Department of Pathology
Moffitt Cancer Center
Tampa, FL
USA

Serhan Alkan
Department of Pathology
Cedars-Sinai Medical Center
Los Angeles, CA
USA

ISBN 978-3-030-37710-6   ISBN 978-3-030-37708-3   (eBook)
https://doi.org/10.1007/978-3-030-37708-3

© Springer Nature Switzerland AG 2020
This work is subject to copyright. All rights are reserved by the Publisher, whether the whole or part of the material is concerned, specifically the rights of translation, reprinting, reuse of illustrations, recitation, broadcasting, reproduction on microfilms or in any other physical way, and transmission or information storage and retrieval, electronic adaptation, computer software, or by similar or dissimilar methodology now known or hereafter developed.
The use of general descriptive names, registered names, trademarks, service marks, etc. in this publication does not imply, even in the absence of a specific statement, that such names are exempt from the relevant protective laws and regulations and therefore free for general use.
The publisher, the authors and the editors are safe to assume that the advice and information in this book are believed to be true and accurate at the date of publication. Neither the publisher nor the authors or the editors give a warranty, expressed or implied, with respect to the material contained herein or for any errors or omissions that may have been made. The publisher remains neutral with regard to jurisdictional claims in published maps and institutional affiliations.

This Springer imprint is published by the registered company Springer Nature Switzerland AG
The registered company address is: Gewerbestrasse 11, 6330 Cham, Switzerland

This book is dedicated to my spouse, Jianmin Huang.
Without his support, this would not be possible.

– Ling Zhang

The book is dedicated to my family.

– Haipeng Shao

This book is dedicated to my wife, Dilek Alkan, who supported me
throughout my career and made this journey possible.

– Serhan Alkan

Preface

The diagnosis of hematopoietic neoplasms in the spleen and liver remains a challenge for many pathologists. Misinterpretation or misdiagnosis could occur due to an incomplete work-up in splenic or hepatic biopsies as well as in specimens post whole splenectomy. Biopsies are not usually obtained for primary diagnosis of hematopoietic neoplasms, as the diagnosis is most frequently made on other tissues, such as lymph nodes, peripheral blood, or bone marrows. Splenectomy is indicated mostly for therapeutic intervention rather than diagnostic purposes. Therefore, many practicing pathologists are challenged with the morphologic features and diagnostic approaches of hematopoietic disorders in the spleen and liver, especially of the rarer entities.

Following the emergence of modern diagnostic technology, e.g., next-generation sequencing (NGS), over the last decades, scientists have new insights into the pathogenesis of many hematopoietic disorders, benign or malignant. Many novel markers have been introduced to diagnosis, risk stratification, and prognostication. With the publication of the revised fourth edition of *WHO Classification of Tumours of Haematopoietic and Lymphoid Tissues* in 2017, we considered it would be timely to compile a new book on the current pathologic diagnosis of hematopoietic neoplasms in the spleen and liver. While a number of books have been published previously on this subject, significant progresses have been made on disease subclassification that requires integration of highly complex immunophenotypic and molecular features of a variety of common and rare hematopoietic neoplasms involving the spleen or liver. The objective of this book is to provide a comprehensive and most up-to-date overview of the pathologic features of common benign and malignant hematopoietic disorders in the spleen and liver for practicing pathologists, hematopathologists, and clinicians.

The authors are from large academic centers, affiliated teaching hospitals, and central referral clinics and are experienced in the diagnosis of hematopoietic disorders, not limited in the spleen and liver. In this book, we tried to cover the majority of diagnosing hematopoietic disorders in the spleen and liver. The book consists of 21 chapters. Chapters 1, 2, and 3 are devoted to normal histologic features, conventional, cytogenetic, and molecular studies necessary for the diagnosis of hematopoietic disorders in the spleen and liver. Chapters 4, 5, 6, 7, 8, 9, 10, 11, 12, 13, 14, 15, 16, and 17 cover the primary and secondary mature B- and T-/NK-cell lymphomas, Hodgkin lymphoma, B- and T-cell lymphoblastic leukemias, myeloid neoplasms, histiocytic and dendritic neoplasms, and common posttransplant disorders including graft versus host disease (GvHD) and posttransplant lymphoproliferative disorders in brief. Chapters 19, 20, and 21 encompass red blood cell disorders, other benign hematologic disorders, and infectious/inflammatory disorders that could mimic hematopoietic neoplasms. The histopathologic, cytogenetic, and molecular features of different disease entities are discussed in detail. To serve as a quick reference for pathologists, we have formatted most chapters on specific hematopoietic neoplasms to comprise epidemiology, etiology, pathogenesis, morphology, immunophenotyping, molecular genetics, prognosis, and brief treatment guidelines. The contents in the book are largely updated according to the most recent publications. Diagnostic caveats are included in the majority of book chapters in order to have a quick review of the key points in each chapter.

Compared with previous books, our book covers most, if not all, of the benign and malignant hematopoietic disorders in the spleen and liver. It is our sincere hope that general pathologists and hematopathologists will find this book practical and useful for their practice. The book would also benefit clinicians and researchers who are interested in hematology and hepatosplenic system.

Tampa, FL, USA   Ling Zhang
Tampa, FL, USA   Haipeng Shao
Los Angeles, CA, USA   Serhan Alkan

Contents

Contributors

Saba Fatima Ali, MD Department of Pathology and Laboratory Medicine, City of Hope National Medical Center, Duarte, CA, USA

Serhan Alkan Department of Pathology and Laboratory Medicine, Cedars-Sinai Medical Center, Los Angeles, CA, USA

Pukhraz Basra, MD Department of Pathology, H. Lee Moffitt Cancer Center and Research Institute, Tampa, FL, USA

Lugen Chen, MD, PhD Department of Pathology, Tampa General Hospital, Tampa, FL, USA

Wei Chen, MD Department of Pathology, Brigham and Women's Hospital, Harvard Medical School, Boston, MA, USA

Ahmet Dogan, MD, PhD Department of Pathology, Memorial Sloan Kettering Cancer Center, Hematopathology Service, New York, NY, USA

Michelle Don, MS, MD Department of Pathology and Laboratory Medicine, Cedars-Sinai Medical Center, Los Angeles, CA, USA

Andrew G. Evans, MD, PhD Department of Pathology and Laboratory Medicine, Strong Memorial Hospital, University of Rochester Medical Center, Rochester, NY, USA

David C. Gajzer, MD Department of Pathology, H. Lee Moffitt Cancer Center and Research Institute, Tampa, FL, USA

Karthik Ganapathi, MBBS, PhD Department of Laboratory Medicine, University of California, San Francisco, CA, USA

Raul S. Gonzalez, MD Department of Pathology, Beth Israel Deaconess Medical Center, Boston, MA, USA

Maha Guindi, MD, FRCPC Department of Pathology and Laboratory Medicine, Cedars-Sinai Medical Center, Los Angeles, CA, USA

Qin Huang, MD, PhD Department of Pathology and Laboratory Medicine, Cedars-Sinai Medical Center, Los Angeles, CA, USA

Mohammad Hussaini, MD Department of Pathology, H. Lee Moffitt Cancer Center and Research Institute, Tampa, FL, USA

Brent K. Larson, DO Department of Pathology and Laboratory Medicine, Cedars-Sinai Medical Center, Los Angeles, CA, USA

Pei Lin, MD Department of Hematopathology, University of Texas MD Anderson Cancer Center, Houston, TX, USA

Elizabeth Margolskee, MD, MPH Department of Pathology and Laboratory Medicine, Weill Cornell Medical College/New York Presbyterian Hospital, New York, NY, USA

Madhu P. Menon, MD, PhD Department of Pathology and Laboratory Medicine, Henry Ford Hospital, Detroit, MI, USA

Lynh Nguyen, MD Department of Pathology and Laboratory Medicine, James A. Haley Veterans' Hospital, Tampa, FL, USA

Attilio Orazi, MD Department of Pathology, Texas Tech University Health Sciences Center El Paso, El Paso, Texas, USA

Deniz Peker, MD Department of Pathology and Laboratory Medicine, Emory University, Atlanta, GA, USA

Xin Qing, MD, PhD Hematopathology and Hematology Laboratory, Department of Pathology, Harbor-UCLA Medical Center, Torrance, CA, USA

Haipeng Shao, MD, PhD Department of Pathology, H. Lee Moffitt Cancer Center and Research Institute, Tampa, FL, USA

Rohit Sharma, MD Diagnostic Molecular Pathology, Memorial Sloan Kettering Cancer Center, New York, NY, USA

Min Shi, MD, PhD Department of Laboratory Medicine and Pathology, Mayo Clinic, Rochester, MN, USA

Jinming Song, MD, PhD Department of Pathology, H. Lee Moffitt Cancer Center and Research Institute, Tampa, FL, USA

Joo Young Song, MD Department of Pathology and Laboratory Medicine, City of Hope National Medical Center, Duarte, CA, USA

Nukhet Tuzuner, MD Department of Pathology, Istanbul University Cerrahpasa Medical Faculty, Fatih-Aksaray, Turkey

Mariko Yabe, MD, PhD Department of Pathology, Memorial Sloan Kettering Cancer Center, Hematopathology Service, New York, NY, USA

Changjun Yue, MD, PhD Department of Medical Affair, Covance Clinical Trial, Los Angeles, Los Angeles, CA, USA

Ling Zhang, MD Department of Pathology, H. Lee Moffitt Cancer Center and Research Institute, Tampa, FL, USA

Xiaohui Zhang, MD, PhD Department of Pathology, H. Lee Moffitt Cancer Center and Research Institute, Tampa, FL, USA

Lynh Nguyen and Ling Zhang

Spleen

Anatomy

The spleen is the largest lymphatic organ in the body and lies just below the diaphragm in the left upper quadrant of the posterior peritoneal cavity adjacent to the left lower ribs, stomach, left kidney, tail of the pancreas, and colon [1]. It is usually not palpable on physical examination, but may be felt in children, adolescents, and thin adults [2]. However, because the spleen moves with respiration it may be best palpated when enlarged at the end of inspiration. The organ is extremely vulnerable to injury especially when the body experiences external trauma. Accessory spleens or spleniculi, in which a small nodule of splenic tissue is found outside the spleen proper, are not uncommon. They can form during embryological development or as a result of trauma and can be visualized and mistaken for a lymph node on imaging or be a site of recurrent disease in cases where treatment requires splenectomy.

The capsule of spleen is composed of thin dense connective tissue lined by mesothelial cells. The trabeculae project from the splenic capsule and cross the splenic parenchyma along with blood vessels and nerves [2]. These trabeculae form a robust framework to support the surrounding fine reticulin meshwork found throughout the splenic parenchyma.

The spleen is supplied by the splenic artery and is drained by the splenic vein [1, 3]. Together the splenic artery, splenic vein, and accompanying nerves and lymphatics enter and leave the spleen through the hilum. The splenic artery branches repeatedly as it pierces the hilum becoming trabecular arteries within the trabecular septum. As the artery leaves the trabeculae, it is infiltrated by a sheath of lymphocytes called the periarterial lymphatic sheath (PALS) and becomes the central artery. The central arteries further subdivide into follicular arterioles that supply the lymphoid nodules of the splenic white pulp or subdivide into penicillar arteries that enter the red pulp, delivering blood to the splenic sinuses. Portions of the penicillar arteries are surrounded by macrophages and are referred to as Schweigger-Seidel sheaths, which are considered the first part of the splenic filtration system [2, 4, 5].

The peculiar cells that line the splenic sinuses have contractile microfilaments that create gaps between the cells and control the passage of erythrocytes. Under normal circumstances, red blood cells are able to pass through these gaps or slits; however, erythrocytes with rigid inclusions or less deformable cell membranes cannot. The splenic sinuses and a loose network of reticular fibers surrounded by macrophages, lymphocytes, and plasma cells known as the splenic cords of Billroth make up the red pulp. These are drained by the small veins, which merge to form the splenic vein and empty into the portal vein [4].

The spleen is rich in reticular cells and reticular fibers similar to those found in lymph nodes and are arranged in concentric layers to support the PALS. This allows for interaction of new antigens with the reticulum and removal of particles from the bloodstream [4].

Embryology

The spleen is derived from the primitive mesoderm on the left side of the dorsal mesogastrium and begins to develop at the fifth week of gestation. During fetal development, the cephalic portion of dorsal mesogastrium bulges to form a lobated spleen at six weeks of gestation [2, 6]. Blood vessels

L. Nguyen (✉)
Department of Pathology and Laboratory Medicine, James A. Haley Veterans' Hospital, Tampa, FL, USA
e-mail: Lynh.Nguyen3@va.gov

L. Zhang
Department of Pathology, H. Lee Moffitt Cancer Center and Research Institute, Tampa, FL, USA

© Springer Nature Switzerland AG 2020
L. Zhang et al. (eds.), *Diagnostic Pathology of Hematopoietic Disorders of Spleen and Liver*,
https://doi.org/10.1007/978-3-030-37708-3_1

appear at approximately nine weeks; however, the red and white pulp cannot be distinguished until the ninth month. The number of lymphocytes also gradually increases with each developmental stage. The human immune system first develops during embryogenesis, but continues well after birth. Follicles and marginal zones, for example, do not appear in the splenic white pulp until after birth.

Normal Function

The spleen plays a critical role in maintenance of normal immunity and hematopoiesis. A major function of the spleen is to filter the blood by removing senescent and poorly deformable red blood cells from the circulation [5]. It also removes particles from circulating red blood cells such as nuclear remnants (Howell-Jolly bodies), insoluble globin precipitates (Heinz bodies), and endocytic vacuoles. In individuals with asplenism or hyposplenism, Howell-Jolly bodies appear more frequently in the peripheral blood [5, 7, 8].

As a major lymphopoietic organ, the spleen plays a major role in antibody formation and T-cell and B-cell proliferation and can quickly enlarge and respond to infection or blood-borne antigens. Macrophages in the spleen have receptors [e.g. class I scavenger receptor macrophage receptor with collagenous structure (MACRO) and C-type lectin SIGN-R1] that can recognize and bind to polysaccharide antigens on some encapsulated bacteria [9–11]. When the spleen is removed, these individuals, particularly children or adolescents, become more susceptible to bacterial sepsis, especially secondary to encapsulated organisms (i.e. *Haemophilus influenzae, Neisseria meningitidis,* and *Streptococcus pneumoniae*) [5, 12]. The spleen can also trap and destroy antibody-coated platelets or red blood cells in patients with immune thrombocytopenia or autoimmune hemolytic anemia [13–15].

The spleen also acts as a reservoir, sequestering approximately a third of the total volume of platelets and a number of granulocytes [2]. In addition, the spleen serves as a hematopoietic organ during fetal development and may resume this function into adulthood if necessary.

Imaging Findings

The average spleen measures 4.0–5.0 cm in width, 11.0 cm in length, and 4.0 cm in thickness although it can vary between individuals [6]. A number of imaging studies can be used to evaluate the spleen. If a spleen is normal in size (<5.0 cm width), it should not be seen on abdominal plain films. On ultrasound and liver-spleen colloid scanning, however, the normal size of the spleen is <13.0 cm in length, while on CT or PET/CT scanning, a spleen is considered enlarged if its length is >10.0 cm.

Gross

The human spleen is a convex, bean-shaped organ with a smooth capsule with overlying visceral peritoneum. It is the second largest lymphoid organ in the body with weight ranging from 150–250 grams in adults, but can be substantially smaller in the elderly [2] (Fig. 1.1).

Cut section of the normal spleen shows a predominantly red beefy parenchyma (red pulp) with interspersed pale gray areas no larger than 2.0 mm in diameter (white pulp or Malpighian corpuscles). Small vessels branching from the splenic artery may be identified grossly.

Microscopic Findings

The spleen is extremely vulnerable to autolysis, which makes histology often times difficult to interpret.

White Pulp

The white pulp is composed of the periarterial lymphatic sheath (PALS) and lymphoid nodules including primary and secondary follicles, together occupying 5–20% of the splenic parenchyma (Fig. 1.2). Similar to lymph nodes, B and T lymphocytes localized to specific regions of the splenic white pulp. PALS, as mentioned, surround the central artery and are predominantly composed of T-cells (T-zone). PALS frequently enclose lymphoid nodules or follicles, which are B-cell rich. Germinal centers in secondary follicles can be seen if the spleen has been exposed to an antigen. Cells in the germinal centers experience somatic hypermutation, isotype switching, and clonal expansion [12]. The intermediate zone between the red and white pulp is called the marginal zone and is composed of

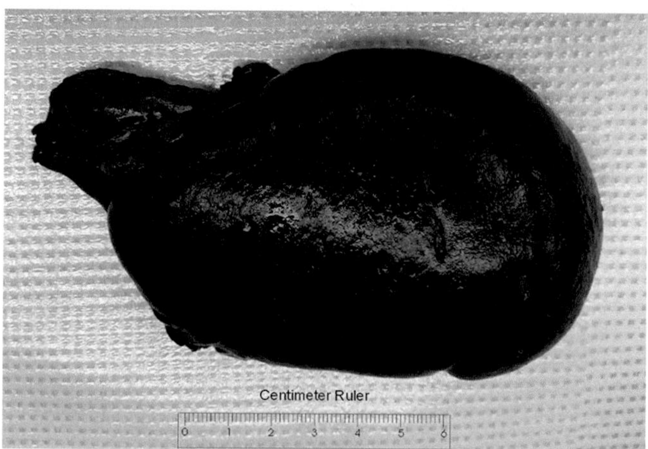

Fig. 1.1 Gross image of normal spleen from an adult. The spleen is bean-shaped and covered by a thin smooth capsule. It measures 12.5 cm × 5.0 cm × 3.5 cm and weighs 220 grams

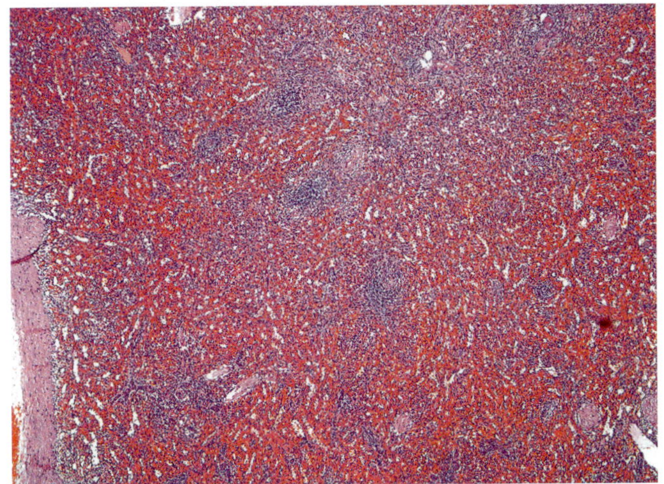

Fig. 1.2 Low-power view of normal spleen. Note the thin fibrous capsule and the trabeculae that carry the arteries, veins, and nerves from the hilum. The white pulp and central arteriole can be easily identified. The red pulp is slightly expanded and is composed of sinuses and cords (H&E, 40x)

B and T lymphocytes, plasma cells, macrophages and interdigitating dendritic cells (Fig. 1.3). A number of vascular channels or marginal sinuses are present in the marginal zone and are fed by vessels radiating from the central arteries [5]. The function of white pulp is similar to those of the lymph node paracortex and superficial cortex. It is here that antigens, particulate matter, and cells within the circulation are exposed to the splenic parenchyma. Antigen-presenting cells search for antigens traveling in the blood while macrophages found in the marginal zone attack microorganisms and elicit an immune response by activating marginal zone B-cells to present epitopes to T-cells [5].

The splenic lymphoid follicles are predominantly composed of B-cells, and like other lymphoid organs have germinal centers with surrounding mantle zone and marginal zone. Germinal centers are composed of B-cells, more specifically a mixture of centrocytes and centroblasts that show polarization with more centroblasts concentrated in the dark zone and centrocytes, macrophages, and plasma cells in the

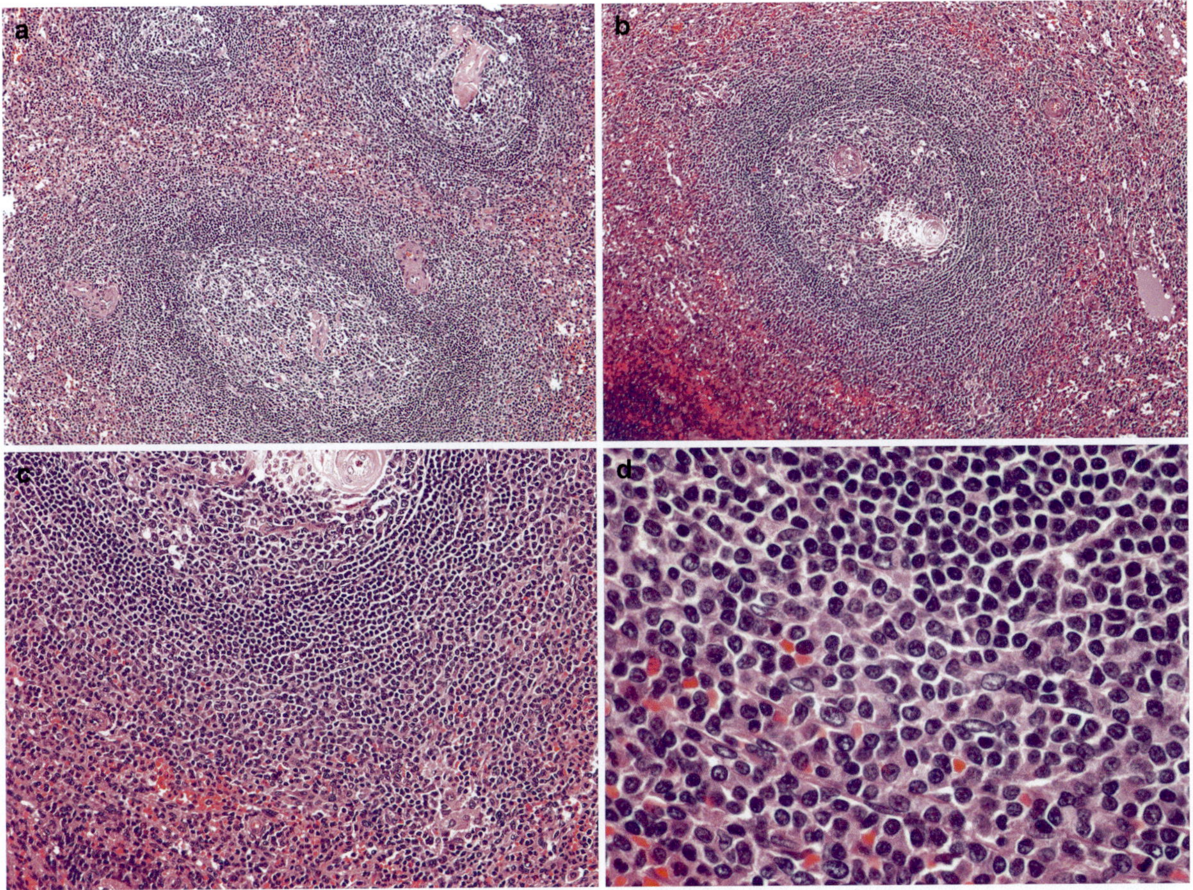

Fig. 1.3 Splenic white pulp. H&E sections from a splenectomy specimen show a normal splenic parenchyma composed of predominantly white pulp. (**a**) It consists of several follicles with reactive germinal centers and identifiable arterioles (H&E ×200). (**b, c**) The white pulp includes a well demarcated mantle zone (inner layer) and marginal zone (outer layer) (H&E, ×200). (**d**) The cells of the mantle zone are smaller in size with more condensed chromatin, while the marginal zone cells show more monocytoid or plasmacytoid differentiation with slightly eccentric nuclei and moderate amount of eosinophilic cytoplasm (H&E, 200×)

light zone. Reactive germinal centers may be diminished or absent as one ages. The germinal centers are supported by stromal cells called follicular dendritic cells that express CD21, CD23, and CD35. The B-lymphocytes of the germinal centers express CD19, CD20, CD10, and CD79a, have a high proliferation index (especially in dark zone), and are negative for BCL2. Mantle and marginal zones are composed of densely packed medium-sized lymphocytes that are supported by a reticulin meshwork. Notably T-cells are located adjacent to surrounding red pulp and merge with the marginal zone. The mantle zone predominantly consists of CD5-positive lymphocytes that are IgM (−), IgD (−), DBA.44 (+), and alkaline phosphatase (−). The splenic marginal zone, in contrast, is composed of B-cell lymphocytes, representative of IgM-positive memory cells that are IgM (+), IgD (+/−), and DBA.44 (−) and alkaline phosphatase (+) [12, 16]. Additionally macrophages are present in the marginal zone and are CD68 (+).

Red Pulp

The red pulp occupies the largest compartment of the spleen and consists of two major components: the venous sinusoids (30%) connected by cords of Billroth and intervening splenic parenchyma (70%) [17] (Fig. 1.2). Reticular fibers, myofibroblasts, plasma cells, plasmablasts, and macrophages together form the splenic cords. The macrophages of sheathed capillaries are a major component in the splenic parenchyma and play a critical role in phagocytosis and removing deformed or aged red blood cells. The macrophages also engulf and accumulate broken-down cellular components such as hemosiderin and lipofuscin. The lymphocytes, mostly T-cells, are located in non-filtering areas of the spleen without sheathed capillaries. Blood enters into venous sinuses from the splenic cords. The venous sinuses are lined by endothelial cells that are elongated or spindled and arranged parallel to the longitudinal axis of the sinuses [5] (Fig. 1.4). The splenic sinusoids

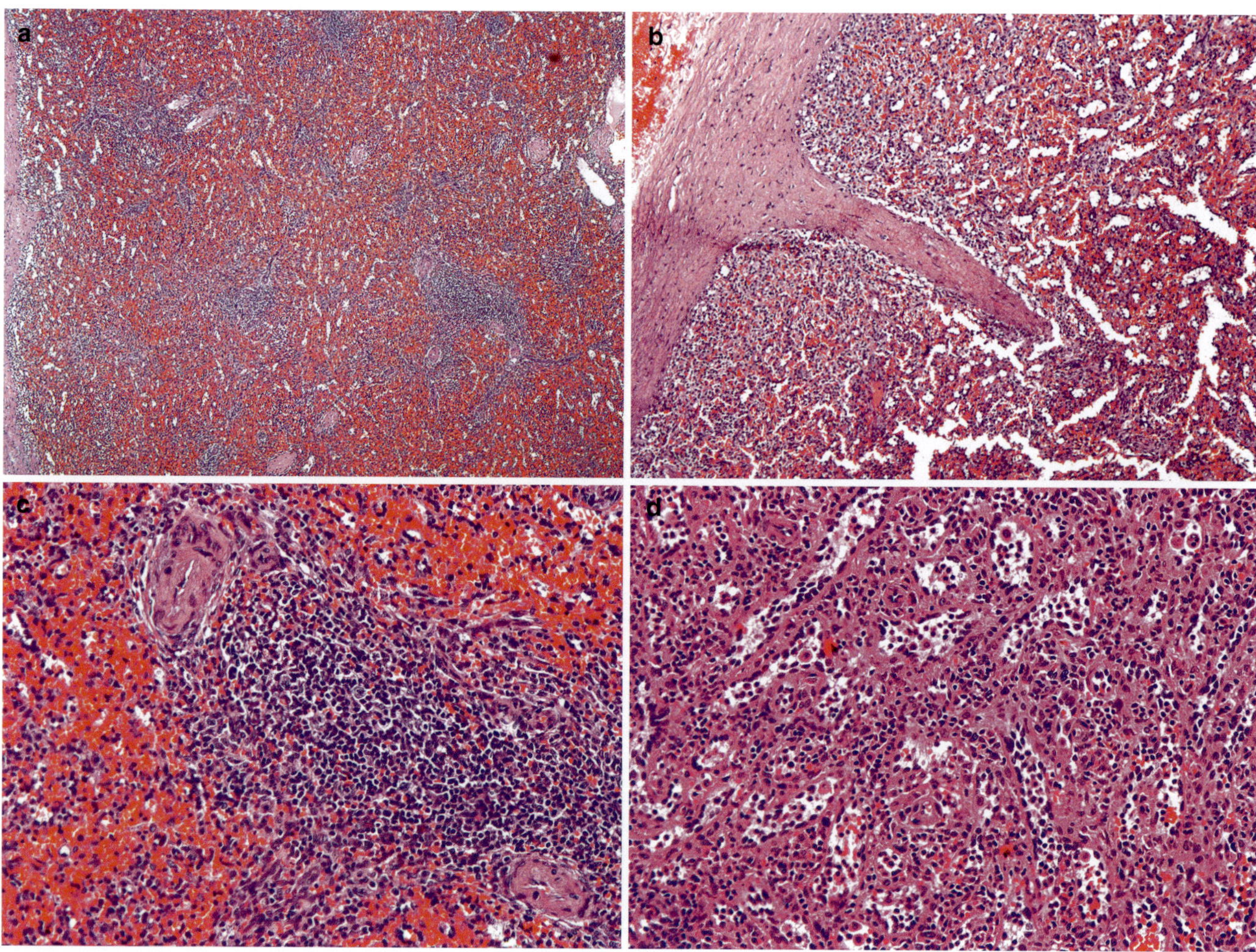

Fig. 1.4 Splenic red pulp. H&E section of a spenectomy specimen demonstrates a normal splenic parenchyma. (**a**) The red pulp is slightly expanded. Small lymphoid follicles (white pulp) are present (H&E, 40×). (**b**) Section shows a slightly thickened splenic capsule with trabecula entending into splenic parenchyma (H&E, 100×). (**c**) The periarterial lymphatic sheath (PALS), lymphoid nodules and adjacent small vessels can be identified here (H&E, 200×). (**d, e**) Low and high power views of the red pulp showing the sinuses and cords (H&E, 200× and 600×, respectively). The sinuses shown in (**e**) are longitudinally arranged and lined by discontinuously spaced endothelial cells. Passing through the splenic cords are peripheral blood elements such as red blood cells, neutrophils, monocytes, and lymphocytes. Some plasma cells and reticular fibroblasts are also present (H&E, 600×). (**f**) Section through the larger branches of splenic arteries and veins with patent vascular lumen (H&E, 200×)

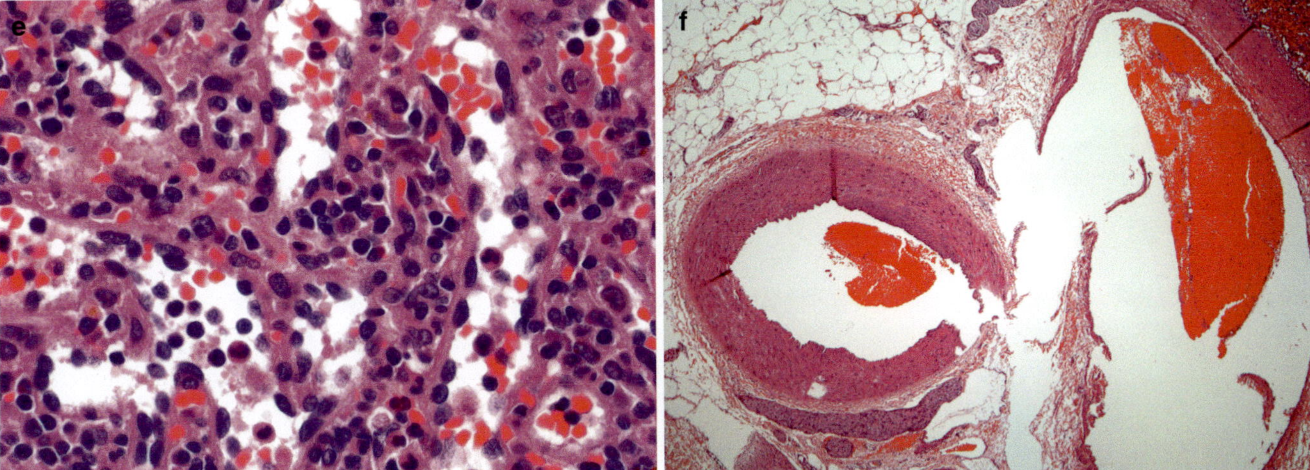

Fig. 1.4 (continued)

stain for vascular markers CD31, CD34, factor VIII, and are strongly positive for CD8 [12]. Underneath the basement membrane of the sinusoidal cells is a layer of fibers with intersecting space that form slits or fenestrations. Red blood cells that are senescent or stiff cannot pass through the fenestrations and as a result are removed by the macrophages in the cords [12]. In splenic biopsies, the architecture of the spleen is largely preserved with intact or partially intact white and red pulp (Fig. 1.5). The red pulp often shows mild to moderate congestion due to biopsy artifact.

Liver

Anatomy

The liver is a wedge-shaped organ located in the right upper quadrant of the abdominal cavity below the diaphragm and is completely protected by the rib cage. It is the largest gland and visceral organ in the body and extends from the right fifth intercostal space down to the right costal margin and to the left as far as the left midclavicular line. The normal adult liver weighs between 1400–1600 grams [18], comprising approximately 2.5% of the body's weight. It measures approximately 10 cm vertically, 12–15 cm in thickness, and 15–20 cm in greatest transverse diameter.

The liver is connected to the diaphragm via the coronary, falciform, and triangular ligaments (right and left) and is almost completely covered by peritoneum and a thin collagenous capsule called the Glisson capsule. The area devoid of peritoneum is small, adjacent to the diaphragm and surrounded by reflections of the coronary ligaments [1, 4]. The Glisson capsule extends into the liver parenchyma to support the biliary and vascular structures.

In contrast to other digestive organs, the liver has a dual blood supply that enters the liver inferiorly at the porta hepatis. It receives 30% of its oxygenated blood from the left and right hepatic arteries. The remaining 70% of oxygenated blood comes from the portal vein, which also transports nutrient-rich blood to the liver. Blood passes through hepatic sinuses and leaves the liver via the hepatic veins that later empty into the inferior vena cava [19].

Embryology

The liver first appears at the third week of gestation as a hollow endodermal outgrowth known as the hepatic diverticulum, which buds from the ventral foregut. The diverticulum then expands and hepatoblasts begin to proliferate and project ventrally into the mesoderm of the septum transversum becoming the hepatic parenchyma [19]. The hepatoblasts rapidly grow and eventually develop into the hepatic cords that are one cell thick. Glisson capsule and the falciform, coronary, and triangular ligaments develop from the mesoderm of the septum transversum. By the fifth week of gestation, the right and left umbilical veins, transverse portal sinus, ductus venosus, and portal vein have developed. Hematopoiesis begins at six weeks of gestation and is most active during the sixth and seventh months. The liver and intrahepatic bile ducts develop from the anterior part of the hepatic diverticulum or liver bud, while the gallbladder and extrahepatic biliary tree are formed from the posterior portion. Membranous infoldings between individual hepatocytes form the biliary system, initially appearing as thin intercellular spaces. Bile canaliculi are formed by the sixth week and start to produce bile by nine weeks of gestation. The intrahepatic bile ducts are not fully formed at birth, but gradually developed after birth until 1 year of age[19, 20].

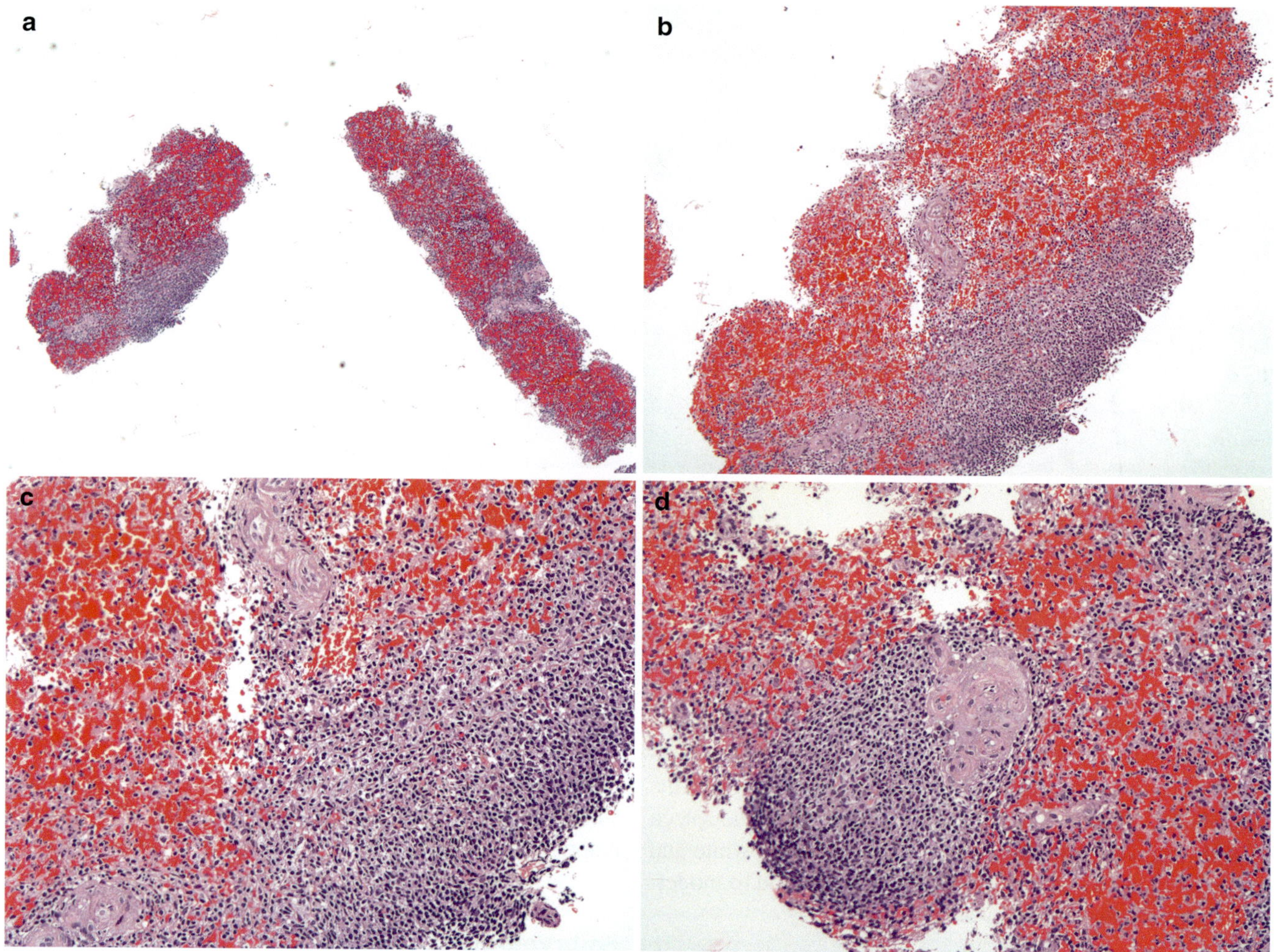

Fig. 1.5 Splenic needle core biopsy. The splenic parenchyma is slightly distorted by congestion and tissue fragmentation. (**a**) Under low-power, both white and red pulp are appreciated (H&E, 40×). (**b**) The white pulp consists of aggregates of small lymphocytes with a cen-trally located vessel and vaguely identifiable germinal centers and mantle and marginal zones (H&E, 100×). (**c, d**) A high-power view shows well-demarcated white pulp and both centrally and peripherally located small vessels (H&E, 200×)

Normal Function

The liver has both endocrine and exocrine functions. It syn-thesizes bile which is delivered via the right and left hepatic ducts to the gallbladder where it is stored, concentrated, and released. In addition, hepatocytes are able to detoxify nox-ious substances and excrete them in the bile. The liver is also responsible for lipid, carbohydrate, and protein metabolism; hormone degradation; and drug detoxification and is an impor-tant source of glycolysis, gluconeogenesis, and blood clotting factors [4, 5]. In addition, it stores the body's largest amount of vitamin A and significant amounts of vitamins D and B_{12} [5].

Kupffer cells are found interposed with the fenestrated endothelial cells of the sinusoids and are positioned as such to help destroy toxic, foreign, and infective substances found in the circulation. Originating from macrophages of the cir-culating blood, Kupffer cells can remove senescent red blood cells by phagocytosis and lysosomal degradation. The result-ing hemosiderin stored in the Kupffer cells can be later recy-cled and made available for hemoglobin production.

Hematopoiesis is also one of the most important functions of the liver during fetal life. It begins during the sixth week of gestation and stops in the third trimester, at which point the liver accounts for approximately 5% of the newborn's body weight [19].

Imaging Findings

Computed tomography (CT) has been used routinely to evaluate the hepatic parenchyma for mass lesions, its bili-ary and vascular anatomy, and volume [21, 22]. Transient elastography can also measure the liver stiffness and give important clinical information regarding liver fibrosis and steatosis. Novel CT fluoroscopy has improved visualization and efficiency of liver biopsies with less radiation exposure [23]. Recently magnetic resonance imaging (MRI) has become the choice imaging technique as it can characterize small lesions more accurately because of its high lesion-to-liver contrast [22]. Gadolinium diethylenetriaminepentaacetic acid (DTPA), similar to contrast agents used in CT, is the most commonly used MRI contrast agent that specifically targets the liver with negligible effects on renal function. Gadolinium DTPA and other new MRI contrast agents have improved detection and characterization of liver tumors so that a definitive diagnosis can be made noninvasively in some cases, having important prognostic and therapeutic implications [24]. There are two other liver-specific contrast mediums available, mangafodipir trisodium (taken up by hepatocytes) and ferumoxide (taken up by Kupffer cells), that are primarily used for detection of liver lesions [24, 25].

Gross

Grossly the liver has multiple lobes that can be identified based on the visible deep fissures and septa. The liver can be divided into two main lobes (left and right) separated by the falciform and round ligments and ligamentum teres anteriorly. Two smaller lobes – caudate and quadrate – that are located inferiorly are not as well-demarcated [19]. The adherent gallbladder and round ligament separate the quadrate lobe from the right and left lobes, while the ductus venosus and inferior vena cava separate the caudate lobe [19]. These divisions are only significant topographically. Functionally, the liver is divided into eight segments based on vascular supply (hepatic artery and portal vein) and biliary drainage. Hepatic veins are located at the periphery of each segment. These segments are clinically important when dissecting out mass lesions or removing portions of the liver for transplantation without disrupting or affecting the blood supply of the remaining hepatic parenchyma. Thus, resection lines should be parallel to the hepatic veins [27].

Cut section through the liver shows pink to brown-tan hepatic parenchyma rich in vasculature with a rubbery consistency. Focally yellow-green discoloration may be seen due to bile staining [18].

Microscopic Findings

Each hepatic lobe is made by many lobules, or acini. The basic unit of the liver is the lobule which can be of three types: classical lobules, portal lobules, and the hepatic acinus (acinus of Rappaport) [4]. The classical hexagonal lobules are centered on the central vein. Hepatocytes radiate from the central vein and are separated from each other by hepatic

sinusoids. The central vein receives blood from all the sinusoids of the lobule. Located between hepatic lobules are the portal triads, which consist of the hepatic artery, portal vein, and intralobular bile ducts [4]. Hepatocytes are normally arranged in anastomosing plates and cords and conduct multiple functions. Hepatocytes are normally polyhedral or cuboidal in shape and contain big round nuclei and single or multiple nucleoli. Chromatin is usually dispersed and in perinuclear distribution. Because it is rich in mitochondria, the cytoplasm of hepatocytes is strongly eosinophilic with a fine basophilic granularity (Fig. 1.6). Lipofuscin pigmentation, the result of lysosomal digestion and aging, is not uncommonly observed [26].

The hepatic parenchyma can also be organized based on the flow of exocrine secretion to an intralobular bile duct – each unit constituting a portal lobule defined as a triangular region centered on a portal area bound by three central veins as the apices of the triangle. Bile travels to the periphery of the lobule, entering the bile canaliculi from the hepatocyte and emptying into the bile duct.

Lastly, the hepatic lobules can be arranged based on blood flow in a diamond or ovoid-shaped lobule known as the hepatic acinus. The hepatic acinus, in contrast, is centered on a distributing artery. Based on the blood flow of the hepatic lobules and order of hypoxic injury, the hepatic parenchyma can be categorized into three zones with zone 3 extending to the central vein as the most oxygen-poor region; zone 1 in close proximity to the portal triads, which are oxygen-rich; and zone 2 in between the two.

Hepatic sinuses are lined by capillaries, which are discontinuous to permit the products synthesized within the liver to be released into the circulation. Kupffer cells are also a part of sinusoidal lining and play important role in ingestion of cellular debris, microorganisms, iron particles, and pigmentation [4].

Hepatocytes stain with CK8, CK18, and CAM5.2 and more intensely in zone 1. Hepatocyte paraffin-1 (Hep-Par1) and thyroid transcription factor-1 (TTF1) stain hepatocytes in diffuse, granular, cytoplasmic pattern. Bile canaliculi can be highlighted using pCEA and CD10. Bile ducts and ductules stain positively for CK7, CK19, CK8, CK18, and AE1/AE3 antibodies [27].

In normal liver, positive staining for CD31 and CD34 is limited to vascular endothelium of portal tract vessels and periportal sinusoids. Sinusoidal endothelial cells, however, do not express factor VIII or CD34 and show low-level CD31 expression if any. However, in chronic liver diseases, such as cirrhosis and hepatocellular carcinoma, the sinusoids may express these markers.

Alpha-1 antitrypsin and fibrinogen immunostains can help identify intracytoplasmic inclusion bodies in alpha-1 antitrypsin deficiency and fibrinogen storage disease, respectively [27].

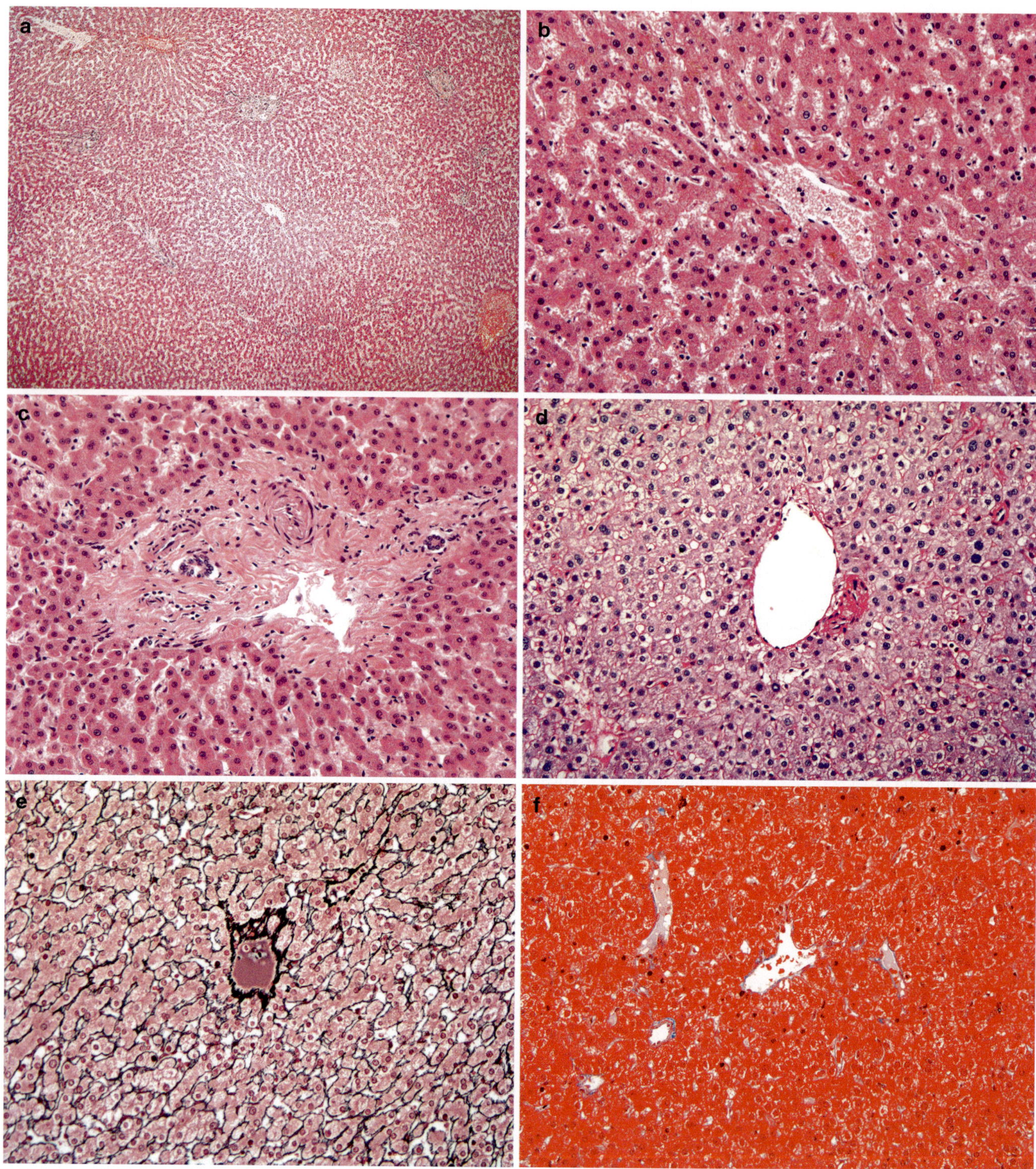

Fig. 1.6 Normal liver parenchyma. (**a**) The micrograph shows multiple normal liver lobules including hepatic acini with bordering portal tracts (H&E, 40x). (**b**) The plates of hepatocyte are in single-cell layers and centered on central vein. The normal hepatocytes are uniform in size, large, polyhedral with round nuclei, prominent nucleoli, and abundant eosinophilic cytoplasm (H&E, 200×). (**c**) Portal tracts or portal triads are composed of a terminal branch of the hepatic portal vein, a terminal branch of the hepatic artery with its slightly more thickened wall, and a small bile duct (H&E, 200X). (**d**) PAS-D stain performed on the hepatic tissue shows no abnormal PAS-positive diastase-resistant globules or microorganisms (PAS-D, 200×). (**e**) Reticulin stain highlights normal distribution of a fine meshwork of reticulin fibers between hepatocytes, sinusoid lining cells, and perivascular areas (reticulin, 200×), and (**f**) trichrome stain shows no collagen fibrosis in the normal parenchyma (trichrome, 200x)

Lipofuscin pigment is produced by lysosomal oxidation of lipids and is a sign of cell aging and is commonly seen in the liver as a light brown, PAS-positive diastase-resistant granules typically within the hepatocytes of zone 3 [27].

Kupffer cells are found attached to the fenestrated hepatic sinusoids. They originate from circulating macrophages and stain similarly with CD68 [27].

References

1. Chung KW. Gross anatomy. Baltimore: Williams & Wilkins; 1991.
2. Hiatt J, Phillips E, Morgenstern L. Surgical diseases of the spleen. Heidelberg: Springer; 2006.
3. Skandalakis J, Colborn GL, Pemberton LB. The surgical anatomy of the spleen. Probl Gen Surg. 1989;55(5):291.
4. Johnson K. Histology and cell biology. Baltimore: Williams & Walkins; 1991.
5. Young B, Heath J. Immune system. In: Young B, Heath J, editors. Wheater's functional histology – a text and colour atlas. London: Churchill Livingstone; 2000. p. 193–221.
6. Skandalakis J, Gray S. Embryology for surgeons. Baltimore: Williams & Walkins; 1994.
7. Resende V, Petroianu A. Functions of the splenic remnant after subtotal splenectomy for treatment of severe splenic injuries. Am J Surg. 2003;185(4):311–5.
8. Harrod VL, Howard TA, Zimmerman SA, Dertinger SD, Ware RE. Quantitative analysis of Howell-Jolly bodies in children with sickle cell disease. Exp Hematol. 2007;35(2):179–83.
9. Geijtenbeek TB, Groot PC, Nolte MA, et al. Marginal zone macrophages express a murine homologue of DC-SIGN that captures blood-borne antigens in vivo. Blood. 2002;100(8):2908–16.
10. Kang YS, Kim JY, Bruening SA, et al. The C-type lectin SIGN-R1 mediates uptake of the capsular polysaccharide of Streptococcus pneumoniae in the marginal zone of mouse spleen. Proc Natl Acad Sci U S A. 2004;101(1):215–20.
11. Elomaa O, Sankala M, Pikkarainen T, et al. Structure of the human macrophage MARCO receptor and characterization of its bacteria-binding region. J Biol Chem. 1998;273(8):4530–8.
12. Medeiros L, O'Malley D, Caraway N, Vega F, Elenitoba-Johnson K, Lim M. Tumors of the lymph nodes and spleen. Washington, D.C.: ARP press; 2017.
13. Sandler SG. The spleen and splenectomy in immune (idiopathic) thrombocytopenic purpura. Semin Hematol. 2000;37(1 Suppl 1):10–2.
14. Barcellini W. New insights in the pathogenesis of autoimmune hemolytic anemia. Transfus Med Hemother. 2015;42(5):287–93.
15. Matsumoto N, Ishihara T, Fujii H, Nakamura H, Uchino F, Miwa S. Fine structure of the spleen in autoimmune hemolytic anemia associated with systemic lupus erythematosus. Tohoku J Exp Med. 1978;124(3):223–32.
16. Pillai S, Cariappa A, Moran ST. Marginal zone B cells. Annu Rev Immunol. 2005;23:161–96.
17. van Krieken JH, Te Velde J, Hermans J, Welvaart K. The splenic red pulp; a histomorphometrical study in splenectomy specimens embedded in methyl methacrylate. Histopathology. 1985;9(4):401–16.
18. Gray H, Lewis W. Gray's anatomy of the human body. Bartleby: New York; 2000.
19. Torbenson M, Zen Y, Yeh M. Tumors of the liver. Washington, D.C.: ARP Press; 2018.
20. Roskams T, Desmet V. Embryology of extra- and intrahepatic bile ducts, the ductal plate. Anat Rec (Hoboken). 2008;291(6):628–35.
21. Francis IR, Cohan RH, McNulty NJ, et al. Multidetector CT of the liver and hepatic neoplasms: effect of multiphasic imaging on tumor conspicuity and vascular enhancement. AJR Am J Roentgenol. 2003;180(5):1217–24.
22. Sahani DV, Kalva SP. Imaging the liver. Oncologist. 2004;9(4):385–97.
23. Bissoli E, Bison L, Gioulis E. Multislice CT fluoroscopy: technical principles, clinical applications and dosimetry. Radiol Med (Torino). 2003;106:201–2.
24. Hahn PF, Saini S. Liver-specific MR imaging contrast agents. Radiol Clin N Am. 1998;36(2):287–97.
25. Kamel IR, Bluemke DA. MR imaging of liver tumors. Radiol Clin N Am. 2003;41(1):51–65.
26. Young B, Heath J. Wheater's functional histology. London: Churchill Livingstone; 2000.
27. Mills S. Histology for pathologists. Wolters Kluwer: Philadelphia; 2019.

Diagnostic Approaches to Hematopoietic Disorders of the Spleen and Liver

Ling Zhang, Pukhraz Basra, and Serhan Alkan

Introduction

The spleen is the largest lymphoid tissue in the human body and is composed of red and white pulp along with the supporting stroma. It is an important organ for filtration, immune regulation, and hematopoiesis during fetal development [1]. Although the intact immune modulation from the spleen would protect human beings from diseases, there are a number of primary and secondary hematologic malignancies that may occur when immunity of the spleen is compromised or overridden by other processes [2]. Additional non-hematopoietic diseases affecting the spleen include, but are not limited to, viral, bacterial, fungal, and parasitic infections, sarcoidosis, and storage disorders (deposition of abnormal metabolic materials); these diseases may sometimes mimic primary hematologic neoplasms [1, 2].

Similar to the spleen, the liver is also involved in hematopoiesis during embryonic development, in addition to playing a role in digestion, metabolism, and intoxication [3]. There are a number of hematopoietic neoplasms that may occur *de novo* or secondarily involve the liver, such as primary or secondary hepatic T- or B-cell lymphomas, Hodgkin lymphoma, myeloproliferative neoplasms (MPN), mixed myelodysplastic/myeloproliferative neoplasms (MDS/MPN), myeloid sarcoma, plasma cell neoplasms, and Langerhans cell histiocytosis. Certain reactive conditions such as hepatic pseudo-lymphoma, follicular cholangitis, and extramedullary hematopoiesis may resemble hematopoietic malignancies; distinguishing between the reactive and neoplastic processes is crucial, given the different treatment strategies and clinical outcomes [4].

There is a broad spectrum of hematopoietic disorders that can involve the liver or the spleen, or both. Understanding the pathogenesis of these diseases has been hindered by several factors [5]. Primarily, diagnostic splenectomy is infrequently performed due to the majority of hematologic disorders being a part of a disseminated or systemic process that can be diagnosed by other convenient methods, for example, peripheral blood examination and bone marrow or lymph node biopsy for histology and ancillary tests. Splenic and liver biopsies are only occasionally performed for diagnosis due to the risk of spontaneous bleeding that could be life-threatening. Tissue from a liver biopsy is usually very limited only allowing for histologic assessment, a restricted panel of immunohistochemical studies, and routine special staining. Therapeutic splenectomy is sometimes performed when conventional cytotoxic chemotherapy, immunomodulation, radiation, and/ or novel drugs have failed to improve the hematopoietic disorders. In such situations, the splenic histology could be altered due to extensive tissue necrosis, vascular occlusion, infarction, or fibrosis to such an extent that it becomes difficult for pathologists/hematopathologists to accurately assess for initial or residual disease in the spleen. Hepatectomies are occasionally performed for therapeutic, not only for diagnostic, purposes, if there is focal disease involvement of the right lobe, potentially followed by liver transplantation. Of note, autolysis frequently occurs in postmortem liver tissue, which may also impair an accurate assessment of liver histopathology [5].

The diagnostic approach to liver and splenic lesions is largely dependent on the size of the specimens obtained. In general, all obtained samples need to be examined grossly and processed through histology including fixation, sectioning, and staining. Microscopic examination of histology can be supplemented with ancillary tests if review of hematoxylin and eosin (H&E) stained sections cannot reach a final diagnosis. Common ancillary tests include flow cytometry, immunohistochemical staining, cytogenetics, and molecular studies. In this chapter, biopsy indications, sample gross-

L. Zhang (✉) · P. Basra
Department of Pathology, H. Lee Moffitt Cancer Center and Research Institute, Tampa, FL, USA
e-mail: ling.zhang@moffitt.org

S. Alkan
Department of Pathology and Laboratory Medicine, Cedars-Sinai Medical Center, Los Angeles, CA, USA
e-mail: serhan.alkan@cshs.org

© Springer Nature Switzerland AG 2020
L. Zhang et al. (eds.), *Diagnostic Pathology of Hematopoietic Disorders of Spleen and Liver*,
https://doi.org/10.1007/978-3-030-37708-3_2

ing, histological processing, microscopic examination, and immunophenotyping will be elaborated and discussed. The cytogenetics and molecular studies will be mentioned in a separate chapter.

Spleen

To be familiar with the diagnostic approaches to hematopoietic disorders of the spleen, the foremost importance is to be aware of the indications of splenic biopsy or surgical removal (partial or total splenectomy).

Indications of Splenectomy

Splenomegaly can be divided into three levels: mild (200–500 grams), moderate (500–1000 grams), and severe (>1000 grams) [6, 7]. Splenectomy is usually indicated when a patient presents with hypersplenism. Hypersplenism is defined as an abnormal hyperfunctioning of the spleen clinically characterized by a triad of splenomegaly, the presence of sustained cytopenia(s) that is/are usually not responsive to conventional therapy, and normal cellularity of the bone marrow [8]. However, not all hypersplenism is associated with splenomegaly. Table 2.1 summarizes the common diseases that are associated with hypersplenism where splenectomy may or may not be necessary.

Splenectomy performed in adults is usually safe without adverse clinical consequences. Conversely, relatively high morbidity (8.6–37%) and mortality (0–2.9%) rates have been reported, which are mainly attributed to secondary infection [7, 9, 10], especially in patients who are older in age or with concomitant malignancy [11]. Recently, splenic artery embolization (SAE) [12, 13] has been widely accepted as an alternative of splenectomy, possibly avoiding some significant complications post splenectomy (e.g., hemorrhage, thrombosis, infection).

Open splenectomy is more frequently adopted, while laparoscopic splenectomy is the choice for some diseases or situations. Although the indications of the both procedures are not different, laparoscopic splenectomy is preferred

Table 2.1 Disorders associated with hypersplenism

Status	Subcategories	Diseases
Congenital	Red blood cell disorders	Hereditary spherocytosis Hereditary elliptocytosis
	Hemoglobinopathy	Thalassemia Sickle cell disease Sickle/thalassemia
	Altered blood flow and cordal macrophages	Banti's syndrome*
Acquired	Red blood cell destruction	Autoimmune hemolytic anemia Infection, e.g., malaria

	Splenic diseases	*Increased phagocytosis:*
		  Storage disease
		  Langerhans cell histocytosis
		  Hemophagocytic lymphohistiocytosis (HLH), primary or secondary
		  Secondary to parasitic infection, e.g., Kala azar
		  Neoplastic histiocytic proliferation
		Splenic occupying lesions:
		  Hematopoietic neoplasms, e.g., leukemia, lymphoma, MDS/MPN, MPN, systemic mastocytosis (SM)
		  Metastatic tumor
		  Microorganisms, e.g., tuberculosis, malaria
		Cystic lesions:
		  True cysts
		  Pseudocysts
		Vascular lesions:
		  Malformation
		  Vascular tumor
		  Peliosis

	Other lesions	Hyperthyroidism Hypogammaglobulinemia Progressive multifocal leukoencephalopathy

Table modified from [5]

*Banti's syndrome a chronic congestion of the spleen resulting in premature destruction of the red blood cells by the spleen. MDS/MPN: myelodysplastic/myeloproliferative neoplasm; MPN: myeloproliferative neoplasm

for patients with normal-sized spleen or for specimens not intended for pathologic diagnosis [5].

Primary splenic masses can be principally divided into two categories: benign or malignant. The benign primary splenic lesions mainly include hemangiomas, angiomas, Littoral cell angioma, lymphangiomas, lipoma, angiomyolipomas, fibromas, and splenic cysts. The malignant splenic lesions are lymphomas, angiosarcomas, and leiomyosarcomas [5].

Table 2.2 [5] lists the common benign and malignant diseases that may require splenectomy or tend to be refractory to standard therapy. For example, in the early phase of idiopathic thrombocytopenic purpura (ITP), administration of a blood transfusion, glucocorticoids, or intravenous immunoglobulin may control disease progression in certain, but not all, patients. Splenectomy is only indicated in ITP when there is persistent thrombocytopenia (<10 k/μL) post 1.5-month conventional therapy, less than 30 k/μL after 3.0 -month therapy, or complicated with intracerebral hemorrhage [14]. Splenectomy can also be used for stabilized thrombotic thrombocytopenic purpura (TTP) [15].

Indications of Splenic Fine Needle Aspirate and Needle Core Biopsy

Spleen fine needle aspirate (FNA) or biopsy is indicated for a refined, unexplainable splenic lesion or known history of hematologic malignancy, most commonly lymphoma, which requires tissue for further pathologic diagnosis or staging [18, 19]. The splenic biopsy is usually an imaging-guided percutaneous intervention, which, though avoids a surgery, has not been widely adopted clinically due to some potential complications [18]. The fresh tissue is feasible for flow cytometric immunophenotyping, cytogenetics, and molecular studies.

Grossing

Spleen from Splenectomy

The processing of splenectomy specimens must follow the laboratory standard manual (Table 2.3). As soon as the specimen is obtained, the first thing is to check if the spleen is intact or fragmented. It is important to weigh (normal spleen is 125–195 grams), measure (outer dimensions), and carefully examine the surface of the specimen (intactness and texture) and the hilar area, including lymph nodes [7, 20]. Any surface abnormality should be documented, e.g., ruptures, laceration, fibrosis, or masses. After completion of the above steps, the intact spleen is bisected along the long axis to expose its largest cut surface. The appearance of the cut surface, with or without lesions or tumors included, is described. The fresh cut surface of a normal spleen is red-tan and juicy with areas of fairly demarcated, small nodules representing the white pulp. Pictures of the surface and cut surface of the spleen should be taken for pathologic records (Fig. 2.1).

The splenic white pulp and red pulp are orderly distributed without discrete nodularities or masses. The corresponding CT scan of the normal spleen can show a mottled pattern of enhancement or homogeneous enhancement [21]. Given that the spleen is an organ rich in blood, it is often associated with hemorrhage during processing, and therefore, appropriate fixation is required. Regardless of an intact or morcellated specimen, the spleen is further sliced in 1.0 cm thickness in

Table 2.2 Indications for splenectomy

	Benign	Neoplastic
Hematologic	Refractory ITP	Hodgkin or non-Hodgkin lymphoma
	TTP	Myeloid neoplasms, e.g., primary myelofibrosis, CML, leukemia
	Hereditary red blood cell disorders, e.g., hereditary spherocytosis, sickle cell disease	Rarely systemic mastocytosis
	Hemoglobinopathy, e.g., thalassemia	Hairy cell leukemia
	Chronic autoimmune hemolytic syndrome	CLL, splenic marginal zone lymphoma
Non-hematologic	Felty's disease (when neutropenia <1000/uL)	Lymphangioma/hemangioma/hemangiopericytoma/ hemangioendothelioma/hamartoma
	Trauma	Littoral cell hemangioma
	Cysts (true or pseudo)	Angiosarcoma
	Abscess	SANT
	Thrombosis (splenic vein)	Metastatic tumors
	Sarcoidosis	
	Gaucher's disease	

Table modified from [5, 16, 17]
ITP idiopathic thrombocytopenia purpura, *TTP* thrombotic thrombocytopenic purpura, *CML* chronic myeloid leukemia, *CLL* chronic lymphocytic leukemia, *SANT* splenic angiomatoid nodular transformation

Table 2.3 The common grossing procedures for total splenectomy[a]

Items	Stepwise processing
General steps	1. Weigh and measure the spleen in three dimensions in centimeter. 2. Examine and document the surface texture of the spleen (smooth, irregular, nodular, plaques, etc.), and identify any laceration, tumor, and foreign body. 3. Serial sections the spleen, every 1.0 cm apart; sample notable nodules. 4. Describe the cut surface of the spleen and lesions including location, color, size, and consistency. 5. Hilar lymph nodes, if any, are dissected and put in to individual cassettes. 6. Sections for histology should be immediately fixed in 10% buffered formalin for optimal morphologic examination.
To gross spleen for trauma or spontaneous spleen rupture	1. Three (3) representative sections are harvested fixed with 10% formalin-saline and stained with H&E. 2. The remaining part kept until a definitive diagnosis is made.
To examine lymphoma or myeloid neoplasms	1. Perform touch imprints (×3) that are stained with a Wright-Giemsa stain, for intraoperative diagnosis and triage. 2. A representative section of neoplasm (1.5 cm × 0.3 cm thickness) from non-necrotic areas should be saved in a tube containing RPMI medium and delivered directly to flow cytometry laboratory as directed by responsible hematopathologist. 3. A representative section of neoplasm (1.5 cm × 0.3 cm thickness) from non-necrotic areas should be saved in a tube containing RPMI medium with antibiotics and delivered directly to sample processing department to process or ship to the outside reference laboratory for cytogenetics or molecular study as directed by responsible hematopathologist. 4. A representative section of neoplasm (1.5 cm × 0.3 cm thickness) from non-necrotic area should be saved in a tube containing RPMI medium with antibiotics and delivered directly to a molecular laboratory for PCR study (e.g., T- or B-cell gene rearrangement) or other tests as directed by responsible hematopathologist. 5. Six to eight representative sections are fixed in 10% formalin-saline for histologic process and subsequently stained with H &E. 6. Additional touch imprints are prepared but unstained in case of future needs for performing FISH or other diagnostic tests, as directed by responsible hematopathologist.
To examine non-hematopoietic tumors	1. Identify tumor and select representative sections for frozen section diagnosis (H&E stain). 2. Perform frozen sections (H&E stain), for intraoperative diagnosis and triage. 3. Six to eight representative sections are fixed in 10% formalin-saline for histologic process and subsequently stained with H&E. 4. Additional touch imprints (unstained) may be needed for performing FISH or other diagnostic tests, as directed by responsible pathologists.

[a]Table modified based on Moffitt splenic grossing protocol (not published)

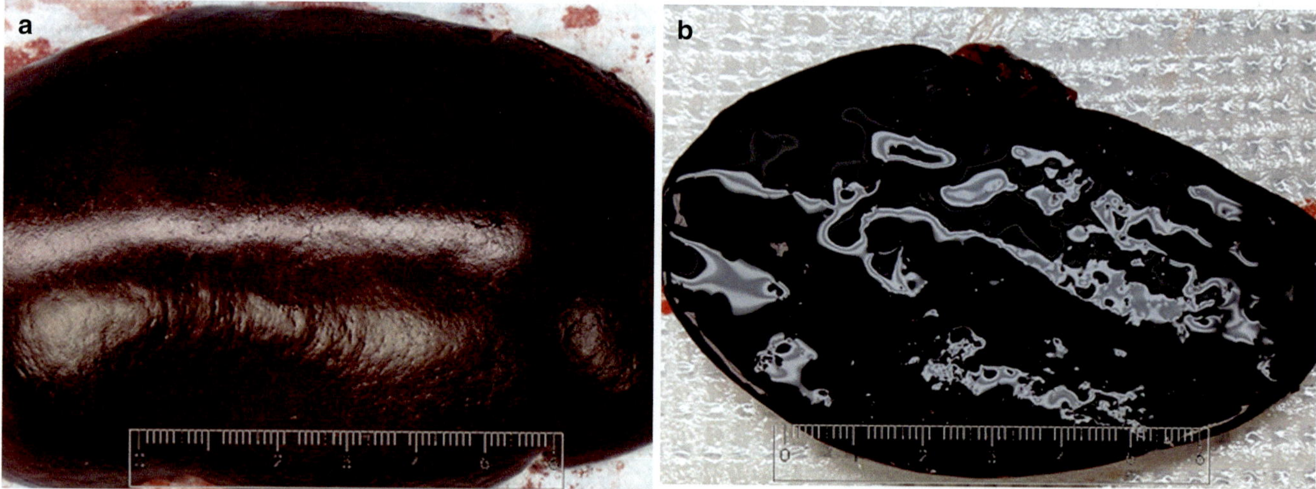

Fig. 2.1 (**a**) The image shows diaphragmatic surface of the spleen, which is convex, smooth, and shining. (**b**) The fresh cut surface of the normal spleen specimen is brown-tan and juicy. The pin-point pink-tan areas (white pulp) can be vaguely seen

order to get better fixation [22]. Studies have shown that the 1.0 cm sections of the spleen increase the exposure of the specimen to more than 10-fold formalin-based fixative. When gross lesions or tumors are identified during processing, additional measurements and descriptions must be carried out. If any white lesions, small to large, are present, these may be pathologic. The color, size, location (distance to the subcapsule), and consistency of each lesion must be documented [7, 23]. It is also critical to enumerate the number of lesions and estimate the percentage of total parenchyma occupied by the lesions [7]. The size, border, number, and nature of lesions are useful for definitive diagnosis. Any hematopoietic neoplasm involving the spleen demonstrates its own unique infiltrating pattern. The gross appearance can fully or partially reflect on its microscopic findings. The uninvolved areas are also described (color, consistency, and percentage) in relationship to the normal counterpart. In general, the cut surface of lymphoma involvement of the spleen is similar to that in lymph node, white-tan and like fresh fish meat. Splenic marginal zone lymphoma (SMZL) grossly shows numerous, small, tan to transparent nodules (3–5 mm in size) due to white pulp hyperplasia (Fig. 2.2). Classic Hodgkin lymphoma involving the spleen often forms a large mass (ranging from 2.0 to 10.0 cm) often associated with dense septal fibrosis (Fig. 2.3). Leukemias usually involve the splenic red pulp. Classically, the cut surface of hairy cell leukemia is diffuse congestion with a dark or beefy red color, and it usually shows focal hemorrhage because the leukemia cells involve predominantly the red pulp of the spleen [24] (Fig. 2.4). The changes adjacent to the lesions or masses such as congestion, hemorrhage, and coagulative necrosis are also potential clues to support the diagnosis [23].

Touch imprints are usually obtained after blotting with a towel to remove excess blood and stained appropriately for microscopic examination.

The lesions involving the spleen show variable gross morphologies, which are subgrouped into single cystic lesions, complex cystic lesions with solid masses, solid mass(es) related or unrelated to hematopoietic disorders, and diffuse red pulp lesions, hematopoietic or non-hematopoietic origin (Table 2.4) (Figs. 2.5, 2.6, 2.7, 2.8, 2.9, 2.10, 2.11, and 2.12). However, identification of the gross lesions must be in con-

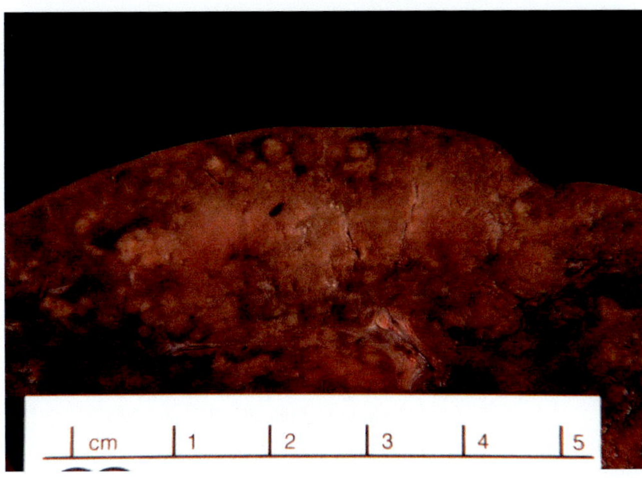

Fig. 2.3 **Classic Hodgkin lymphoma involving the spleen**. Grossly, the cut surface of the spleen shows multiple variable-sized, firm, white-tan nodules associated with fibrosis becoming a big mass

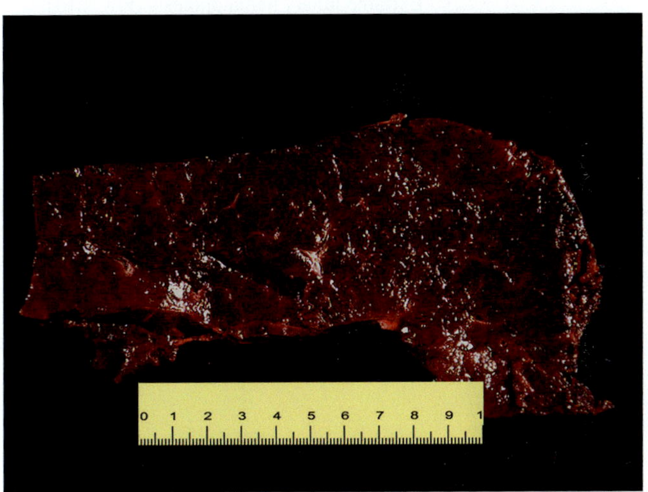

Fig. 2.4 **Hairy cell leukemia involving the spleen**. The cut surface of the spleen is beefy red-tan in color, which is due to an overt expansion of red pulp, while the normal pinpoint white pulp nodules of the spleen are diminished

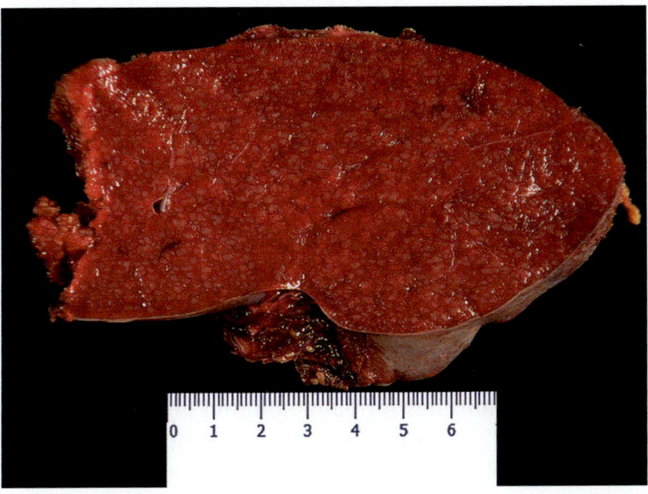

Fig. 2.2 **Splenic marginal zone lymphoma involving the spleen**. The cut surface of the spleen from a patient with splenic marginal zone lymphoma shows increased pink-tan, slightly transparent small nodules (white pulp) and relatively reduced red pulp

junction with microscopic examination and ancillary studies to attain final interpretation.

Of note, touch imprint of the cut surface of the spleen and lymph nodes before fixation is routinely performed. The hematopathologist who is on-call will examine the H&E or Wright-Giemsa-stained touch preparations of the spleen and lymph nodes and render a preliminary diagnosis. Alternatively, aspiration of cells by inserting a needle with a syringe into the fresh, unfixed spleen can be performed. The smear of cells is prepared and stained with H&E or Wright-Giemsa for review. A representative portion of fresh tissue of the spleen is placed in RPMI medium for further flow cytometry or molecular studies if there is suspicion for lymphoma, leukemia, or other

Table 2.4 Gross findings of common splenic lesions

Subcategory	Differential Dx
Single cystic lesions	Pseudocyst (post-traumatic) (Fig. 2.5) True cyst Congenital cyst Echinococcosis (initial phase)
Complex cystic lesions including solid mass	Hemangioma or hemorrhagic cyst Hematoma Lymphangioma Littoral cell angioma (Fig. 2.6) Angiosarcoma (Fig. 2.7)
Solid mass – hematopoietic related	Lymphomas (Hodgkin lymphoma, diffuse large B-cell lymphoma (DLBCL), mantle cell lymphoma, splenic marginal zone lymphoma) (Figs. 2.2, 2.3, and 2.8)
Solid mass – non-hematopoietic	Metastatic carcinoma, sarcoma, or melanoma (Figs. 2.9 and 2.10) Sarcoidosis (Fig. 2.11)
Diffuse red pulp lesions – hematopoietic related	Hairy cell leukemia (Fig. 2.4) T-cell large granular lymphocytic leukemia Hepatosplenic T-cell lymphoma Myeloid neoplasms (Fig. 2.12) Extramedullary hematopoiesis (Fig. 2.13)
Diffuse red pulp lesions – non-hematopoietic	Infections

Table modified from [25, 26]

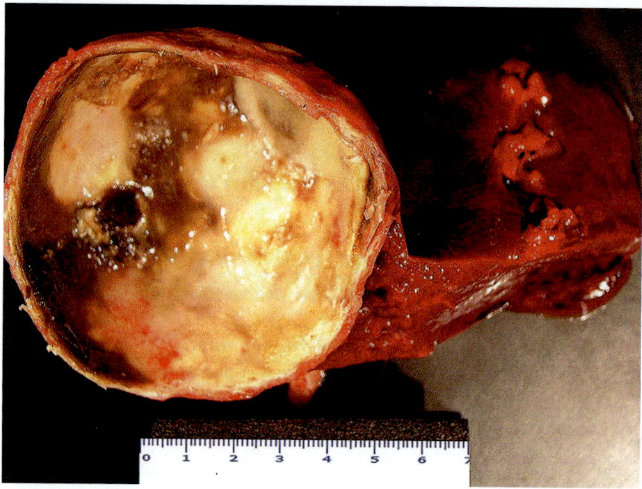

Fig. 2.5 **Benign splenic cyst**. Received is a big splenic pseudocyst with thickened capsule associated with calcification. The cystic space contains mucinous and yellow-white creamy materials. The attached part of the normal spleen appears red-brown-tan and visceral surface is concave with some impressions

hematologic disorders or neoplasms. Given the tendency of fixative to slowly penetrate the splenic tissue, the sections prepared for paraffin blocks should be thin, allowing for adequate fixation.

Splenic Biopsy

Percutaneous image-guided biopsy of the spleen is a recently emerging procedure and can be used for initial diagnosis of splenic lesions. The procedure has been proven for its diagnostic accuracy [27]. The main concerns revolve around the risk of hemorrhage and the diagnostic challenges to pathologists when the sample obtained may be insufficient or too minute to perform ancillary studies [7, 9, 10, 28–32]. Recent studies have attempted to select a needle size equal to or less than 18 gauge, similar to that used for kidney or liver biopsy [29, 30, 33]. According to a meta-analysis of 13 published studies, the procedure was performed on arm A-639 patients evaluated for diagnosis and arm B-741 patients were evaluated for complications and showed a sensitivity of 87.0% (95% confidence interval [CI], 80.7%, 91.4%) and a specificity of 96.4% (95% CI, 81.4%, 99.4%). The overall complication rate was 2.2% (95% CI, 0.8%, 5.6%); a lower rate of 1.3% (95% CI, 0.6%, 2.5%) was found when only analyzing those using a needle smaller than 18 gauge [27].

Laparoscopic Splenectomy

This type of surgery is preferred for idiopathic thrombocytopenic purpura (ITP) and other hematopoietic diseases with normal splenic size, for example, hereditary spherocytosis, autoimmune hemolytic anemia, staging for Hodgkin lymphoma, some subtypes of lymphoma/leukemia (Fig. 2.14), thrombocytopenic thrombotic purpura (TTP), splenic abscess, Gaucher's disease, splenic infarct, and AIDS-induced thrombocytopenia [5]. The major concerns included a large volume of blood loss, splenosis, and variable technical skills, however, all of which have been recently enhanced by technical improvement [34, 35]. The sample from laparoscopic splenectomy should be handled similar to whole splenectomy including weighing, measuring, gross examination, and identification of lesions, if any. Representative sections are similarly submitted.

Sample Processing

Adequate fixation is an important step for preparation of good-quality H&E slides for microscopic examination. The spleen is routinely fixed in a container filled with 10% neutral buffered formalin solution consisting of 4% formaldehyde or alternatively in acetic acid-zinc-formalin (AZF) [36]. B5, a previously used fixative, is no longer adopted because of mercuric chloride content (toxicity/

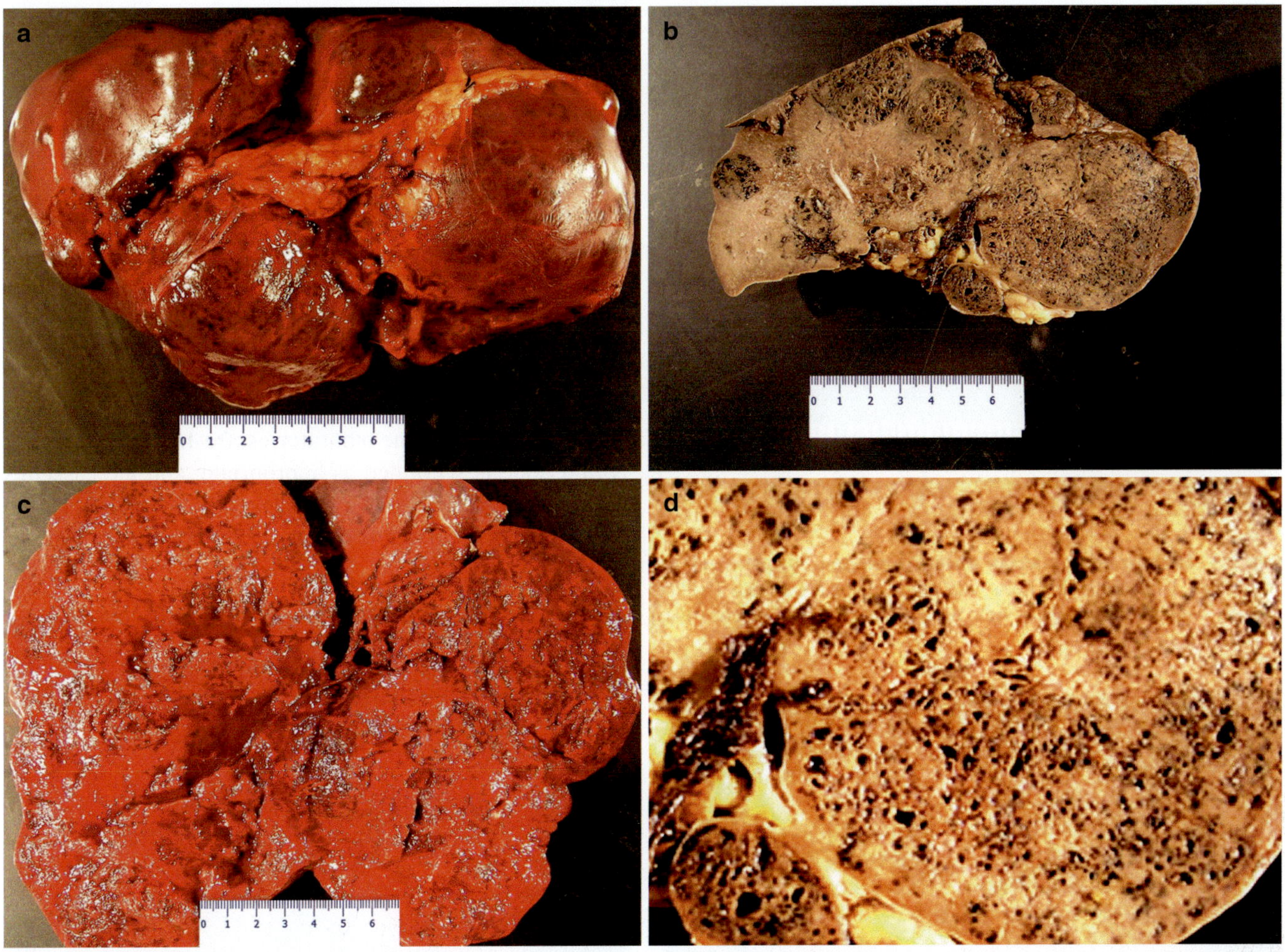

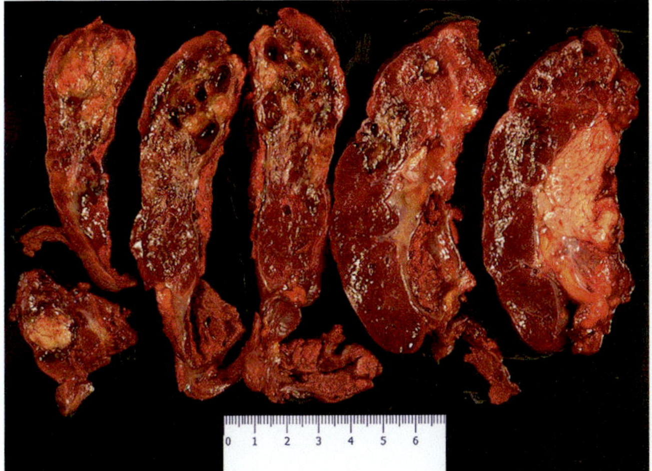

Fig. 2.6 Littoral cell angioma. (**a**) Splenectomy specimen is well encapsulated and enlarged in size. (**c**) The fresh bisected spleen with red-tan irregular cut surface. (**b, d**) After overnight formalin fixation, the cut surface of the spleen reveals multiple nodular lesions with spongy appearance

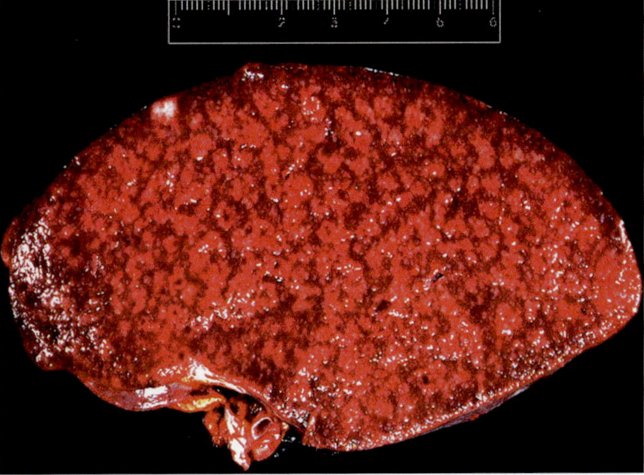

Fig. 2.7 Angiosarcoma. A series of sections through the splenectomy specimen consist of multiple lesions which are yellow or dark-red in color associated with hemorrhage, necrosis, and cystic changes

Fig. 2.8 Mantle cell lymphoma involving the spleen (post splenectomy specimen). The cut surface shows numerous small white-tan nodules indicating white pulp expansion and relative red pulp reduction

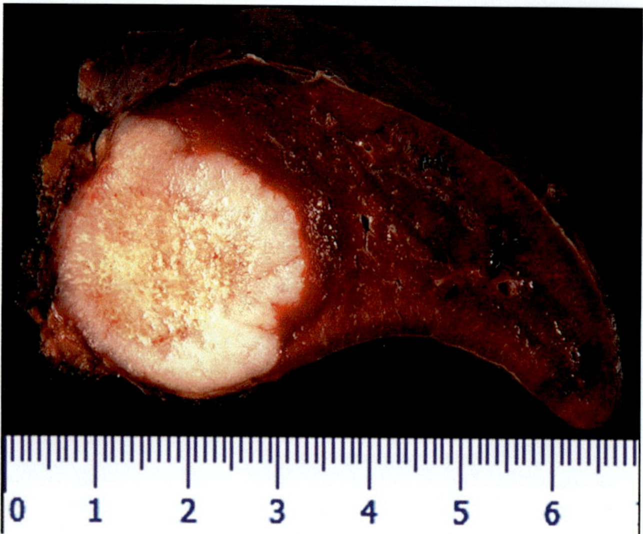

Fig. 2.9 High-grade mullerian serous carcinoma metastasized to the spleen. It contains a big mass with slightly irregular border. The cut surface is white-tan to slightly light yellow-tan with focal mucous-like discoloration

safety issue) and other concerns about unsuitability for molecular studies or antigen retrieval due to overfixation [36]. As suggested, after 24-hour fixation in 10% neutral buffered formalin solution, the spleen specimen is rinsed in tap water for 1–2 minutes. The representative sections (usually 2–3 mm in thickness) of normal spleen and lesions are sampled and placed in the prepared cassettes. One to three sections of each representative lesion are cut, sized slightly smaller than cassette. Only one lesion per cassette should be submitted, but the total number of cassettes per lesion is usually <10. In addition, five sections from the uninvolved spleen are cut in similarly sized sections and submitted. All hilar lymph nodes are bisected and submitted. In some laboratories, fresh splenic tissue or lymph node is sectioned as appropriate, and the cassettes with representative tissue are soaked in a container with formalin-related fixative overnight. Touch imprint slides

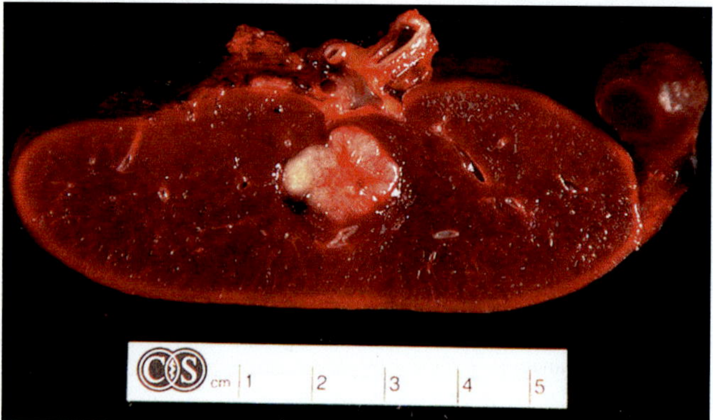

Fig. 2.10 Metastatic melanoma. Melanoma metastasized to the spleen shows the lesion white to focally pink in color, an with irregular or lobulated border

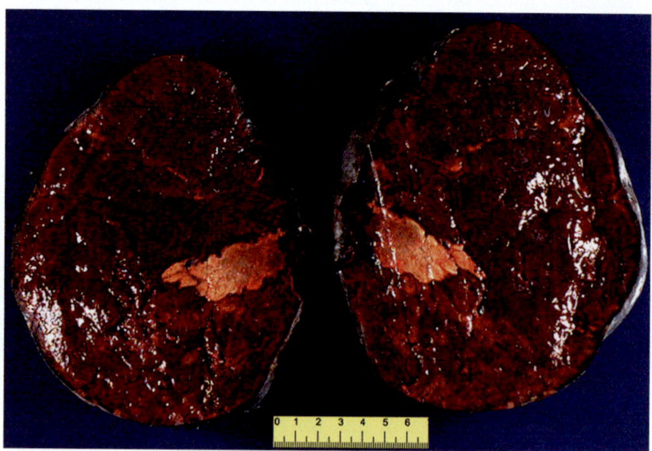

Fig. 2.12 Acute myeloid leukemia/myeloid sarcoma involving the spleen. The splenectomy specimen from a patient with acute myeloid leukemia shows diffuse red pulp expansion, which makes the cut surface of the spleen appear to be dark reddish to brown-tan in color

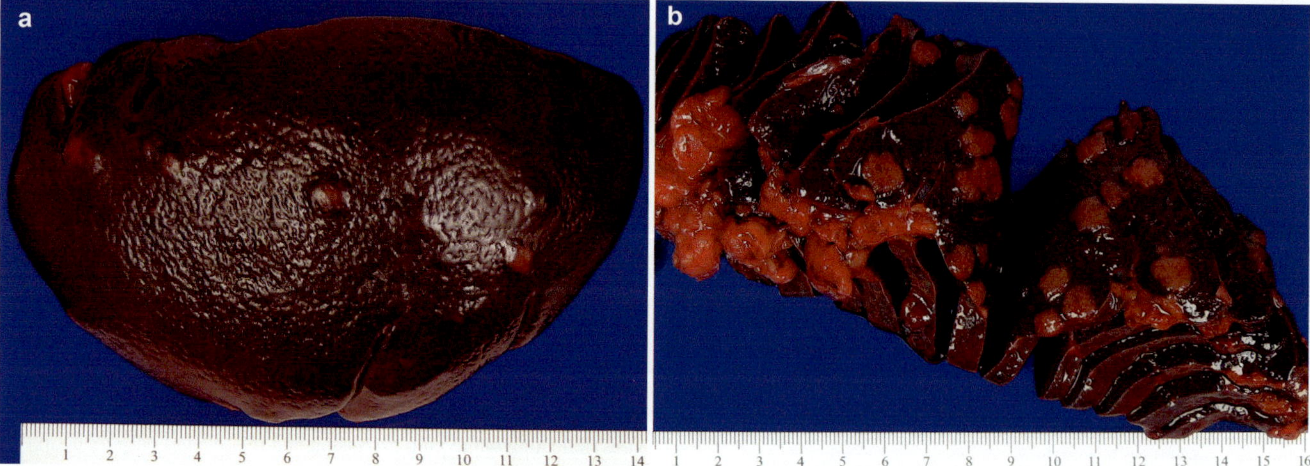

Fig. 2.11 Sarcoidosis. The spleen is enlarged with subcapsular visible nodules (**a**). The cut surface of the spleen shows multiple well-separated white-tan nodules (**b**)

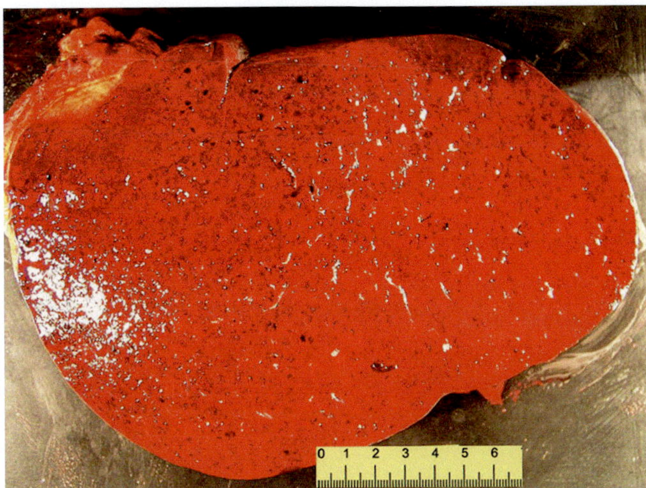

Fig. 2.13 Extramedullary hematopoiesis. The spleen specimen is from a patient with a massive splenomegaly due to extramedullary hematopoiesis. The cut surface reveals diffuse red-pulp expansion with multiple small cystic bloody lakes

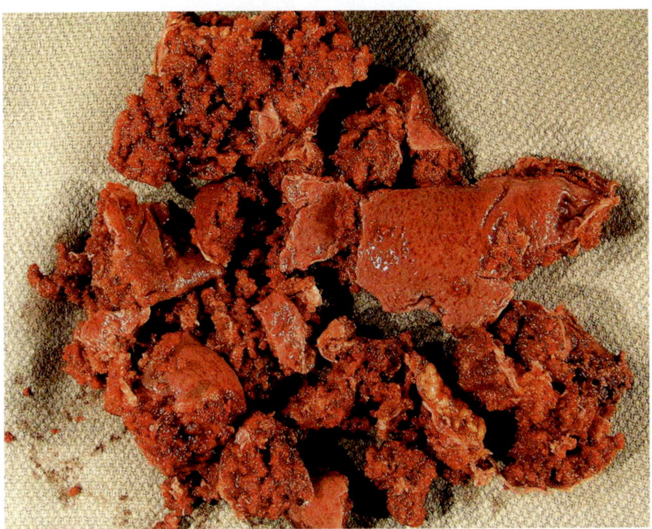

Fig. 2.14 Sample from laparoscopic splenectomy Laparoscopic splenectomy specimen from a patient with small lymphocytic lymphoma shows multiple fragmented splenic tissues, brown-tan in color, roughly granular, and focally bloody in nature. The surface appears thin and smooth

or fine needle aspirate smears are stained with Wright-Giemsa. Paraffin-embedded splenic tissue sections are stained with hematoxylin and eosin (H&E) [22].

Microscopy

Microscopic examination of the normal spleen shows both red pulp and white pulp with orderly distribution [37]. A trabecular branch arising from the splenic capsule is found to extend into normal splenic red pulp. The white pulp is constituted by lymphoid cells: T-cells usually form the peri-arteriolar lymphoid sheath and B-cells form the primary or secondary follicles. Different from primary follicles, the secondary follicles include a germinal center, in addition to mantle and marginal zones. Malpighian corpuscles, lymphoid follicles with a central artery, can often be identified. The normal red pulp contains many T-cells. The splenic cords are composed of red blood cells, macrophages, and lymphoid cells, which locate between sinusoids, and the splenic sinuses are thin-walled venous vessels lined by endothelial cells [21, 37] (Fig. 2.15).

Splenic lesions can be identified based on the changes involving the red pulp, white pulp, mixed red and white pulp, or diffuse pattern (Figs. 2.16, 2.17, 2.18, 2.19, and 2.20). Expansion of white pulp is seen with many types of B-cell non-Hodgkin lymphomas, while atrophy of white pulp can be observed in the following conditions: post-chemotherapy, post-radiation therapy, or immune suppressants [5]. In elderly patients, reactive germinal centers are more prominent, which may be secondary to self-limited antigen exposure and considered within normal physiologic range [5]. In contrast to lymphoma, leukemias and myeloid neoplasms are usually involving the red pulp. Slow-growing low-grade lymphomas, e.g., small lymphocytic lymphoma (SLL)/chronic lymphocytic leukemia (CLL) and SMZL, show both white and red pulp involvement. Examination of primary or secondary splenic tumors can also be based on three subclassifications including lymphoid tumors, non-hematolymphoid tumors including mostly vascular tumors, and tumor-like lesions [21]. Identification of granulomatous changes is helpful for further differential diagnosis. Granulomatous changes can often be associated with bacterial, fungal, and protozoal infection, sarcoidosis, classic Hodgkin lymphoma, or other malignant lymphomas [38]. A primary splenic lymphoma can be incidentally found in post-traumatic splenectomy without overt splenomegaly [39]. A low-level involvement by low-grade non-Hodgkin lymphoma could be missed without additional immunohistochemical staining, as the majority of them usually are uniformly distributed in a miliary pattern. Aggressive lymphomas are rarely identified in the spleen except for systemic involvement, which frequently present with single to multiple masses. Table 2.5 lists a number of benign and malignant hematopoietic neoplasms with the different histologic patterns when they involve the spleen.

Ancillary Studies

Immunohistochemistry Study

Immunocytochemistry is effective and usually concordant with flow cytometric findings for a majority of lymphoplasmacytic disorders identified in the spleen or lymph nodes [41]. It is important to perform immunohistochemical studies on splenic tissue because certain markers are not available via flow cytometry study [40]. For example,

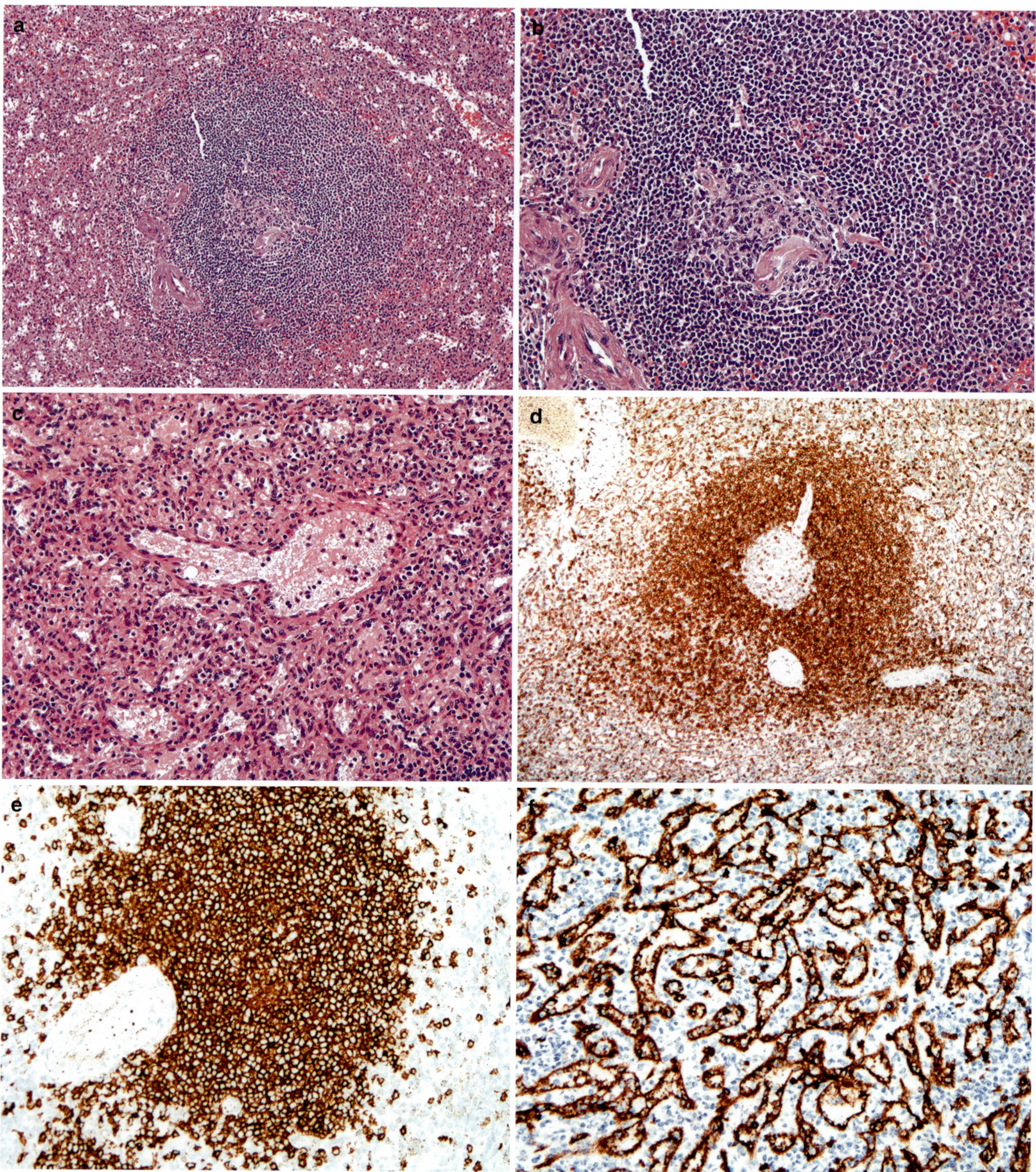

Fig. 2.15 Spleen histology. Normal splenic white and red pulp. (**a–c**) The normal splenic parenchyma is composed of mixed white pulp (lymphoid aggregate with or without identifiable germinal centers) and red pulp, including splenic cords and sinuses (H&E, 100×, 200×, and 200×). (**d–e**) Immunohistochemical stains were performed on the spleen sections. (**d**) BCL-2 highlights T- and B-cells surrounding germinal centers. The germinal center cells are negative for BCL- 2 (100×). (**e**) CD20 highlights B-cell follicles (200×). (**f**) The sinus lining cells show immunoreactivity to CD8 (200×)

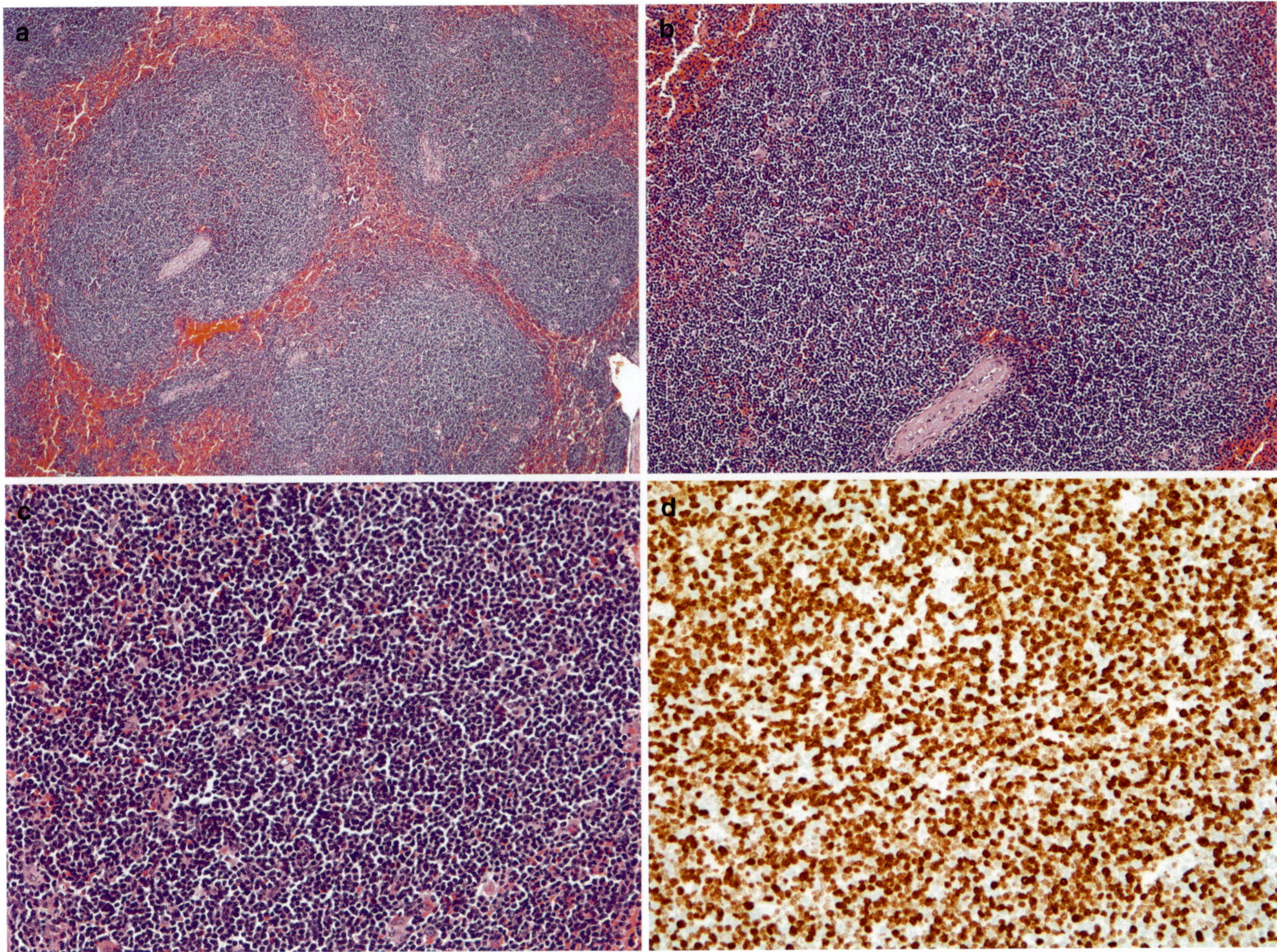

Fig. 2.16 **Microscopic findings of mantle cell lymphoma**. (**a**, **b**, **c**) Low-power review of H&E section from a splenectomy specimen shows expanded white pulp and reduced red pulp spaces. There are no identifiable germinal centers. The mantle zones are expanded, which are composed of small mature lymphoid cells with condense chromatin (40×, 100×, 300×). (**d**) Cyclin D1 immunostain highlights the mantle cell lymphoma cells (200×)

Annexin 1, VE1 (BRAF V600E), and tartrate-resistant acid phosphatase (TRAP) immunohistochemical stains are performed to distinguish between classic hairy cell leukemia and hairy cell leukemia variant as well as splenic marginal zone lymphoma [42]. However, it can sometimes be challenging for pathologists to interpret immunostaining on splenic tissue due to different histologic and staining patterns from other lymphoid or hematopoietic tissues. Thus, recognition of the normal splenic architecture is necessary before accurate interpretation of IHC findings. It is well known that many hematopoietic disorders primarily involve the white pulp, while others are found in red pulp or both (Table 2.5). Familiarity with splenic stromal and vascular compartments along with corresponding IHC staining markers is also helpful for diagnosis of related diseases. There are four splenic stromal parts: the vascular part, the reticuloendothelial part, the monocyte/macrophage part, and the remaining part including extracellular matrix and supporting mesenchymal cells [43]. The endothelial cells and vasculature are positive for CD31, CD34, and factor VIII. The monocytic/histiocytic components stain positive for CD4, CD68, CD163, and lysozyme [22, 40]. It is noted that many diseases involving the spleen not only show unique infiltrating compartments but also particular immunohistochemical staining patterns. Littoral cell angioma stains positive for vascular markers such as CD31, factor VIII, ERG, and FLI-1, as well as histiocytic marker (CD68, lysozyme) and dendritic cell marker (CD21) but

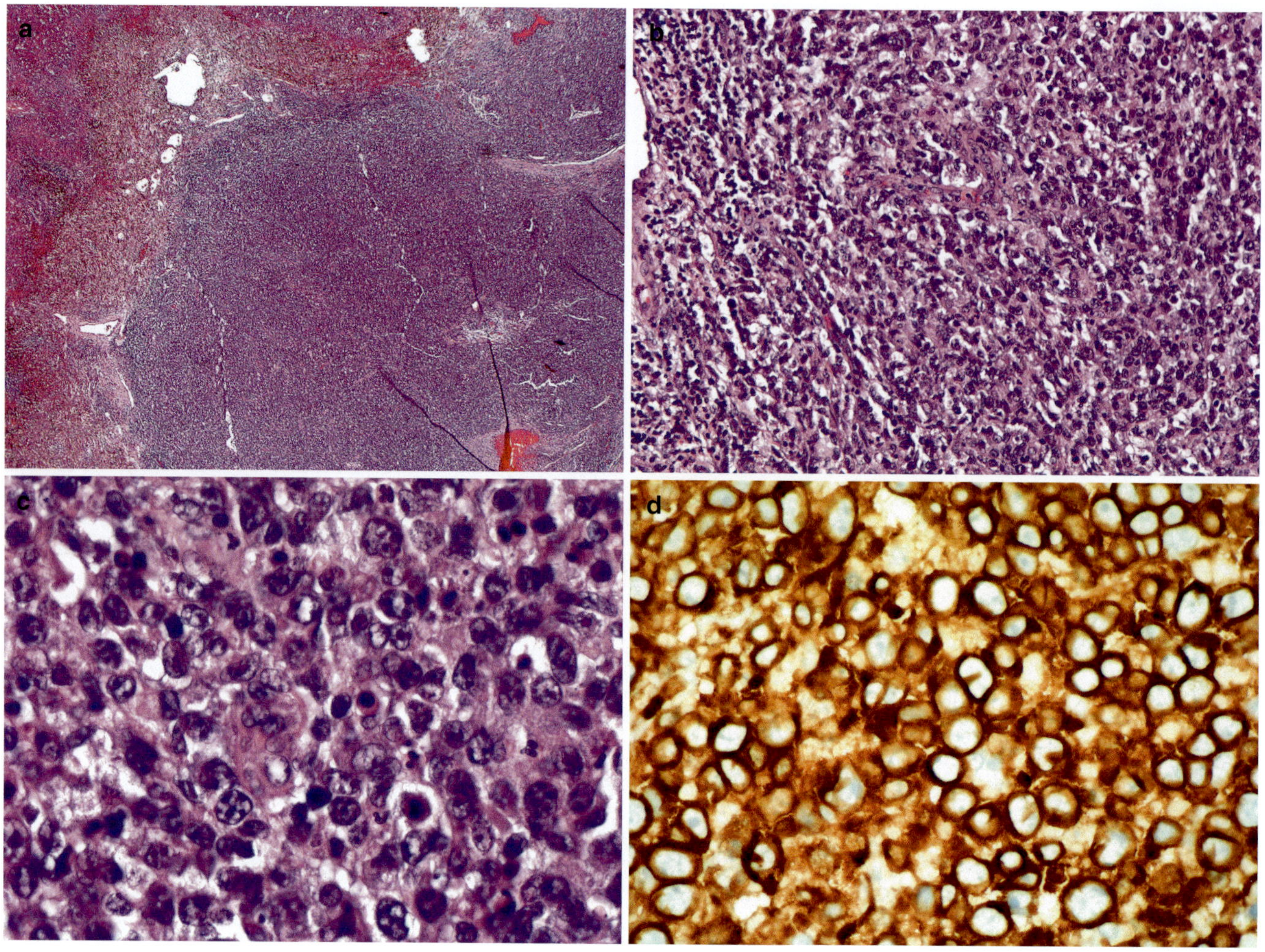

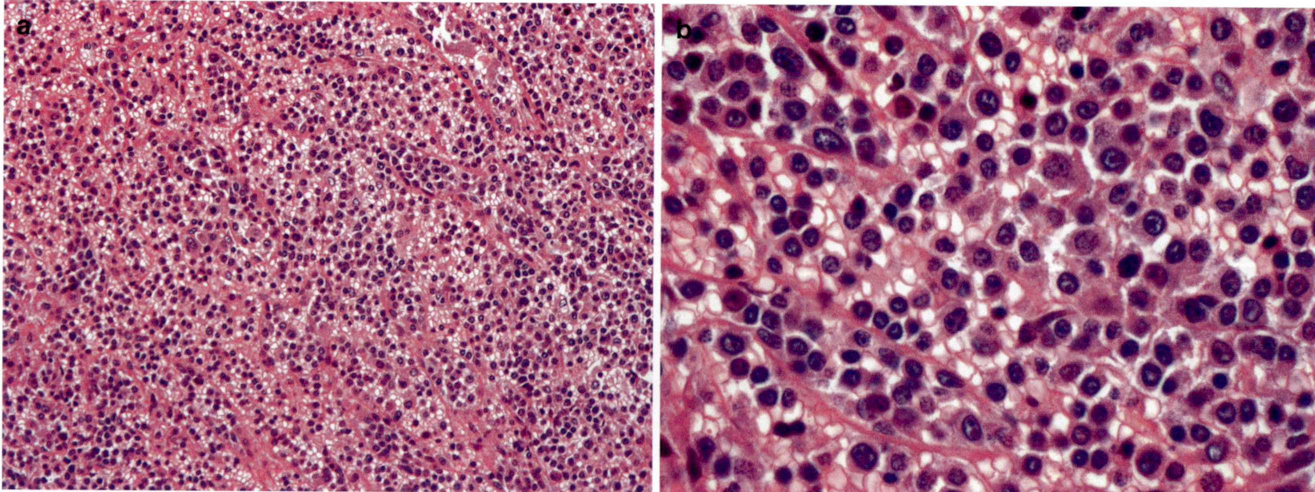

Fig. 2.17 Diffuse large B-cell lymphoma involving the spleen. It often shows a vague nodular pattern. (**a**) Under a very low power, the image showed nodular proliferation of lymphoid cells that are separated from the normal splenic parenchyma by a fibrotic border secondary to fibrohistiocytic reaction (H&E, 20×). (**b** and **c**) Medium- to higher-power views demonstrate the atypical cellular infiltrate is composed of large atypical lymphoid cells with vesicular chromatin and small visible nucleoli with increased apoptosis in the background (H&E, 200× and 600×). (**d**) Immunostain highlights these large atypical lymphoid cells to be positive for CD20 (immunoperoxidase, 600×)

Fig. 2.18 Splenic diffuse red pulp small B-cell lymphoma. (**a** and **b**). Representative H&E sections of splenic diffuse red pulp small B-cell lymphoma (200× and 600×). These red pulps are overtly expanded and composed of small atypical lymphoid cells with a moderate amount of eosinophilic cytoplasm intermingling with rare histiocytes

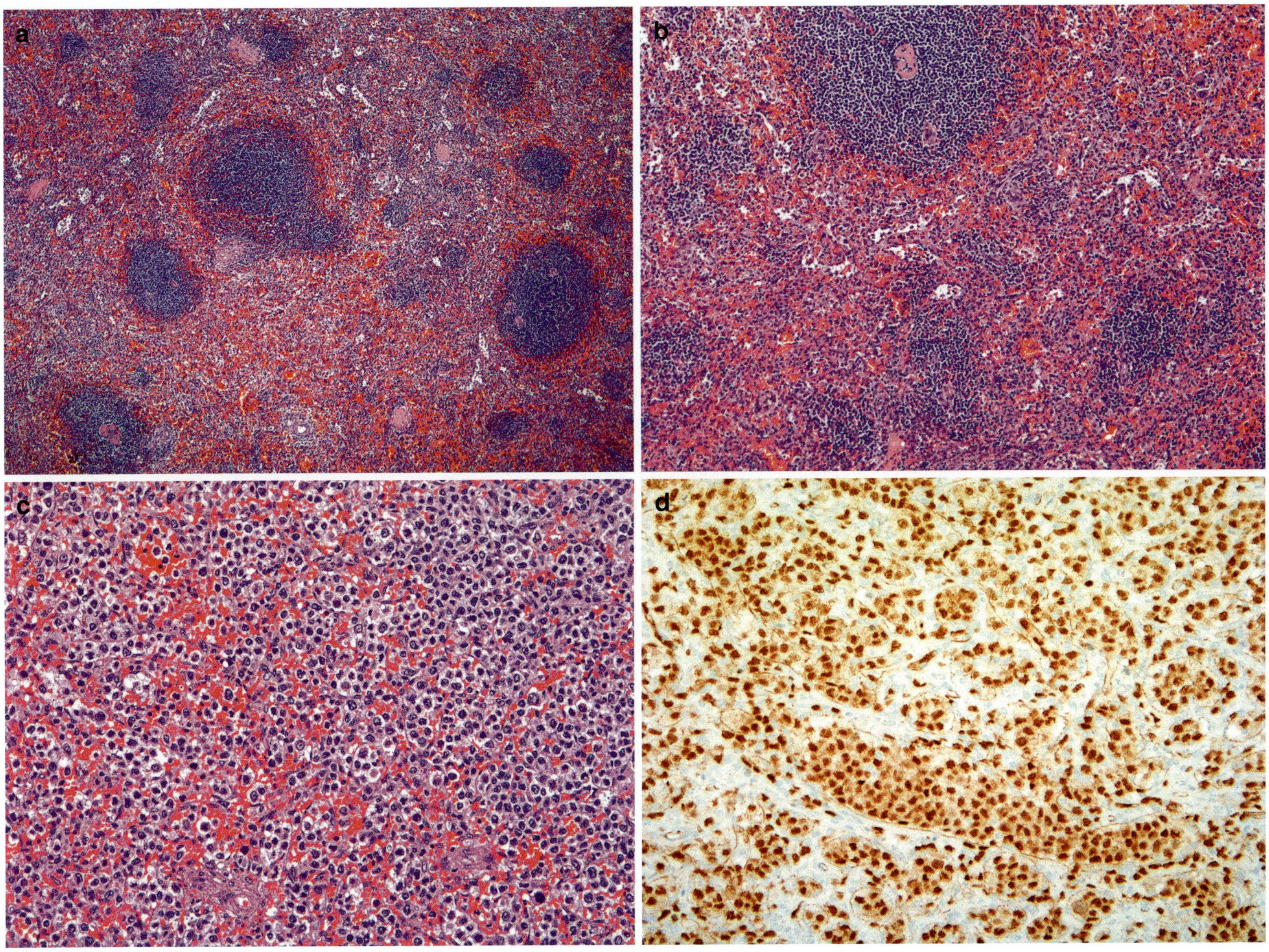

Fig. 2.19 **Splenic marginal zone lymphoma with large cell transformation**. The images demonstrate mixed white and red pulp infiltrating (**a** and **b**, H&E, 100× and 100×, early phase) and diffuse infiltrating pattern (**c**, H&E, 200×, late transformed phase) of splenic marginal zone lymphoma. (**d**) The lymphoma cells are highlighted by PAX-5 (immunoperoxidase, 200×)

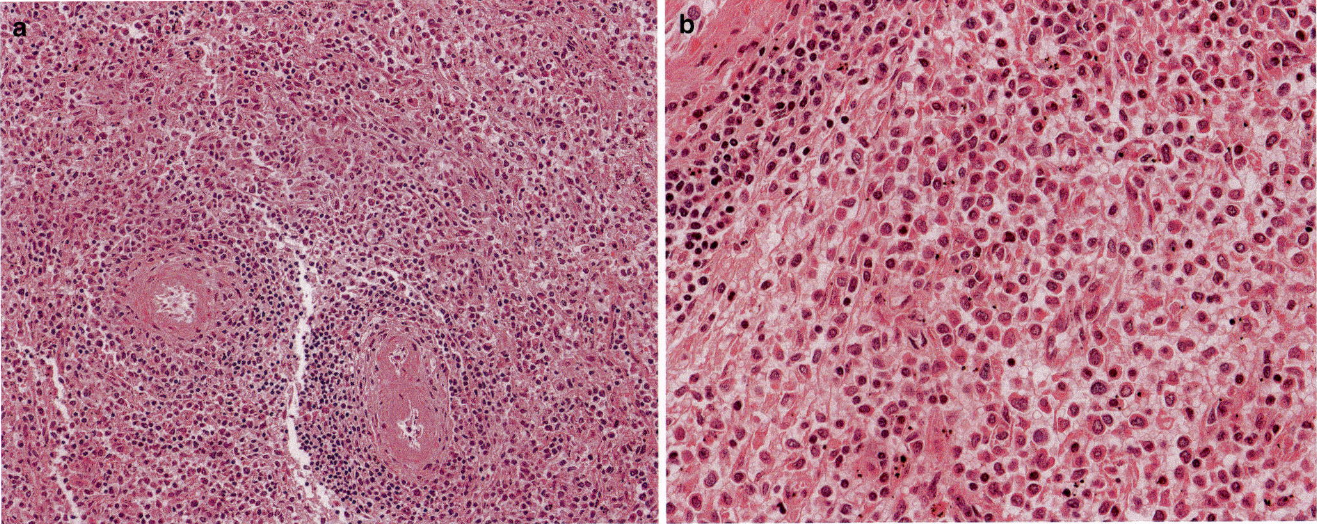

Fig. 2.20 **AML involving the spleen**. Myeloid sarcoma (AML involving the spleen) mainly shows blasts in the red pulp while the white pulp is spared (H&E, **a** and **b**, 200× and 600×). The blasts are medium to large in size with round to oval nuclei and dispersed chromatin and abundant cytoplasm

Table 2.5 Microscopic pattern of benign and malignant splenic disorders

Histologic distribution of splenic disorders		
Predominantly in white pulp	Predominantly in red pulp	Combined white and red pulp
NEOPLASTIC DISORDERS		
Early small lymphocytic lymphoma (SLL)	Hairy cell leukemia	Splenic marginal zone lymphoma
Mantle cell lymphoma	Hairy cell leukemia variant	Chronic lymphocytic leukemia/small lymphocytic lymphoma (mixed or diffuse pattern)
Follicular lymphoma	Splenic diffuse red pulp lymphoma (SDRPL)	Angioimmunoblastic T-cell lymphoma
Burkitt lymphoma	T-cell large granular lymphocytic leukemia	Primary amyloidosis
Diffuse large B-cell lymphoma	Hepatosplenic T-cell lymphoma	
High-grade B-cell lymphoma	Peripheral T-cell lymphoma, NOS	
Classic Hodgkin lymphoma	Acute myeloid leukemia	
	Myeloproliferative neoplasms	
	Myelodysplastic/myeloproliferative neoplasms (MDS/MPN)	
	Plasma cell neoplasm	
COMMON BENIGN DISORDERS		
Reactive follicular hyperplasia	Sinus histiocytosis	Infectious mononucleosis
Castleman disease	Rosai-Dorfman disease	Drug-related hypersensitivity
Progressive transformation of germinal centers	Langerhans cell histiocytosis	Granulomatous lymphadenitis
	Hemophagocytic lymphohistocytosis (HLH)	Kikuchi-Fujimoto lymphadenitis
	Extramedullary hematopoiesis	Systemic lupus lymphadenitis
	Kaposi sarcoma	Angioimmune lymphoproliferative syndrome
		EBV-associated inflammatory pseudotumor

Table modified from [22, 40]

negative for CD34, CD8, D2-40, and factor XIIIa [22, 40, 44, 45]. Littoral cells also stain positive for periodic acid–schiff (PAS)[44]. It is unique that normal splenic sinusoidal endothelial lining cells express CD8, a marker for cytotoxic T-cells; therefore, CD8 becomes a very useful maker to highlight splenic sinusoidal space as well as a subset of T-cells with cytotoxic function [22, 40].

It is helpful to subclassify lymphomas or myeloid neoplasms based on a panel of immunohistochemical staining patterns and antibody expression level. The following Table 2.6 summarizes the common panels of immunohistochemical (IHC) antibodies/in situ hybridization (ISH) implicated in diagnosis of splenic involvement by hematopoietic neoplasms.

If splenectomy is performed after chemo-immunotherapy, interpretation of immunohistochemical markers should be done with caution. For example, hairy cell leukemia cells are typically positive for tartrate-resistant acid phosphatase (TRAP), DBA44 (CD72), CD25, CD123, cyclin D1, and Annexin A1 by IHC study. However, when a patient has been treated with a BRAF inhibitor, staining for cyclin D1 and CD25 has been reported to be downregulated or results in weak expression [24]. Administration of rituximab (Rituxan, target CD20), brentuximab (target CD30), and epratuzumab (target CD22) as well as recent chimeric antigen receptor (CAR) T-cell therapy will lead to loss of particular surface antigen expression [46, 47]. Other potential diagnostic pitfalls could occur due to inappropriate fixation, loss of antigenicity during antigen retrieval

or specimen processing, inadequate assessment, or incorrect interpretation [48]. Recently, following the wide utilization of molecular diagnosis, combined IHC study and molecular markers help to lead to a more accurate diagnosis of lymphomas. Table 2.7 summarizes the IHC and molecular studies applied for common hematopoietic malignancies involving the spleen.

Flow Cytometry

Flow cytometry has been widely adopted for detection of abnormal population of T-cells, B-cells, NK cells, plasma cells, and blasts in the specimen from splenectomy or splenic biopsy [62]. Flow cytometry identifies the cell size (forward scatter, FSC) and internal complexity (side scatter) and evaluates different antigen expressions on the cell surface or cytoplasm by implication of multiple [4–10] fluorescence parameters in order to determine a normal versus abnormal cell population, even if the latter is in very low events [62–64]. A screening panel includes antibodies against T-, B-, and NK cells including CD19, CD20, CD5, CD10, CD23, CD11c, CD25, CD103, FMC-7, surface kappa light chain, surface lambda light chain, CD2, CD3, CD4, CD7, CD8, CD16, CD56, CD57, TCRαβ, and TCRγδ. The antibody panels can be modified according to the preview of morphologic findings and the patient's preexisting disorder(s). A modified small panel of flow cytometric parameters (CD45, CD3, CD5, CD10, CD19, CD20,

Table 2.6 Immunohistochemical staining panels and in situ hybridization selected for common hematopoietic neoplasms involving the liver and spleen

Type of lymphoma	IHC/ISH screening panel
DLBCL, Burkitt lymphoma, high-grade B-cell lymphoma	CD20, CD3, CD5, CD10, CD30, BCL-2, BCL-6, MUM1, MYC, Ki67, EBER
MZL, SLL, FL, MALToma	CD20, CD3, CD5, CD10, CD23, BCL-1, BCL2, BCL-6
HCL, HCLv, SRPD	CD8, CD68, CD34, DBA44, Annexin A1, VE1(*BRAF* V600E), CD25, TRAP
Plasmacytoma	CD20, CD138, CD56, CD117, kappa, lambda (monoclonal process)
Classic Hodgkin lymphoma	CD15, CD30, PAX-5, CD45, CD20
Mature T-cell lymphoma	CD2, CD3, CD5, CD7, CD4, CD8, CD10, CD21, CD25, CD30, PD1, CXCL13, granzyme B, TIA, perforin, CD56, CD57, Ki67
NK cell leukemia/lymphoma	CD2, CD3, CD4, CD5, CD7, CD8, EBER, TIA1, granzyme B, CD30, CD56, CD57
T-lymphoblastic lymphoma	CD3, CD1a, CD4, CD8, CD5, CD7, CD34, CD99, TdT
B-lymphoblastic lymphoma	CD19, CD10, CD20, CD79a, PAX-5, TdT, CD34
Myeloid sarcoma	CD43, lysozyme, CD117, CD68, CD163, MPO
Blastic plasmacytoid dendritic neoplasm	CD123, CD4, CD56, TCF4, TCL1, CD34, CD117, MPO
Systemic mastocytosis	CD117, mast cell tryptase, CD25, CD2, CD3
Inflammatory pseudotumor	CD20, CD138, kappa, lambda (polyclonal process)
Langerhans cell histiocytosis and other histiocytic or dendritic cell proliferation	CD21, CD23, CD35, clusterin, EBER, CD68, CD163, CD4, S100 protein, CD1a, langerin, CD3
Vascular tumor	ERG, CD31, CD34, factor VIII, D2-40, CD68, CD163, CD8
Metastatic carcinoma/melanoma	Cytokeratin, Melan A, SMB45, SOX10

Table modified from [22, 40]

IHC immunohistochemical staining, *ISH* in situ hybridization, *DLBCL* diffuse large B-cell lymphoma, *EBER* Epstein-Barr virus-encoded RNA probe, *HCL* hairy cell leukemia, *HCLv* hairy cell leukemia variant, *MZL* marginal zone lymphoma, *SLL* small lymphocytic lymphoma, *FL* follicular lymphoma, *MALToma* Lymphoma involving the mucosa-associated lymphoid tissue

Table 2.7 IHC and molecular studies used in diagnosis of common hematologic neoplasms involving the spleen

Diseases	IHC/FCM markers	Special staining, specific cytogenetics/ molecular markers
Hairy cell leukemia [24, 42, 49, 50]	CD20 (+), PAX5 (+), DBA44/CD72 (+), CD11c (+), CD25 (+), CD103 (+), CD123 (+), cyclin D1 (subset+), VE1(*BRAF* V600E) (+), and Annexin A1 (+)	TRAP (+) *BRAF* V600E mutation (nearly 100%) [51, 52] *IgHV4–34* (10%) [53]
Splenic marginal zone lymphoma [54, 55]	CD5 (−), CD10 (−), CD23 (−) ANXA1 (−), CD123 (−); CD11c (−/rare+), CD25 (−/rare+), and CD103 (−/rare+)	Lacks recurrent chromosomal translocations
Atypical hairy cell leukemia [50, 56]	Similar to HCL, CD20 (+), PAX5 (+), CD11c (+), CD103 (+), TRAP (+), Annexin A1 (−), CD123 (−), and CD25 (−)	*MAP2K1* [57, 58] (17–42%) *IgHV4–34* (40–50%) *BRAF* V600E mutation NOT detected
Splenic diffuse red pulp B-cell lymphoma (SDRPL) [50, 59, 60]	CD20 (+), PAX-5 (+), CD123 (+), or 103(+), but Annexin A1 (−)	*CCND3* PEST domain mutation (77%) [61]
T-large granular lymphocytic leukemia	Surface CD3 (+), dim CD5 (+), or CD5 (−), CD7 (+), CD8 (+), CD57 (+), CD16 (−/+), TIA (+), granzyme B (+), perforin (+), and commonly TCR βF1 (+) and less frequently TCR γδ (+)	*STAT3* mutation (approximately 30%)
Hepatosplenic T-cell lymphoma	Surface CD3 (+), CD5 (+), CD7 (+), CD8 (−/+), TIA (+), granzyme B (−), perforin (−), Less commonly TCRβ F1 (+) and frequently TCR gamma or delta (+)	Isochromosome 7

TRAP tartrate-resistant acid phosphatase, *FCM* flow cytometry

κ, λ, FMC7, CD23) is selected when only a small amount of tissue from splenic fine needle aspirate or needle core biopsy is obtained [65]. An anti-CD45 antibody must be included for gating. The splenic cell suspension in RPMI culture medium (usually 0.5 to 1-million cells/tube) is stained with selected fluorescein dyes. Cellular viability is measured to ensure the testing results are accurate. Using the above panel, it is very easy to differentiate splenic marginal zone lymphoma (Fig. 2.21) from hairy cell leukemia (Fig. 2.22) as well as other hematopoietic neoplasms. The

Fig. 2.21 Flow cytometric analysis of splenic marginal zone lymphoma (gating on lymphocyte region, blue for abnormal B-cells and green for reactive T-cells) shows the lymphoma cells expressing CD19, CD20, dim CD11c, and FMC7. They are "triple negative" for CD5, CD10, and CD23 as well as negative for CD25 and CD103

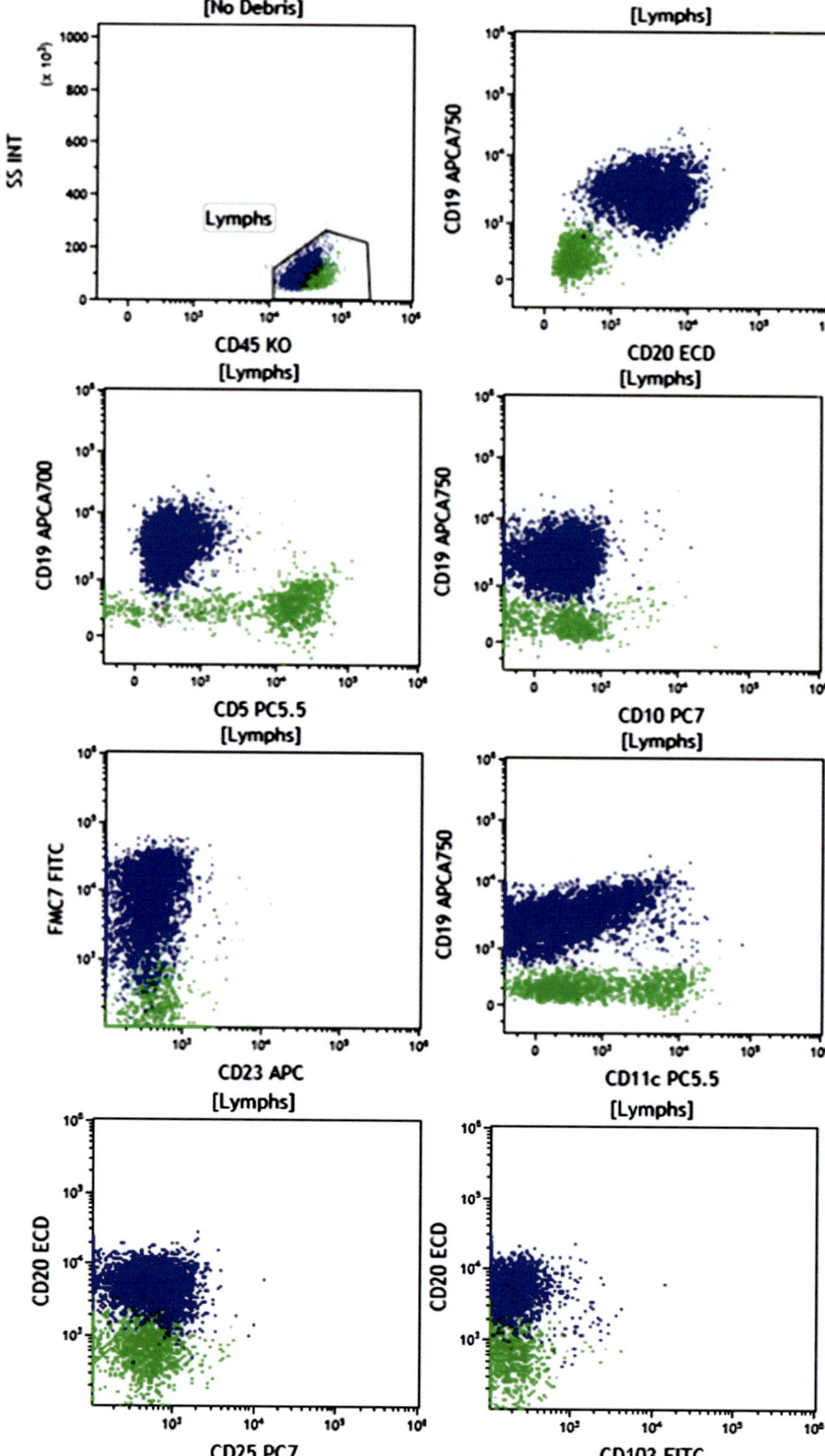

Fig. 2.22 Flow cytometric analysis of hairy cell leukemia by gating on monocyte region (in blue) exhibits a distinct population of lambda clonal B-cells co-expressing CD19, CD20, CD11c, CD25, CD103, and FMC7

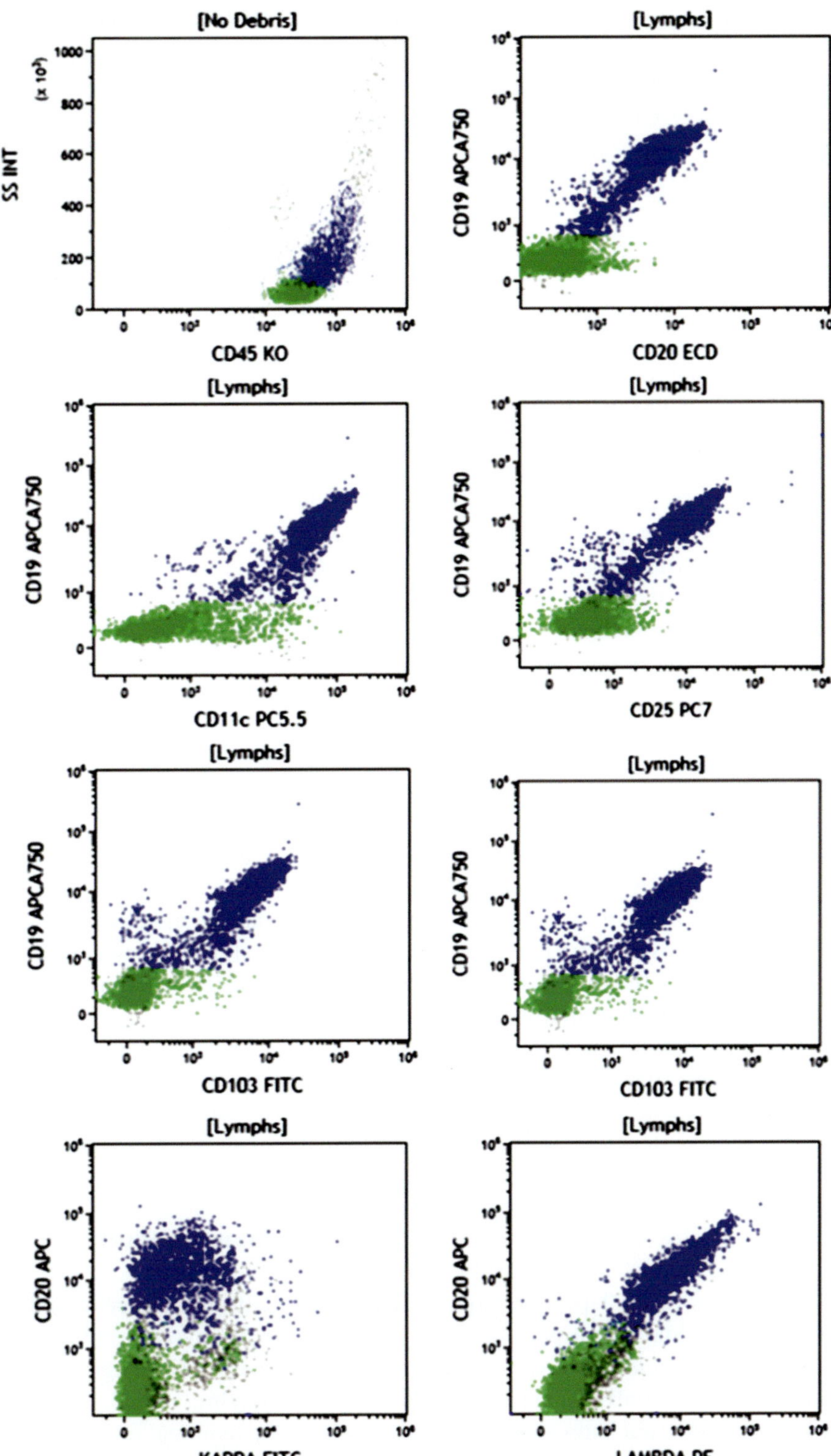

characteristic immunophenotype of HCL cells is positive for CD19, CD20, CD22, CD103, CD25, and CD11c with kappa or lambda light chain restriction. SMZL cells phenotypically express CD19, CD20, CD22, and kappa or lambda light chain and are usually negative for CD5, CD10, CD23, CD43, CD103, and CD25.

Liver

The liver is the largest solid organ and gland in our body. It executes many important functions, including producing bile, absorbing and metabolizing bilirubin to help digestion, and synthesis and metabolism of lipid, carbohydrates, protein, angiotensinogen, and clotting factors and vitamin and mineral storage. In addition, the liver filtrates and removes certain blood components, e.g., alcohol, medications, and hormones. Many diseases, most commonly non-neoplastic disorders, can involve the liver. Neoplastic disorders, in particular hematopoietic malignancies, are identified but less frequently. To identify the nature of these neoplastic or non-neoplastic diseases, further subclassification, and prognostication, a biopsy of the liver is necessary.

Indications for Liver Biopsy

Liver biopsy is an invasive procedure and is associated with post-procedure bleeding that may lead to a lethal consequence when it is severe. A recent study from a British group revealed that liver biopsy is principally used for evaluation of liver disease in a diffuse pattern (67%) while a subset is implicated for diagnosis of localized lesions per imaging study [66]. Whether it is necessary to perform a biopsy to diagnose a hematopoietic neoplasm largely depends on the patient's clinical presentation. Albeit many hematologic neoplasms are often manifested by hepatosplenomegaly, liver biopsy is not the first choice when an alternative specimen is available. For example, hepatomegaly is a common feature for patients with T-prolymphocytic leukemia (T-PLL); however, obtaining a peripheral blood specimen for morphologic and ancillary diagnoses is more convenient than a potentially dangerous liver biopsy as these T-PLL patients often show marked lymphocytosis [67]. The specimens from liver biopsies are commonly applied for diagnosis, staging, and infrequently for treatment. The indications are broad and the common ones are summarized in Table 2.8.

Hepatic tissue can be obtained by performing needle core biopsy or lobectomy. The needle core biopsy is indicated when it is necessary to assess non-neoplastic liver disease

Table 2.8 Indications for liver biopsy

	Benign	Neoplastic
Non-hematologic	Hepatitis B, C	HCC
	Autoimmune hepatitis	LCA
	Primary sclerosing cholangitis	Metastatic tumors
	Primary biliary cirrhosis	
	Nutritional-toxic/ alcoholic steatohepatitis	
	NAFLD/NASH	
	Iatrogenic toxic	
	Hemochromatosis	
	Post liver transplantation-related disorders	
Hematologic	Graft-versus-host disease	B- or T-cell lymphomas
		B- or T-ALL
		Myeloid sarcoma/AML/ myeloid neoplasms
		Plasma cell neoplasm/ amyloidosis
		Post-transplant lymphoproliferative disorders

Table modified from [68, 69]
NAFLD nonalcoholic fatty liver disease, *NASH* nonalcoholic steatohepatitis, *HCC* hepatocellular carcinoma, *LCA* liver cell adenoma, *ALL* acute lymphoblastic leukemia, *AML* acute myeloid leukemia

that has affected the liver function, as well as to confirm clinical or radiologic suspicions of primary or secondary malignancies including metastatic carcinomas and hematopoietic neoplasms.

Hepatic lobectomy is not indicated for any hematopoietic neoplasm but can be suitable for certain benign lesions or tumors, e.g., adenomas and focal nodular hyperplasia or sometimes isolated single metastatic colon carcinoma.

Imaging Study

Ultrasound performed on a patient with hepatic involvement by a mass-forming lymphoma shows a hypoechoic mass. CT imaging is commonly adopted for lymphoma staging, which usually detects hyper-enhancement of lymphoma in the liver, when compared with the surrounding normal hepatic parenchyma [70]. However, neither CT nor ultrasound findings are specific to distinguish lymphoma from hepatocellular carcinoma (HCC). ^{18}FDG PET/CT is more widely used for diagnosis, detection of degree of involvement, and assessment of treatment response. It is also more useful in identifying hepatic lymphoma by showing hypermetabolic lesions

[70–72]. Ultimately, image-guided liver biopsy is necessary to reach a pathologic diagnosis and subclassification of hepatic lymphoma [73].

Grossing

There are two methods for obtaining liver biopsy: fine needle core biopsy and wedge biopsy.

Liver Biopsy

When tissue is obtained for grossing, documentation of the size, color, and texture of biopsy tissue is necessary. Normal liver biopsy appears tan-brown, soft, and threadlike cores (intact or fragmented). Attention to the lesion(s) in the biopsy should be paid and documentation of the identified lesion(s) is required. The needle cores are arranged in parallel, laid on a sponge, and placed in a cassette for fixation [23].

Resection/Lobectomy

First, the specimen must be weighed and measured. Thin-sliced wedge biopsies (usually 0.5 cm in thickness) are carefully examined including the appearance, color, cut surface, and included lesions. The capsule of normal liver is thin, smooth, and glistening and the cut surface is homogeneous red-brown-tan (Fig. 2.23). Abnormal findings include central scar, hemorrhage, nodularity, necrosis, cystic changes, and bulging masses. The size, shape, and relationship to the capsules, uninvolved liver, adjacent main organ/tissue, and surgical margin of any abnormal findings must be well documented. All surgical margins at the closest approach of the tumor, representative sections of tumor (one to multiple depending upon the size), and uninvolved liver parenchyma

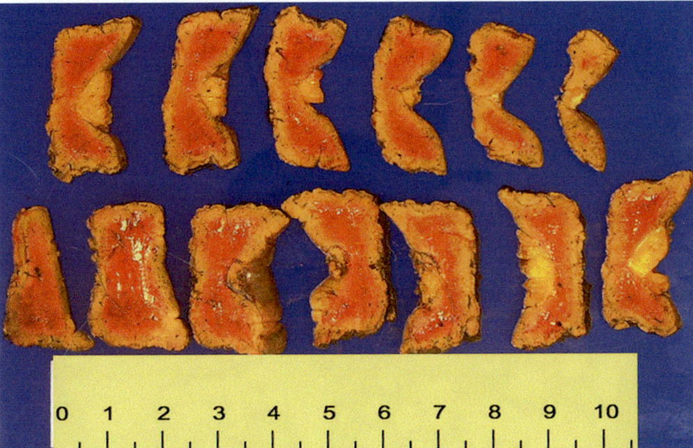

Fig. 2.23 A series of sections of partially fixed hepatic parenchyma show yellow-tan on the peripheral and brown-tan in the center with overt abnormal gross findings

(in two cassettes) are submitted and adequately fixed similar to the needle core biopsy [23].

Sample Processing

Fixation, Routine, and Special Staining

Liver tissue is fixed in 10% neutral buffered formalin solution. Hematoxylin and eosin stain is routinely performed in liver biopsy tissue, which highlights the nuclei of hepatocytes in deep blue and the cytoplasm of hepatocytes in pink. Extracellular matrix is also stained in a shade of pink. The special stains including periodic acid-Schiff (PAS), PAS-D (PAS with diastase), Prussian blue, reticulin, and Masson's trichrome are also included in the routine panel for liver biopsy assessment [23]. Prussian blue is used to assess iron storage. PAS is used to detect polysaccharides such as glycogen and mucosubstances, e.g., glycolipids, glycoproteins, and mucins. Adding diastase (PAS-D) is able to identify AAT polymer inclusion in a patient with alpha-1 antitrypsin deficiency disease [74]. Reticulin stain highlights normal vasculature and the presence of any abnormal portal or lobular fibrosis. The unique features of Masson's trichrome stain are to highlight collagen in blue, nuclei in black, and fibrin, cytoplasm, erythrocytes, or smooth muscle bundles in red. Trichrome stain highlights severe collagen fibrosis. Although the aforementioned special staining may not be indispensable for diagnosis of hematologic neoplasms involving the liver, they are routinely performed for assessment of hepatic lesions such as cirrhosis, alcoholism, or nonalcoholic fatty liver disease (NAFLD) (Fig. 2.24) by gastrointestinal (GI) pathologists. Therefore, evaluation of non-hematopoietic neoplasms in the liver should be carried on at the same time when evaluating for lymphomas or myeloid neoplasms.

Microscopic Examination

Lymphomas involving the liver are mostly T- or B-cell non-Hodgkin lymphomas, although occasionally classic Hodgkin lymphoma is reported. The histologic pattern can be divided into two: nodular or diffuse. Diffuse large B-cell lymphoma is considered one of the most common primary hepatic lymphomas (Fig. 2.25) followed by extranodal marginal zone lymphoma of the mucosa-associated lymphoid tissue (MALT). Other primary hepatic lymphomas are Burkitt lymphoma, lymphoblastic lymphoma/leukemia, follicular lymphoma, mantle cell lymphoma, T-cell/histiocyte-rich B-cell lymphoma, hepatosplenic T-cell lymphoma, and anaplastic large cell lymphoma (null type) [75, 76]. The infiltrating pattern is variable and summarized in Table 2.9. Primary hepatosplenic T-cell lymphoma

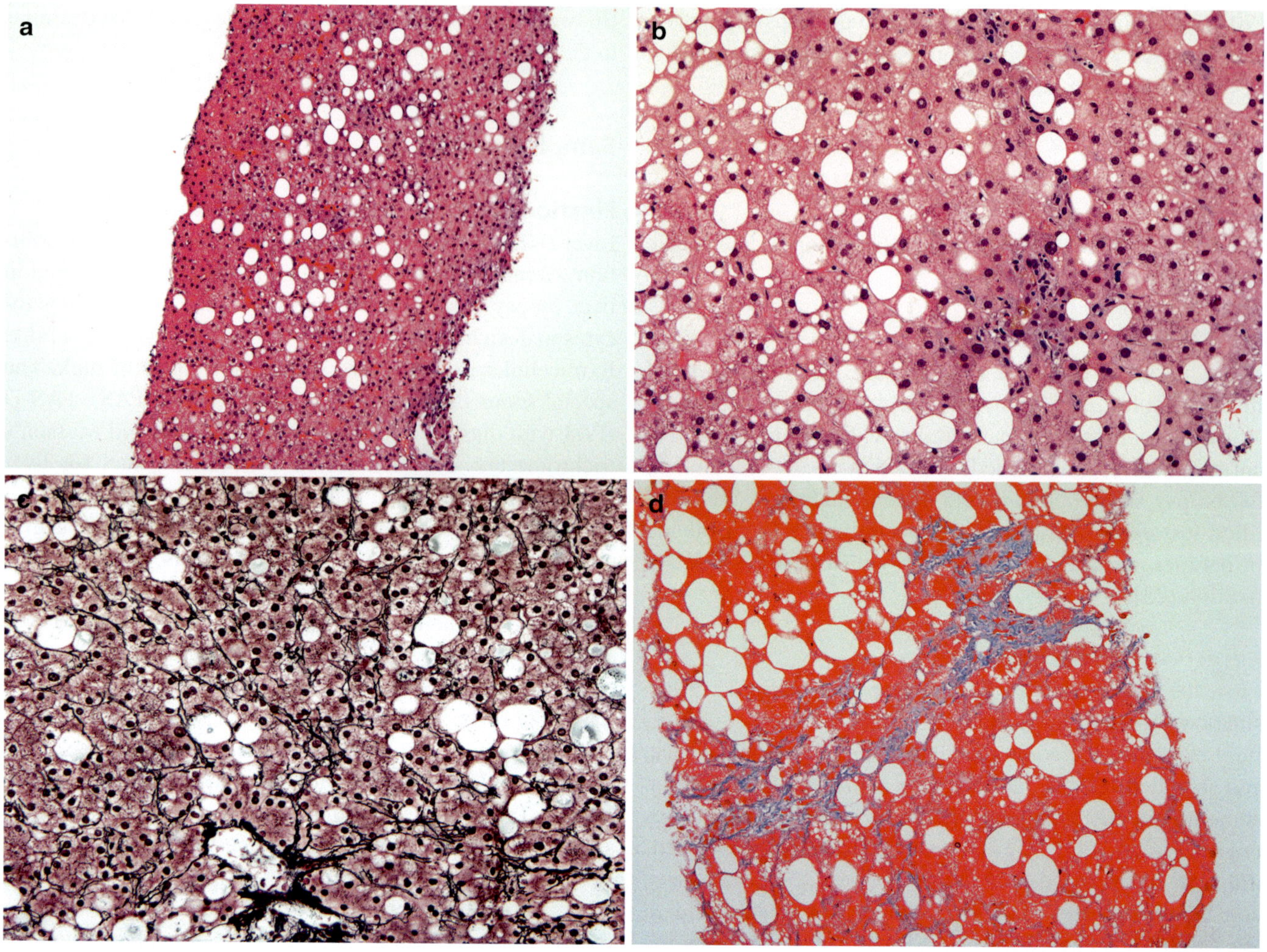

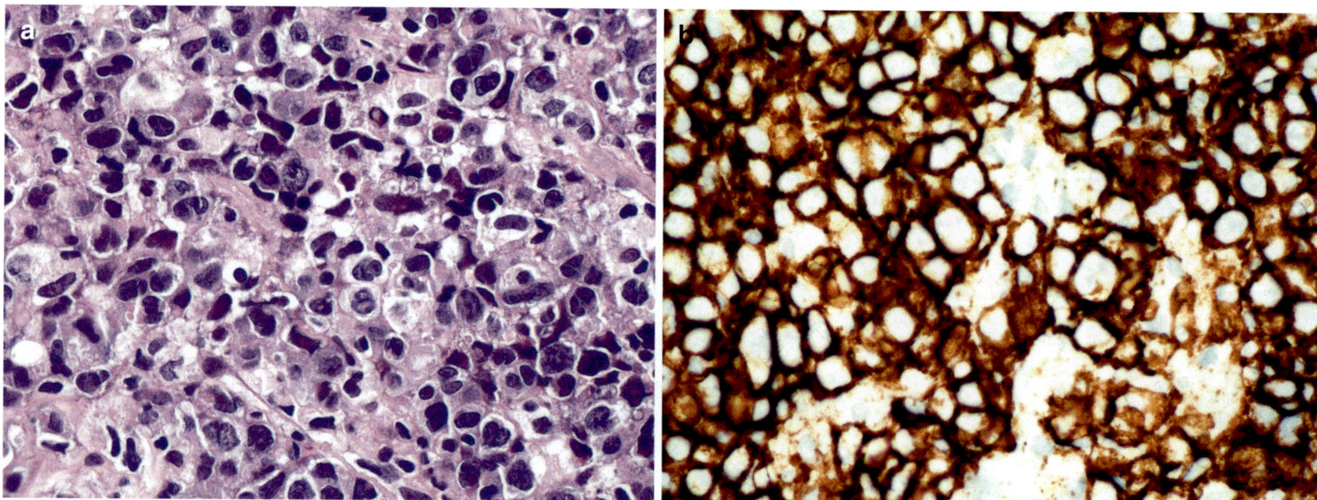

Fig. 2.24 Microscopic examination of liver biopsy. The liver biopsy from a patient with nonalcoholic fatty liver disease (NASH) shows overt steatosis predominantly macrovesicular pattern admixed with few microvesicles (H&E, **a** and **b,** 100× and 600×). Marked reticulin fibrosis is present (**c,** reticulin stain, 600x) and septal collagen fibrosis is highlighted by trichrome staining (**d,** 600×)

Fig. 2.25 Diffuse large B-cell lymphoma involving the liver. High-power view of diffuse large B-cell lymphoma involving the liver (**a** H&E, 600×). CD20 highlights the neoplastic B-cells (**b** immunoperoxidase, 600×)

Table 2.9 Histologic findings of common lymphoplasmacytic and myeloid neoplasms involving the liver

Type of diseases	Cytohistological findings
Primary hepatic diffuse large B-cell or secondary lymphoma (Fig. 2.26)	Large atypical lymphoid cells with vesicular chromatin and prominent nuclei, arranged in sheets, with or without necrosis
Burkitt lymphoma	Uniformly medium-sized atypical lymphoid cells with disperse chromatin, two to three small prominent nucleoli, increased apoptosis and macrophages, arranged in "starry sky" pattern
Extranodal marginal zone lymphoma of mucosa-associated lymphoid tissue	Nodular to diffuse proliferation of small- to medium-sized atypical lymphoid cells with hyperchromatic nuclei, identifiable germinal centers, periductal lymphoepithelial lesion
Mantle cell lymphoma	Nodular and periportal lymphoid infiltrate consisting of small-sized lymphoid cells with hyperchromasia and visible nucleoli
Plasma cell neoplasm	Sinusoidal or portal involvement by plasma cells in aggregates
Hodgkin lymphoma	Involves portal track associated with Hodgkin cells and background of inflammatory cells
Hepatosplenic T-cell lymphoma (Fig. 2.27)	Predominantly intra-sinusoidal atypical lymphoid infiltrate composed of small- to medium-sized lymphoid cells with mild nuclear irregularity, arranged in cords or small clustering; hemophagocytic lymphohistocytosis (HLH) may present
T-large granular lymphocytic leukemia or NK cell lymphoma/leukemia	Predominantly intra-sinusoidal atypical lymphoid infiltrate composed of small- to medium-sized lymphoid cells with mild nuclear irregularity, devoid of portal areas
Adult T-cell lymphoma/leukemia	Mainly found in periportal region and rarely involved in sinusoidal spaces
Leukemia/myeloid sarcoma	Involves both portal tract and sinuses. AML cells show more sinusoidal infiltration pattern, while ALL/LBL frequently invades into portal region
Pseudolymphoma	Infiltrating pattern could be similar to extranodal marginal zone lymphoma of MALT
Extramedullary hematopoiesis (Fig. 2.28)	Predominantly sinusoidal and perivascular infiltrating pattern

Table modified from [4]

AML acute myeloid leukemia, *ALL/LBL* acute lymphoblastic leukemia/lymphoblastic lymphoma, *MALT* mucosal-associated lymphoid tissue

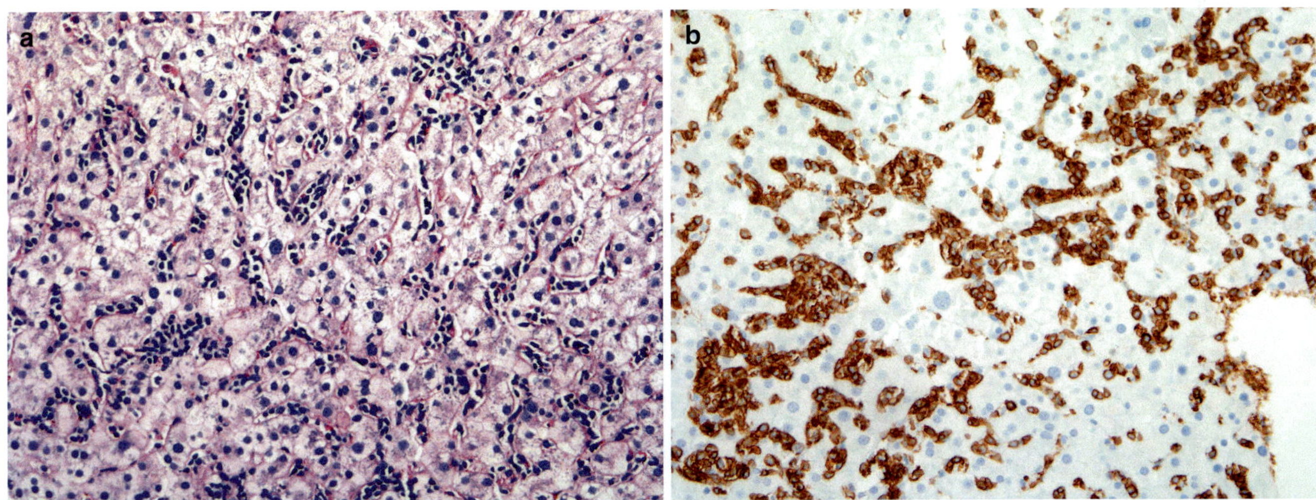

Fig. 2.26 Hepatosplenic T-cell lymphoma. The image shows sinusoidal atypical lymphoid infiltrate consisting of small forms with irregular nuclear contours and high N:C ratio (**a,** PAS, 200×). The CD3 staining highlights the neoplastic T-cells in characteristic sinusoidal infiltrating pattern (**b,** immunoperoxidase 200x)

frequently involves intra-sinusoidal spaces [76, 77] (Fig. 2.26). Diffuse portal infiltration is commonly observed while lymphoma cells spread into the hepatic parenchyma resulting in "erosion of the hepatic cords" or "spillover to sinusoids" [70, 76]. Extramedullary hematopoiesis in the liver shows sinusoidal hematopoietic precursors e.g. erythroid precursors (Fig. 2.27.). Some non-hematopoietic neoplasms involving the liver shows cytic changes secondary to abnormal proliferation of endothelial cells e.g., Kaposi sarcoma (Fig. 2.28.)

Ancillary Studies

Flow Cytometry

Flow cytometry is infrequently used for diagnosis of lymphomas involving the liver due to limited liver biopsy tissue.

Immunohistochemistry Study

Immunohistochemical stains have been popularly performed on the liver biopsy to differentiate benign

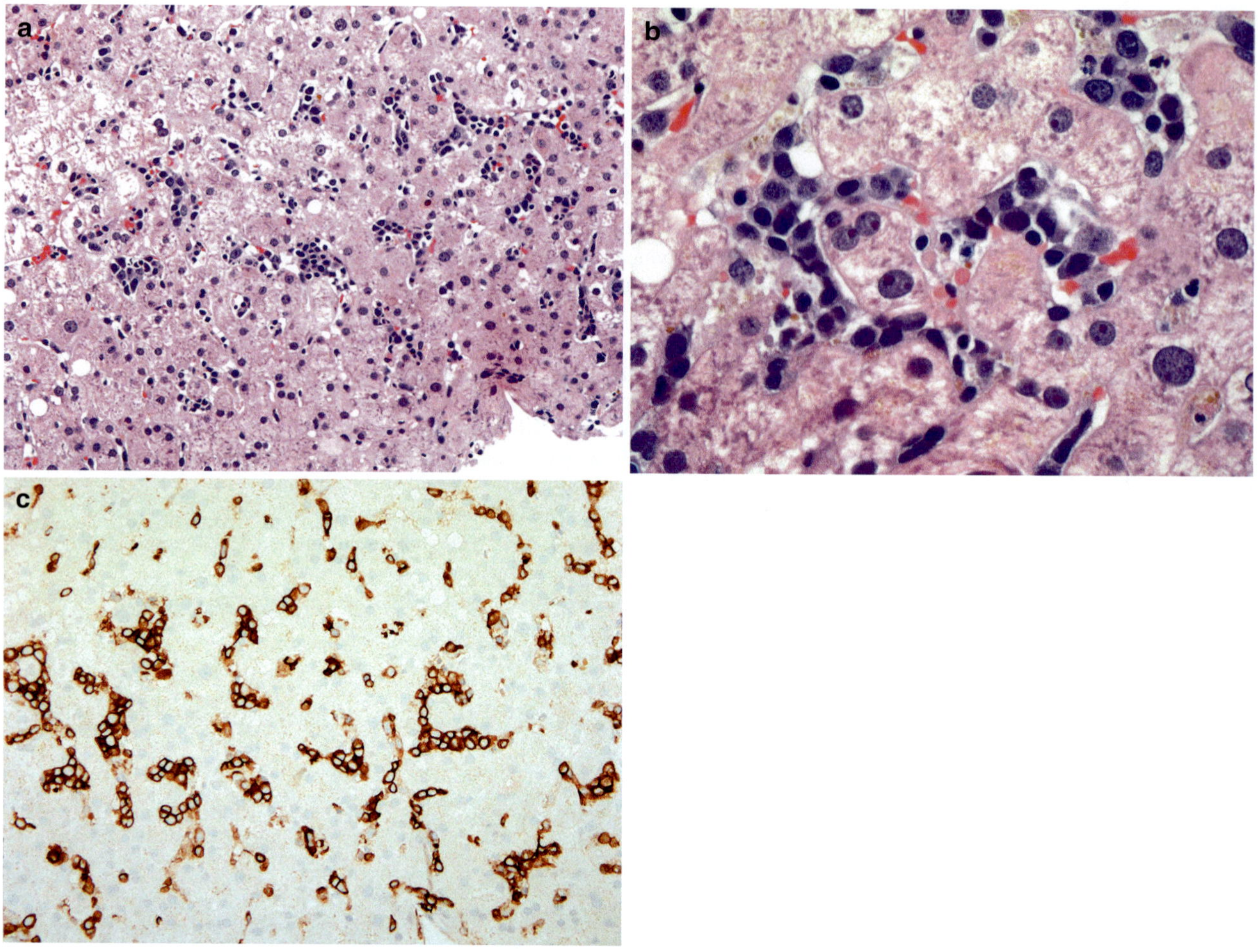

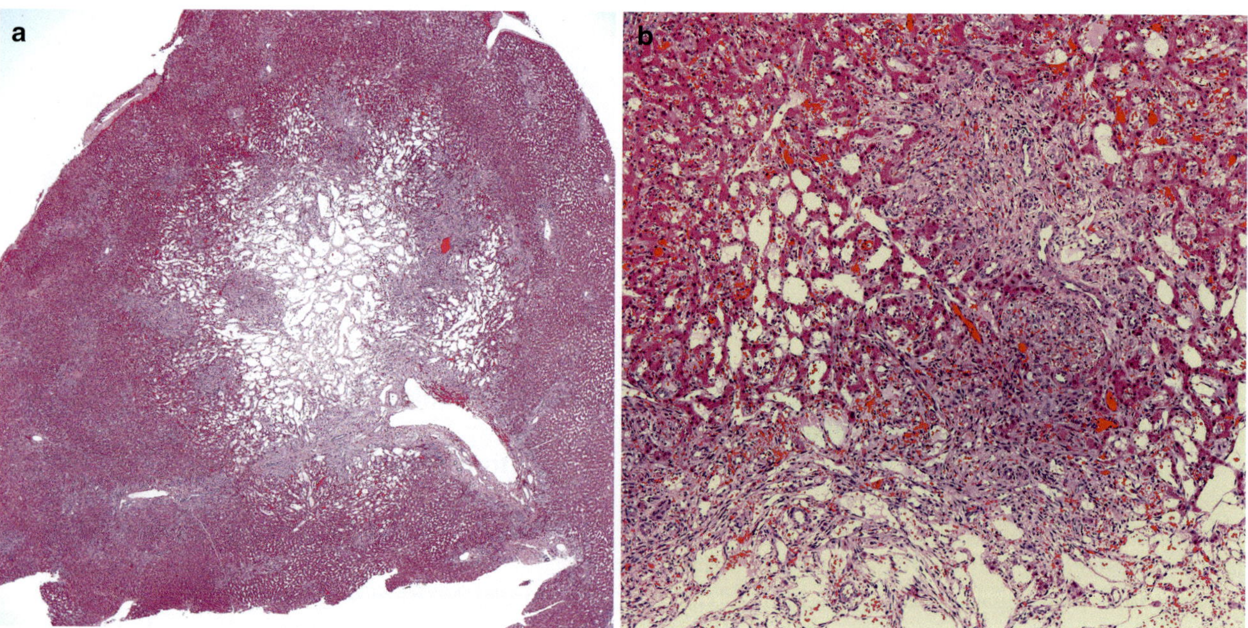

Fig. 2.27 The liver is involved by extramedullary hematopoiesis (**a** and **b**) with the presence of sinusoidal erythroid precursors (H&E, 200× and 600×), which are highlighted by immunohistochemical stain (**c**) with anti-spectrin antibody (immunoperoxidase 200×)

Fig. 2.28 **Kaposi sarcoma**. (**a**) The H&E section (20×) shows a portion of the liver with multiple lesions in the center associated with small cystic changes. (**b–d**) Medium- to high-power views reveal the lesions are constituted with a spindle cell proliferation of endothelial cells forming slit-like sinusoidal spaces with extravascular red blood cells (H&E, 100×, 200× and 600×)

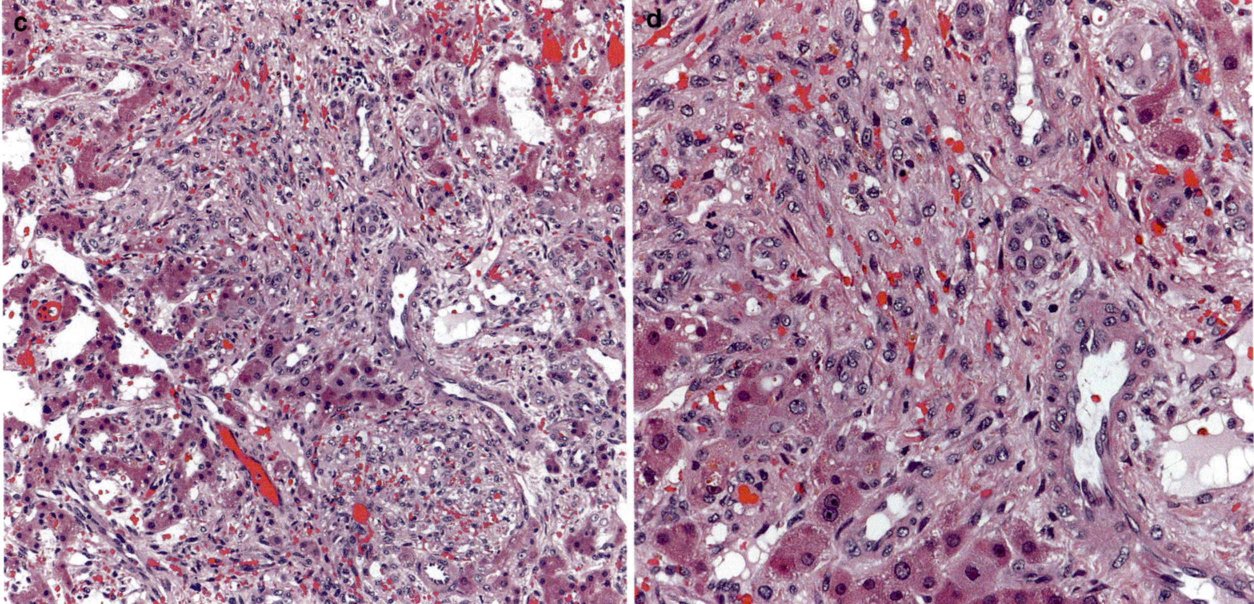

Fig. 2.28 (continued)

lymphoplasmacytic proliferations from malignant lymphoma or plasma cell myeloma. Some immunohistochemical markers show unique staining patterns in the hepatobiliary tissue that must be kept in mind. For example, liver injury often leads to prominent Kupffer cell proliferation with phagocytosis of cellular debris. Interpretation should be performed with caution as they are similar to HLH and also stain positive for CD68 [4]. CD10 stains positive for canalicular structures between the hepatocytes. A small panel of immunohistochemical stains is applied due to limited biopsy tissue. The following table includes the common IHC panels used for diagnosis of the subtype of T- or B-cell lymphoma [78, 79].

In summary, there are a variety of hematopoietic or non-hematopoietic disorders identified in the spleen or liver or both. They may share some similarities in morphology leading to diagnostic challenges. It is important to carefully examine the submitted spleen and liver tissue, adequately sample the representative sections, and make a differential diagnosis in accordance with histologic, immunophenotypic, and possible cytogenetic/molecular findings.

References

1. Mebius RE, Kraal G. Structure and function of the spleen. Nat Rev Immunol. 2005;5(8):606–16.
2. Bronte V, Pittet MJ. The spleen in local and systemic regulation of immunity. Immunity. 2013;39(5):806–18.
3. Corless JK, Middleton HM 3rd. Normal liver function. A basis for understanding hepatic disease. Arch Intern Med. 1983;143(12):2291–4.
4. Torbenson M, Zen Y, Yeh M. Tumors of the liver. Washington, D.C.: ARP Press; 2018.
5. Hiatt J, Phillips E, Morgenstern L. Surgical diseases of the spleen. Heidelberg: Springer; 1997.
6. Johnson HA, Deterling RA. Massive splenomegaly. Surg Gynecol Obstet. 1989;168(2):131–7.
7. Lehne G, Hannisdal E, Langholm R, Nome O. A 10-year experience with splenectomy in patients with malignant non-Hodgkin's lymphoma at the Norwegian Radium Hospital. Cancer. 1994;74(3):933–9.
8. Lv Y, Lau WY, Li Y, et al. Hypersplenism: history and current status. Exp Ther Med. 2016;12(4):2377–82.
9. Cadili A, de Gara C. Complications of splenectomy. Am J Med. 2008;121(5):371–5.
10. Machado NO, Grant CS, Alkindi S, et al. Splenectomy for haematological disorders: a single center study in 150 patients from Oman. Int J Surg. 2009;7(5):476–81.
11. Dendle C, Sundararajan V, Spelman T, Jolley D, Woolley I. Splenectomy sequelae: an analysis of infectious outcomes among adults in Victoria. Med J Aust. 2012;196(9):582–6.
12. Alzen G, Basedow J, Luedemann M, Berthold LD, Zimmer KP. Partial splenic embolization as an alternative to splenectomy in hypersplenism–single center experience in 16 years. Klin Padiatr. 2010;222(6):368–73.
13. Amin MA, el-Gendy MM, Dawoud IE, Shoma A, Negm AM, Amer TA. Partial splenic embolization versus splenectomy for the management of hypersplenism in cirrhotic patients. World J Surg. 2009;33(8):1702–10.
14. George JN, Woolf SH, Raskob GE, et al. Idiopathic thrombocytopenic purpura: a practice guideline developed by explicit methods for the American Society of Hematology. Blood. 1996;88(1):3–40.
15. Kappers-Klunne MC, Wijermans P, Fijnheer R, et al. Splenectomy for the treatment of thrombotic thrombocytopenic purpura. Br J Haematol. 2005;130(5):768–76.
16. Bonnet S, Guedon A, Ribeil JA, Suarez F, Tamburini J, Gaujoux S. Indications and outcome of splenectomy in hematologic disease. J Visc Surg. 2017;154(6):421–9.
17. Katz SC, Pachter HL. Indications for splenectomy. Am Surg. 2006;72(7):565–80.

18. Singh AK, Shankar S, Gervais DA, Hahn PF, Mueller PR. Image-guided percutaneous splenic interventions. Radiographics. 2012;32(2):523–34.

19. Patel N, Dawe G, Tung K. Ultrasound-guided percutaneous splenic biopsy using an 18-G core biopsy needle: our experience with 52 cases. Br J Radiol. 2015;88(1055):20150400.

20. Libepathology.org/wiki/splenectomy-grossing. In: Patholog L, ed 2019.

21. Abbott RM, Levy AD, Aguilera NS, Gorospe L, Thompson WM. From the archives of the AFIP: primary vascular neoplasms of the spleen: radiologic-pathologic correlation. Radiographics. 2004;24(4):1137–63.

22. O'Malley DP, George T, Orazi A, Abbondanzo S. Benign and reactive conditions of lymph node and spleen, vol. 7. Washington, D.C.: American Registery of Pathology; 2009.

23. Lester. Manual of surgical pathology. Philadelphia: Churchill Livingstone; 2001.

24. Wotherspoon A, Attygalle A, Mendes LS. Bone marrow and splenic histology in hairy cell leukaemia. Best Pract Res Clin Haematol. 2015;28(4):200–7.

25. Urrutia M, Mergo PJ, Ros LH, Torres GM, Ros PR. Cystic masses of the spleen: radiologic-pathologic correlation. Radiographics. 1996;16(1):107–29.

26. Morgenstern L. Nonparasitic splenic cysts: pathogenesis, classification, and treatment. J Am Coll Surg. 2002;194(3):306–14.

27. McInnes MD, Kielar AZ, Macdonald DB. Percutaneous image-guided biopsy of the spleen: systematic review and meta-analysis of the complication rate and diagnostic accuracy. Radiology. 2011;260(3):699–708.

28. Keogan MT, Freed KS, Paulson EK, Nelson RC, Dodd LG. Imaging-guided percutaneous biopsy of focal splenic lesions: update on safety and effectiveness. AJR Am J Roentgenol. 1999;172(4):933–7.

29. Civardi G, Vallisa D, Berte R, et al. Ultrasound-guided fine needle biopsy of the spleen: high clinical efficacy and low risk in a multicenter Italian study. Am J Hematol. 2001;67(2):93–9.

30. Tam A, Krishnamurthy S, Pillsbury EP, et al. Percutaneous image-guided splenic biopsy in the oncology patient: an audit of 156 consecutive cases. J Vasc Interv Radiol. 2008;19(1):80–7.

31. Friedlander MA, Wei XJ, Iyengar P, Moreira AL. Diagnostic pitfalls in fine needle aspiration biopsy of the spleen. Diagn Cytopathol. 2008;36(2):69–75.

32. Ramdall RB, Cai G, Alasio TM, Levine P. Fine-needle aspiration biopsy for the primary diagnosis of lymphoproliferative disorders involving the spleen: one institution's experience and review of the literature. Diagn Cytopathol. 2006;34(12):812–7.

33. Gomez-Rubio M, Lopez-Cano A, Rendon P, et al. Safety and diagnostic accuracy of percutaneous ultrasound-guided biopsy of the spleen: a multicenter study. J Clin Ultrasound. 2009;37(8):445–50.

34. Phillips EH, Carroll BJ, Fallas MJ. Laparoscopic splenectomy. Surg Endosc. 1994;8(8):931–3.

35. Poulin EC, Thibault C, Mamazza J. Laparoscopic splenectomy. Surg Endosc. 1995;9(2):172–6; discussion 176–7

36. Bonds LA, Barnes P, Foucar K, Sever CE. Acetic acid-zinc-formalin: a safe alternative to B-5 fixative. Am J Clin Pathol. 2005;124(2):205–11.

37. Medeiros L, O'Malley DP, Caraway N, Vega F, Elenitoba-Johnson K, Lim M. Tumors of the lymph nodes and spleen. Washington, D.C.: ARP Press. 2017

38. Neiman RS. Incidence and importance of splenic sarcoid-like granulomas. Arch Pathol Lab Med. 1977;101(10):518–21.

39. Rosso R, Neiman RS, Paulli M, et al. Splenic marginal zone cell lymphoma: report of an indolent variant without massive splenomegaly presumably representing an early phase of the disease. Hum Pathol. 1995;26(1):39–46.

40. Borch WR, Aguilera NS, Brissette MD, O'Malley DP, Auerbach A. Practical applications in immunohistochemistry: an immunophenotypic approach to the spleen. Arch Pathol Lab Med. 2019;143(9):1093–105.

41. Grimm K, Barry T, Omarrley D, Weiss L. Immunophenotypic markers useful in the diagnosis and classification of hematopoietic and lymphoid neoplasms. In: Knowles' neoplasmitc hematopathology. Philadelphia: Wolters Kluwer/Lippincott Williams & Wilkins; 1992. p. 91–118.

42. Sherman MJ, Hanson CA, Hoyer JD. An assessment of the usefulness of immunohistochemical stains in the diagnosis of hairy cell leukemia. Am J Clin Pathol. 2011;136(3):390–9.

43. Neiman R, Orazi A. Hematopmathologic manifestation of lymphoproliferative and myeloproliferative disorders involving the spleen. In: DM K, editor. Neoplastic hematopathology. Baltimore: Lipplincott Williams & Wilkins; 2000.

44. Du J, Shen Q, Yin H, Zhou X, Wu B. Littoral cell angioma of the spleen: report of three cases and literature review. Int J Clin Exp Pathol. 2015;8(7):8516–20.

45. Peckova K, Michal M, Hadravsky L, et al. Littoral cell angioma of the spleen: a study of 25 cases with confirmation of frequent association with visceral malignancies. Histopathology. 2016;69(5):762–74.

46. Ujjani C, Cheson BD. The current status and future impact of targeted therapies in non-Hodgkin lymphoma. Expert Rev Hematol. 2013;6(2):191–202; quiz 203

47. Miliotou AN, Papadopoulou LC. CAR T-cell therapy: a new era in cancer immunotherapy. Curr Pharm Biotechnol. 2018;19(1):5–18.

48. Werner M, Chott A, Fabiano A, Battifora H. Effect of formalin tissue fixation and processing on immunohistochemistry. Am J Surg Pathol. 2000;24(7):1016–9.

49. Sharpe RW, Bethel KJ. Hairy cell leukemia: diagnostic pathology. Hematol Oncol Clin North Am. 2006;20(5):1023–49.

50. Foucar K, Catovsky D, et al. Hairy cell leukemia. In: Swedlow S, Harris N, et al., editors. WHO classification of tumors of haematopoietic and lymphoid tissue. Lyon: LARC; 2008. p. 188–90.

51. Tiacci E, Trifonov V, Schiavoni G, et al. BRAF mutations in hairy-cell leukemia. N Engl J Med. 2011;364(24):2305–15.

52. Arcaini L, Zibellini S, Boveri E, et al. The BRAF V600E mutation in hairy cell leukemia and other mature B-cell neoplasms. Blood. 2012;119(1):188–91.

53. Xi L, Arons E, Navarro W, et al. Both variant and IGHV4-34-expressing hairy cell leukemia lack the BRAF V600E mutation. Blood. 2012;119(14):3330–2.

54. Thieblemont C, Davi F, Noguera ME, et al. Splenic marginal zone lymphoma: current knowledge and future directions. Oncology (Williston Park). 2012;26(2):194–202.

55. Matutes E, Morilla R, Owusu-Ankomah K, Houliham A, Meeus P, Catovsky D. The immunophenotype of hairy cell leukemia (HCL). Proposal for a scoring system to distinguish HCL from B-cell disorders with hairy or villous lymphocytes. Leuk Lymphoma. 1994;14(Suppl 1):57–61.

56. Jones G, Parry-Jones N, Wilkins B, Else M, Catovsky D, British Committee for Standards in H. Revised guidelines for the diagnosis and management of hairy cell leukaemia and hairy cell leukaemia variant∗. Br J Haematol. 2012;156(2):186–95.

57. Mason EF, Brown RD, Szeto DP, et al. Detection of activating MAP 2K1 mutations in atypical hairy cell leukemia and hairy cell leukemia variant. Leuk Lymphoma. 2017;58(1):233–6.

58. Waterfall JJ, Arons E, Walker RL, et al. High prevalence of MAP 2K1 mutations in variant and IGHV4-34-expressing hairy-cell leukemias. Nat Genet. 2014;46(1):8–10.

59. Traverse-Glehen A, Baseggio L, Bauchu EC, et al. Splenic red pulp lymphoma with numerous basophilic villous lymphocytes: a distinct clinicopathologic and molecular entity? Blood. 2008;111(4):2253–60.

60. Mendes LS, Attygalle A, Matutes E, Wotherspoon A. Annexin A1 expression in a splenic diffuse red pulp small B-cell lymphoma: report of the first case. Histopathology. 2013;63(4):590–3.

61. Curiel-Olmo S, Mondejar R, Almaraz C, et al. Splenic diffuse red pulp small B-cell lymphoma displays increased expression of cyclin D3 and recurrent CCND3 mutations. Blood. 2017;129(8):1042–5.

62. Colovai AI, Giatzikis C, Ho EK, et al. Flow cytometric analysis of normal and reactive spleen. Mod Pathol. 2004;17(8):918–27.

63. Imashuku S, Obayashi M, Hosoi G, et al. Splenectomy in haemophagocytic lymphohistiocytosis: report of histopathological changes with CD19+ B-cell depletion and therapeutic results. Br J Haematol. 2000;108(3):505–10.

64. Lucio P, Parreira A, van den Beemd MW, et al. Flow cytometric analysis of normal B cell differentiation: a frame of reference for the detection of minimal residual disease in precursor-B-ALL. Leukemia. 1999;13(3):419–27.

65. Zeppa P, Anniciello A, Vetrani A, Palombini L. Fine needle aspiration biopsy of hepatic focal fatty change. A report of two cases. Acta Cytol. 2002;46(3):567–70.

66. Howlett DC, Drinkwater KJ, Lawrence D, Barter S, Nicholson T. Findings of the UK national audit evaluating image-guided or image-assisted liver biopsy. Part I. Procedural aspects, diagnostic adequacy, and accuracy. Radiology. 2012;265(3):819–31.

67. Laribi K, Lemaire P, Sandrini J, Baugier de Materre A. Advances in the understanding and management of T-cell prolymphocytic leukemia. Oncotarget. 2017;8(61):104664–86.

68. Tannapfel A, Dienes HP, Lohse AW. The indications for liver biopsy. Dtsch Arztebl Int. 2012;109(27–28):477–83.

69. Grant A, Neuberger J. Guidelines on the use of liver biopsy in clinical practice. British Society of Gastroenterology. Gut. 1999;45 Suppl 4:IV1–IV11.

70. Mastoraki A, Stefanou MI, Chatzoglou E, et al. Primary hepatic lymphoma: dilemmas in diagnostic approach and therapeutic management. Indian J Hematol Blood Transfus. 2014;30(3):150–4.

71. Elsayes KM, Menias CO, Willatt JM, Pandya A, Wiggins M, Platt J. Primary hepatic lymphoma: imaging findings. J Med Imaging Radiat Oncol. 2009;53(4):373–9.

72. Gota VS, Purandare NC, Gujral S, Shah S, Nair R, Rangarajan V. Positron emission tomography / computerized tomography evaluation of primary Hodgkin's disease of liver. Indian J Cancer. 2009;46(3):237–9.

73. El-Sharkawi D, Ramsay A, Cwynarski K, et al. Clinico-pathologic characteristics of patients with hepatic lymphoma diagnosed using image-guided liver biopsy techniques. Leuk Lymphoma. 2011;52(11):2130–4.

74. Fu DA, Campbell-Thompson M. Periodic acid-Schiff staining with diastase. Methods Mol Biol. 2017;1639:145–9.

75. Agmon-Levin N, Berger I, Shtalrid M, Schlanger H, Sthoeger ZM. Primary hepatic lymphoma: a case report and review of the literature. Age Ageing. 2004;33(6):637–40.

76. Anthony PP, Sarsfield P, Clarke T. Primary lymphoma of the liver: clinical and pathological features of 10 patients. J Clin Pathol. 1990;43(12):1007–13.

77. Swerdlow S, Campo E, Harris N, et al. *WHO classification of tumours of haematopoietic and lymphoid tissues.* Lyon: IARC; 2017.

78. Salmon JS, Thompson MA, Arildsen RC, Greer JP. Non-Hodgkin's lymphoma involving the liver: clinical and therapeutic considerations. Clin Lymphoma Myeloma. 2006;6(4):273–80.

79. Zucca E, Gregorini A, Cavalli F. Management of non-Hodgkin lymphomas arising at extranodal sites. Ther Umsch. 2010;67(10):517–25.

Molecular and Genetic Diagnostic Approaches of Hematopoietic Disorders of the Spleen and Liver

Jinming Song, Rohit Sharma, and Mohammad Hussaini

Introduction

Hematopoietic disorders, benign or malignant, involving the liver and/or spleen are heterogenous in clinical, biological, genetic, and molecular aspects. It is widely accepted that these hematopoietic diseases are mostly driven by genetic alterations including gene deletion, amplification, translocation, karyotypic rearrangements, mutations, or epigenetic changes. Understanding the gene profiles of a hematopoietic disorder helps us to have better insights into disease pathogenesis, make accurate diagnosis and subclassification, perform risk stratification, predict clinical outcome and treatment response, and moreover develop novel targeted therapy for patients with the disorder. In addition to traditional cytogenetic analyses [karyotype analysis, fluorescence in situ hybridization (FISH)], emerging molecular technologies have introduced a number of laboratory methods, e.g., next-generation sequencing (NGS), ultra-deep polymerase chain reaction (PCR), whole genome sequencing, and exome sequencing that have given us unprecedented view into the genomics of hematopoietic malignancies. These newer molecular methods are slowing being incorporated into daily practice. This chapter will focus on the most common cytogenetic and molecular methodologies used in the diagnosis and classification of malignant hematologic disorders that involve the liver and spleen. Less common technologies are briefly discussed.

Cytogenetics

Cytogenetic abnormalities have been detected in many hematopoietic disorders, including both myeloid and lymphoid neoplasms. Similar to solid tumors, hematopoietic neoplasms involving the liver or spleen can develop due to an inherited genetic predisposition followed by acquisition of somatic mutations. Certain malignancies, e.g., chronic lymphocytic leukemia/small lymphocytic lymphoma (CLL/SLL), are associated with considerable inheritability and family predisposition [1, 2]. Accordingly, DNA changes at nucleotide or chromosomal level are the common features in these diseases. These genetic abnormalities include numerical and structural chromosomal changes such as aneuploidy, translocations, inversions, deletions or insertions, single-nucleotide polymorphisms (SNP), loss of heterozygosity (LOH, regional loss as a part or whole), and gene amplifications. The net result of these genomic aberrations is activation of oncogenes or loss of tumor suppressor genes, which ultimately alter normal cellular signaling pathways leading to uncontrolled cell growth. Cytogenetic studies have proven to be essential in the diagnosis, prognosis, and therapeutic target identification of hematologic malignancies.

Certain cytogenetic aberrations may be submicroscopic or cryptic. For such changes, specific testing methods have been developed to provide greater resolution beyond conventional methods. Currently, there are multiple methods available for cytogenetic analysis, including conventional karyotyping (most commonly G-banding), fluorescence in situ hybridization (FISH), comparative genomic hybridization (CGH), array-based CGH (aCGH), single-nucleotide polymorphism array (SNP array), and cytogenetic interrogation by advanced molecular methods.

J. Song · M. Hussaini (✉)
Department of Pathology, H. Lee Moffitt Cancer Center and Research Institute, Tampa, FL, USA
e-mail: mohammad.hussaini@moffitt.org

R. Sharma
Diagnostic Molecular Pathology, Memorial Sloan Kettering Cancer Center, New York, NY, USA

© Springer Nature Switzerland AG 2020
L. Zhang et al. (eds.), *Diagnostic Pathology of Hematopoietic Disorders of Spleen and Liver*,
https://doi.org/10.1007/978-3-030-37708-3_3

Conventional Karyotyping

Karyotype is defined as the number and visual appearance of the chromosomes in cell nuclei of an organism or species. There are 22 autosomal chromosomes and one pair of sex chromosomes in human beings, totaling 23 pairs. Each chromosome has two copies resulting in either a 46, XX (female) or 46, XY (male) karyotype in normal human cells (Fig. 3.1). However, in tumor cells from lymphomas or myeloid neoplasms, an abnormal karyotype may be observed. For example, isochromosome 7q (Fig. 3.2) is identified in a subset of patients diagnosed with hepatosplenic T-cell lymphoma (HSTCL). This unique chromosomal aberration is therefore helpful in the diagnosis of this entity. Overall, cytogenetic abnormalities include three major subtypes: balanced translocation or inversion, gain or loss of whole or part of chromosomes, and loss of heterozygosity (LOH).

The principle behind conventional karyotyping is to harvest dividing cells and analyze them. Appropriate cell culture, preparation, banding, and interpretation are the key steps. The technology involves growing fresh cells in culture, using hypotonic solution (commonly 0.075 M KCl) to cause the cells to swell and to spread the chromosomes apart, arresting mitosis in metaphase by reagents such as colchicine, staining the chromosomes with a suitable dye (usually Giemsa), transfering the chromosomes onto a slide, taking photos, cutting up the photomicrograph, and finally mapping them into a karyogram. Any tissue with nucleated cells undergoing division can be used for chromosomal study. Similar to bone marrow cells, tissue post splenectomy and fluids collected from ascites and pleural effusions are also

suitable for cytogenetic study [3]. In general, a minimum of 16–24 hour unstimulated culture is required for the majority of cases. However, in cases of acute lymphoblastic leukemia (ALL) or CLL/SLL, mitogens are needed and culture might take 3–5 days [3]. Almost all conventional karyotyping is done at metaphase. In this phase of the cell cycle, the chromosomes are maximally contracted, and hence, their banding patterns are easier to observe and analyze. Staining of the chromosomes with dye results in a reproducible banding pattern. Chromosomal banding patterns are used to identify each individual chromosome, to assess whether the correct number of each chromosome is present, and to assess if every chromosome has the normal length and/or structures. The most frequently used banding technique is G-banding with trypsin and Giemsa. Alternative banding techniques [(reverse banding pattern (R-bands), a fluorescence banding technique using quinacrine derivatives (Q-bands), or centromeric staining (C-bands)] are also available [4].

In contrast to the probe-based cytogenetic techniques described below, the advantages of conventional karyotyping include the following [5]:

1. It allows for the analysis of the entire genome and every chromosome at one time. It can detect changes in the number of the chromosomes, large translocations, and large deletions or insertions.
2. It can detect unknown cytogenetic abnormalities for which probes are not available.

The disadvantages of conventional karyotyping compared with other probe-based techniques are the following [5]:

Fig. 3.1 The normal karyotype of human cells (female, 46, XX)

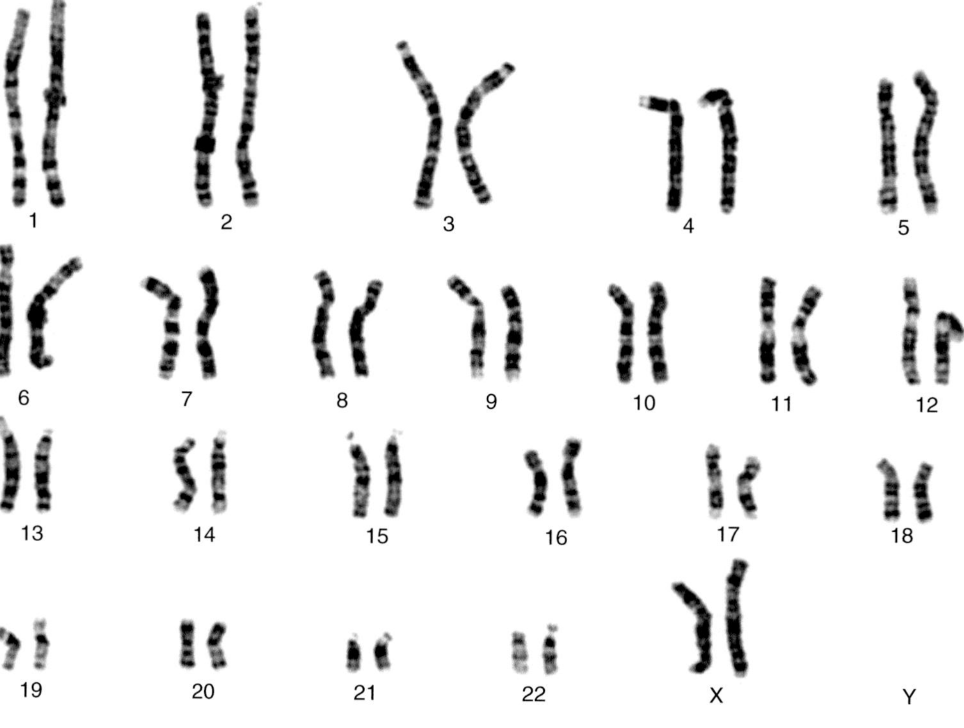

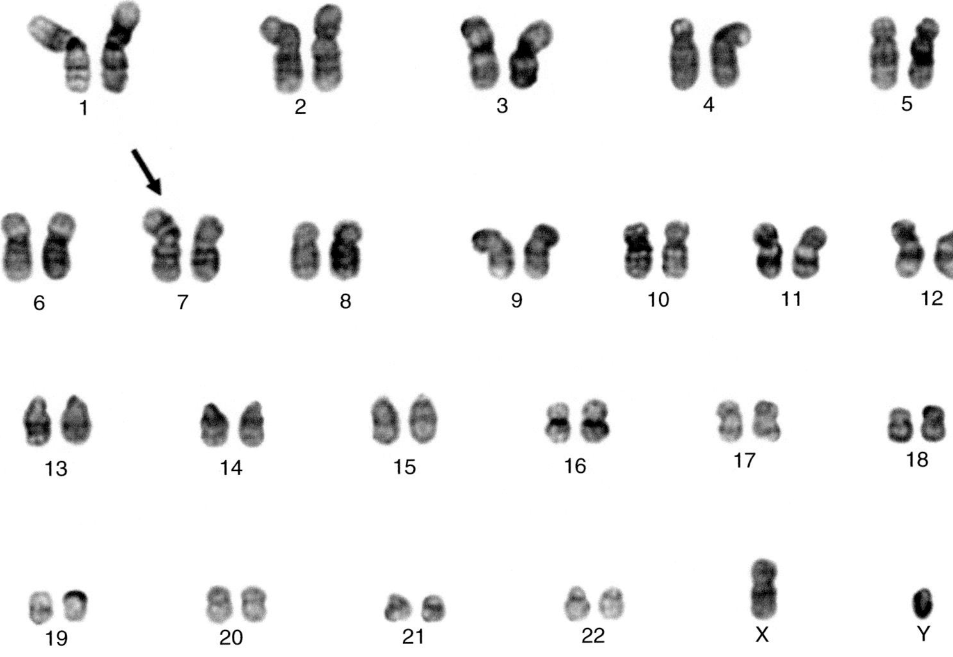

Fig. 3.2 Isochromosome 7q as seen in splenic tissue from a patient with hepatosplenic T-cell lymphoma

- It requires the use of fresh cells or tissue specimens.
- It has high failure rate in indolent lymphomas (e.g., SLL), because the tumor cells may fail to grow and only normal cells will be present.
- Conventional karyotype is a slow procedure with a turn-around time of 7 days or more, which may not be fast enough for clinical lymphoma diagnosis in urgent situations.
- It can only detect major structural abnormalities and will not detect smaller regions of DNA gain or loss. Conventional karyotyping using G-banding technique can detect chromosome changes that are approximately 400–500 bands per haploid genome providing a resolution of about 10 Mb [6, 7]. This might be inadequate for some diseases where shorter regions are involved. However, high-resolution banding might be available to study smaller chromosomal rearrangements [5]. In high-resolution banding cell cycles can be synchronized and all cells be arrested in prometaphase (yeilding 550 bands/haploid genome) or even prophase (approximately 800 bands/haploid genome). The increased number of bands allows for greater resolution in detecting smaller changes.
- Interpretation is labor-intensive and highly dependent on the experience and the skills of lab technicians, especially for complex karyotypes.

Fluorescence In Situ Hybridization (FISH)

FISH studies use fluorescence-labeled DNA probes to target specific chromosome positions or sequences in the genome. It involves binding of fluorescence-labeled fragments of single-stranded DNA to complementary target sequence in target cells. Most of the probes are commercially available. The standard FISH protocol includes sample pretreatment using proteolytic enzymes to prepare for efficient hybridization, denaturation of the double-stranded DNA of both the probes and the samples to single-stranded DNA, hybridization of single-stranded DNA probe to the complementary DNA sequence in target cells, washing to remove the unbounded or imperfectly bounded probes, and finally detecting signals from the flourescently-labeled probes using fluorescence microscopy [8]. FISH can be performed on metaphase chromosomes or interphase nuclei (most common) and therefore can be done on paraffin-embedded tissues, smears, or cytospin preparations. For metaphase FISH, cells are arrested in mitosis similar to chromosomal banding in conventional karyotyping.

FISH probes produce a fluorescent signal on the chromosome to which they hybridize. Normally, every pair of chromosomes produces two signals. Cells that are monosomic for the targeted chromosomal region would show only a single signal per nucleus, while trisomy cells would show three signals. When there are translocations, two separated loci might fuse together, and these two signals (when labeled with two different color probes) will fuse to form one hybrid signal. For example, when one red and one green signal fuse together with each other, a yellow signal will be produced. Alternatively, the translocation can be detected by break-apart probes.

FISH probes can be used to detect translocations or copy number changes in chromosomes.

1. Probes to detect translocations. Two types of FISH probes can be used to detect translocations, dual-fusion probes and break-apart probes [9] (Fig. 3.3).

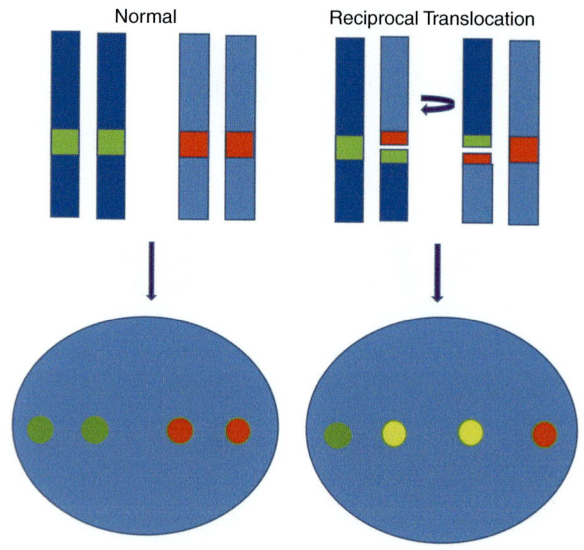

Fig. 3.3 Illustration of dual-fusion probes

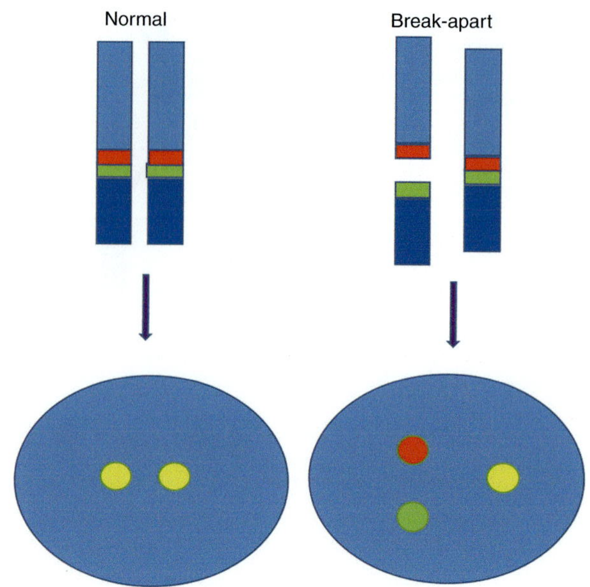

Fig. 3.4 Illustration of the break-apart probes

Dual-fusion probes use a pair of probes labeled with two different fluorescent colors and target two different loci involved in the translocation. For example, to detect t(11;14)(q13;q32)/*IgH-CCND1* in mantle cell lymphoma, a red-colored probe targeting q13 of chromosome 11 and a green-colored probe targeting chromosome 14q32 will be used. Two red signals and two green signals will be seen in normal cells because of the diploidy of the cells. When there is a reciprocal t(11;14)(q13;q32) translocation, one red and one green signal will split in a half and be exchanged, resulting in two fusion signals of red and green, which will appear yellow in color. The remaining uninvolved loci will show as one red and one green signal. This is the typical translocation pattern. When there are chromosome amplifications or deletions, the patterns could look different and should also be reported as abnormal. The advantage of dual-fusion probes is that they can clearly identify the translocation when the translocation partners are known. The disadvantage and/or limitations of this approach is that it cannot be used when translocation partners are not know or are numerous (e.g., *MLL*) and in some cases pairing probes cannot be designed.

Dual-color, break-apart probes (Fig. 3.4) operate on the opposite principle. They also use a pair of probes targeting gene regions upstream and downstream of the translocation focus of one of the gene partners. One of the probes is labeled with red color and one with green color. In a normal diploid cell, these two probes are close to each other and show two fusion signals (yellow). When there is reciprocal translocation, one locus will be split apart, generating one red and one green signal, while the intact locus will remain as a yellow signal. The advantage of break-apart

probes is that they do not require apriori information about translocation partners. In addition, the break-apart signals, which yield one red and one green signal, are easier to read than the yellow fusion signals of dual-fusion probes. The disadvantage is that they cannot detect very small insertions and do not yield information about translocation partners. Break-apart signals also have the caveat of appearing as separated in a normal cell because of the secondary structures of the chromosomes leading to false positivity. In principle, dual-fusion probes are more specific than break-apart signals because of less false positives [9]. Dual-color, break-apart probes are commonly used to detect genes with multiple translocation partners, e.g., *MLL/KMT2A*, *IgH*, or *MYC*.

2. Probes to detect copy number changes. Copy number changes include aneusomies, deletions, or amplifications. Probes to detect copy number changes target a specific region in a chromosome or the centromeric or pericentromeric satellites (chromosome enumeration probes). These probes are usually labeled in one color. One caveat in using these probes to detect deletions in paraffin-embedded tissue is the occurrence of false positives due to partial chromosome loss during tissue sectioning [9]. Therefore, it is recommended to use thicker sections than conventional histology when doing FISH on paraffin-embedded blocks. However, this might introduce difficulty in interpretation because of cells lying in multiple planes of section.

When a new FISH test is first implemented, validation should include sensitivity, accuracy, precision, and specificity. The report threshold should be established to ensure that FISH results are clear and interpretable. Furthermore, ongoing monitoring of interobserver reproducibility, accomplished in part by having two laboratory personnel read in every case, should be a routine practice to ensure the validity of the results. It is also important to establish all the signal patterns for every test. Hematologic malignancies can have very complex cytogenetic abnormalities, especially when hematologic malignancies occur as secondary events. So atypical or variant patterns should not be ignored and should be reported and explained in the context of pathology reports and patient history.

Compared with conventional karyotyping, FISH has the following advantages [5]:

- It offers higher resolution. FISH can detect cytogenetic abnormalities 2 megabases (Mb) or greater, compared to around 10 Mb for conventional karyotyping. It can also detect cryptic or subtle chromosomal changes.
- It is applicable to both dividing (metaphase) and nondividing (interphase) cells and therefore can be used on formalin-fixed and paraffin-embedded (FFPE) blocks. However, identification and counting of signals per cell on fresh-frozen paraffin-embedded (FFPE) tissue might be impeded by many factors such as cutting artifact, nuclear overlap, and fixation. If low levels of gains and losses are targeted, FISH on isolated nuclei, either prepared from intact cell suspension or nuclear suspensions from paraffin blocks, is preferable.
- The protocol is simpler than conventional karyotyping.
- It has a shorter turnaround time, usually 2–3 days, in comparison with 1 week or more for conventional karyotyping.

Disadvantages/limitations of FISH studies include the following [5]:

- It cannot be used for detection of unknown cytogenetic abnormalities or cytogenetic abnormalities for which probes are not available or cannot be designed.
- It cannot detect very small deletions or insertions and point mutations.
- It cannot resolve uniparental disomy (UPD) (inheritance of both copies of a chromosome from the same parent).
- Probe and reagent costs can prevent its application to genome-wide survey. For example, the diagnosis of Burkitt lymphoma requires the presence of *MYC* rearrangement but also the absence of other cytogenetic abnormalities to distinguish it from high grade B-cell lymphoma, with *MYC* and *BCL2* and/or *BCL6* rearrangements [10, 12–14].

Finally, genome-wide genetic changes might be studied by more esoteric methodologies such as multiplex FISH, spectral karyotyping, or COBRA FISH (combined binary ratio labeling FISH) [11, 14–17]. In these methods, multiple labels are generated by using mixtures of different fluorochromes to bind to multiple genomic regions of the chromosomes. Complex structural abnormalities can be visualized readily and the chromosomal origin of abnormal structures such as marker chromosomes can be identified much more easily than by conventional cytogenetics. However, these methods require specific interpretative skills and complex equipment. Therefore they are accessible to only a limited number of investigators.

Cytogenetic Abnormalities Detectable by Conventional Karyotyping or FISH in Lymphomas

Many cytogenetic abnormalities have been detected in lymphomas by conventional karyotyping or FISH studies. Some are specific for a lymphoma, such as t(14;18)(q32;q21) for follicular lymphoma (FL) and t(11;14)(q13;q32) for mantle cell lymphoma (MCL), and therefore, these changes are diagnostic. Other cytogenetic abnormalities can occur in either lymphoid or myeloid neoplasms and are not specific. Thus, it is important to know which cytogenetic abnormalities are specific to disease, to avoid misinterpretation. Of note, the absence of a specific cytogenetic abnormality cannot be used to exclude the particular type of disease given that all patients with a given hematologic neoplasm might not harbor said cytogenetic abnormality. For example, t(14;18)(q32;q21) translocation is observed in about 85% of follicular lymphomas. This means a small portion of the patients with follicular lymphoma may not be positive for the translocation [18]. However, the presence of cytogenetic abnormalities, even when nonspecific, can be helpful to at least confirm the clonal or neoplastic nature of the process and to distinguish it from reactive conditions. In addition, some nonspecific cytogenetic abnormalities might provide prognostic value for lymphoma. For example, the t(8;14)(q24;q32) translocation is a primary cytogenetic abnormality in Burkitt lymphoma. When it becomes a secondary aberration in a patient with follicular lymphoma, the translocation is associated with a poor prognosis in this setting [9, 19].

The most common cytogenetic abnormalities detected in all lymphomas that could typically involve the spleen or liver are summarized in Table 3.1.

Cytogenetic study has also applied for myeloid neoplasms involving liver and spleen. For disease-specific cytogenetic aberrations please see the corresponding chapters.

Table 3.1 The most common cytogenetic abnormalities detected in lymphomas

Lymphoma	Cytogenetics	References
CLL/SLL	Deletion of 13q, trisomy 12, deletion of 11q, deletion of 17p	[20], 2120A
B-PLL	Complex cytogenetic abnormalities, deletion of 17p, deletion of 13q, deletion of 11q, *MYC* amplification or translocation	[20–22]
SMZL	Lack recurrent cytogenetic abnormalities, rarely t(2;7)(p12;q21), heterozygous deletion of 7q, gain of 3q	[20, 23–25]
HCL	No specific abnormalities, rarely numerical abnormalities of chromosome 5 or chromosome 7	[20]
Splenic diffuse red pulp small B-cell lymphoma	Complex cytogenetic alterations, including t(9;14)(p13;q32) (*PAX5/IGH*)	[20]
LPL	No specific abnormalities, trisomy 4 (~20%), very rarely t(9;14)(p13;q32) (*IGH/PAX5*), del(6q)	[20, 26–33]
MALT	t(11;18)(q21;q21) (pulmonary and gastric), t(1;14)(p22;q32), t(14;18)(q32;q21) (ocular adnexa, orbit, and salivary gland lesions), t(3;14)(p14.1;q32) (thyroid, ocular adnexa, orbit, and skin), Trisomy 3 or 18	[20, 34]
NMZL	Gains of chromosome 3 and chromosome 18, losses of 6q23–24	[20]
FL	t(14;18)(q32;q21)(*IGH/BCL2*)∗, abnormalities of 3q27 and/or *BCL6* rearrangement, losses of 1p, 6q, 10q, and 17p and gains of chromosomes 1, 6p, 7, 8, 12q, X, and 18q, rarely t(8;14)(q24;q32)	[20, 35–42]
Large B-cell lymphoma with *IRF4* rearrangement	Cryptic rearrangement of *IRF4* with an *IGH* locus, *BCL6* locus breakpoints	[20, 43, 44]
DLBCL NOS	Rearrangement of 3q27 (*BCL6*), t(14;18)(q32;q21.3)(*IGH/BCL2*), or *MYC* alone	[20, 45–57]
MCL	t(11;14)(q13;q32) (*CCND1/IGH*)∗, secondary abnormalities in 3q26, 7p21, 8q24 (*MYC*), losses of 1 p13-31, 6q23-27 (*TNFAIP3*), 9p21(*CDKN2A*), 11q22-23 (*ATM*), 13q11-13, 13q14-34, 17p13 (*TP53*), trisomy 12, rarely t(8;14)(q24;q32)(*MYC/BCL2*) or *BCL6* (3q27)	[58–63]
ALK + LBCL	t(2;17)(p23;q23) (*CLTC/ALK*)∗, rarely t(2;5)(p23;q35) (*NPM/ALK*)	[20]
PBL	Complex abnormalities, *MYC* rearrangement	[20]
BL	t(8;14)(q24;q32) (*MYC/IGH*), less commonly t(2;8)(p12;q32) or t(8;22)(q24;q11), gains of 1 q, 7, and 12, and losses of 6q, 13q32–34, and 17p	[20]
BL with 11q aberration	Interstitial gains including a minimal region of gain in 11 q23.2–23.3 and losses of 11 q24.1-ter	[64–66]
High-grade B-cell lymphoma with *MYC* and *BCL2* and/or *BCL6* rearrangements (double or triple-hit)	Rearrangements of *MYC* and *BCL2* and/or *BCL6*, and usually complex karyotype	[20]
B-cell lymphoma, unclassifiable, with features intermediate between diffuse large B-cell lymphoma and classic Hodgkin lymphoma (gray zone lymphoma)	Gains and amplification of 9p24.1 (*JAK2* and *PDCD1LG2*), breaks at 16p13.13, gains in *MYC*	[20, 67]
High-grade B-cell lymphoma NOS	*MYC* rearrangement at 8q24 or rarely amplification of 18q21 involving *BCL2*	[68–70]
T-PLL	Inv (14)(q11q32), t(14;14)(q11;q32) (*TCL1A/TCL1B*), t(X;14)(q2S;q11) (*MTCP1*), idic(S)(p11), t(S;S)(p11-12;q12), trisomy 8q, gain of *MYC*, deletions at 12p13 and 22q, amplification of 5p, deletion of 11 q23 (*ATM*)	[20, 71, 72]
Extranodal NK/T-cell lymphoma, nasal type	del(6)(q21q25) or i (6)(p10)	[20, 73–76]
HSTCL	Isochromosome 7q in most cases, ring chromosomes leading to 7q amplification, trisomy 8	[20, 77]
PTCL NOS	Complex karyotypes, recurrent chromosomal gains and losses	[20, 78–81]
AITL	Trisomy of chromosomes 3, 5, and 21, gain of X, loss of 6q	[20]
Follicular T-cell lymphoma	t(5;9)(q33;q22) (*ITK/SYK*)	[20, 82, 83]
ALCL ALK+	t(2;5)(p23;q35) *NPM1/ALK*∗, variant translocations involving t(1;2)(q25;p23)(TPM3), inv(2)(p23q35) (*ATIC*), t(2;3)(p23;q12.2)(TFG), t(2;17)(p23;q23)(CLTC), t(X;2)(q11–12;p23)(MSN), t(2;19)(p23;p13.1)(TPM4), t(2;22)(p23;q11.2)(*MYH9*), t(2;17)(p23;q25) (*RNF213*)	[20, 84–92]
ALCL ALK-	Rearrangement in 6p25.3 (*DUSP22*), inv(3)(q26q28) (*TP63/TBL1XR1*)	[20, 93]

CLL/SLL chronic lymphocytic leukemia/small lymphocytic lymphoma, *B-PLL* B-cell prolymphocytic lymphoma, *SMZL* splenic marginal zone lymphoma, *HCL* hairy cell leukemia, *LPL* lymphoplasmacytic lymphoma, *MALT* extranodal marginal zone lymphoma of mucosa-associated lymphoid tissue, *NMZL* nodal marginal zone lymphoma, *FL* follicular lymphoma, *DLBCL* diffuse large B-cell lymphoma, *MCL* mantle cell lymphoma, *ALK+ LBCL* ALK+ large B-cell lymphoma, *PBL* plasmablastic lymphoma, *BL* Burkitt lymphoma, *T-PLL* T-cell prolymphocytic leukemia, *HSTCL* hepatic splenic T-cell lymphoma, *PTCL-NOS* peripheral T-cell lymphoma, not otherwise specified, *AITL* angioimmunoblastic T-cell lymphoma, *ALCL ALK+* or ALK− anaplastic large cell lymphoma, ALK+ or ALK−

∗The cytogenetic abnormalities that are specific for and diagnostic of the corresponding lymphomas

Array-Based Comparative Genomic Hybridization (aCGH) and Single-Nucleotide Polymorphism (SNP) Array

Comparative genomic hybridization (CGH) labels the tumor and normal cells with different fluorescent colors, which allows them to bind to the reference chromosomes in a 1:1 ratio, and then compares the density of hybridization from these two groups of cells along the whole chromosomes. Higher density of tumor DNA hybridization in one region indicates gain of DNA for tumor cells, while higher density hybridization in normal cells indicates loss of DNA in the tumor cells. CGH can detect amplifications or deletions of smaller regions of DNA along the lengths of all of the chromosomes. It has a resolution of around 5–10 Mb. Array-based comparative genomic hybridization (aCGH) is a modification of CGH in which the comparator DNA, RNA, or tissue is arrayed on a glass slide or glass beads [5, 94]. aCGH is a quick cytogenetic method to compare copy number variations (CNVs) in the genome of tumor and normal cells. aCGH can detect unbalanced chromosome abnormalities, but not balanced translocations because they do not affect copy numbers.

Single-nucleotide polymorphism (SNP), a change at a single site in DNA, is the most frequent type of genetic changes. An SNP array allows a library of immobilized whole genome allele-specific oligonucleotide (ASO) probes to bind fluorescence-labeled fragmented tumor cell DNA to detect which SNP is present in the tumor cells. It is a powerful method to study whole genome cytogenetic abnormalities. Most SNP-based arrays now also include single locus probes (a DNA or RNA sequence that is able to hybridize with DNA or RNA from a specific restriction fragment on the Southern blot) as well as SNPs [5]. This technology was reported to be able to detect genetic abnormalities that are as small as 35 kb [6, 95, 96] and has been applied to cancer genomics, including lymphomas [6, 97–99].

Both aCGH and SNP arrays can detect CNVs, but only SNP arrays can be used to detect the absence or loss of heterozygosity (AOH or LOH) in the presence of normal copy numbers of chromosomes [5, 100]. AOH is the inheritance of either paternal or maternal alleles alone. The absence of parental inheritance can be seen in uniparental disomy (UPD), in which two different homologous chromosomes from the same parent (either maternal or paternal) are inherited, instead of one chromosome from each parent. UPD can also occur when there are two identical copies from a single parental chromosome (isodisomy). SNP arrays can only detect UPDs secondary to isodisomies [5, 100]. UPD is important to detect, because regions of UPD may harbor one or more genes with inactivating mutations of tumor suppressor genes [14, 101–103]. When both alleles have

the mutation in a region with UPD, the Knudson two-hit rule for tumor suppressor genes is fulfilled, and the tumor suppressor gene is inactivated. Alternatively, regions with UPD may contain biallelic hypermethylated and thus silenced candidate tumor suppressor genes.

The major difficulty in SNP analysis is the distinction between acquired abnormalities and germline polymorphisms. This can only be resolved conclusively by analyzing paired germline (e.g., cells from a buccal swab) and tumor cells from the same patient [14, 104]. Comparing the data from a lymphoma sample with large SNP databases of germline mutations to correct for all potential polymorphisms is still not reliable and often results in the exclusion of many regions smaller than 250 kb [14]. Therefore, if germline DNA is not available, SNP analysis is not superior to aCGH for the genome-wide assessment of structural abnormalities.

The advantages of aCGH or SNP arrays include the following [5]:

- Only DNA is required, so both viable cells and formalin-fixed and paraffin-embedded (FFPE) blocks are suitable specimens.
- It shows much higher resolution than FISH on the order of <50–100 kb [14] depending upon the type of array used and the average spacing of the "probes" on the array. SNP arrays can even detect single-nucleotide changes.
- SNP array is the only technology that can detect UPDs.

The disadvantages of aCGH or SNP arrays include the following [5]:

- It cannot detect balanced structural rearrangements (i.e., balanced translocations, inversions, insertions), when there is no change in copy numbers. However, due to the fact that many structural abnormalities such as chromosomal breakpoints in lymphomas are associated with mutations and also small deletions or duplications of several nucleotides, such abnormalities might be detectable by SNP analysis.
- It cannot detect mosaicism (i.e., copy number changes in some, but not all, cells) with less than 20% tumor cells.
- It is difficult to identify copy number changes when the phenotypically normal controls also carry the same changes.
- It is relatively expensive, so it is not routinely applicable.

Until now, approximately 65 publications have appeared on the application of aCGH in mature B-cell and T-cell lymphomas [14, 105–108], which show distinct patterns of gain and loss characteristic of particular lymphoma subtypes. For example, activated B-cell (ABC) type DLBCL has a different pattern from the germinal center B-cell

(GCB) type, with recurrent trisomy 3, gains of 18q and 19q, and loss of 6q in ABC type and gain/amplification of 2p and losses of 1p and 13q in GCB type [14, 109]. These DLBCL subtypes have different prognosis. Similarly, distinct features were found between different types of T-cell lymphomas. aCGH is also applicable to myeloid neoplasms, but this lies beyond the scope of this chapter.

A large number of clinically significant CNVs and UPD have been identified in lymphomas and are summarized in Table 3.2.

Table 3.2 Common genetic abnormalities detected by SNP array in lymphomas

Disease	CNVs/CNAs and/or associated genes	LOH/UPD and/or associated genes	Prognostic association	References
cHL	Gain of *MAP3K14*	14q (*TRAF3*)		[110]
DLBCL	Frequent gains and deletions; gains *HDAC7A* on chromosome 12 predominantly in GCB-DLBCL, losses of *BACH2* and *CASP8AP2* on chromosome 6 predominantly in ABC-DLBCL; potential tumor suppressor genes, *CASP3*, *IL5RA ARID1B*, *ROBO2*, and *MRS1*; potential oncogenes, *KLHL6*, *IL31*, and *LRP1*	11p11.2 (*PTPRJ*)	Worse prognosis: loss of 8p23.1	[111–114]
FL	*CDKN2A*, *CDKN2B*, *FHIT*, *KIT*, *PEX14*, and *PTPRD*	1p36 (*TNFRSF14*), 6p, 6q, 9p (*CDKN2A*), 10q, 12q, 16p, and 17p (*TP53*)	Worse prognosis when > 3 SNP abnormalities; aUPD and deletion of 1p36, or aUPD of 16p are identified	[102, 103]
CLL	Deletion of 17p13 (*TP53*), 11q22 (*ATM*) and 13q14 (*DLEU1* and *DLEU2*), 2p16.1-2p15, 8q24.21, 6q21 (*AIM1*) Gains of 12, 2p16 (*REL*, *BCL11A*)	13q, 13 (*miR-15a/miR-16-1*),17p, and 11q	Worse prognosis when genomic complexity, large genomic aberrations, or large (type II) 13q14 deletions are identified	[115–118]
MCL	Deletion of *INK4A/ARF*, *ATM*, *TP53*, 1p, 6q, *CDKN2C*, *BCL2L11*, *CDKN2A*, and *RB1*, *FAF1*, *MAP2*, *SP100*, *MOBKL2B*, *ZNF280A*, and *PRAME* Amplification of *MYC*, 11q13(*cyclin D1*), 13q (*miR17-92,C13orf25*), dup(3q), 18q (*BCL2*)	9p, 9, 17p (*TP53*)		[101, 119]
MZL	Deletion of 6q23 (*TNFAIP3, A20*), 9p Gains of 3, 18, 6p, and 21q Gains of *REL*, *BCL11A*, *ETS1*, *PTPN1*, *PTEN*, and *KRAS* in transformation to DLBCL	6q (*A20*), 3q		[120–122]
BL	Losses of 6q14.1–q22.33, 9p21.3 (*CDKN2A*), and 13q14.2–q14.3 Gains of 1q23.3–q31.3, 7, 13q31.3	6p12.2-pter, 9p23-pter, and 17p11.2-pter (*TP53*)		[123]
MM	Genomic alterations at 1p, 1q, 6q, 8p, 13, and 16q	1q, 16q (*CYLD*), and X	Worse prognosis when amplifications in 1q and deletions in 1p, 12p, 14q, 16q, and 22q or UPD of 16q (*CYLD*) are identified Favorable prognosis when amplifications of 5, 9, 11, 15, and 19 are detected	[124–127]
PTCL, NOS	Losses of 1p35–36, 3q, 5q33, 6p22, 6q16, 6q21–22, 8p21–23, 9p21, 10p11–12, 10q11–22, 10q25–26, 13q14, 15q24, 16q22, 16q24, 17p11, 17p13, and Xp22 Gains of 1q32–43, 2p15–16 (*REL*), 7, 8q24, 11q14–25, 17q11–21 and 21q11–21, 9p and 19q	2q32.3		[78]
AILT	Losses of 3q and 9p Gains of 8q, 9p, and 19q	2q32.3	Worse prognosis when the presence of CNAs and overexpression of *CARMA1* at 7p22 or *MYCBP2* at 13q22 are found	[128]
ATLL	Deletion of 10p11.2 (*TCF8*)			[129]
T-PLL	Losses of 6q, 8p, 10p, 11q (*microRNA 34b/c*, *ETS1*, and *FLI1*), and 18p and gains of 6p and 8q Aberrations in 5p, 12p, 13q, 17, and 22 (*DNAH5*, *ETV6*, *miR-15a* and *miR-16-1*, *p53*, *BIRC5*, and *SOCS3*)	3q, 17q		[130, 131]

CNVs copy number variations, *CNAs* copy number aberrations, *LOH* loss of heterozygosity, *UPD* uniparental disomy, *cHL* classic Hodgkin lymphoma, *DLBCL* diffuse large B-cell lymphoma, *FL* follicular lymphoma, *CLL* chronic lymphocytic leukemia, *MCL* mantle cell lymphoma, *MZL* marginal zone lymphoma, *BL* Burkitt lymphoma, *MM* multiple myeloma, *PTCL NOS* peripheral T-cell lymphoma, NOS, *AILT* angioimmunoblastic T-cell lymphoma, *ATLL* adult T-cell leukemia/lymphoma, *T-PLL* T-cell prolymphocytic leukemia

Since multiple cytogenetic study methods are available, a decision tree was proposed by Song et al. [6]. If unknown cytogenetic abnormalities are suspected and micro-alterations are not suspected, conventional karyotyping is recommended. If known cytogenetic abnormalities are suspected and specific probes are available, FISH studies are preferable. If unknown cytogenetic abnormalities are suspected or important for patient care or small unknown cytogenetic abnormalities or LOH are suspected or important, aCGH is the best option.

Finally, as the cost of next-generation sequencing (NGS) continues to drop, NGS will be increasingly applied in clinical laboratories. As a result, SNP array will likely gradually phase out. However, as a mature technology with fully developed data analysis algorithm and relatively low cost, SNP array may continue to play a limited role in clinical laboratories, especially in situations where diagnostic and prognostic significance of SNP lesions are well established.

Polymerase Chain Reaction

Polymerase chain reaction (PCR) was invented in 1983 by Dr. Kary Mullis for which he received a Nobel Award 10 years later in 1993, rightfully so, given that the advent of PCR drastically revolutionized the study of human biology, genomics, and disease. In simple terms, PCR is a method to amplify nucleic acid(s) (i.e., DNA or RNA). If there is sufficient nucleic acid present, then it becomes easy to further analyze it by other laboratory techniques such as sequencing. Understandably, a single molecule of DNA would be exceedingly difficult to study. However, if we had say a million copies of the same DNA molecule, then it would be much easier to detect and analyze genomic changes therein. PCR is extremely sensitive, cost-effective, and rapid [132].

PCR is basically an enzymatic reaction. It involves addition of four main ingredients: (1) DNA polymerase, (2) nucleotides (adenosine, thymine, cytosine, and guanine), (3) template DNA (the DNA that we are trying to amplify), and (4) primers (short oligonucleotides that flank the region of interest that we want to amplify). These ingredients are mixed in small test tube-like structures (namely, wells) on a plate. The primers are short, manufactured segments of DNA complementary to the sequence that flanks the region of interest on the template DNA. When the ingredients are mixed, the primers will bind complementary regions on the template DNA. Then the DNA polymerase will extend the primers by incorporating nucleotides complementary to the template DNA in the region of interest.

Procedurally, once the mixture is made, the mixture in the well is placed in a thermocycler machine that heats and cools the wells in the plate in a precise and controlled manner. When the well is heated, the DNA strands in the mixture separate (denature). When it cools, it allows the template DNA to bind to the primers (and then the DNA polymerase to extend the primer subsequently).

If initially we have two strands of template DNA (plus and minus strand), one cycle of PCR would allow for the primers flanking the region of interest to bind DNA polymerase, to extend the primer over the region of interest, and then the strands (now four strands) to separate. The next cycle would allow primers to bind to each of the four strands and double the amount of DNA. In each cycle, the amount of DNA is doubled, and thus, there is exponential increase in the amount of DNA.

Once we have amplified our DNA (PCR product), we will still need to visualize the product in other to analyze it. There are two main methods in this respect. Both involve the labeling of the PCR product by some type of tag (fluorescent) and separation of the PCR product(s) to allow for observation and analysis.

The simpler of the two typically involves labeling the PCR product with a dye like ethidium bromide. Then the PCR product is loaded onto an agarose gel and subjected to electrophoresis, which separates products based on size and charge. The PCR product will be run alongside a standardized mix of labeled products that create a ladder (labeled axis) of known size to help determine the size of our PCR product. The other common method is that of Sanger sequencing, which is further described below.

PCR can be both qualitative and quantitative. Qualitative analysis tells us if the product is there or not. Quantitative analysis tells us how much of the product is present. An example of a quantitative analysis is the PCR assay for p190 *BCR/ABL1* transcripts in Philadelphia chromosome-positive B lymphoblastic leukemia/lymphoma. Real-time PCR uses newer thermal cycler methods to measure the number of amplicons as it amplifies and quantities the fluorescent-labeled elongated products. Reverse transcription (RT)-PCR is used to amplify RNA targets by using reverse transcriptase to generate complimentary DNA (cDNA) followed by conventional PCR of the cDNA products [133]. For unique or specific applications and/or to circumvent certain pitfalls, the basic PCR technique can be modified. These modifications include nested PCR, whole genome amplification, inverse PCR, hot-start PCR, and allele-specific PCR.

Overall, PCR offers a simple, highly sensitive, and potentially quantitative method to enable robust analysis of scant or degraded samples, to produce millions to billions of copies of a particular nucleic acid template. The amplified PCR product allows for cloning, sequencing, or other analyses. The drawback of this technique is that a small amount of contamination can result in spurious product and incorrect results. One of other limitations and technical pitfalls of this method is that prior knowledge of the sequence of the targeted gene is needed [133]. With regard to hematopoietic malignancies in particular B- or T-cell lymphoma, perhaps the most common application of PCR technology is in the performance of gene rearrangement clonality studies of immunoglobulin (IG) (B-cell) and T-cell receptor (TCR). These are discussed below.

B- and T-Cell Receptor Studies

The immune system uses B- and T-cells to recognize foreign antigens. B- and T-cells do this by the use of surface antigen receptors, immunoglobulin (IG), and T-cell receptor (TCR), respectively (Figs. 3.5 and 3.6).

Antigen receptors are, in effect, proteins that are encoded by a limited number of genes. Each gene encodes for a portion of the receptor, and the portions are assembled to give the final antigen receptor. Given the wide diversity of potential antigens and the need to recognize them, the immune system overcomes this challenge through the process of gene rearrangement. The genes encoding antigen receptors comprise of various segments, namely, variable (V), diversity (D), and J (joining; present only in some antigen receptors). Shuffling and recombination of these segments allow for receptor diversity to facilitate the recognition of multitudinous potential antigens. Assessment for antigen receptor is useful in assigning lineage (not 100% due to lineage infidelity) and in establishing clonality in lymphoid malignancies.

Rearrangement is sequential. First D and J segments are rearranged, followed by the V segment. These are then joined to the constant region. In B-cells, immunoglobulin heavy chain (IGH) is first rearranged. Since each B-cell has two alleles, if the first allele rearrangement is nonfunc-

tional, the second allele is rearranged. This is followed by rearrangement of kappa light chain, which can only occur if IGH rearrangement has been previously successful. If kappa light chain rearrangement is nonproductive, it is deleted and

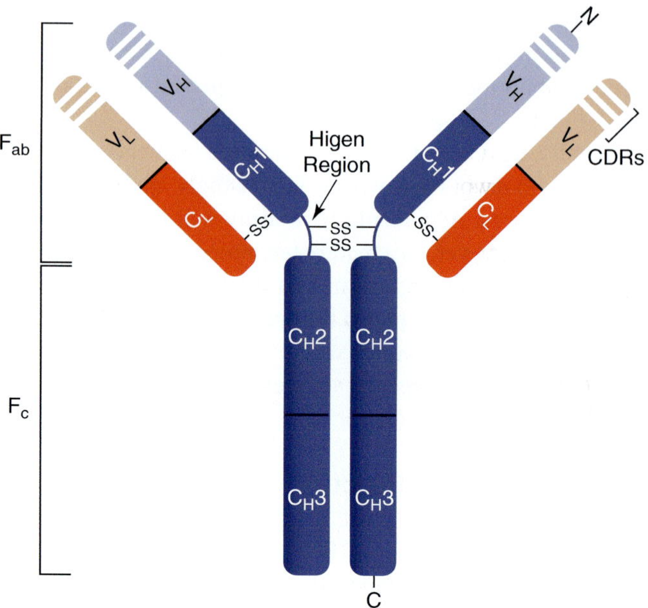

Fig. 3.5 Schematic representation of an immunoglobulin G (IgG) mAb structure. The IgG molecule is composed of constant (C) and variable (V) domains for each light (L) or heavy (H) chain. The heavy chain comprises of three constant domains (CH) and one variable (VH) region. (https://www.researchgate.net/figure/Schematic-representation-of-an-immunoglobulin-G-IgG-mAb-structure-The-IgG-molecule-is_fig 2_280879734)

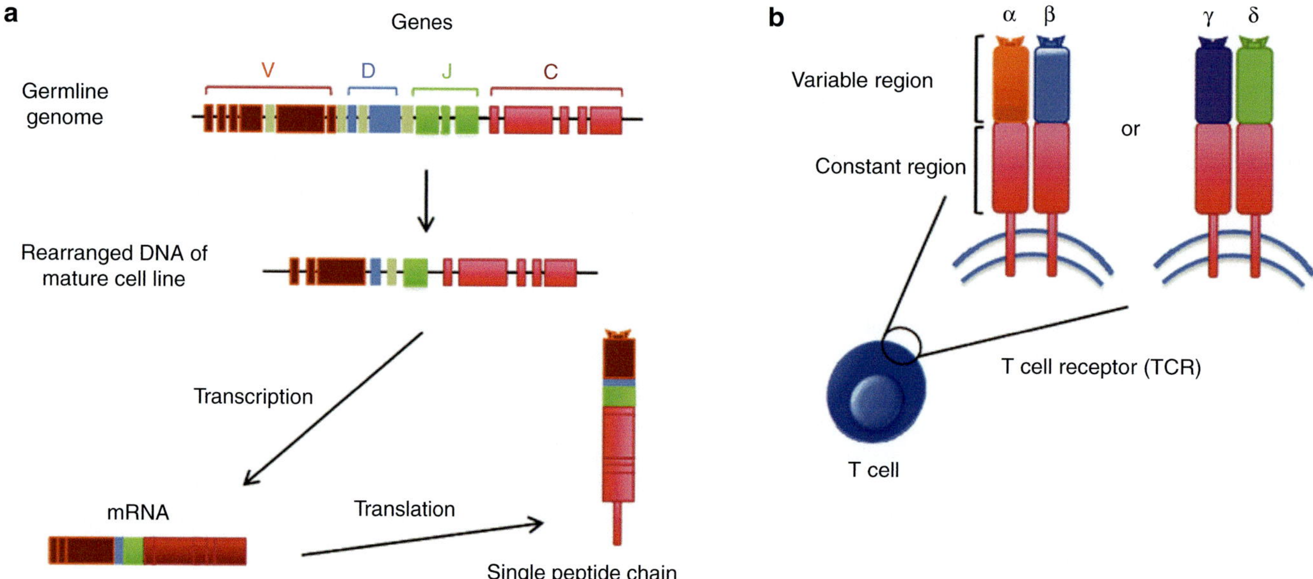

Fig. 3.6 Schematic representation of T-cell receptor. (**a**) Transcription and translation of TCR. (**b**) Schema of final protein TCR product on cell surface (https://www.researchgate.net/figure/The-T-cell-receptor-TCR-can-function-as-a-unique-identifying-bar-code-of-T-cells-a_fig 2_317155934)

lambda light chain will undergo recombination. Among the T-cells, T-cell receptor gamma and delta first undergo recombination. The majority of T cells however have a nonfunctional TCR gamma delta antigen receptor, and thus, TCR alpha/beta undergoes recombination.

The immunoglobulin heavy chain variable region can be further divided into three framework regions (FR1–FR3) and three complementarity determining regions (CDRs). Framework regions demonstrate a high degree of sequence homology, and therefore, forward consensus primers for PCR target these regions. The reverse universal primer targets the framework region in the J region of the heavy chain (FR4). Alternatively, incomplete DJ rearrangement may be utilized. Additional primers can be used for evaluation of light chain in addition to heavy chain to increase the likelihood of detecting a clonal rearrangement. The theory is that if VDJ rearrangement is a random process, this will result in the generation of randomly sized PCR product fragments that will result in an electropherogram demonstrating a Gaussian distribution. However, if a clonal population of the cells exist, they all should theoretically share the identical IGH configuration and generate a single PCR product, which would be recognized as a single strong clonal peak on an electropherogram vs. polyclonality (Figs. 3.7 and 3.8).

Several limitations and caveats to antigen receptor testing exist that should be kept in mind. First of all, post-germinal center B-cell lymphomas may be negative for clonality studies due to somatic hypermutation, which occurs in the germinal center. These alterations can affect the VJ region resulting in loss of homology for the consensus primers and a negative result. Another potential pitfall, as previously alluded to, is lineage infidelity. Immunoglobulin gene rearrangements can be seen in AML (up to approximately 20%), T-cell lymphomas (up to approximately 15%), and T lymphoblastic leukemia (up to ~20%). So the presence of a B-cell receptor clonal rearrangement does not always correlate with a B-cell lymphoma, just as a clonal T-cell gene rearrangement is not necessarily indicative of a T-cell lymphoma. Another caveat is that DNA extracted from formalin-fixed paraffin-embedded tissues may be degraded or old. If the fragments are less than 200 base pairs, lower detection rates by PCR may be expected. False positive results can also occur (pseudo-clonality) due to the presence of a small number of B-cells or T-cells, respectively. This results in a restricted B- or T-cell repertoire, which may be erroneously interpreted as a clonal population. This can be avoided by running the sample in duplicate [134].

Sanger Sequencing

Sanger sequencing leverages the labeling of nucleotides to allow for reading a sequence of a DNA. Template DNA is denatured to unwind the double helix and to allow for a primer to bind to the sequence located proximal to the region of interest. In the reaction mix, there are numerous deoxynucleotide triphosphates (dNTPs, A, C, T, and G) and small of amount of dideoxynucleotide triphosphates (ddNTPs, A, C, T and G). These ddNTPs are labeled with a fluorescent probe. Just as we saw in PCR, the DNA polymerase extends the primer to reform double-stranded DNA using nucleotides (dNTPs) complementary to the template strand. When a ddNTP binds though, the DNA polymerase cannot extend the sequence any further, which results in chain termination. Since ddNTPs compete with dNTPs for binding at any given spot, they will randomly bind at different locations resulting in chain termination and generation of different-sized DNA fragments. These fragments are then subjected to electrophoresis, which allows separation of the DNA fragments with single-nucleotide precision. Smaller fragments will move faster and larger fragments will move slower. In the capillary of the electrophoresis machine, it is as if the DNA fragments form a single file line in order from smallest to largest, even if the fragments differ by one nucleotide in length. When the fragment travels in a capillary and moves past a laser, a fluorescent signal is generated and recorded. Since each ddNTP has its own color fluorescent label, we are able to visualize the nucleotide (A, T, C, or G) at each position (Fig. 3.9).

Next-Generation Sequencing

Next-generation sequencing (NGS) does not refer to a particular technology or test but rather to the aggregate of post-Sanger sequencing technologies. All of these have certain features in common such a high throughput, markedly lower cost, and massively parallel sequencing. The advent of NGS was enabled by various technological advances such as those in computing power, bioinformatic methods, and optics. The major advantages of NGS come from multiplexing, which does away with the limitation of one reaction per well seen in Sanger sequencing. In NGS, all template DNA of interest is immobilized on a surface and subjected to a single volume of reagents. In effect, this allows for millions of sequencing reactions to occur in parallel. Also, sequencing products need not be subjected to electrophoretic analysis. Instead, as the DNA polymerase or ligase incorporates each nucleotide, a signal (fluorescent, pH change, etc.) is generated and recorded, thus, the moniker, "sequencing-by-synthesis."

Furthermore, instead of prior amplification of nucleic acid by PCR, immobilized DNA template can be clonally amplified in vitro on a two-dimensional surface such as a lawn of oligonucleotides, beads, or nanoballs.

A sample simplified NGS workflow would first involve generation of a DNA library. This library would contain all of the regions of interest that we would like to sequence in the

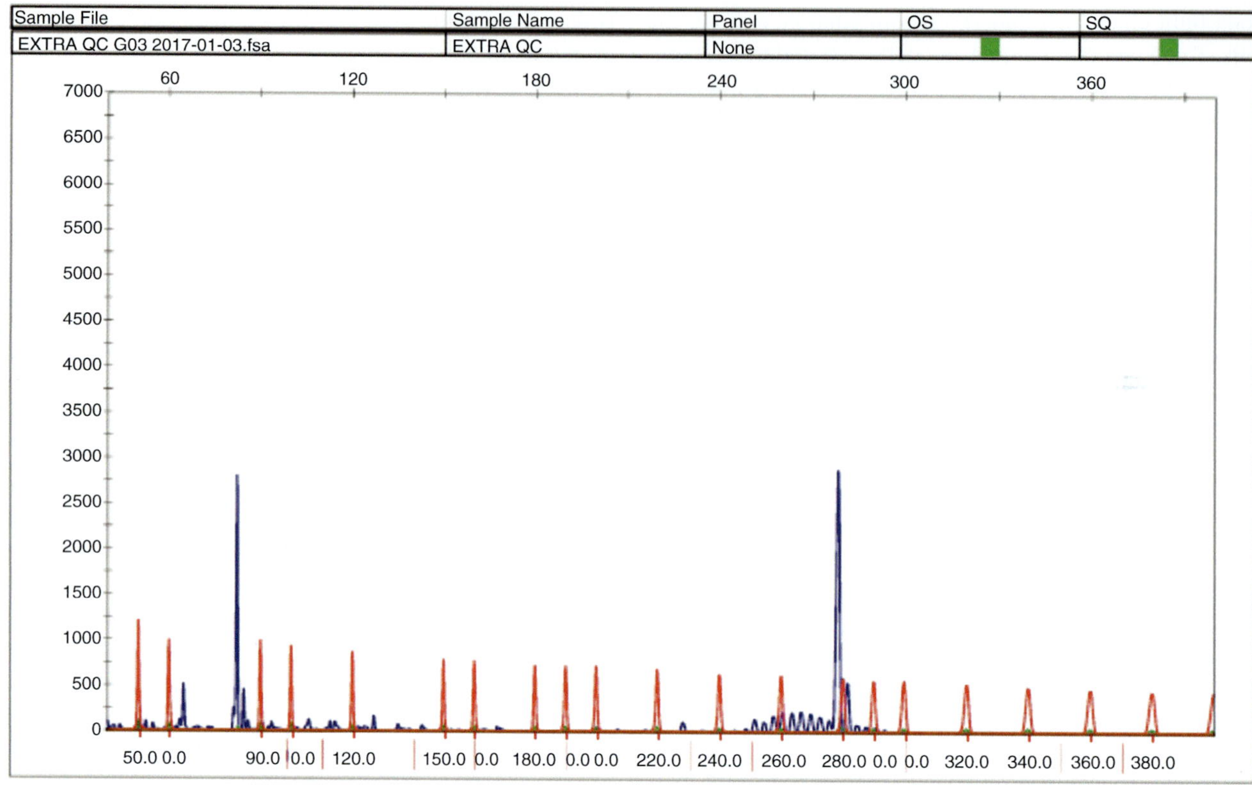

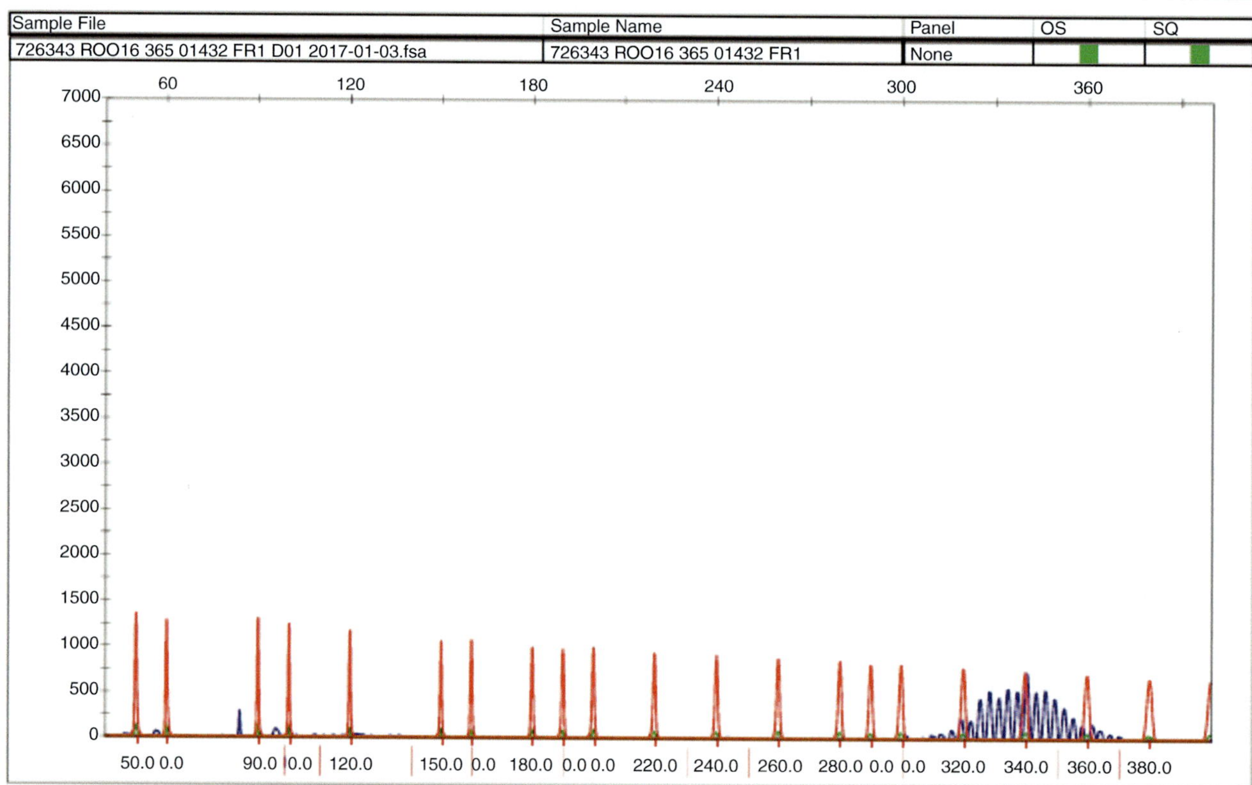

Figs. 3.7 and 3.8 Examples of different IGH Ig clonality electrophe-rogram patterns. Laboratory PCR testing for TCR typically focuses on TCR gamma and TCR beta.

TCR gamma is less complex than TCR beta so some labs will only test for TCR gamma, but addition of TCR beta increases sensitivity. Similar to immunoglobulin testing, PCR analysis for TCR involves consensus primers that amplify the VJ coding sequence of TCR. In the normal state, different-sized PCR product fragments are generated, which when separated by electrophoresis result in a Gaussian distribution on electropherogram. However, if there is a clonal population, a single prominent PCR product is generated, which is reflected as a monoclonal peak on the electropherogram readout

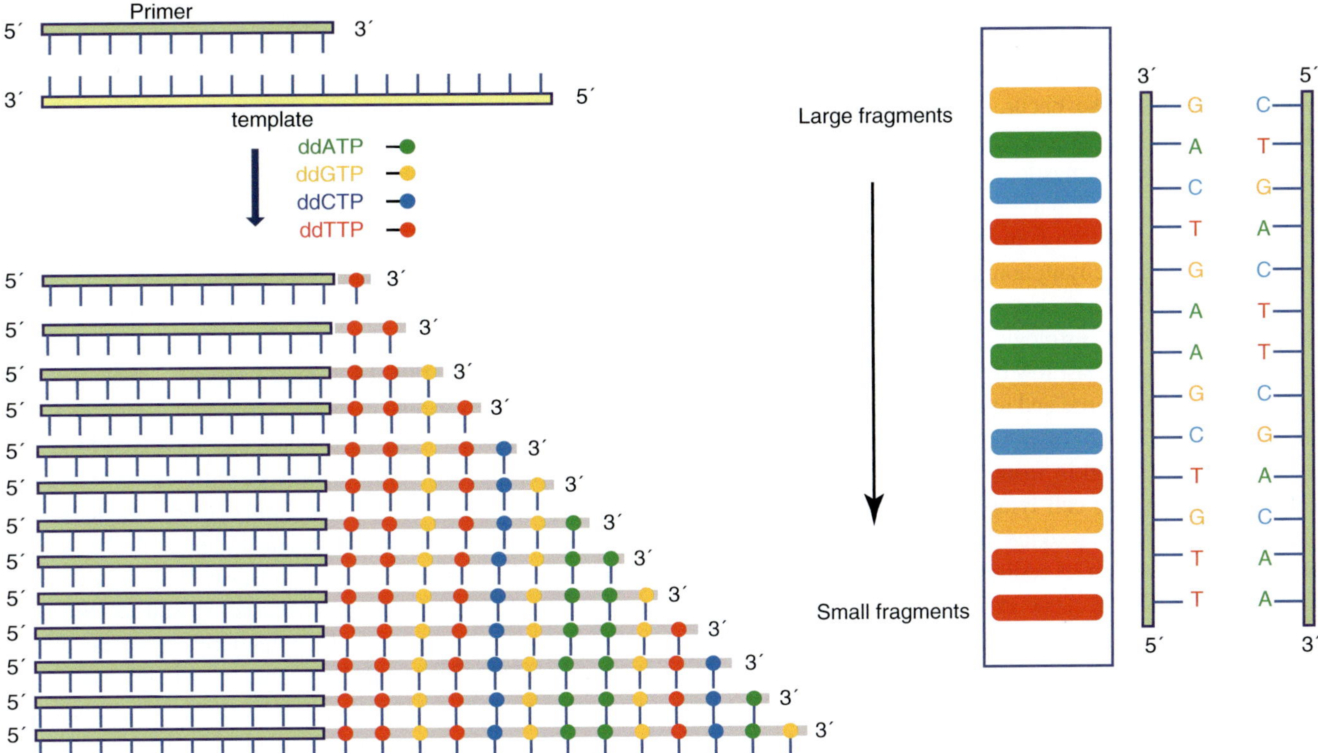

Fig. 3.9 Schematic representation of Sanger sequencing. (Courtesy of http://www.anmjournal.com/viewimage.asp?img=AnnNigerian Med_2014_8_2_51_153352_f1.jpg). The drawbacks of Sanger sequencing have limited sensitivity (at least 20% mutant DNA is required) and the fact that it is comparatively expensive, time-consuming, and labor-intensive

genome in the same way that an individual's personal library contains all of the books that they are interested in reading. These regions of interest will have "book-ends" added to them (primers) to facilitate immobilization on a lawn with complementary oligonucleotides to the primers. The template DNA is then immobilized on the surface of the lawn and amplified. Reversibly-terminating, reversibly-fluorescent dNTPs are added and incorporate to the complementary sequence on the immobilized template DNA via a DNA polymerase, which stalls after the incorporation of one nucleotide. The fluorescent tag of the dNTP (unique for A, C, T, and G) is imaged. The blocking and fluorescent groups are removed allowing for incorporation of a new set of reversibly-terminating, reversibly-fluorescent dNTPs. Another dNTP will get incorporated at each locus on the lawn (each locus corresponds to a strand of template DNA) and will be imaged at the end of that cycle. The cycle is repeated until the template DNA is sequenced. There are millions of loci on each lawn, so millions of DNA sequences (reads) are generated.

Now, these stretches of sequenced DNA are referred to as "reads." These reads are aligned against the reference genome. The more reads that support the presence of a particular nucleotide at a particular position, the more sure we are that the sequence of the read is correct. If the sequenced DNA on the read does not match the reference genome, then we understand that there is a potential mutation at this locus.

If many, many reads show this discrepancy, then we have increased surety that the mutation is real.

Next-generation sequencing can be used to evaluate for single-nucleotide variants, insertions and deletions, copy number changes, and even translocations. Depending on the depth of coverage, the limit of detection for NGS is approximately 1%. In clinical use, a cutoff of 2–5% is more typical. However, the use of molecular bar codes has enabled detection at much lower levels, 10^{-5}, opening up the potential use of this technology in minimal residual disease applications [135].

The advent of NGS has dramatically revolutionized our understanding of the molecular biology of hematologic malignancies by exponentially increasing the rate of genomic discovery in cancer [136]. This in turn has facilitated translation of these discoveries into several clinical arenas: diagnosis, prognosis, disease monitoring, targetable mutations, and/or resistance mutations.

Genetic Mutations in Splenic and Hepatic Lymphomas

Primary involvement of the spleen by lymphoma is rare (2%) and typically will involve diffuse large B-cell lymphoma, hairy cell leukemia (or variant), splenic marginal zone lymphoma, follicular lymphoma, or splenic diffuse red pulp small B-cell lymphoma [137]. Primary hepatic lymphomas are even rarer (0.4%) and most commonly of diffuse large B-cell lymphoma type. However, other lymphoma types can also occur, such as lymphoblastic lymphoma, Burkitt lymphoma, follicular lymphoma, marginal zone lymphoma, anaplastic large cell lymphoma, mantle cell lymphoma, and hepatosplenic T-cell lymphoma [138, 139]. Of course, either of these organs can be secondarily involved by systemic lymphoma.

With regard to lymphomas, traditionally, these have been diagnosed based on histologic and immunophenotypic categorization. Over the last few decades, detection of translocation involving oncogenes and tumor suppression genes (*MYC*, *CCND1*, *BCL2*, *BCL6*, etc.) has offered us new insight into these lymphomas, and in many a case, they are lymphoma-defining (e.g., mantle cell lymphoma and "double-hit" lymphoma). Biologically speaking, lymphoma progression occurs with the accumulation of additional "hits" in key genes such as *TP53* or *CDKN2A*. Gene expression profiling studies and miRNA signatures have elucidated pathways or constellation of genes that are dysregulated in lymphoma. While some genes, such as *ID3* in Burkitt lymphoma, show definite specificity for a single lymphoma subtype, most genes are mutated in more than one lymphoma subtype, often with a range of frequencies (e.g., *TET2*, *TP53*, and *STAT3*). This underlies the "long-tail distribution" of genetic alterations in lymphomas, which has limited the diagnostic utility of mutational profiling in lymphomas. Moreover, this has led investigator to pay attention to clustering of mutations along cellular pathways that may be targeted. Elucidation of frequently dysregulated pathways in lymphoma has in turn facilitated targeted therapeutic intervention: nuclear factor-κB (NF-κb) pathway (bortezomib), PI3K/MTOR pathway (idelalisib, everolimus), NOTCH pathway (gamma secretase inhibitors), JAK-STAT pathway (ruxolitinib), B-cell receptor signaling pathway (ibrutinib), apoptosis pathway (venetoclax), splicing, and focal adhesion [140, 141]. That being said, response and prognosis can be variable in any given case of lymphoma, and they cannot always be easily explained or predicted based on genetic profiling. Furthermore, options with regard to targetable therapy are somewhat limited, and cytotoxic therapy and/or immunotherapy remain the mainstay of clinical management. This should not dampen enthusiasm with regard to the promise of NGS in lymphomas. According to a recent study, 82% of lymphomas tested had a potentially actionable alterations using FDA-approved drugs and/or experimental therapies (clinical trials) [142, 143]. Hereunder, we summarize some of the major mutational findings of clinical import in lymphomas involving the liver and spleen (Tables 3.3, 3.4, 3.5, 3.6, 3.7, and 3.8).

Table 3.3 Genetic alterations seen in small lymphocytic lymphoma/chronic lymphocytic leukemia and mantle cell lymphoma

Gene name	Mutation	Frequency	Reference
ATM	Mutations	Second most commonly mutated gene in CLL; frequency rises from less than 10% early in the course of disease to greater than 25% in relapse disease 50% of mantle cell lymphomas	[144]
BIRC3	Mutations	<5% of CLL cases	[145]
	Inactivating mutations and/or deletions	24% of fludarabine-refractory CLL; 4% of CLL; 0% of monoclonal B-cell lymphocytosis High-risk disease warranting p53-independent drugs or transplant; potentially reduced response to ibrutinib	[146–148]
	Mutations>deletions	Affected in 11% of SMZL (matched germline DNA extracted from saliva for control)	[149]
CCND1	Mutations	35% of mantle cell lymphoma	
DDX3X	Mutation	3% of CLL vs. matched normal tissue in these patients	[150]
FBXW7	Mutation	4% of CLL vs. matched normal tissue in these patients	[150, 151]
VH CD3	Stereotyped B-cell receptor	Significantly more common in clonally related Richter syndrome (50%) than in clonally unrelated Richter syndrome (7.6%) (*p* = 0.009)	[152]
KLHL6	Mutation: F49 L/L65PL90FL58P/T64A/Q81P (mutations between residues 49 and 90)	Overall found in 1.8% of CLL cases (4.5% of IGVH mutated vs. 0 of unmutated)	[151]
MAPK1	Mutation	3% of CLL vs. matched normal tissue in these patients	[150]
MEFV	Five most common MEFV gene mutations (M694 V, M680I, V726A, M694I, and E148Q)	High-frequency of mutation carriers seen in MM (60%), ALL (33.3%) vs. CLL (9%), and NHL (5%). No mutations seen in HL. None had history or family history of family Mediterranean fever	[153]
miR-16-1, miR-15A	Mutations	Germline or somatic mutations were found in 5 of 42 sequenced microRNAs in 11 of 75 patients with CLL, but no such mutations were found in 160 subjects without cancer (*p* < 0.001); Removes repression of bcl2 and ZAP70	[154]

Table 3.3 (continued)

Gene name	Mutation	Frequency	Reference
MYD88	Mutations	50% of cases of primary CNS lymphoma vs. 9% of gastric MALT 3–10% of CLL that present at more advanced clinical stage; although no differences were observed in progression or survival rates. *MYD88* p.L265P mutation associated with *IGHV*-mutated group 5% of Burkitt lymphoma 29% of ABC-DLBCL vs. 6% of the germinal center B-cell DLBCL; rare or absent in other DLBCL and Burkitt	[150, 151, 155, 156]
NOTCH1	Mutations	Observed in 8–15% of CLL (one series cites 1.5%) Detected at significantly higher frequency during disease progression toward Richter transformation (31.0%) as well as in chemo-refractory CLL (20.8%) 3.77-fold increase in the hazard of death and to shorter overall survival (OS; $p < 0.001$) Also associated with +12 and confers worse prognosis in this group (2.4 times increased risk of death) and in this subgroup is more commonly associated with unmutated *IGVH*	[145, 150, 151, 157–159]
	Mutations resulting in premature stop codon	12% of CLL, mostly *IGHV* unmutated Adverse prognostic indicator 12% of patients (14/121) with MCL; associated with shorter survival Poor prognosis in mantle cell lymphoma; may be amenable to gamma-secretase inhibitors	[151, 160–162]
PLEKHG5	Mutations	<5% of CLL cases	[145]
SF3B1	Somatically mutated	10–15% of CLL cases and associated with faster disease progression and poor overall survival 10 of 59 (17%) fludarabine-refractory cases, with a frequency significantly greater than that observed in a consecutive CLL cohort sampled at diagnosis (17/301, 5%; $p = 0.002$)	[150, 163, 164]
TP53	Mutation and/or deletion	Most common molecular abnormality in Richter's syndrome (47%). More common in clonally related Richter's syndrome. Associated with bad prognosis: 10 m vs. 27 m ($p = 0.008$; 10 m vs. 35.8 months ($p < 0.001$) Clonally unrelated Richter's syndrome has significantly lower prevalence of TP53 abnormalities (23%) and better prognosis (similar clinically and molecularly to de novo DLBCL) than clonally related Richter's syndrome	[152]
TGM7	Mutations	<5% of CLL cases	[145]
IGHV	Unmutated	Same in CLL: unmutated signature worse prognosis in CLL/SLL vs. mutated Recurrent genomic lesions, including poor prognostic markers, were more common in unmutated IGHV cases vs. mutated IGHV in splenic marginal zone lymphomas	[165], 11733577
XPO1 (*CRM1*)	Mutation	Found in 2.4% of CLL cases but more common in unmutated *IGVH* vs. mutated *IGVH* (5% vs. 1.5%)	[159]
	Mutations: p.E571K and p.E571G	Rare in CLL; all *IGHV* unmutated	[151]
ZMYM3	Mutation	4% of CLL vs. matched normal tissue in these patients	[150]
TERT-CLPTM1L	Chromosome 5p; translocations to IG and non-IG partners	Occurs rarely in B-cell neoplasms (ALL, CLL, MCL, and SMZL) (no % given)	[166]
IGH@	t(14;19)(q32;q13)	0.1% of all B-cell neoplasms usually classified as atypical CLL with more aggressive course	[167]
HIST1H1C	Mutations	Novel candidate driver; chromatin regulator	[144]
CHD2	Mutations	Novel candidate driver; chromatin regulator	[144]
EGR2	Mutations	Novel candidate driver; B-cell transcription factors	[144]
IKZF3	Mutations	Novel candidate driver; B-cell transcription factors	[144]
RANBP2	Mutations	Novel candidate driver; RNA export factor	[144]
POT1	Mutations	Novel candidate driver; telomere-associated protein	[144]
MAP2K1	Mutations	Novel candidate driver; signal transducer	[144]
MAP2K3	Mutations	Novel candidate driver; signal transducer	[144]
RPS15	Mutations	Novel candidate driver; ribosomal protein	[144]
MLL2	Mutation	10–15% of mantle cell lymphoma (epigenetic histone modifier)	
WHSC1	Mutation	10–15% of mantle cell lymphoma (epigenetic histone modifier)	

MM multiple myeloma, *CLL/SLL* chronic lymphocytic leukemia/small lymphocytic lymphoma, *MCL* mantle cell lymphoma, *CNS* central nerve system, *MALT* extranodal marginal zone lymphoma with mucosa-associated lymphoid tissue, *ALL* acute lymphoblastic leukemia, *ABC-DLBCL* activated B-cell-like diffuse large B-cell lymphoma, *SMZL* splenic marginal zone lymphoma

Table 3.4 Genetic alterations seen in marginal zone lymphoma and follicular lymphoma

Gene name	Mutation	Frequency	Reference
6p	rs10484561 and rs6457327	rs10484561 ($p = 3.5 \times 10^{-9}$) and rs6457327 ($p = 0.008$) are associated with risk of FL rs6457327 predicts both time to ($p = 0.02$) and risk of ($p < 0.01$) FL transformation independently of clinical variables	[168]
C6orf15 (STG)	rs6457327	Risk for developing FL, robust statistical significance on this observation, with a combined allelic P value of $4.7 \times 10^{\wedge}-11$	[169, 170]
CREBBP	Deletions and/or somatic mutations	29% of DLBCL; more frequent in GCB subtype 42% vs. 17% ABC type 32.6% of FL	[171]
EP300	Nineteen sequence variants leading to amino acid changes ($n = 11$), in-frame deletions ($n = 2$), and premature stop codons due to frame shift deletions, aberrant splicing or nonsense mutations ($n = 6$)	10% of DLBCL and 8.7% of FL vs. virtually absent other B-NHL	[171]
EZH2	Heterozygous missense mutation at amino acid Y641, within the SET domain, and other mutations	Seen in 21.7% of GCB DLBCLs and 22% of FL and are absent from ABC DLBCLs, primary CNS lymphoma, and splenic marginal zone lymphoma In immunodeficient patients: seen in 3/116 (2.6%) immunodeficiency-related NHL including non-GC cases (cases included 90 HIV-NHL, 22 PTLD, 2 methotrexate (MTX)-related DLBCL, and 2 common variable immunodeficiency-related DLBCL) albeit at low frequency Potential for anti-EZH2 (GSK126)	[172–178]
FBXO11	Deletions and mutations	Seen in DLBCL (8–15%), FL (2%), MALTs (7%) vs. 0% of CLL	[179]
FOXO1	Mutations	GCB, 5% of DLBCL, and 25% of FL	[180]
FOXP1	t(3;14)	Extranodal MZL (MALT): ocular, stomach, thyroid, and skin sites DLBCL	[181–183]
GNA13	Mutations	Only in GCB DLBCL cases, 15% DLBCL, and 25% of FL	[180, 184]
HDAC7	Mutations	6% of DLBCL and 10% of FL	[180]
HIST1H4I	Translocation between 6p21.3 and BCL6	Reported as a translocation partner for *BCL6* in NHL (overall 12 cases of *BCL6* rearranged B-NHL)	[185]
MEF2B	Mutations	15% of DLBCL and 15% of FL	[180, 184, 186]
MLL2	Mutations	89% of FL and 24–32% of DLBCL	[180, 186]
PIM1	Mutation	15% of FL and 15–30% of DLBCL, ABC	[115, 180, 184, 186]
	Aberrant somatic hypermutation	Along with MYC, RHOH/TTF(ARHH), and PAX5, seen in 50% of DLBCL	[187]
SOCS1	Inactivating mutations	Described in PMBL but also present in ~25% of DLBCL and FL; rare mutations were observed in Burkitt lymphoma, plasmacytoma, and MCL, but not in tumors of a non-B-cell origin	[188]
TP53	Disruption (mutation)	FL; associated with worse prognosis	[169]
	Mutation (also isochromosome 17, deletion, translocations)	Worse prognosis and shorter time to transformation in FL The presence at diagnosis of a chromosome break at 6q23–26 or 17p defined a subgroup of 16 patients with a very poor prognosis ($p < .000\,1$) and a shorter time to transformation ($p < 0.001$). Significant in multivariate analysis	[40, 189]
	Mutation	Frequent in splenic diffuse red pulp small B-cell lymphoma	[190]
TNFAIP3 (A20)	Mutation and/or deletions	5% of DLBCL and 10% of FL	[180, 186]
	Somatic mutation	Affected in 13% of SMZLs (matched germline DNA extracted from saliva for control); also seen in other B-NHLs	[149, 191]

Table 3.4 (continued)

Gene name	Mutation	Frequency	Reference
TNFRSF14	1p36 gene mutations; nonsynonymous mutations	Seen in 18.3% of FL cases vs. not seen in normal; the most common mutation target so far described in the disease Associated with inferior clinical outcomes Multivariate analysis: OS and DSS after adjustment for the IPI in rituximab-treated patients (hazard ratios of 4.54 (1.80–11.44; $p = 0.001$) and 3.97 (1.50–10.51; $p = 0.006$), respectively; however, conflicting data with subsequent study showing better prognosis In all patients in multivariate analysis, cases with both aberrations (1p36 deletion and *TNFRSF14* mutation) remained a significant predictor of OS independent of the IPI compared with the group of no aberrations (HR, 3.65; 95% CI, 1.35–9.878; $p = 0.011$) and also displayed a significantly inferior DSS compared with those without either alteration	[192]
	Mutations	GCB, 15–20% of DLBCL and 20–30% of FL	[180, 184]
MYC	t(8;14)	Seen rarely in FL and can occur with t(14;18); aggressive course	[41, 42]
RHOH (ARHH, TTF)	Translocation with 4p13 and BCL6; t(3;4)(q27;p11) with ARHH/TTF	Seen in FL; those with *BCL6* translocation were more likely to transform ($p = 0.0048$)	[193]
LCP	Translocation between 13q14.1–q14.3 and BCL6; t(3;13)(q27;q14)	0.02% of B-NHL (5/210): DLBCL (3), FL (1), and Burkitt lymphoma (1); *LCP* involved in two cases	[194, 195]
BCL6	Translocations and deletions	Seen in FL; translocations in ~14%; higher risk of transformation to aggressive lymphoma	[193, 196]
	Rearrangement with various partners	*BCL6* breakpoints are more common in large cell component of composite lymphoma (large cell with MZL) and large cell variant of MZL vs. MZL (30% vs. 9%; not statistically significant) *BCL6-SFRS3* identified in DLBCL (1) and FL (1)	[197–200]
MYD88	Mutations	9% of gastric MALT lymphoma	[150, 151, 155, 156]
NOTCH2	Mutation	2/69 (3%) of MZL 5/63 (8%) DLBCL 25% of SMZL 20% NMZL	[201–203]
BCL10	t(1;14)(p22;q32)	One of the known translocations in extranodal MZL (MALT) lymphoma	[34]
		MALTs that usually do not respond to *Helicobacter pylori* eradication	[204]
BIRC3 (API2)/ MALT1	t(11;18)(q21;q21)	45% of pulmonary MALT lymphoma vs. reactive LN (as negative controls)	[205]
		Extranodal MZL (MALT) lymphoma, mainly pulmonary and gastric sites	[206]
		MALT lymphoma that usually does not respond to *Helicobacter pylori* eradication	[204]
IGH@	Rearrangement	5% of pulmonary MALT lymphoma vs. reactive LN (as negative controls)	[205]
	t(14;18)(q32;q21); IGH-MALT1	MALTs that usually do not respond to *Helicobacter pylori* eradication	[204]
MALT1	Rearrangement or amplification	65% of pulmonary MALT vs. reactive LN (as negative controls)	[205]
	Translocation; *BIRC3/MALT1* or *IGHV/MALT1*	Most common translocation of MALT lymphoma	[207]
	t(14;18)(q32;q21)	Extranodal MZL (MALT): ocular and salivary gland sites	[208]
PTPRD	Mutations	20% NMZL	[209]
KLF2	Mutation	70% NMZL	[209]

OS overall survival, *DSS* disease-specific survival, *FL* follicular lymphoma, *GCB-DLBCL* germinal center B-cell like diffuse large B-cell lymphoma, *LN* lymph node, *MZL* marginal zone lymphoma, *MALT lymphoma* extranodal marginal zone lymphoma with mucosa-associated lymphoid tissue, *NMZL* nodal marginal zone lymphoma

Table 3.5 Genetic alterations seen in splenic marginal zone lymphoma, lymphoplasmacytic lymphoma, and hairy cell leukemia

Gene name	Mutation	Frequency	Reference
BIRC3	Mutations>deletions	Affected in 11% of SMZL (matched germline DNA extracted from saliva for control)	[149]
BRAF	K601E mutations	Detected in a single case of SMZL vs. all cases of hairy cell leukemia	[210]
CARD11	Somatic mutation	(3/34 = 8.8%) splenic MZL but also seen in other B-NHLs	[191]
IKBKB	Mutation and copy number alterations	Affected in 3% of SMZLs (matched germline DNA extracted from saliva for control) In another study activated in 10% SMZL L265P in 91% of LPL vs. 7% of marginal zone lymphoma	[149, 211]
CDK6	Translocations involving 7q31–32	−40% of SMZL Reported in six cases of low-grade B-cell lymphoma	[23, 212]
	t(2;7)	Reported in a case of CD5(−) B-cell lymphocytosis but also reported in SMZL (see above)	[213]
MYD88	Somatic mutation	6/46 (13%) of SMZL but also seen in other B-NHLs 87–100% of LPL; involved in innate and adaptive immune response	[191, 211]
NOTCH2	Mutation	25% of SMZL; 2/69 (3%) of MZL; 5/63 (8%) DLBCL	[201–203]
TNFAIP3 (A20)	Somatic mutation	Affected in 13% of SMZLs (matched germline DNA extracted from saliva for control); also seen in other B-NHLs	[149, 191]
TRAF3	Mutation and copy number alterations	Affected in 10% of SMZL (matched germline DNA extracted from saliva for control)	[149]
MYD88	L265P mutations	*MYD88* L265P was specifically associated with WM/LPLs. WM/LPL may thus be functionally associated with constitutive nuclear factor-κB activation	[214]
CXCR4	Mutation	36% of LPL cases	[215]
TERT-CLPTM1L	Chromosome 5p; translocations to IG and non-IG partners	Occurs rarely in B-cell neoplasms (ALL, CLL, MCL, and SMZL) (no % given)	[166]
BRAF	BRAF V600E mutation	100% patients with HCL vs. none of 195 other peripheral B-cell lymphoma/leukemias Treatment with vemurafenib	[216, 217]
	K600E mutations	Detected in a single case of SMZL vs. all cases of hairy cell leukemia	[210]
	V600E mutation	All cases of HCL. Rare in other CLPD including HCL variant	[218–220]

NHLs non-Hodgkin lymphomas, *WM/LPL* Waldenstrom's macroglobulinemia/lymphoplasmacytic lymphoma, *ALL* acute lymphoblastic leukemia, *CLL* chronic lymphocytic leukemia, *MCL* mantle cell lymphoma, *SMZL* splenic marginal zone B-cell lymphoma, *MZL* marginal zone lymphoma, *CLPD* chronic lymphoproliferative disorders, *HCL* hairy cell leukemia

Table 3.6 Genetic alterations seen in classic Hodgkin lymphoma

Gene name	Mutation	Frequency	Reference
TNFAIP3 (A20)	Mutations and deletions	44% of CHL 36% of PMBL	[221]
	Deletion or mutation	By FISH, A20 deletion in 18% and by IHC, A20 mutations in 16% of AIDS-related lymphomas (ARLs) vs. no control data	[222]
	Inactivating deletions or mutations	16/36 (44%) cases of CHL. Clearly inactivating mutations found only in EBV-negative cases, suggesting that EBV and TNFAIP3 inactivation are alternative ways of activating NF-κB	[223]
6q21	Two intergenic SNP variants close to *PRDM1*; rs4946728 and rs1040411 mapped to chromosome 6q21, intergenic between *ATG5* and *PRDM1*. The strongest evidence for association in this region was for rs4946728 ($p = 1.09 \times 10^{-8}$, $OR_{allelic} = 4.22$ [95% CI = 2.53–7.05]). rs8083533 mapped to 18q11.2, intronic to *TAF4B* ($p = 4.98 \times 10^{-8}$, $OR_{allelic} = 3.78$ [95% CI = 2.31–6.18]	Increased incidence of therapy-induced second malignancies after HL; rs4946728 ($p = 0.002$) and rs1040411 ($p = 0.03$)	[224]
BCL6	Translocation	48% of NLPHL cases; not detected in CHL	[45, 48, 225–228]

Table 3.6 (continued)

Gene name	Mutation	Frequency	Reference
CIITA (*MHC2TA*)	Recurrent rearrangement, translocation partners include C16orf75 on 16p13.13, 9p24 (cd273, cd274), FLJ27352, RALGDS, RUNDC2A, BCL6	Seen in PMBL (38%) and CHL (15%) vs. 3% of DLBCL ($p < 0.0001$)	[229]
IKBKB	Deleterious mutations (particularly IκBα)	10–20% of CHL	[223]
SOCS1	Mutations/small deletions	~50% of CHL microdissected cells	[230]
JAK2	Rearrangements	2% of CHL cases	[231]
NPAT	Truncating germline mutation/germline deletion of serine 724	First gene implicated in NLPHL predisposition (odds ratio = 4.11; $p = 0.018$	[232]
	Replacement mutation in codon 724	NLPHL and CHL at a significantly higher frequency than in healthy controls	[233]
	Germline deletion c. 2437-2438delAG of 2 bp, resulting in frame shift	Seen in family with NLPHL (four of four patients)	[232]
OTC	p.R277W mutation	Associated with OTC deficiency with hyperammonemic crisis after treatment for HL	[234]
SEC31A-JAK2	t(4;9)(q21;p24)	Characteristic of CHL (two cases reported); may be responsive to JAK inhibitors	[231]

IHC immunohistochemistry, *AIDS* acquired immune deficiency syndrome, *EBV* Epstein-Barr virus, *CHL* classic Hodgkin lymphoma, *PMBCL* primary mediastinal B-cell lymphoma, *HL* Hodgkin lymphoma, *NLPHL* nodal lymphocytic predominant Hodgkin lymphoma

Table 3.7 Genetic alterations seen in diffuse large B-cell lymphoma

Gene name	Mutation	Frequency	Reference
BCL2	t(14;18)	20–30% of DLBCL	[235, 236]
	Translocation BCL2/NFATC1	Specific for ABC-DLBCL	[14]
	Structural rearrangements/mutations	GCB enrichment	[180]
BCL6	Abnormality 3q27 +/− BCL6 rearrangement	30% of DLBCL; can involve *BCL6* (most common translocation in DLBCL) BCL6 rearrangement was associated with better prognosis; patients with *BCL6* rearrangement had a relative risk of death of 0.09 (95% confidence interval, 0.02–0.42), as compared with patients without *BCL6* rearrangement, after the other prognostic variables in the model had been controlled for ($p = 0.002$)	[47, 50, 237]
	Translocation, ~50% of the time with Ig, of which 75% is IgH. Major breakpoint cluster in 5'UTR of BCL6, minor cluster ~250 kb upstream	24% of ABC DLBCL; 10% of GCB DLBCL; 33% of PMBL Non-IG translocation partners associated with worse prognosis in DLBCL ($p = 0.0440$); the estimated 2-year overall survival rates were 58.3% vs. 17.6% ($p = 0.005$) Rearrangement of the *BCL6* gene correlated with a favorable clinical outcome in diffuse lymphomas with large cell component 48% of NLPHL cases; not detected in CHL	[45, 48, 225–228]
	Mutations	61% of DLBCL cases, significantly higher frequency in GCB subtype and PMBL (>70%) than in ABC subtype (44%). Exon 1 mutations mostly in GCB subtype	[48]
CARD11	Missense mutations, all within exons encoding the coiled-coil domain	In ~10% ABC DLBCL biopsies (9.6%). Rare in GCB-DLBCL	[238–242]
CD79A	Somatic mutations affecting the immunoreceptor tyrosine-based activation	Along with CD79b mutations, frequently seen in ABC DLBCL biopsy samples but rarely in other DLBCLs and never in Burkitt lymphoma or MALT; also absent in immunodeficiency-related NHL (the study included: 90 HIV-NHL, 22 PTLD, 2 methotrexate (MTX)-related DLBCL, and 2 common variable immunodeficiency-related DLBCL)	[174, 243]
CD79B	Somatic mutations affecting the immunoreceptor tyrosine-based activation	Along with CD79a mutations, frequently seen in ABC DLBCL biopsy samples but rarely in other DLBCLs and never in Burkitt lymphoma or MALT; also absent in immunodeficiency-related NHL (the study included: 90 HIV-NHL, 22 PTLD, 2 methotrexate (MTX)-related DLBCL, and 2 common variable immunodeficiency-related DLBCL)	[174, 243]

(continued)

Table 3.7 (continued)

Gene name	Mutation	Frequency	Reference
	Mutations: the first ITAM tyrosine mutated; less common were missense mutations in other ITAM residues and deletions that disrupted all or part of the motif	18% of ABC DLBCLs, overall, the frequency of CD79B ITAM mutations was significantly higher in ABC DLBCL (21.1%) than in GCB DLBCL (3.1%) ($p = 8.9 \times 10^{-4}$). No CD79B ITAM mutations in Burkitt or gastric MALT	[240, 242, 243]
CREBBP	Deletions and/or somatic mutations	29% of DLBCL, more frequent in GCB subtype 42% vs. 17% ABC type 32.6% of FL	[171]
EZH2	Heterozygous missense mutation at amino acid Y641, within the SET domain, and other mutations	Seen in 21.7% of GCB DLBCLs and 7.2–12% of follicular lymphomas and are absent from ABC DLBCLs and primary CNS lymphoma Absent from ABC DLBCLs and splenic marginal zone lymphoma In immunodeficient patients: seen in 3/116 (2.6%) immunodeficiency-related NHL including non-GC cases (cases included 90 HIV-NHL, 22 PTLD, 2 methotrexate (MTX)-related DLBCL, and 2 common variable immunodeficiency-related DLBCL) albeit at low frequency Also seen in poor prognosis myelodysplasia-myeloproliferative neoplasms (10 to 13%), myelofibrosis (13%), and various subtypes of myelodysplastic syndromes (6%)	[172] [173–180]
EP300	Inactivating mutation	Seen in 5% of DLBCL; acyltransferase	[244]
FAS (CD95; TNFRSF6)	Mutation	Can be seen in FL; also associated with worse prognosis in FL; 5% of FL and 15% of GCB-DLBCL	[169, 180, 184]
FOXO1	Mutations	GCB restricted, 5% of DLBCL, and 25% of FL	[180]
GNA13	Mutations	Only in GCB DLBCL cases, 15% DLBCL, and 25% of FL	[180, 184]
GSTT1	Null genotype and double-null genotype	In de novo DLBCL treated with RCHOP: GSTT1 null genotype: more frequent grade III–IV chemotherapy-related toxicities (OR 3.1; $p = 0.025$) GSTM1/T1 double-null genotype: shorter event-free survival period ($p = 0.02$) in males	[245]
LCP	Translocation between 13q14.1-q14.3 and BCL6; t(3;13)(q27;q14)	0.02% of B-NHL (5/210): DLBCL (3), FL (1), and Burkitt lymphoma (1); LCP involved in two cases	[194, 195]
MEF2B	Mutations	11.4% of DLBCL and 13.4% of follicular lymphoma; GCB restricted, 15% of DLBCL, and 15% of FL	[180, 184, 186]
MLL2	Mutations	24–30% of DLBCL, 32% of DLBCL, and 89% of follicular lymphoma One of the most commonly mutated genes in FL and DLBCL	[180, 186]
MYC	Rearrangement	Poor prognostic indicator in DLBCL	[246]
	8q24 translocation; partner is IG (60%)	10% of diffuse large B-cell lymphoma; very unfavorable outcome	[235]
MYD88	Mutations	29% of ABC-DLBCL vs. 6% of the GCB- DLBCL; rare or absent in other DLBCL and Burkitt lymphoma	[156, 241]
NOTCH2	Mutation	2/69 (3%) of MZL 5/63 (8%) DLBCL 25% of SMZL	[201–203]
PAX5	Aberrant somatic hypermutation	Along with MYC, RHOH/TTF(ARHH), and PIMI, seen in 50% of DLBCL; however, rare in other NHL except for MYC in Burkitt lymphoma	[187]
	t(9;14)(p13;q32) With PAX5 and IGH@	Reported in THR-BCL (four cases) and PTLD-DLBCL (two cases) Associated with a subset of de novo DLBCL presenting with advanced disease and adverse prognosis Has also been described in FL, SLL with plasmacytoid morphology, PEL (1), and alpha heavy chain disease (1), SMZL (3)	[247–251]

Table 3.7 (continued)

Gene name	Mutation	Frequency	Reference
PIM1	Mutation	ABC, 15–30% of DLBCL, and 15% of FL	[115, 180, 184, 186]
	Aberrant somatic hypermutation	Along with MYC, RHOH/TTF(ARHH), and PAX5, seen in 50% of DLBCL; however, rare in other NHL except for MYC in Burkitt lymphoma	[187]
PRDM1 (BLIMP)	Homozygous deletions, truncating or missense mutations, and transcriptional repression by constitutively active BCL6	Seen in 10% DLBCL; seen in ~51% of ABC and non-GC type DLBCL vs. none of the GC subtype of DLBCL	[184, 186, 252]
RECQL4	Mutations, e.g., c.1919_1924delTCACAG, p.L640_A642delinsP in exon 12 of the *RECQL4* gene and mutation c.1704 + 1G > A in intron 10 of the *RECQL4* gene	A patient with Rothmund-Thomson syndrome developed large cell anaplastic T-cell lymphoma at the age of 9 years, DLBCL and osteosarcoma when he was 14 years old, and finally ALL when he was 21 years old; there was spontaneous remission of DLBCL. Lymphomas also reported in Rapadilino and Baller-Gerold syndrome (BGS)	[253–255]
RHOH (ARHH, TTF)	Aberrant somatic hypermutation	Along with MYC, PIMI, and PAX5, seen in 50% of DLBCL; however, rare in other NHL except for MYC in Burkitt lymphoma	[187]
SMARCA1	Mutation	2% DLBCL	[186]
SOCS1	Inactivating mutations	Described in PMBL but also present in 1/4 of diffuse large B-cell lymphoma and follicular lymphomas; rare mutations were observed in Burkitt lymphoma, plasmacytoma, and MCL, but not in tumors of a non-B-cell origin	[188]
SGK1	Mutations	DLBCL and FL; only GCB	[180]
TNFAIP3 (A20)	Mutations	3% (1/32) of primary CNS lymphoma (DLBCL) vs. spinal DLBCL 20% (2/10)	[256]
	Mutation and/or deletions	5% of DLBCL and 10% of follicular lymphoma	[180, 186]
	Somatic mutation	Found in 17% of gastrointestinal DLBCL and associated with worse 5-year OS (0 vs. 0.654; $p = 0.001$) and EFS (0 vs. 0.57; $p = 0.002$)	[257]
	Mutations and/or deletions	32% of ABC-DLBCL and 34% of non-GC/nonclassified (NC)-DLBCL; almost exclusively segregating with an ABC/non-GC phenotype (24% ABC-DLBCL and 20% non-GC/NC-DLBCL, vs. 3% GCB-DLBCL)	[238, 240]
	Mutations	ABC enriched, 15–20% of DLBCL, and 20–30% of FL	[180, 184]
TNFRSF14	Mutations	GCB, 15–20% of DLBCL, and 20–30% of FL	[180, 184]
TP53	Mutation	70% of DLBCL associated with CI	[258]
	Mutation and/or deletion	Poor prognostic indicator in DLBCL; the presence of a p53 gene mutation affected survival ($p = 0.01$), with a 6-year survival rate estimated to be 44% in mutated patients, compared with 79% in non-mutated ones; GCB restricted	[259, 260]
	Inactivation (mutations)	Reported in PMBL (13% of cases; $n = 27$)	[261]
TRAF2	Missense mutations	3% of DLBCL	[238]
TRAF5	Missense mutations	5% of DLBCL	[238]

GCB or ABC-DLBCL germinal center B-cell-like or activated B-cell-like diffuse large B-cell lymphoma, *NLPHL* nodular lymphocyte predominant Hodgkin lymphoma, *THR-BCL* T-cell-/histiocyte-rich B-cell lymphoma, *MALT* extranodal marginal zone lymphoma with mucosa-associated lymphoid tissue, *PTLD* posttransplant lymphoproliferative disorder, *SMZL* splenic marginal zone lymphoma, *PEL* primary effusion lymphoma, *MCL* mantle cell lymphoma, *NHL* non-Hodgkin lymphoma, *ALL* acute lymphoblastic leukemia, *OS* overall survival, *EFS* event-free survival, *FL* follicular lymphoma, *PMBL* primary mediastinal B-cell lymphoma

Table 3.8 Genetic alterations seen in natural killer cell and T-cell lymphomas

Gene name	Mutation	Frequency	Reference
IDH2	Mutation	20–45% of AITL cases; not found in other PTCL	[262]
ITK/SYK	t(5;9)(q33;q22)	17% of unspecified PTCL This aberration was not found in AITL or ALK(−)-ALCL	[83]
TET2	Mutations	Most common genetic lesion in AITL Associated with *DNMT3A mutations* Treatment with demethylating agents may be considered	[262, 263]
RECQL4	Mutations, e.g., c.1919_1924delTCACAG, p.L640_A642delinsP in exon 12 of the RECQL4 gene and mutation c.1704 + 1G > A in intron 10 of the RECQL4 gene	A patient with Rothmund-Thomson syndrome developed ALCL at the age of 9 years, DLBCL and osteosarcoma when he was 14 years old, and finally acute lymphatic leukemia when he was 21 years old; there was spontaneous remission of DLBCL. Lymphomas also reported in Rapadilino and Baller-Gerold syndrome (BGS)	[253–255]
ALK	Translocation; partners for ALK are 1, 2, 3, 17, 19, 22, and X	ALCL, ALK(+) 85% have t(2;5)(p23;q35) and 15% have variant translocations	[264–266]
DUSP22/ FRA7H	t(6;7)(p25.3;q32.3)	11/29 cases of ALK(−) ALCL vs. none of 108 PTCL cases showed 7q32.3 break	[267]
DNMT3A	Mutation	Eleven of the 96 patients (11%) had a *DNMT3A* mutation Nine AITLs and two PTCL, NOS Consider treating with demethylating agents Associated with *TET2* mutations	[263]
IRF4	Translocations (break-apart FISH)	Specific for cutaneous ALCL as opposed to LyP, systemic ALCL, or other T-cell or NK cell lymphomas	[268]
JAK3	Somatic mutation	3.3% of cutaneous T-cell lymphomas; if there is a mutation, it is unlikely to be ATLL	[269]
FARP2 (FERM)	Mutation	Induces gain of function of JAK3 Found in 4/36 ATLL patients (11%) Inhibited by kinase inhibitors in clinical testing stage	[270]
HTLV1	Monoclonal integration of	ATLL; no clonal integration is seen in healthy carriers	[271]
NOTCH1	Activating mutations	>30% of ATLL	[272]
EBV	Clonal	EBV+ T-cell lymphoproliferative disorder of childhood	[273]
HLA-DQA1 and HL-DRB1	In celiac patients: HLADQA1∗0501, DQB1∗0201; DRB 1∗03,04 heterozygotes	90% of EATL vs. 23–21% of 151 normal controls (respectively) DRB 1∗0304 heterozygotes was significantly increased in the EATL group (16 of 40, 40%) compared with both control individuals (3 of 151, 2%; $p < 10$ m6, RR = 32.9) and uncomplicated CD patients (6 of 9 1, 7%; $p = 0.04$, RR = 9.4)	[274]
PTPN2	Biallelic inactivation (deletion and mutation)	Seen in 2 out of 39 cases of PTCL, NOS, but not in Hodgkin's lymphoma	[275]
FGFR3	t(4;12)(p16;p13)	Reported in a case of PTCL, NOS	[276]
X	t(X;14)	Less common in T-PLL than t(14;14)	[277]
TCLA1	inv14(q11;q32) or t(14;14) (q11;q32)	80% of T-PLL; most frequent chromosomal abnormality in T-PLL	[71, 278]
ATM	Missense mutations	Seen in 63% of T-PLL	[279]
TRA@ and TCL1A and B	t(14;14)	10% of T-PLL	[280]
KRAS	(G13D) mutation	Cutaneous T-cell lymphoma: described in one mycosis fungoides and one pleomorphic CTCL Decreased overall survival in stage IV CTCL patients	[281]
NRAS	Mutations (Q61K)	CTCL: described in one MF and one pleomorphic CTCL Decreased overall survival in stage IV patients *NRAS*(Q61K) mutation sensitized Hut78 cells toward growth inhibition by the MEK inhibitors U0126, AZD6244, and PD0325901	[281]
CDKN2A (p16)	Inactivation (deletion and methylation)	Common in Sezary; 44% and 78% in plaque and tumor stages of MF, respectively ($n = 9$)	[282, 283]

Table 3.8 (continued)

Gene name	Mutation	Frequency	Reference
Beta catenin	Mutation	Found in extranodal NK/TCL, nasal type with a higher percentage in Japanese vs. Korean cases Overall, found in 30% (6/20) of extranodal NK/TCL, nasal type	[284, 285]
KIT	Mutation	Extranodal NK/TCL, nasal type (5%, 1/20), and other PTCL	[284, 286]
KRAS	Mutation	Extranodal NK/TCL, nasal type (5%, 1/20)	[284]
TP53	Mutation	Extranodal NK/TCL, nasal type (31% and 62% in Korea and Japan, respectively) Overall, found in 40% (8/20)of extranodal NK/TCL, nasal type Cases with p53 mutations were associated with large cell morphology ($p = 0.0162$) and presented more often with advanced stage disease	[284, 285, 287]
SETD2	Mutation	25% of HSTCL; chromatin modifier, chromatin-modifying genes are mutated in 62% of HSTCL	[288]
INO80	Mutation	21% of HSTCL chromatin modifier, chromatin-modifying genes are mutated in 62% of HSTCL	[288]
TET3	Mutation	15% of HSTCL; chromatin modifier, chromatin-modifying genes are mutated in 62% of HSTCL	[288]
SMARCA2	Mutation	10% of HSTCL; chromatin modifier, chromatin-modifying genes are mutated in 62% of HSTCL	[288]
STAT5B	Mutation	31% of HSTCL 2% LGLL	[288, 289]
STAT3	Mutation	9% of HSTCL 40% T-cell LGLL	[288, 290]
PIK3CD	Mutation	9% of HSTCL	[288]
7q	Isochromosome	Most cases of HSTCL	[291]
TP63	Rearrangements	8% of ALK-negative ALCL, poorer survival	[93]
DUSP22	Rearrangements	30% of ALK-negative ALCL, 85% 5-year OS	[93]

AITL angioimmunoblastic T-cell lymphoma, *ALK(+) or ALK(−) ALCL* ALK(+) or ALK(−) anaplastic large cell lymphoma, *LyP* lymphomatoid papulosis; *ATLL* adult T-cell lymphoma/leukemia, *EATL* enteropathy-associated T-cell lymphoma; *PTCL, NOS* peripheral T-cell lymphoma, not otherwise specified, *T-PLL* T-cell prolymphocytic leukemia, *CTCL* cutaneous T-cell lymphoma, *MF* mycosis fungoides, *Extranodal NK/TCL nasal type* extranodal NK/T-cell lymphoma, nasal type, *LGL* large granular lymphocytic leukemia, *HSTCL* hepatosplenic T-cell lymphoma, *OS* overall survival

Key signaling pathways implicated in CLL/SLL include inflammation (e.g., POT1NFk-B), WNT signaling, Notch signaling, and B-cell receptor signaling.

Dysregulated pathways in splenic marginal zone lymphoma (SMZL) include NOTCH signaling, NF-κB, and TRAF3/MAP 3 K14-TRAF2/BIRC3-negative regulatory complex [292]

Some 150 driver genes have been identified in DLBCL. Genetic lesions and DLBCL involve histone/chromatin modifiers (85%), MLL2 inactivation, inactivation of acetyl transferases, deregulation of BCL6, and evasion of immune surveillance [244]. A recent study has provided a molecular classification of diffuse large B-cell lymphoma beyond the traditional germinal center B-cell (GCB) type and activated B-cell-like (ABC) type classification. Genetic subtypes were termed MCD (*MYD88*[L265P] and *CD79B* mutations), BN2 (*BCL6* fusions and *NOTCH2* mutations), N1 (*NOTCH1* mutations), and EZB (*EZH2* mutations and *BCL2* translocations). Survival in the BN2 and EZB subtypes was favorable, and outcomes in the MCD and N1 subtypes were inferior [293].

References

1. Goldin LR, Pfeiffer RM, Li X, Hemminki K. Familial risk of lymphoproliferative tumors in families of patients with chronic lymphocytic leukemia: results from the Swedish Family-Cancer Database. Blood. 2004;104(6):1850–4.
2. Golomb HM, Rowley JD, Vardiman JW, Testa JR, Butler A. "Microgranular" acute promyelocytic leukemia: a distinct clinical, ultrastructural, and cytogenetic entity. Blood. 1980;55(2):253–9.
3. Rao N. Principles of cytogenetics. In: Naeim F, Rao N, Grody W, editors. Hematopathology- morphology, immunophenotype, cytogenetics and molecular approaches. Amsterdam: Elsevier; 2008. p. 56–64.
4. Veerabhadrappa SK, Chandrappa PR, Roodmal SY, Shetty SJ, Gunjiganur MS, Karyotyping PMKK. Current perspectives in diagnosis of chromosomal disorders. Sifa Med J. 2016;3(2):6.
5. Schrijver I, Zehnder JL, Cherry AM. Tools for genetics and genomics: cytogenetics and molecular genetics. 2017. https://www.uptodate.com/contents/tools-for-genetics-and-genomics-cytogenetics-and-molecular-genetics.
6. Song J, Shao H. SNP Array in hematopoietic neoplasms: a review. Microarrays (Basel). 2015;5(1):1.
7. Bayani J, Squire J. Traditional banding of chromosomes for cytogenetic analysis. Curr Protoc Cell Biol. 2004;23(1):7.
8. Wan TSK. Cancer cytogenetics: an introduction. Humana Press; 2017.

9. Ventura RA, Martin-Subero JI, Jones M, et al. FISH analysis for the detection of lymphoma-associated chromosomal abnormalities in routine paraffin-embedded tissue. J Mol Diagn. 2006;8(2):141–51.

10. Hummel M, Bentink S, Berger H, et al. A biologic definition of Burkitt's lymphoma from transcriptional and genomic profiling. N Engl J Med. 2006;354(23):2419–30.

11. Tanke HJ, Wiegant J, van Gijlswijk RP, et al. New strategy for multi-colour fluorescence in situ hybridisation: COBRA: COmbined binary RAtio labelling. Eur J Human Genet EJHG. 1999;7(1):2–11.

12. Boerma EG, Siebert R, Kluin PM, Baudis M. Translocations involving 8q24 in Burkitt lymphoma and other malignant lymphomas: a historical review of cytogenetics in the light of todays knowledge. Leukemia. 2009;23(2):225–34.

13. Seegmiller AC, Garcia R, Huang R, Maleki A, Karandikar NJ, Chen W. Simple karyotype and bcl-6 expression predict a diagnosis of Burkitt lymphoma and better survival in IG-MYC rearranged high-grade B-cell lymphomas. Mod Pathol. 2010;23(7):909–20.

14. Kluin P, Schuuring E. Molecular cytogenetics of lymphoma: where do we stand in 2010? Histopathology. 2011;58(1):128–44.

15. Speicher MR, Gwyn Ballard S, Ward DC. Karyotyping human chromosomes by combinatorial multi-fluor FISH. Nat Genet. 1996;12(4):368–75.

16. Veldman T, Vignon C, Schrock E, Rowley JD, Ried T. Hidden chromosome abnormalities in haematological malignancies detected by multicolour spectral karyotyping. Nat Genet. 1997;15(4):406–10.

17. Kearney L. Multiplex-FISH (M-FISH): technique, developments and applications. Cytogenet Genome Res. 2006;114(3–4):189–98.

18. Horsman DE, Okamoto I, Ludkovski O, et al. Follicular lymphoma lacking the t(14;18)(q32;q21): identification of two disease subtypes. Br J Haematol. 2003;120(3):424–33.

19. Johansson B, Mertens F, Mitelman F. Cytogenetic evolution patterns in non-Hodgkin's lymphoma. Blood. 1995;86(10):3905–14.

20. Swerdlow SH, Campo E, Harris NL, et al. WHO classification of Tumours of Haematopoietic and lymphoid tissues. 4th edn. WHO International Agency for Research on Cancer (IARC); 2017.

21. Del Giudice I, Davis Z, Matutes E, et al. IgVH genes mutation and usage, ZAP-70 and CD38 expression provide new insights on B-cell prolymphocytic leukemia (B-PLL). Leukemia. 2006;20(7):1231–7.

22. Flatley E, Chen AI, Zhao X, et al. Aberrations of MYC are a common event in B-cell prolymphocytic leukemia. Am J Clin Pathol. 2014;142(3):347–54.

23. Corcoran MM, Mould SJ, Orchard JA, et al. Dysregulation of cyclin dependent kinase 6 expression in splenic marginal zone lymphoma through chromosome 7q translocations. Oncogene. 1999;18(46):6271–7.

24. Rinaldi A, Mian M, Chigrinova E, et al. Genome-wide DNA profiling of marginal zone lymphomas identifies subtype-specific lesions with an impact on the clinical outcome. Blood. 2011;117(5):1595–604.

25. Salido M, Baro C, Oscier D, et al. Cytogenetic aberrations and their prognostic value in a series of 330 splenic marginal zone B-cell lymphomas: a multicenter study of the Splenic B-Cell Lymphoma Group. Blood. 2010;116(9):1479–88.

26. Braggio E, Fonseca R. Genomic abnormalities of Waldenstrom macroglobulinemia and related low-grade B-cell lymphomas. Clin Lymphoma Myeloma Leuk. 2013;13(2):198–201.

27. Terre C, Nguyen-Khac F, Barin C, et al. Trisomy 4, a new chromosomal abnormality in Waldenstrom's macroglobulinemia: a study of 39 cases. Leukemia. 2006;20(9):1634–6.

28. Cook JR, Aguilera NI, Reshmi S, et al. Deletion 6q is not a characteristic marker of nodal lymphoplasmacytic lymphoma. Cancer Genet Cytogenet. 2005;162(1):85–8.

29. George TI, Wrede JE, Bangs CD, Cherry AM, Warnke RA, Arber DA. Low-grade B-cell lymphomas with plasmacytic differentiation lack PAX5 gene rearrangements. J Mol Diagn. 2005;7(3):346–51.

30. Mansoor A, Medeiros LJ, Weber DM, et al. Cytogenetic findings in lymphoplasmacytic lymphoma/Waldenstrom macroglobulinemia. Chromosomal abnormalities are associated with the polymorphous subtype and an aggressive clinical course. Am J Clin Pathol. 2001;116(4):543–9.

31. Cook JR, Aguilera NI, Reshmi-Skarja S, et al. Lack of PAX5 rearrangements in lymphoplasmacytic lymphomas: reassessing the reported association with t(9;14). Hum Pathol. 2004;35(4):447–54.

32. Ocio EM, Schop RF, Gonzalez B, et al. 6q deletion in Waldenstrom macroglobulinemia is associated with features of adverse prognosis. Br J Haematol. 2007;136(1):80–6.

33. Schop RF, Van Wier SA, Xu R, et al. 6q deletion discriminates Waldenstrom macroglobulinemia from IgM monoclonal gammopathy of undetermined significance. Cancer Genet Cytogenet. 2006;169(2):150–3.

34. Streubel B, Simonitsch-Klupp I, Mullauer L, et al. Variable frequencies of MALT lymphoma-associated genetic aberrations in MALT lymphomas of different sites. Leukemia. 2004;18(10):1722–6.

35. Horsman DE, Gascoyne RD, Coupland RW, Coldman AJ, Adomat SA. Comparison of cytogenetic analysis, southern analysis, and polymerase chain reaction for the detection of t(14;18) in follicular lymphoma. Am J Clin Pathol. 1995;103(4):472–8.

36. Rowley JD. Chromosome studies in the non-Hodgkin's lymphomas: the role of the 14;18 translocation. J Clin Oncol. 1988;6(5):919–25.

37. Finn LS, Viswanatha DS, Belasco JB, et al. Primary follicular lymphoma of the testis in childhood. Cancer. 1999;85(7):1626–35.

38. Hoglund M, Sehn L, Connors JM, et al. Identification of cytogenetic subgroups and karyotypic pathways of clonal evolution in follicular lymphomas. Genes Chromosomes Cancer. 2004;39(3):195–204.

39. Offit K, Parsa NZ, Gaidano G, et al. 6q deletions define distinct clinico-pathologic subsets of non-Hodgkin's lymphoma. Blood. 1993;82(7):2157–62.

40. Tilly H, Rossi A, Stamatoullas A, et al. Prognostic value of chromosomal abnormalities in follicular lymphoma. Blood. 1994;84(4):1043–9.

41. Au WY, Horsman DE, Gascoyne RD, Viswanatha DS, Klasa RJ, Connors JM. The spectrum of lymphoma with 8q24 aberrations: a clinical, pathological and cytogenetic study of 87 consecutive cases. Leuk Lymphoma. 2004;45(3):519–28.

42. Voorhees PM, Carder KA, Smith SV, Ayscue LH, Rao KW, Dunphy CH. Follicular lymphoma with a burkitt translocation–predictor of an aggressive clinical course: a case report and review of the literature. Arch Pathol Lab Med. 2004;128(2):210–3.

43. Quintanilla-Martinez L, Sander B, Chan JK, et al. Indolent lymphomas in the pediatric population: follicular lymphoma, IRF4/MUM1+ lymphoma, nodal marginal zone lymphoma and chronic lymphocytic leukemia. Virchows Arch. 2016;468(2):141–57.

44. Salaverria I, Philipp C, Oschlies I, et al. Translocations activating IRF4 identify a subtype of germinal center-derived B-cell lymphoma affecting predominantly children and young adults. Blood. 2011;118(1):139–47.

45. Akasaka T, Ueda C, Kurata M, et al. Nonimmunoglobulin (non-Ig)/BCL6 gene fusion in diffuse large B-cell lymphoma results in worse prognosis than Ig/BCL6. Blood. 2000;96(8):2907–9.

46. Barrans SL, O'Connor SJ, Evans PA, et al. Rearrangement of the BCL6 locus at 3q27 is an independent poor prognostic factor in nodal diffuse large B-cell lymphoma. Br J Haematol. 2002;117(2):322–32.

47. Bastard C, Deweindt C, Kerckaert JP, et al. LAZ3 rearrangements in non-Hodgkin's lymphoma: correlation with histology, immunophenotype, karyotype, and clinical outcome in 217 patients. Blood. 1994;83(9):2423–7.

48. Iqbal J, Greiner TC, Patel K, et al. Distinctive patterns of BCL6 molecular alterations and their functional consequences in different subgroups of diffuse large B-cell lymphoma. Leukemia. 2007;21(11):2332–43.

49. Lossos IS, Jones CD, Warnke R, et al. Expression of a single gene, BCL-6, strongly predicts survival in patients with diffuse large B-cell lymphoma. Blood. 2001;98(4):945–51.

50. Offit K, Lo Coco F, Louie DC, et al. Rearrangement of the bcl-6 gene as a prognostic marker in diffuse large-cell lymphoma. N Engl J Med. 1994;331(2):74–80.

51. Barrans SL, Evans PA, O'Connor SJ, et al. The t(14;18) is associated with germinal center-derived diffuse large B-cell lymphoma and is a strong predictor of outcome. Clin Cancer Res. 2003;9(6):2133–9.

52. Shustik J, Han G, Farinha P, et al. Correlations between BCL6 rearrangement and outcome in patients with diffuse large B-cell lymphoma treated with CHOP or R-CHOP. Haematologica. 2010;95(1):96–101.

53. Huang JZ, Sanger WG, Greiner TC, et al. The t(14;18) defines a unique subset of diffuse large B-cell lymphoma with a germinal center B-cell gene expression profile. Blood. 2002;99(7):2285–90.

54. Iqbal J, Sanger WG, Horsman DE, et al. BCL2 translocation defines a unique tumor subset within the germinal center B-cell-like diffuse large B-cell lymphoma. Am J Pathol. 2004;165(1):159–66.

55. Visco C, Tzankov A, Xu-Monette ZY, et al. Patients with diffuse large B-cell lymphoma of germinal center origin with BCL2 translocations have poor outcome, irrespective of MYC status: a report from an international DLBCL rituximab-CHOP Consortium Program Study. Haematologica. 2013;98(2):255–63.

56. Tzankov A, Xu-Monette ZY, Gerhard M, et al. Rearrangements of MYC gene facilitate risk stratification in diffuse large B-cell lymphoma patients treated with rituximab-CHOP. Mod Pathol. 2014;27(7):958–71.

57. Savage KJ, Johnson NA, Ben-Neriah S, et al. MYC gene rearrangements are associated with a poor prognosis in diffuse large B-cell lymphoma patients treated with R-CHOP chemotherapy. Blood. 2009;114(17):3533–7.

58. Li JY, Gaillard F, Moreau A, et al. Detection of translocation t(11;14)(q13;q32) in mantle cell lymphoma by fluorescence in situ hybridization. Am J Pathol. 1999;154(5):1449–52.

59. Rosenberg CL, Wong E, Petty EM, et al. PRAD1, a candidate BCL1 oncogene: mapping and expression in centrocytic lymphoma. Proc Natl Acad Sci U S A. 1991;88(21):9638–42.

60. Vaandrager JW, Schuuring E, Zwikstra E, et al. Direct visualization of dispersed 11q13 chromosomal translocations in mantle cell lymphoma by multicolor DNA fiber fluorescence in situ hybridization. Blood. 1996;88(4):1177–82.

61. Vandenberghe E, De Wolf-Peeters C, van den Oord J, et al. Translocation (11;14): a cytogenetic anomaly associated with B-cell lymphomas of non-follicle centre cell lineage. J Pathol. 1991;163(1):13–8.

62. Williams ME, Swerdlow SH, Rosenberg CL, Arnold A. Chromosome 11 translocation breakpoints at the PRAD1/cyclin D1 gene locus in centrocytic lymphoma. Leukemia. 1993;7(2):241–5.

63. Vaishampayan UN, Mohamed AN, Dugan MC, Bloom RE, Palutke M. Blastic mantle cell lymphoma associated with Burkitt-type translocation and hypodiploidy. Br J Haematol. 2001;115(1):66–8.

64. Aukema SM, Theil L, Rohde M, et al. Sequential karyotyping in Burkitt lymphoma reveals a linear clonal evolution with increase in karyotype complexity and a high frequency of recurrent secondary aberrations. Br J Haematol. 2015;170(6):814–25.

65. Pienkowska-Grela B, Rymkiewicz G, Grygalewicz B, et al. Partial trisomy 11, dup(11)(q23q13), as a defect characterizing lymphomas with Burkitt pathomorphology without MYC gene rearrangement. Med Oncol. 2011;28(4):1589–95.

66. Salaverria I, Martin-Guerrero I, Wagener R, et al. A recurrent 11q aberration pattern characterizes a subset of MYC-negative high-grade B-cell lymphomas resembling Burkitt lymphoma. Blood. 2014;123(8):1187–98.

67. Eberle FC, Salaverria I, Steidl C, et al. Gray zone lymphoma: chromosomal aberrations with immunophenotypic and clinical correlations. Mod Pathol. 2011;24(12):1586–97.

68. Li S, Seegmiller AC, Lin P, et al. B-cell lymphomas with concurrent MYC and BCL2 abnormalities other than translocations behave similarly to MYC/BCL2 double-hit lymphomas. Mod Pathol. 2015;28(2):208–17.

69. Lin P, Dickason TJ, Fayad LE, et al. Prognostic value of MYC rearrangement in cases of B-cell lymphoma, unclassifiable, with features intermediate between diffuse large B-cell lymphoma and Burkitt lymphoma. Cancer. 2012;118(6):1566–73.

70. Perry AM, Crockett D, Dave BJ, et al. B-cell lymphoma, unclassifiable, with features intermediate between diffuse large B-cell lymphoma and burkitt lymphoma: study of 39 cases. Br J Haematol. 2013;162(1):40–9.

71. Brito-Babapulle V, Catovsky D. Inversions and tandem translocations involving chromosome 14q11 and 14q32 in T-prolymphocytic leukemia and T-cell leukemias in patients with ataxia telangiectasia. Cancer Genet Cytogenet. 1991;55(1):1–9.

72. Maljaei SH, Brito-Babapulle V, Hiorns LR, Catovsky D. Abnormalities of chromosomes 8, 11, 14, and X in T-prolymphocytic leukemia studied by fluorescence in situ hybridization. Cancer Genet Cytogenet. 1998;103(2):110–6.

73. Siu LL, Chan V, Chan JK, Wong KF, Liang R, Kwong YL. Consistent patterns of allelic loss in natural killer cell lymphoma. Am J Pathol. 2000;157(6):1803–9.

74. Siu LL, Wong KF, Chan JK, Kwong YL. Comparative genomic hybridization analysis of natural killer cell lymphoma/leukemia. Recognition of consistent patterns of genetic alterations. Am J Pathol. 1999;155(5):1419–25.

75. Tien HF, Su IJ, Tang JL, et al. Clonal chromosomal abnormalities as direct evidence for clonality in nasal T/natural killer cell lymphomas. Br J Haematol. 1997;97(3):621–5.

76. Wong KF, Zhang YM, Chan JK. Cytogenetic abnormalities in natural killer cell lymphoma/leukaemia–is there a consistent pattern? Leuk Lymphoma. 1999;34(3–4):241–50.

77. Wlodarska I, Martin-Garcia N, Achten R, et al. Fluorescence in situ hybridization study of chromosome 7 aberrations in hepatosplenic T-cell lymphoma: isochromosome 7q as a common abnormality accumulating in forms with features of cytologic progression. Genes Chromosomes Cancer. 2002;33(3):243–51.

78. Hartmann S, Gesk S, Scholtysik R, et al. High resolution SNP array genomic profiling of peripheral T cell lymphomas, not otherwise specified, identifies a subgroup with chromosomal aberrations affecting the REL locus. Br J Haematol. 2010;148(3):402–12.

79. Rizvi MA, Evens AM, Tallman MS, Nelson BP, Rosen ST. T-cell non-Hodgkin lymphoma. Blood. 2006;107(4):1255–64.

80. Thorns C, Bastian B, Pinkel D, et al. Chromosomal aberrations in angioimmunoblastic T-cell lymphoma and peripheral T-cell lymphoma unspecified: a matrix-based CGH approach. Genes Chromosomes Cancer. 2007;46(1):37–44.

81. Zettl A, Rudiger T, Konrad MA, et al. Genomic profiling of peripheral T-cell lymphoma, unspecified, and anaplastic large T-cell lymphoma delineates novel recurrent chromosomal alterations. Am J Pathol. 2004;164(5):1837–48.

82. Huang Y, Moreau A, Dupuis J, et al. Peripheral T-cell lymphomas with a follicular growth pattern are derived from follicular helper T cells (TFH) and may show overlapping features with angioimmunoblastic T-cell lymphomas. Am J Surg Pathol. 2009;33(5):682–90.

83. Streubel B, Vinatzer U, Willheim M, Raderer M, Chott A. Novel t(5;9)(q33;q22) fuses ITK to SYK in unspecified peripheral T-cell lymphoma. Leukemia. 2006;20(2):313–8.

84. Cools J, Wlodarska I, Somers R, et al. Identification of novel fusion partners of ALK, the anaplastic lymphoma kinase, in anaplastic

large-cell lymphoma and inflammatory myofibroblastic tumor. Genes Chromosomes Cancer. 2002;34(4):354–62.

85. Falini B, Pulford K, Pucciarini A, et al. Lymphomas expressing ALK fusion protein(s) other than NPM-ALK. Blood. 1999;94(10):3509–15.

86. Feldman AL, Vasmatzis G, Asmann YW, et al. Novel TRAF1-ALK fusion identified by deep RNA sequencing of anaplastic large cell lymphoma. Genes Chromosomes Cancer. 2013;52(11): 1097–102.

87. Hernandez L, Pinyol M, Hernandez S, et al. TRK-fused gene (TFG) is a new partner of ALK in anaplastic large cell lymphoma producing two structurally different TFG-ALK translocations. Blood. 1999;94(9):3265–8.

88. Touriol C, Greenland C, Lamant L, et al. Further demonstration of the diversity of chromosomal changes involving 2p23 in ALK-positive lymphoma: 2 cases expressing ALK kinase fused to CLTCL (clathrin chain polypeptide-like). Blood. 2000;95(10):3204–7.

89. Tort F, Pinyol M, Pulford K, et al. Molecular characterization of a new ALK translocation involving moesin (MSN-ALK) in anaplastic large cell lymphoma. Lab Investig. 2001;81(3):419–26.

90. Rosenwald A, Ott G, Pulford K, et al. t(1;2)(q21;p23) and t(2;3) (p23;q21): two novel variant translocations of the t(2;5)(p23;q35) in anaplastic large cell lymphoma. Blood. 1999;94(1):362–4.

91. Stein H, Foss HD, Durkop H, et al. CD30(+) anaplastic large cell lymphoma: a review of its histopathologic, genetic, and clinical features. Blood. 2000;96(12):3681–95.

92. Lamant L, Gascoyne RD, Duplantier MM, et al. Non-muscle myosin heavy chain (MYH9): a new partner fused to ALK in anaplastic large cell lymphoma. Genes Chromosomes Cancer. 2003;37(4):427–32.

93. Parrilla Castellar ER, Jaffe ES, Said JW, et al. ALK-negative anaplastic large cell lymphoma is a genetically heterogeneous disease with widely disparate clinical outcomes. Blood. 2014;124(9):1473–80.

94. Aradhya S, Cherry AM. Array-based comparative genomic hybridization: clinical contexts for targeted and whole-genome designs. Genet Med. 2007;9(9):553–9.

95. Kallioniemi A, Kallioniemi OP, Sudar D, et al. Comparative genomic hybridization for molecular cytogenetic analysis of solid tumors. Science. 1992;258(5083):818–21.

96. de Ravel TJ, Devriendt K, Fryns JP, Vermeesch JR. What's new in karyotyping? The move towards array comparative genomic hybridisation (CGH). Eur J Pediatr. 2007;166(7):637–43.

97. Kennedy GC, Matsuzaki H, Dong S, et al. Large-scale genotyping of complex DNA. Nat Biotechnol. 2003;21(10):1233–7.

98. Lindblad-Toh K, Tanenbaum DM, Daly MJ, et al. Loss-of-heterozygosity analysis of small-cell lung carcinomas using single-nucleotide polymorphism arrays. Nat Biotechnol. 2000;18(9):1001–5.

99. Wong KK, Tsang YT, Shen J, et al. Allelic imbalance analysis by high-density single-nucleotide polymorphic allele (SNP) array with whole genome amplified DNA. Nucleic Acids Res. 2004;32(9):e69.

100. Papenhausen P, Schwartz S, Risheg H, et al. UPD detection using homozygosity profiling with a SNP genotyping microarray. Am J Med Genet Part A. 2011;155A(4):757–68.

101. Bea S, Salaverria I, Armengol L, et al. Uniparental disomies, homozygous deletions, amplifications, and target genes in mantle cell lymphoma revealed by integrative high-resolution whole-genome profiling. Blood. 2009;113(13):3059–69.

102. O'Shea D, O'Riain C, Gupta M, et al. Regions of acquired uniparental disomy at diagnosis of follicular lymphoma are associated with both overall survival and risk of transformation. Blood. 2009;113(10):2298–301.

103. Fitzgibbon J, Iqbal S, Davies A, et al. Genome-wide detection of recurring sites of uniparental disomy in follicular and transformed follicular lymphoma. Leukemia. 2007;21(7):1514–20.

104. Heinrichs S, Li C, Look AT. SNP array analysis in hematologic malignancies: avoiding false discoveries. Blood. 2010;115(21):4157–61.

105. Seto M, Honma K, Nakagawa M. Diversity of genome profiles in malignant lymphoma. Cancer Sci. 2010;101(3):573–8.

106. Booman M, Szuhai K, Rosenwald A, et al. Genomic alterations and gene expression in primary diffuse large B-cell lymphomas of immune-privileged sites: the importance of apoptosis and immunomodulatory pathways. J Pathol. 2008;216(2):209–17.

107. Schraders M, Jares P, Bea S, et al. Integrated genomic and expression profiling in mantle cell lymphoma: identification of gene-dosage regulated candidate genes. Br J Haematol. 2008;143(2):210–21.

108. Wessendorf S, Barth TF, Viardot A, et al. Further delineation of chromosomal consensus regions in primary mediastinal B-cell lymphomas: an analysis of 37 tumor samples using high-resolution genomic profiling (array-CGH). Leukemia. 2007;21(12):2463–9.

109. Lenz G, Wright GW, Emre NC, et al. Molecular subtypes of diffuse large B-cell lymphoma arise by distinct genetic pathways. Proc Natl Acad Sci U S A. 2008;105(36):13520–5.

110. Otto C, Giefing M, Massow A, et al. Genetic lesions of the TRAF3 and MAP 3K14 genes in classical Hodgkin lymphoma. Br J Haematol. 2012;157(6):702–8.

111. Scholtysik R, Kreuz M, Hummel M, et al. Characterization of genomic imbalances in diffuse large B-cell lymphoma by detailed SNP-chip analysis. Int J Cancer. 2015;136(5):1033–42.

112. Aya-Bonilla C, Green MR, Camilleri E, et al. High-resolution loss of heterozygosity screening implicates PTPRJ as a potential tumor suppressor gene that affects susceptibility to non-Hodgkin's lymphoma. Genes Chromosomes Cancer. 2013;52(5):467–79.

113. Trifonov V, Pasqualucci L, Dalla Favera R, Rabadan R. MutComFocal: an integrative approach to identifying recurrent and focal genomic alterations in tumor samples. BMC Syst Biol. 2013;7:25.

114. Scandurra M, Mian M, Greiner TC, et al. Genomic lesions associated with a different clinical outcome in diffuse large B-cell lymphoma treated with R-CHOP-21. Br J Haematol. 2010;151(3):221–31.

115. Pfeifer D, Pantic M, Skatulla I, et al. Genome-wide analysis of DNA copy number changes and LOH in CLL using high-density SNP arrays. Blood. 2007;109(3):1202–10.

116. Lehmann S, Ogawa S, Raynaud SD, et al. Molecular allelokaryotyping of early-stage, untreated chronic lymphocytic leukemia. Cancer. 2008;112(6):1296–305.

117. Edelmann J, Holzmann K, Miller F, et al. High-resolution genomic profiling of chronic lymphocytic leukemia reveals new recurrent genomic alterations. Blood. 2012;120(24):4783–94.

118. Ouillette P, Collins R, Shakhan S, et al. The prognostic significance of various 13q14 deletions in chronic lymphocytic leukemia. Clin Cancer Res. 2011;17(21):6778–90.

119. Kawamata N, Ogawa S, Gueller S, et al. Identified hidden genomic changes in mantle cell lymphoma using high-resolution single nucleotide polymorphism genomic array. Exp Hematol. 2009;37(8):937–46.

120. Flossbach L, Holzmann K, Mattfeldt T, et al. High-resolution genomic profiling reveals clonal evolution and competition in gastrointestinal marginal zone B-cell lymphoma and its large cell variant. Int J Cancer. 2013;132(3):E116–27.

121. Novak U, Rinaldi A, Kwee I, et al. The NF-{kappa}B negative regulator TNFAIP3 (A20) is inactivated by somatic mutations and genomic deletions in marginal zone lymphomas. Blood. 2009;113(20):4918–21.

122. Takahashi H, Usui Y, Ueda S, et al. Genome-wide analysis of ocular adnexal lymphoproliferative disorders using high-resolution single nucleotide polymorphism Array. Invest Ophthalmol Vis Sci. 2015;56(6):4156–65.

123. Lundin C, Hjorth L, Behrendtz M, Ehinger M, Biloglav A, Johansson B. Submicroscopic genomic imbalances in Burkitt lymphomas/leukemias: association with age and further evidence that 8q24/MYC translocations are not sufficient for leukemogenesis. Genes Chromosomes Cancer. 2013;52(4):370–7.

124. Walker BA, Leone PE, Jenner MW, et al. Integration of global SNP-based mapping and expression arrays reveals key regions, mechanisms, and genes important in the pathogenesis of multiple myeloma. Blood. 2006;108(5):1733–43.

125. Walker BA, Leone PE, Chiecchio L, et al. A compendium of myeloma-associated chromosomal copy number abnormalities and their prognostic value. Blood. 2010;116(15):e56–65.

126. Kamada Y, Sakata-Yanagimoto M, Sanada M, et al. Identification of unbalanced genome copy number abnormalities in patients with multiple myeloma by single-nucleotide polymorphism genotyping microarray analysis. Int J Hematol. 2012;96(4):492–500.

127. Jenner MW, Leone PE, Walker BA, et al. Gene mapping and expression analysis of 16q loss of heterozygosity identifies WWOX and CYLD as being important in determining clinical outcome in multiple myeloma. Blood. 2007;110(9):3291–300.

128. Fujiwara SI, Yamashita Y, Nakamura N, et al. High-resolution analysis of chromosome copy number alterations in angioimmunoblastic T-cell lymphoma and peripheral T-cell lymphoma, unspecified, with single nucleotide polymorphism-typing microarrays. Leukemia. 2008;22(10):1891–8.

129. Hidaka T, Nakahata S, Hatakeyama K, et al. Down-regulation of TCF8 is involved in the leukemogenesis of adult T-cell leukemia/lymphoma. Blood. 2008;112(2):383–93.

130. Durig J, Bug S, Klein-Hitpass L, et al. Combined single nucleotide polymorphism-based genomic mapping and global gene expression profiling identifies novel chromosomal imbalances, mechanisms and candidate genes important in the pathogenesis of T-cell prolymphocytic leukemia with inv(14)(q11q32). Leukemia. 2007;21(10):2153–63.

131. Nowak D, Le Toriellec E, Stern MH, et al. Molecular allelokaryotyping of T-cell prolymphocytic leukemia cells with high density single nucleotide polymorphism arrays identifies novel common genomic lesions and acquired uniparental disomy. Haematologica. 2009;94(4):518–27.

132. Garibyan L, Avashia N. Polymerase chain reaction. J Invest Dermatol. 2013;133(3):1–4.

133. Grody W, Nao N, Naeim F. Principles of molecular techniques. In: Grody W, Nao N, Naeim F, editors. Hematopathology -morphology, immunophenotype, cytogenetics and molecular approaches. Amsterdam: Elsevier; 2008. p. 65–79.

134. Hodges E, Krishna MT, Pickard C, Smith JL. Diagnostic role of tests for T cell receptor (TCR) genes. J Clin Pathol. 2003;56(1):1–11.

135. Roloff GW, Lai C, Hourigan CS, Dillon LW. Technical advances in the measurement of residual disease in acute myeloid leukemia. J Clin Med. 2017;6(9):E87.

136. Koboldt DC, Steinberg KM, Larson DE, Wilson RK, Mardis ER. The next-generation sequencing revolution and its impact on genomics. Cell. 2013;155(1):27–38.

137. Ingle SB, Hinge Ingle CR. Primary splenic lymphoma: current diagnostic trends. World J Clin Cases. 2016;4(12):385–9.

138. Myoteri D, Dellaportas D, Arkoumani E, Marinis A, Zizi-Sermpetzoglou A. Primary hepatic lymphoma: a challenging diagnosis. Case Rep Oncol Med. 2014;2014:212598.

139. Ugurluer G, Miller RC, Li Y, et al. Primary hepatic lymphoma: a retrospective, Multicenter Rare Cancer Network Study. Rare Tumors. 2016;8(3):6502.

140. Bose P, Gandhi V, Konopleva M. Pathways and mechanisms of venetoclax resistance. Leuk Lymphoma. 2017;58(9):1–17.

141. Aalipour A, Advani RH. Bruton's tyrosine kinase inhibitors and their clinical potential in the treatment of B-cell malignancies: focus on ibrutinib. Ther Adv Hematol. 2014;5(4):121–33.

142. Goodman AM, Choi M, Wieduwilt M, et al. Next generation sequencing reveals potentially actionable alterations in the majority of patients with lymphoid malignancies. JCO Precis Oncol. 2017;1(1):1–13.

143. Dubois S, Viailly PJ, Mareschal S, et al. Next-generation sequencing in diffuse large B-cell lymphoma highlights molecular divergence and therapeutic opportunities: a LYSA study. Clin Cancer Res. 2016;22(12):2919–28.

144. Guieze R, Wu CJ. Genomic and epigenomic heterogeneity in chronic lymphocytic leukemia. Blood. 2015;126(4):445–53.

145. Fabbri G, Rasi S, Rossi D, et al. Analysis of the chronic lymphocytic leukemia coding genome: role of NOTCH1 mutational activation. J Exp Med. 2011;208(7):1389–401.

146. Rossi D, Fangazio M, Rasi S, et al. Disruption of BIRC3 associates with fludarabine chemorefractoriness in TP53 wild-type chronic lymphocytic leukemia. Blood. 2012;119(12):2854–62.

147. Puiggros A, Blanco G, Espinet B. Genetic abnormalities in chronic lymphocytic leukemia: where we are and where we go. Biomed Res Int. 2014;2014:435983.

148. Rahal R, Frick M, Romero R, et al. Pharmacological and genomic profiling identifies NF-kappaB-targeted treatment strategies for mantle cell lymphoma. Nat Med. 2014;20(1):87–92.

149. Rossi D, Deaglio S, Dominguez-Sola D, et al. Alteration of BIRC3 and multiple other NF-kappaB pathway genes in splenic marginal zone lymphoma. Blood. 2011;118(18):4930–4.

150. Wang L, Lawrence MS, Wan Y, et al. SF3B1 and other novel cancer genes in chronic lymphocytic leukemia. N Engl J Med. 2011;365(26):2497–506.

151. Puente XS, Pinyol M, Quesada V, et al. Whole-genome sequencing identifies recurrent mutations in chronic lymphocytic leukaemia. Nature. 2011;475(7354):101–5.

152. Rossi D, Spina V, Deambrogi C, et al. The genetics of Richter syndrome reveals disease heterogeneity and predicts survival after transformation. Blood. 2011;117(12):3391–401.

153. Celik S, Erikci AA, Tunca Y, et al. The rate of MEFV gene mutations in hematolymphoid neoplasms. Int J Immunogenet. 2010;37(5):387–91.

154. Calin GA, Ferracin M, Cimmino A, et al. A MicroRNA signature associated with prognosis and progression in chronic lymphocytic leukemia. N Engl J Med. 2005;353(17):1793–801.

155. Montesinos-Rongen M, Godlewska E, Brunn A, Wiestler OD, Siebert R, Deckert M. Activating L265P mutations of the MYD88 gene are common in primary central nervous system lymphoma. Acta Neuropathol. 2011;122(6):791–2.

156. Ngo VN, Young RM, Schmitz R, et al. Oncogenically active MYD88 mutations in human lymphoma. Nature. 2011;470(7332):115–9.

157. Rossi D, Rasi S, Fabbri G, et al. Mutations of NOTCH1 are an independent predictor of survival in chronic lymphocytic leukemia. Blood. 2012;119(2):521–9.

158. Del Giudice I, Rossi D, Chiaretti S, et al. NOTCH1 mutations in +12 chronic lymphocytic leukemia (CLL) confer an unfavorable prognosis, induce a distinctive transcriptional profiling and refine the intermediate prognosis of +12 CLL. Haematologica. 2012;97(3):437–41.

159. Balatti V, Bottoni A, Palamarchuk A, et al. NOTCH1 mutations in CLL associated with trisomy 12. Blood. 2012;119(2):329–31.

160. Sportoletti P, Baldoni S, Cavalli L, et al. NOTCH1 PEST domain mutation is an adverse prognostic factor in B-CLL. Br J Haematol. 2010;151(4):404–6.

161. Parekh S. Taking it up a notch in MCL. Blood. 2012;119(9):1957–8.

162. Lopez-Guerra M, Xargay-Torrent S, Rosich L, et al. The gamma-secretase inhibitor PF-03084014 combined with fludarabine antagonizes migration, invasion and angiogenesis in NOTCH1-mutated CLL cells. Leukemia. 2015;29(1):96–106.

163. Quesada V, Conde L, Villamor N, et al. Exome sequencing identifies recurrent mutations of the splicing factor SF3B1 gene in chronic lymphocytic leukemia. Nat Genet. 2012;44(1):47–52.

164. Rossi D, Bruscaggin A, Spina V, et al. Mutations of the SF3B1 splicing factor in chronic lymphocytic leukemia: association with progression and fludarabine-refractoriness. Blood. 2011;118(26):6904–8.

165. Rinaldi A, Forconi F, Arcaini L, et al. Immunogenetics features and genomic lesions in splenic marginal zone lymphoma. Br J Haematol. 2010;151(5):435–9.

166. Nagel I, Szczepanowski M, Martin-Subero JI, et al. Deregulation of the telomerase reverse transcriptase (TERT) gene by chromosomal translocations in B-cell malignancies. Blood. 2010;116(8):1317–20.

167. Huh YO, Schweighofer CD, Ketterling RP, et al. Chronic lymphocytic leukemia with t(14;19)(q32;q13) is characterized by atypical morphologic and immunophenotypic features and distinctive genetic features. Am J Clin Pathol. 2011;135(5):686–96.

168. Wrench D, Leighton P, Skibola CF, et al. SNP rs6457327 in the HLA region on chromosome 6p is predictive of the transformation of follicular lymphoma. Blood. 2011;117(11):3147–50.

169. Wrench D, Montoto S, Fitzgibbon J. Molecular signatures in the diagnosis and management of follicular lymphoma. Curr Opin Hematol. 2010;17(4):333–40.

170. Skibola CF, Bracci PM, Halperin E, et al. Genetic variants at 6p21.33 are associated with susceptibility to follicular lymphoma. Nat Genet. 2009;41(8):873–5.

171. Pasqualucci L, Dominguez-Sola D, Chiarenza A, et al. Inactivating mutations of acetyltransferase genes in B-cell lymphoma. Nature. 2011;471(7337):189–95.

172. Chase A, Cross NC. Aberrations of EZH2 in cancer. Clin Cancer Res. 2011;17(9):2613–8.

173. Cerchietti LC, Hatzi K, Caldas-Lopes E, et al. BCL6 repression of EP300 in human diffuse large B cell lymphoma cells provides a basis for rational combinatorial therapy. J Clin Invest. 2010;120(12):4569–82.

174. Capello D, Gloghini A, Martini M, et al. Mutations of CD79A, CD79B and EZH2 genes in immunodeficiency-related non-Hodgkin lymphomas. Br J Haematol. 2011;152(6):777–80.

175. Morin RD, Johnson NA, Severson TM, et al. Somatic mutations altering EZH2 (Tyr641) in follicular and diffuse large B-cell lymphomas of germinal-center origin. Nat Genet. 2010;42(2):181–5.

176. Pellissery S, Richter J, Haake A, Montesinos-Rongen M, Deckert M, Siebert R. Somatic mutations altering Tyr641 of EZH2 are rare in primary central nervous system lymphoma. Leuk Lymphoma. 2010;51(11):2135–6.

177. Bodor C, O'Riain C, Wrench D, et al. EZH2 Y641 mutations in follicular lymphoma. Leukemia. 2011;25(4):726–9.

178. Salido M, Martinez-Aviles L, Adema V, et al. Absence of mutations of the histone methyltransferase gene EZH2 in splenic b-cell marginal zone lymphoma. Leuk Res. 2011;35(3):e23–4.

179. Duan S, Cermak L, Pagan JK, et al. FBXO11 targets BCL6 for degradation and is inactivated in diffuse large B-cell lymphomas. Nature. 2012;481(7379):90–3.

180. Morin RD, Mendez-Lago M, Mungall AJ, et al. Frequent mutation of histone-modifying genes in non-Hodgkin lymphoma. Nature. 2011;476(7360):298–303.

181. Sagaert X, De Wolf-Peeters C, Noels H, Baens M. The pathogenesis of MALT lymphomas: where do we stand? Leukemia. 2007;21(3):389–96.

182. Zheng W, Guan M, Zhu L, et al. Bortezomib therapeutic effect is associated with expression and mutation of FGFR3 in human lymphoma cells. Anticancer Res. 2010;30(6):1921–30.

183. Streubel B, Vinatzer U, Lamprecht A, Raderer M, Chott A. T(3;14)(p14.1;q32) involving IGH and FOXP1 is a novel recurrent chromosomal aberration in MALT lymphoma. Leukemia. 2005;19(4):652–8.

184. Lohr JG, Stojanov P, Lawrence MS, et al. Discovery and prioritization of somatic mutations in diffuse large B-cell lymphoma (DLBCL) by whole-exome sequencing. Proc Natl Acad Sci U S A. 2012;109(10):3879–84.

185. Ohshima A, Miura I, Hashimoto K, et al. Rearrangements of the BCL6 gene and chromosome aberrations affecting 3q27 in 54 patients with non-Hodgkin's lymphoma. Leuk Lymphoma. 1997;27(3–4):329–34.

186. Pasqualucci L, Trifonov V, Fabbri G, et al. Analysis of the coding genome of diffuse large B-cell lymphoma. Nat Genet. 2011;43(9):830–7.

187. Pasqualucci L, Neumeister P, Goossens T, et al. Hypermutation of multiple proto-oncogenes in B-cell diffuse large-cell lymphomas. Nature. 2001;412(6844):341–6.

188. Mottok A, Renne C, Seifert M, et al. Inactivating SOCS1 mutations are caused by aberrant somatic hypermutation and restricted to a subset of B-cell lymphoma entities. Blood. 2009;114(20):4503–6.

189. Levine EG, Arthur DC, Frizzera G, Peterson BA, Hurd DD, Bloomfield CD. Cytogenetic abnormalities predict clinical outcome in non-Hodgkin lymphoma. Ann Intern Med. 1988;108(1):14–20.

190. Mollejo M, Algara P, Mateo MS, et al. Splenic small B-cell lymphoma with predominant red pulp involvement: a diffuse variant of splenic marginal zone lymphoma? Histopathology. 2002;40(1):22–30.

191. Yan Q, Huang Y, Watkins AJ, et al. BCR and TLR signaling pathways are recurrently targeted by genetic changes in splenic marginal zone lymphomas. Haematologica. 2012;97(4):595–8.

192. Cheung KJ, Johnson NA, Affleck JG, et al. Acquired TNFRSF14 mutations in follicular lymphoma are associated with worse prognosis. Cancer Res. 2010;70(22):9166–74.

193. Akasaka T, Lossos IS, Levy R. BCL6 gene translocation in follicular lymphoma: a harbinger of eventual transformation to diffuse aggressive lymphoma. Blood. 2003;102(4):1443–8.

194. Galiegue-Zouitina S, Quief S, Hildebrand MP, et al. Nonrandom fusion of L-plastin(LCP1) and LAZ3(BCL6) genes by t(3;13)(q27;q14) chromosome translocation in two cases of B-cell non-Hodgkin lymphoma. Genes Chromosomes Cancer. 1999;26(2):97–105.

195. Lai JL, Daudignon A, Kerckaert JP, et al. Translocation (3;13)(q27;q14): a nonrandom and probably secondary structural change in non-Hodgkin lymphomas. Cancer Genet Cytogenet. 1998;103(2):140–3.

196. Diaz-Alderete A, Doval A, Camacho F, et al. Frequency of BCL2 and BCL6 translocations in follicular lymphoma: relation with histological and clinical features. Leuk Lymphoma. 2008;49(1):95–101.

197. Flossbach L, Antoneag E, Buck M, et al. BCL6 gene rearrangement and protein expression are associated with large cell presentation of extranodal marginal zone B-cell lymphoma of mucosa-associated lymphoid tissue. Int J Cancer. 2011;129(1):70–7.

198. Hosokawa Y, Maeda Y, Ichinohasama R, Miura I, Taniwaki M, Seto M. The Ikaros gene, a central regulator of lymphoid differentiation, fuses to the BCL6 gene as a result of t(3;7)(q27;p12) trans-

location in a patient with diffuse large B-cell lymphoma. Blood. 2000;95(8):2719–21.

199. Ueda C, Akasaka T, Kurata M, et al. The gene for interleukin-21 receptor is the partner of BCL6 in t(3;16)(q27;p11), which is recurrently observed in diffuse large B-cell lymphoma. Oncogene. 2002;21(3):368–76.

200. Miura I, Ohshima A, Takahashi N, et al. A new non-random chromosomal translocation t(3;6)(q27;p21.3) associated with BCL6 rearrangement in two patients with non-Hodgkin's lymphoma. Int J Hematol. 1996;64(3–4):249–56.

201. Lee SY, Kumano K, Nakazaki K, et al. Gain-of-function mutations and copy number increases of Notch2 in diffuse large B-cell lymphoma. Cancer Sci. 2009;100(5):920–6.

202. Rossi D, Trifonov V, Fangazio M, et al. The coding genome of splenic marginal zone lymphoma: activation of NOTCH2 and other pathways regulating marginal zone development. J Exp Med. 2012;209(9):1537–51.

203. Kiel MJ, Velusamy T, Betz BL, et al. Whole-genome sequencing identifies recurrent somatic NOTCH2 mutations in splenic marginal zone lymphoma. J Exp Med. 2012;209(9):1553–65.

204. Hamoudi RA, Appert A, Ye H, et al. Differential expression of NF-kappaB target genes in MALT lymphoma with and without chromosome translocation: insights into molecular mechanism. Leukemia. 2010;24(8):1487–97.

205. Xia H, Nakayama T, Sakuma H, et al. Analysis of API2-MALT1 fusion, trisomies, and immunoglobulin VH genes in pulmonary mucosa-associated lymphoid tissue lymphoma. Hum Pathol. 2011;42(9):1297–304.

206. Dierlamm J, Baens M, Wlodarska I, et al. The apoptosis inhibitor gene API2 and a novel 18q gene, MLT, are recurrently rearranged in the t(11;18)(q21;q21) associated with mucosa-associated lymphoid tissue lymphomas. Blood. 1999;93(11):3601–9.

207. Kwee I, Rancoita PM, Rinaldi A, et al. Genomic profiles of MALT lymphomas: variability across anatomical sites. Haematologica. 2011;96(7):1064–6.

208. Remstein ED, Dogan A, Einerson RR, et al. The incidence and anatomic site specificity of chromosomal translocations in primary extranodal marginal zone B-cell lymphoma of mucosa-associated lymphoid tissue (MALT lymphoma) in North America. Am J Surg Pathol. 2006;30(12):1546–53.

209. Spina V, Khiabanian H, Messina M, et al. The genetics of nodal marginal zone lymphoma. Blood. 2016;128(10):1362–73.

210. Blombery PA, Wong SQ, Hewitt CA, et al. Detection of BRAF mutations in patients with hairy cell leukemia and related lymphoproliferative disorders. Haematologica. 2012;97(5):780–3.

211. Monge J, Braggio E, Ansell SM. Genetic factors and pathogenesis of Waldenstrom's macroglobulinemia. Curr Oncol Rep. 2013;15(5):450–6.

212. Chen D, Law ME, Theis JD, et al. Clinicopathologic features of CDK6 translocation-associated B-cell lymphoproliferative disorders. Am J Surg Pathol. 2009;33(5):720–9.

213. Parker E, Macdonald JR, Wang C. Molecular characterization of a t(2;7) translocation linking CDK6 to the IGK locus in CD5(−) monoclonal B-cell lymphocytosis. Cancer Genet. 2011;204(5):260–4.

214. Gachard N, Parrens M, Soubeyran I, et al. IGHV gene features and MYD88 L265P mutation separate the three marginal zone lymphoma entities and Waldenstrom macroglobulinemia/lymphoplasmacytic lymphomas. Leukemia. 2013;27(1):183–9.

215. Schmidt J, Federmann B, Schindler N, et al. MYD88 L265P and CXCR4 mutations in lymphoplasmacytic lymphoma identify cases with high disease activity. Br J Haematol. 2015;169(6):795–803.

216. Tiacci E, Trifonov V, Schiavoni G, et al. BRAF mutations in hairy-cell leukemia. N Engl J Med. 2011;364(24):2305–15.

217. Cornet E, Damaj G, Troussard X. New insights in the management of patients with hairy cell leukemia. Curr Opin Oncol. 2015;27(5):371–6.

218. Arcaini L, Zibellini S, Boveri E, et al. The BRAF V600E mutation in hairy cell leukemia and other mature B-cell neoplasms. Blood. 2011;119(1):188–91.

219. Tiacci E, Schiavoni G, Forconi F, et al. Simple genetic diagnosis of hairy cell leukemia by sensitive detection of the BRAF-V600E mutation. Blood. 2011;119(1):192–5.

220. Shao H, Calvo KR, Gronborg M, et al. Distinguishing hairy cell leukemia variant from hairy cell leukemia: development and validation of diagnostic criteria. Leuk Res. 2013;37(4):401–9.

221. Schmitz R, Hansmann ML, Bohle V, et al. TNFAIP3 (A20) is a tumor suppressor gene in Hodgkin lymphoma and primary mediastinal B cell lymphoma. J Exp Med. 2009;206(5):981–9.

222. Giulino L, Mathew S, Ballon G, et al. A20 (TNFAIP3) genetic alterations in EBV-associated AIDS-related lymphoma. Blood. 2011;117(18):4852–4.

223. Farrell K, Jarrett RF. The molecular pathogenesis of Hodgkin lymphoma. Histopathology. 2011;58(1):15–25.

224. Best T, Li D, Skol AD, et al. Variants at 6q21 implicate PRDM1 in the etiology of therapy-induced second malignancies after Hodgkin's lymphoma. Nat Med. 2011;17(8):941–3.

225. Ye BH, Chaganti S, Chang CC, et al. Chromosomal translocations cause deregulated BCL6 expression by promoter substitution in B cell lymphoma. EMBO J. 1995;14(24):6209–17.

226. Butler MP, Iida S, Capello D, et al. Alternative translocation breakpoint cluster region 5′ to BCL-6 in B-cell non-Hodgkin's lymphoma. Cancer Res. 2002;62(14):4089–94.

227. Akasaka H, Akasaka T, Kurata M, et al. Molecular anatomy of BCL6 translocations revealed by long-distance polymerase chain reaction-based assays. Cancer Res. 2000;60(9):2335–41.

228. Wlodarska I, Nooyen P, Maes B, et al. Frequent occurrence of BCL6 rearrangements in nodular lymphocyte predominance Hodgkin lymphoma but not in classical Hodgkin lymphoma. Blood. 2003;101(2):706–10.

229. Steidl C, Shah SP, Woolcock BW, et al. MHC class II transactivator CIITA is a recurrent gene fusion partner in lymphoid cancers. Nature. 2011;471(7338):377–81.

230. Weniger MA, Melzner I, Menz CK, et al. Mutations of the tumor suppressor gene SOCS-1 in classical Hodgkin lymphoma are frequent and associated with nuclear phospho-STAT5 accumulation. Oncogene. 2006;25(18):2679–84.

231. Van Roosbroeck K, Cox L, Tousseyn T, et al. JAK2 rearrangements, including the novel SEC31A-JAK2 fusion, are recurrent in classical Hodgkin lymphoma. Blood. 2011;117(15):4056–64.

232. Saarinen S, Aavikko M, Aittomaki K, et al. Exome sequencing reveals germline NPAT mutation as a candidate risk factor for Hodgkin lymphoma. Blood. 2011;118(3):493–8.

233. Kuppers R. NPAT mutations in Hodgkin lymphoma. Blood. 2011;118(3):484–5.

234. Ritter E, Husain RA, Hinderhofer K, et al. Ornithine transcarbamylase (OTC) deficiency based on a hemizygous p.R277W mutation causing life-threatening hyperammonemic crisis during treatment for Hodgkin's lymphoma. Ann Hematol. 2010;90(7):857.

235. Tomita N. BCL2 and MYC dual-hit lymphoma/leukemia. J Clin Exp Hematopathol JCEH. 2011;51(1):7–12.

236. Weiss LM, Warnke RA, Sklar J, Cleary ML. Molecular analysis of the t(14;18) chromosomal translocation in malignant lymphomas. N Engl J Med. 1987;317(19):1185–9.

237. Ohno H, Fukuhara S. Significance of rearrangement of the BCL6 gene in B-cell lymphoid neoplasms. Leuk Lymphoma. 1997;27(1–2):53–63.

238. Compagno M, Lim WK, Grunn A, et al. Mutations of multiple genes cause deregulation of NF-kappaB in diffuse large B-cell lymphoma. Nature. 2009;459(7247):717–21.

239. Lenz G, Davis RE, Ngo VN, et al. Oncogenic CARD11 mutations in human diffuse large B cell lymphoma. Science. 2008;319(5870):1676–9.

240. de Jong D, Balague Ponz O. The molecular background of aggressive B cell lymphomas as a basis for targeted therapy. J Pathol. 2011;223(2):274–82.

241. Jeelall YS, Horikawa K. Oncogenic MYD88 mutation drives toll pathway to lymphoma. Immunol Cell Biol. 2011;89(6):659–60.

242. Staudt LM. Oncogenic activation of NF-kappaB. Cold Spring Harb Perspect Biol. 2010;2(6):a000109.

243. Davis RE, Ngo VN, Lenz G, et al. Chronic active B-cell-receptor signalling in diffuse large B-cell lymphoma. Nature. 2010;463(7277):88–92.

244. Pasqualucci L, Dalla-Favera R. Genetics of diffuse large B-cell lymphoma. Blood. 2018;131(21):2307–19.

245. Cho HJ, Eom HS, Kim HJ, Kim IS, Lee GW, Kong SY. Glutathione-S-transferase genotypes influence the risk of chemotherapy-related toxicities and prognosis in Korean patients with diffuse large B-cell lymphoma. Cancer Genet Cytogenet. 2010;198(1):40–6.

246. Barrans S, Crouch S, Smith A, et al. Rearrangement of MYC is associated with poor prognosis in patients with diffuse large B-cell lymphoma treated in the era of rituximab. J Clin Oncol. 2010;28(20):3360–5.

247. Ohno H, Ueda C, Akasaka T. The t(9;14)(p13;q32) translocation in B-cell non-Hodgkin's lymphoma. Leuk Lymphoma. 2000;36(5–6):435–45.

248. Kelly RJ, O'Connor SJ, Barrans SL, Johnson RJ, Owen RG. The t(9;14)(p13;q32) is a recurrent but rare abnormality in splenic marginal zone lymphoma. Leuk Lymphoma. 2007;48(8):1636–7.

249. Ohno H, Nishikori M, Haga H, Isoda K. Epstein-Barr virus-positive diffuse large B-cell lymphoma carrying a t(9;14) (p13;q32) translocation. Int J Hematol. 2009;89(5):704–8.

250. Poppe B, De Paepe P, Michaux L, et al. PAX5/IGH rearrangement is a recurrent finding in a subset of aggressive B-NHL with complex chromosomal rearrangements. Genes Chromosomes Cancer. 2005;44(2):218–23.

251. Baro C, Salido M, Domingo A, et al. Translocation t(9;14) (p13;q32) in cases of splenic marginal zone lymphoma. Haematologica. 2006;91(9):1289–91.

252. Mandelbaum J, Bhagat G, Tang H, et al. BLIMP1 is a tumor suppressor gene frequently disrupted in activated B cell-like diffuse large B cell lymphoma. Cancer Cell. 2010;18(6):568–79.

253. Simon T, Kohlhase J, Wilhelm C, Kochanek M, De Carolis B, Berthold F. Multiple malignant diseases in a patient with Rothmund-Thomson syndrome with RECQL4 mutations: case report and literature review. Am J Med Genet Part A. 2010;152A(6):1575–9.

254. Siitonen HA, Sotkasiira J, Biervliet M, et al. The mutation spectrum in RECQL4 diseases. Eur J Human Genet EJHG. 2009;17(2):151–8.

255. Debeljak M, Zver A, Jazbec J. A patient with Baller-Gerold syndrome and midline NK/T lymphoma. Am J Med Genet A. 2009;149A(4):755–9.

256. Montesinos-Rongen M, Schmitz R, Brunn A, et al. Mutations of CARD11 but not TNFAIP3 may activate the NF-kappaB pathway in primary CNS lymphoma. Acta Neuropathol. 2010;120(4):529–35.

257. Dong G, Chanudet E, Zeng N, et al. A20, ABIN-1/2, and CARD11 mutations and their prognostic value in gastrointestinal diffuse large B-cell lymphoma. Clin Cancer Res. 2011;17(6):1440–51.

258. Hongyo T, Kurooka M, Taniguchi E, et al. Frequent p53 mutations at dipyrimidine sites in patients with pyothorax-associated lymphoma. Cancer Res. 1998;58(6):1105–7.

259. Stefancikova L, Moulis M, Fabian P, et al. Prognostic impact of p53 aberrations for R-CHOP-treated patients with diffuse large B-cell lymphoma. Int J Oncol. 2011;39(6):1413–20.

260. Leroy K, Haioun C, Lepage E, et al. p53 gene mutations are associated with poor survival in low and low-intermediate risk diffuse large B-cell lymphomas. Ann Oncol. 2002;13(7):1108–15.

261. Scarpa A, Moore PS, Rigaud G, et al. Molecular features of primary mediastinal B-cell lymphoma: involvement of p16INK4A, p53 and c-myc. Br J Haematol. 1999;107(1):106–13.

262. Cairns RA, Iqbal J, Lemonnier F, et al. IDH2 mutations are frequent in angioimmunoblastic T-cell lymphoma. Blood. 2012;119(8):1901–3.

263. Couronne L, Bastard C, Bernard OA. TET2 and DNMT3A mutations in human T-cell lymphoma. N Engl J Med. 2012;366(1): 95–6.

264. Medeiros LJ, Elenitoba-Johnson KS. Anaplastic large cell lymphoma. Am J Clin Pathol. 2007;127(5):707–22.

265. Lamant L, Meggetto F, al Saati T, et al. High incidence of the t(2;5)(p23;q35) translocation in anaplastic large cell lymphoma and its lack of detection in Hodgkin's disease. Comparison of cytogenetic analysis, reverse transcriptase-polymerase chain reaction, and P-80 immunostaining. Blood. 1996;87(1):284–91.

266. Falini B, Shein H, Lamant-Rochaix L, et al. Anaplastic large cell lymphoma, ALK-positive. In: Swerdlow SH, Campo E, Harris M, et al., editors. *WHO classification of tumors of haematopoietic and lymphoid tissues.* Lyon: IARC Press; 2017. p. 418–21.

267. Feldman AL, Dogan A, Smith DI, et al. Discovery of recurrent t(6;7)(p25.3;q32.3) translocations in ALK-negative anaplastic large cell lymphomas by massively parallel genomic sequencing. Blood. 2011;117(3):915–9.

268. Wada DA, Law ME, Hsi ED, et al. Specificity of IRF4 translocations for primary cutaneous anaplastic large cell lymphoma: a multicenter study of 204 skin biopsies. Mod Pathol. 2011;24(4):596–605.

269. Kameda T, Shide K, Shimoda HK, et al. Absence of gain-of-function JAK1 and JAK3 mutations in adult T cell leukemia/lymphoma. Int J Hematol. 2010;92(2):320–5.

270. Elliott NE, Cleveland SM, Grann V, Janik J, Waldmann TA, Dave UP. FERM domain mutations induce gain of function in JAK3 in adult T-cell leukemia/lymphoma. Blood. 2011;118(14):3911–21.

271. Tsukasaki K, Tsushima H, Yamamura M, et al. Integration patterns of HTLV-I provirus in relation to the clinical course of ATL: frequent clonal change at crisis from indolent disease. Blood. 1997;89(3):948–56.

272. Pancewicz J, Taylor JM, Datta A, et al. Notch signaling contributes to proliferation and tumor formation of human T-cell leukemia virus type 1-associated adult T-cell leukemia. Proc Natl Acad Sci U S A. 2010;107(38):16619–24.

273. Jones JF, Shurin S, Abramowsky C, et al. T-cell lymphomas containing Epstein-Barr viral DNA in patients with chronic Epstein-Barr virus infections. N Engl J Med. 1988;318(12):733–41.

274. Howell WM, Leung ST, Jones DB, et al. HLA-DRB, -DQA, and -DQB polymorphism in celiac disease and enteropathy-associated T-cell lymphoma. Common features and additional risk factors for malignancy. Hum Immunol. 1995;43(1):29–37.

275. Kleppe M, Tousseyn T, Geissinger E, et al. Mutation analysis of the tyrosine phosphatase PTPN2 in Hodgkin's lymphoma and T-cell non-Hodgkin's lymphoma. Haematologica. 2011;96(11):1723–7.

276. Yagasaki F, Wakao D, Yokoyama Y, et al. Fusion of ETV6 to fibroblast growth factor receptor 3 in peripheral T-cell lymphoma with a t(4;12)(p16;p13) chromosomal translocation. Cancer Res. 2001;61(23):8371–4.

277. Stern MH, Soulier J, Rosenzwajg M, et al. MTCP-1: a novel gene on the human chromosome Xq28 translocated to the T cell receptor alpha/delta locus in mature T cell proliferations. Oncogene. 1993;8(9):2475–83.

278. Yokohama A, Saitoh A, Nakahashi H, et al. TCL1A gene involvement in T-cell prolymphocytic leukemia in Japanese patients. Int J Hematol. 2012;95(1):77–85.

279. Stilgenbauer S, Schaffner C, Litterst A, et al. Biallelic mutations in the ATM gene in T-prolymphocytic leukemia. Nat Med. 1997;3(10):1155–9.

280. Pekarsky Y, Hallas C, Isobe M, Russo G, Croce CM. Abnormalities at 14q32.1 in T cell malignancies involve two oncogenes. Proc Natl Acad Sci U S A. 1999;96(6):2949–51.

281. Kiessling MK, Oberholzer PA, Mondal C, et al. High-throughput mutation profiling of CTCL samples reveals KRAS and NRAS mutations sensitizing tumors toward inhibition of the RAS/RAF/MEK signaling cascade. Blood. 2011;117(8):2433–40.

282. Navas IC, Ortiz-Romero PL, Villuendas R, et al. p16(INK4a) gene alterations are frequent in lesions of mycosis fungoides. Am J Pathol. 2000;156(5):1565–72.

283. Scarisbrick JJ, Woolford AJ, Calonje E, et al. Frequent abnormalities of the p15 and p16 genes in mycosis fungoides and sezary syndrome. J Invest Dermatol. 2002;118(3):493–9.

284. Hongyo T, Hoshida Y, Nakatsuka S, et al. p53, K-ras, c-kit and beta-catenin gene mutations in sinonasal NK/T-cell lymphoma in Korea and Japan. Oncol Rep. 2005;13(2):265–71.

285. Hoshida Y, Hongyo T, Jia X, et al. Analysis of p53, K-ras, c-kit, and beta-catenin gene mutations in sinonasal NK/T cell lymphoma in northeast district of China. Cancer Sci. 2003;94(3):297–301.

286. Choe YS, Kim JG, Sohn SK, et al. c-kit expression and mutations in peripheral T cell lymphomas, except for extra-nodal NK/T cell lymphomas. Leuk Lymphoma. 2006;47(2):267–70.

287. Quintanilla-Martinez L, Kremer M, Keller G, et al. p53 Mutations in nasal natural killer/T-cell lymphoma from Mexico: association with large cell morphology and advanced disease. Am J Pathol. 2001;159(6):2095–105.

288. McKinney M, Moffitt AB, Gaulard P, et al. The genetic basis of hepatosplenic T-cell lymphoma. Cancer Discov. 2017;7(4):369–79.

289. Rajala HL, Eldfors S, Kuusanmaki H, et al. Discovery of somatic STAT5b mutations in large granular lymphocytic leukemia. Blood. 2013;121(22):4541–50.

290. Koskela HL, Eldfors S, Ellonen P, et al. Somatic STAT3 mutations in large granular lymphocytic leukemia. N Engl J Med. 2012;366(20):1905–13.

291. Alonsozana EL, Stamberg J, Kumar D, et al. Isochromosome 7q: the primary cytogenetic abnormality in hepatosplenic gammadelta T cell lymphoma. Leukemia. 1997;11(8):1367–72.

292. Arcaini L, Rossi D, Paulli M. Splenic marginal zone lymphoma: from genetics to management. Blood. 2016;127(17):2072–81.

293. Schmitz R, Wright GW, Huang DW, et al. Genetics and pathogenesis of diffuse large B-cell lymphoma. N Engl J Med. 2018;378(15):1396–407.

Hairy Cell Leukemia, Hairy Cell Leukemia Variant, and Splenic Diffuse Red Pulp Small B-Cell Lymphoma

4

Wei Chen and Qin Huang

Introduction

Hairy cell leukemia (HCL) and hairy cell leukemia-like neoplasms including HCL variant (HCL-V) and Splenic diffuse red pulp small B-cell lymphoma (SDRPL) are a group of small mature B-cell lymphomas that often involved the spleen, blood, and bone marrow. HCL accounts for only 2% of lymphoid leukemias and HCL-V and SDRPL are even rare. HCL shows characteristic morphology of kidney-bean-shaped nuclei and abundant clear cytoplasm with cytoplasmic hairy projection and phenotypically coexpresses CD19, CD20, CD11c, CD25, and CD103. Nearly 100% of patients with HCL harbor *BRAF* V600E mutation. Given the differences in infiltrating pattern, phenotype, clinical course, and molecular profiles, both HCL-V and SDRPL are subcategorized under splenic B-cell lymphoma/leukemia, unclassifiable as provisional entities according to the 2017 World Health Organization classification. The clinicopathologic features of all rare lymphomas involving spleen will be discussed in this chapter.

Hairy Cell Leukemia

Definition

Hairy cell leukemia (HCL) is an uncommon hematopoietic disorder characterized by the accumulation of small mature lymphoid cells with abundant cytoplasm and radiated "hairy" projections within the peripheral blood, bone marrow, and splenic red pulp [1, 2]. It is different from hairy cell

leukemia variant (HCL-V), a rare clinicopathologic entity, and was initially identified as a prolymphocytic variant of HCL [3]. HCL-V is, however, no longer considered to be biologically related to HCL and is included as an individual provisional entity under splenic B-cell lymphoma/leukemia, unclassifiable according to the World Health Organization (WHO) classification 2008 [4].

Cell Origin

Studies of the cell origin showed that most cases of HCL are postulated to arise from a late, activated memory B-cell [5] which acquired *BRAF* V600E mutation [6]. The *BRAF* mutation is identified in almost all cases.

Epidemiology

HCL represents approximately 2–3% of all adult leukemias and less than 1% of lymphoid neoplasms. In the United States, the estimated incidence rate is two to three cases per million persons per year [7]. HCL is usually diagnosed in adults with a median age of 50–55 years and is almost never seen in children. There is a strong male predominance with a male to female ratio of approximately 4:1 [8, 9]. Compared to African Americans, the incidence rate is approximately three times higher in Caucasian population among both males and females [10].

Etiology and Pathogenesis

Up to date, the etiopathogenesis of HCL is not fully understood. Two high risks of developing HCL are exposure to radiation or industrial and agricultural chemicals. Genetic alteration is considered the leading mechanism to the development of HCL. In 2011, a clonal somatic *BRAF V600E*-activating

W. Chen
Department of Pathology, Brigham and Women's Hospital, Harvard Medical School, Boston, MA, USA

Q. Huang (✉)
Department of Pathology and Laboratory Medicine, Cedars-Sinai Medical Center, Los Angeles, CA, USA
e-mail: Qin.Huang@cshs.org

© Springer Nature Switzerland AG 2020
L. Zhang et al. (eds.), *Diagnostic Pathology of Hematopoietic Disorders of Spleen and Liver*,
https://doi.org/10.1007/978-3-030-37708-3_4

mutation in the serine/threonine kinase is identified in virtually all cases of classic HCL [11]. Studies using sensitive molecular assays including next-generation sequencing (NGS) and allele-specific polymerase chain reaction (PCR) identified the *BRAF* single codon V600E mutation in the entire tumor clone of classic HCL but appears to be not in other small B-cell lymphoid neoplasms [11–13]. The resultant aberrant activation of the RAF-MEK-ERK signaling pathway leads to a distinct phenotype and enhanced cell survival, which is believed to be essential in HCL featured by a very low proliferative index [14]. The second most common mutation in classic HCL is histone methyltransferase *KMT2C (MLL3)*, which was seen in 15% cases. *KMT2C* was affected by predicted loss-of-function mutations throughout the coding region [15]. In addition, heterozygous loss of chromosome 7q was also reported, the minimally deleted region of which targeted wild-type *BRAF*, subdividing classic HCL into those hemizygous versus heterozygous for the *BRAF* V600E mutation [15]. Other possible causes of HCL include exposures to pesticides, ionizing radiation, and farming [16, 17]. Cigarette smoke is reported to be inversely associated with HCL [16]. In addition, several familial cases have been described [18].

Clinical Presentations

The bone marrow and spleen are primary sites involved by HCL. Typically, a small number of circulating cells are seen in peripheral blood. Clinically, the most common symptoms include general weakness, fatigue, fullness of abdomen, infections of variable degree, and hemorrhagic episodes, which are usually secondary to splenomegaly and cytopenias. The most common clinical finding is splenomegaly (100%). Fevers, night sweats, and weight losses are usually not associated with HCL. Approximately 25% of patients remain nonsymptomatic. Sixty to eighty percent of patients present with pancytopenia, with hematocrits in the range of 20–35% and platelet counts in the range of $20–100 \times 10^9$/L [9, 19]. Monocytopenia is common as well. However, leukocytosis was also reported in 10–20% patients [8]. Hepatomegaly and lymphadenopathy are present in approximately 20% and 10% of patients, respectively.

Morphology

Gross Features

On gross exam, when the spleen is involved by HCL, it demonstrates marked enlargement with diffuse expansion of the red pulp and atrophy of the white pulp [6] (Fig. 4.1).

Microscopic Features

Peripheral Blood

The peripheral blood smear usually demonstrates pancytopenia and circulating neoplastic cells. The HCL cell is

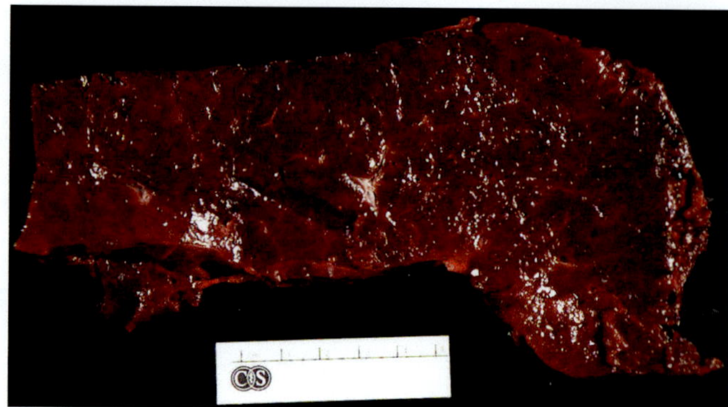

Fig. 4.1 Spleen gross. The gross appearance of the spleen involved by HCL. The spleen is markedly enlarged, with diffuse expansion of the red pulp. Numerous blood lakes of varying size are visible

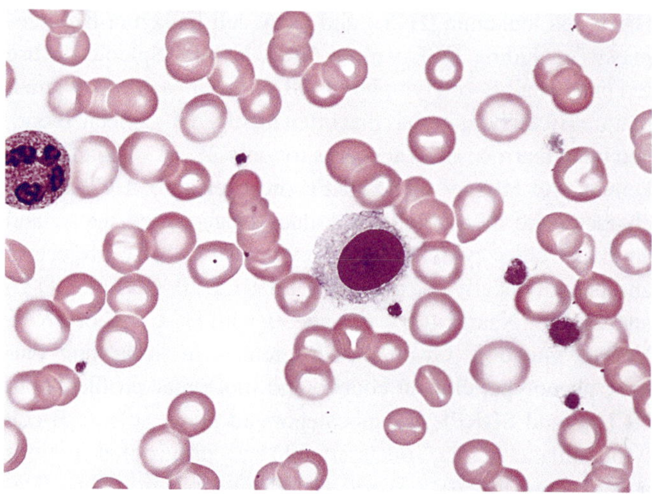

Fig. 4.2 Peripheral blood smear shows medium-sized leukemic cells with ovoid nucleus and homogeneous chromatin and inconspicuous nucleoli. The cytoplasm is usually fairly abundant, pale blue to blue-gray in color. The presence of varying numbers of radiated cytoplasmic projections gives the cell a "hairy" appearance. (Giemsa stain, magnification 500×)

a mononuclear cell that is usually small- to medium-sized lymphoid cells with ovoid or kidney-bean-shaped/indented nucleus. The chromatin is homogeneous and spongy with ground-glass appearance and typically absent nucleoli. The cytoplasm is variable in amount but usually fairly abundant, pale blue to blue-gray in color, and occasionally described as "fluffy." The cytoplasmic outline is often indistinct due to the presence of varying numbers of projections, giving the cell a "hairy" appearance when the projections are thin and a "ruffled" appearance when they are wider and they are notably circumferential (Fig. 4.2). The hairy projections are readily evident on electron microscopic examination and particularly on scanning electron microscopy [20].

Bone Marrow

In bone marrow, the primary pattern of tumor is interstitial or patchy involvement with some preservation of hematopoietic elements. The hairy cell nuclei are widely separated from each other by virtue of the cell's abundant cytoplasm, producing a perinuclear halo or "fried egg" appearance in bone marrow biopsy and tissue (Fig. 4.3). Extravasated red cells are frequently seen. Mitotic figures are uncommon.

Necrosis or apoptosis of tumor cells is absent. In patients with advanced disease, a diffuse solid infiltrate may be evident. However, nodular patterns of marrow infiltration occur rarely. A minority of patients, approximately 10–20%, exhibit a hypocellular bone marrow with only small numbers

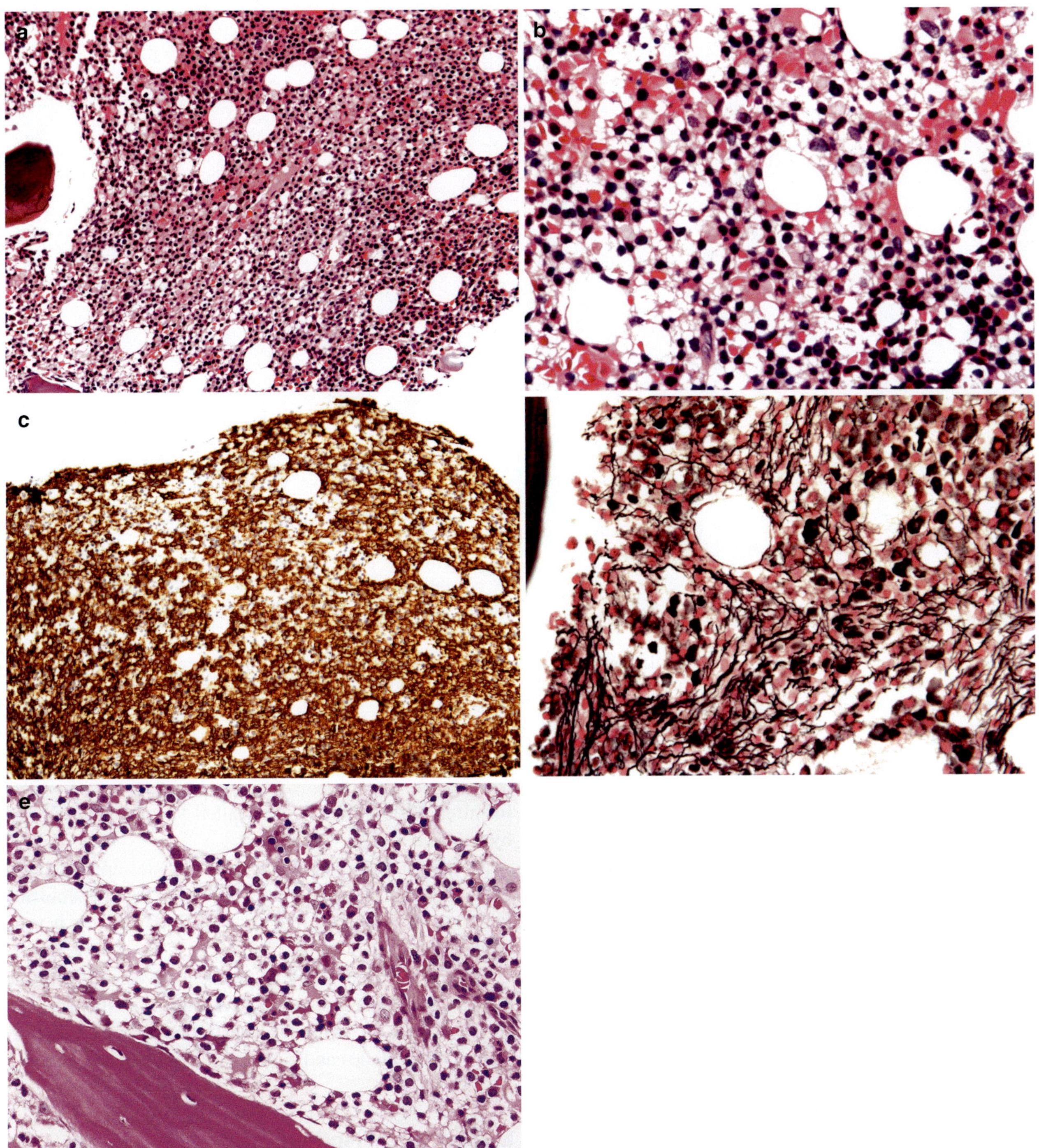

Fig. 4.3 Bone marrow biopsy. (**a, b**) Low- and high-power view of the bone marrow reveals large sheets of leukemic cells with typical "fried egg" appearance (small round nuclei, smooth nuclear contour, and abundant clear cytoplasm) (H&E stain, 200× and 600× respectively). (**c**) Immunostain highlights this atypical infiltrate to be positive for CD20 (immunoperoxidase, 200×). (**d**) HCL is usually associated with marked reticulin fibrosis in bone marrow (myelofibrosis score 3+ of 3, MF3) (reticulin, 600×). (**e**) Higher magnification shows the HCL cells with round to oval nuclei, containing clear cytoplasm and low N:C ratio in a bone marrow core biopsy (H&E, 1000×)

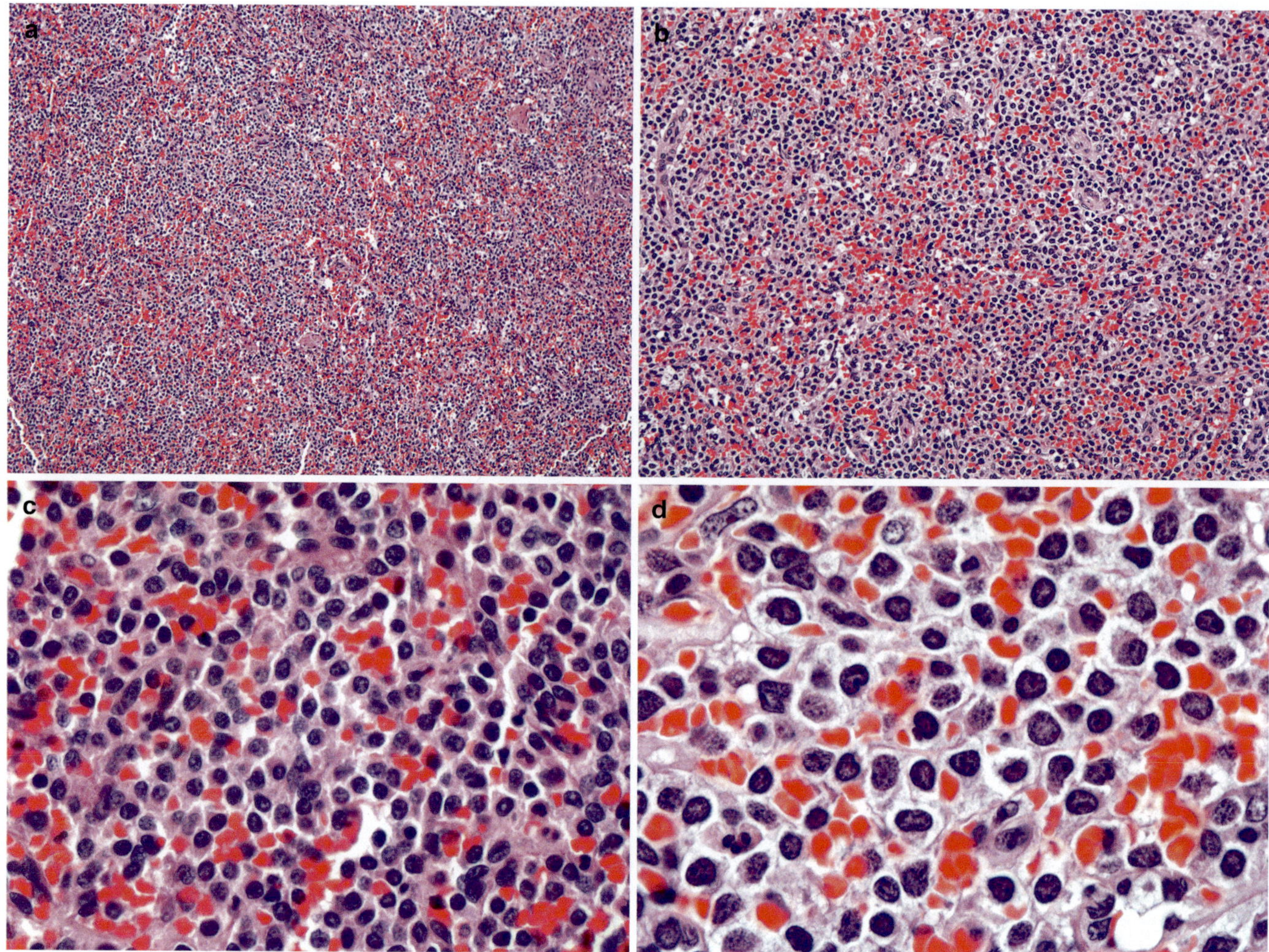

Fig. 4.4 (**a–d**) Diffuse splenic infiltrate by HCL. It demonstrates an extensive expansion of the red pulp interspaced with blood lakes and diminished white pulp (**a** and **b**. 100× and 200×, respectively). View under higher magnification shows these atypical lymphoid cells with round to kidney-shaped nuclei, dense chromatin, inconspicuous nucleoli, and abundant clear cytoplasm (**c** and **d**, 600× and 1000×, respectively)

of hairy cells infiltrating around fat cells, which could be a diagnostic pitfall [21]. Staining of the bone marrow biopsy for reticulin almost always shows a moderate to marked increase in reticulin fibers. Osteosclerosis has been reported. Rarely, convoluted, multilobulated, blastic, prolymphocytic, and spindled variants of hairy cells have been described.

Spleen, Liver, and Lymph Nodes

Histologic examination of the spleen will demonstrate tumor infiltration in virtually all cases. Microscopically, the cords and sinuses of the red pulp are infiltrated by neoplastic cells with a similar morphology compared to those in bone marrow. The tumor infiltrate is comprised of a monotonous population of medium-sized cells with clear cytoplasm that may have interlocking cell borders, producing a "fried egg" appearance [22]. Dilated sinuses may be filled with red cells,

forming "blood lakes" (also called "pseudosinuses") lined by hairy cells (Fig. 4.4).

In rare instances in which liver biopsies are obtained for other indications, patchy involvement of hepatic sinusoids is not unusual, but hepatomegaly is distinctly rare. It is usually confined to sinusoids [6].

Lymph nodes are typically not involved, but infiltration can be seen in patients with advanced HCL [6]. The tumor cells variably involve the interfollicular and paracortical zones. The follicles and sinuses are typically spared.

Cytochemical Findings and Immunophenotyping

Historically, demonstration of tartrate-resistant acid phosphatase (TRAP) activity was routinely used to confirm the diagnosis of HCL. Virtually, all cases of HCL will contain

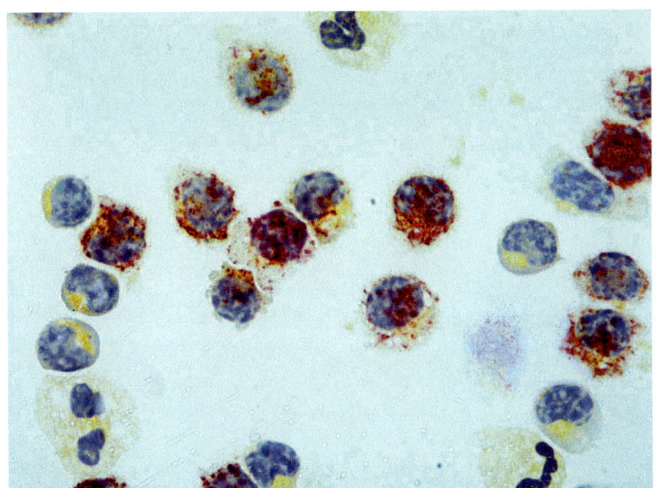

Fig. 4.5 Cytochemical stain with TRAP performed on the patient's peripheral blood shows identifiable cytoplasmic rough brownish granules in atypical lymphoid cells, indicating positive chemical reaction to TRAP, a marker specific for HCL (TRAP stain, 1000×)

at least some cells with strong, granular cytoplasmic TRAP positivity [23] (Fig. 4.5). However, TRAP is a technically challenging cytochemical stain and, while sensitive for HCL, is not as specific as other markers that can be identified by flow cytometry or immunohistochemistry, which has made the use of TRAP staining obsolete.

Classic HCL tumor cells exhibit a mature B-cell phenotype, including bright monotypic surface immunoglobulins, CD19, CD20, and CD22, and usually lack expression of CD5, CD10, CD21, CD23, and CD27 [24]. CD11c, a marker associated with myelomonocytic cells, and CD25, the alpha chain of the interleukin-2 receptor, are also strongly expressed in HCL neoplastic cells [25, 26]. The mucosal lymphocyte antigen, CD103, is a sensitive marker for HCL [27]. CD103 is also present on mucosa-associated T-cells and some activated lymphocytes. Coexpression of CD103 with other pan B-cell markers is highly suggestive of HCL [28]. Annexin A1, a member of the annexin family of Ca^{2+}-dependent phospholipid-binding proteins, was reportedly expressed in 74% cases, which is commonly not found in any other B-cell lymphoma subtype [24]. However, annexin A1 staining must be interpreted in conjunction with staining for a B-cell antigen since it is also expressed by myeloid cells and by some T-cells [24]. In addition, HCL neoplastic cells characteristically express CD123 [24], CD25, and BCL-1 (Fig. 4.6). Staining for CD200 expression is reported to be intense [29].

Flow cytometric demonstration in combination with morphology is a cornerstone of HCL diagnosis. HCL expresses CD45 (at bright intensity) and the B-cell markers CD19, CD20 (at bright intensity), FMC7, CD22 (at bright intensity), and CD79a, and it is usually negative for CD5, CD10, and CD79b [30, 31]. HCL expresses monotypic surface immunoglobulin at high intensity. Bright expression of CD11c, CD25, and CD103 is characteristic of HCL (Fig. 4.7). However, there is no absolutely specific immunophenotypic marker for HCL.

Cytogenetics

The most recurrent copy number alterations in classic HCL were deletions of chromosome 7q and 13q and gains of chromosome 5. Heterozygous loss of chromosome 7q, the minimally deleted region of which targeted wild-type *BRAF*, subdivided HCL into those hemizygous versus heterozygous for the *BRAF V600E* mutation [15]. Abnormalities of chromosome 5 were reported in approximately 40% patients, most commonly trisomy 5 [32]. Analysis of the immunoglobulin variable region genes shows somatic mutations in approximately 85% of cases [33, 34].

Molecular Findings

BRAF V600E, located at chromosome 7q24, is reported in virtually all the cases of classic type HCL. While highly sensitive in HCL, this mutation alone is not specific for diagnosis of HCL since it has also been detected in other entities, including Erdheim-Chester disease and Langerhans cell histiocytosis, as well as in subsets of solid tumors (e.g., melanoma and colonic adenocarcinoma) [35]. An antibody specific for *BRAF* V600E has been developed and may serve as a surrogate marker of this mutation detected by immunohistochemistry (IHC) (Fig. 4.8). The next most commonly mutated genes in classic type HCL were the *KMT2C* (*MLL3*) and *CDKN1B* occurring in 15% (8/53) and 11% (6/53) of patients, respectively [15]. Other recurrent mutations in HCL affected genes involved in transcriptional regulation (*BRD4*, *CEBPA*, *CREBBP*, *RUNX1*, *EP300*, and *MED12*), Notch signaling (*NOTCH1* and *NOTCH2*), and DNA repair (*RAD50*) [15].

The prototypic features of classic HCL are summarized in Table 4.1.

Differential Diagnosis

It is important to distinguish HCL from its morphologic mimickers when they are involved in the spleen. Table 4.2 summarizes the pathologic and molecular features of these lymphomas/leukemias.

Hairy Cell Leukemia Variant (HCL-V)

HCL-V exhibits morphologic features intermediate between hairy cells and prolymphocytes. Unlike HCL,

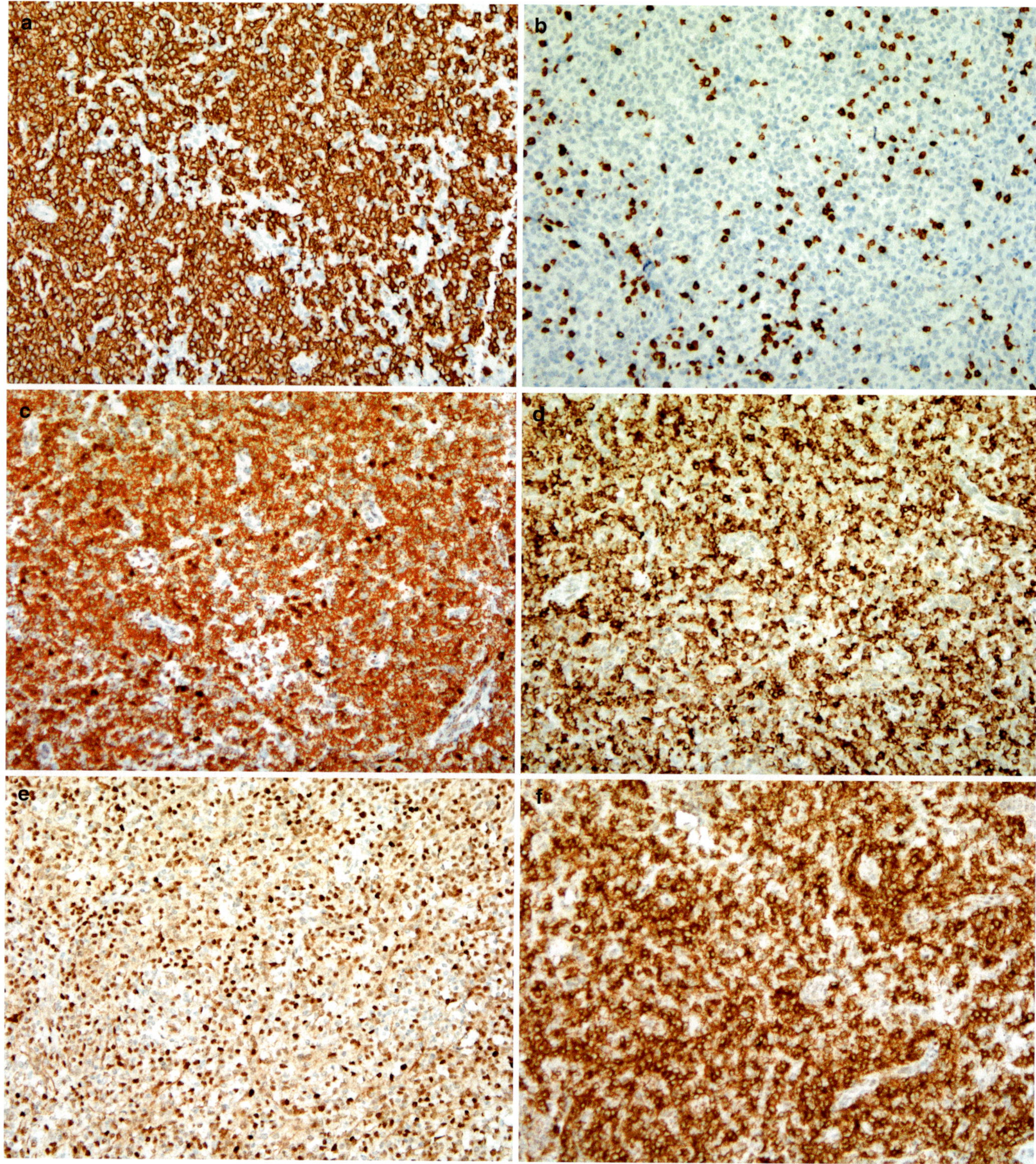

Fig. 4.6 Immunohistochemical stains are performed on the splenic sections which show the neoplastic HCL cells to be immuno-reactive to CD20 (**a**), annexin 1 (**c**), TRAP (**d**), cyclin D1 (**e**), and CD25 (**f**) and negative for CD3 (**b**) (immunoperoxidase, 200× for all)

HCL-V typically has prominent nucleoli with elevated white cell counts including predominance of atypical lymphocytes (Fig. 4.9). It involves the spleen with red pulp expansion and filling in dilated sinusoidal spaces (Fig. 4.10). Bone marrow involvement is infrequent. Immunophenotypically, HCL-V does not express CD25 and is usually dim or negative for CD123. Annexin A1 is expressed in approximately 75% of HCL cases and is universally negative in HCL-V. Importantly, HCL-V lacks the *BRAF V600E* mutation.

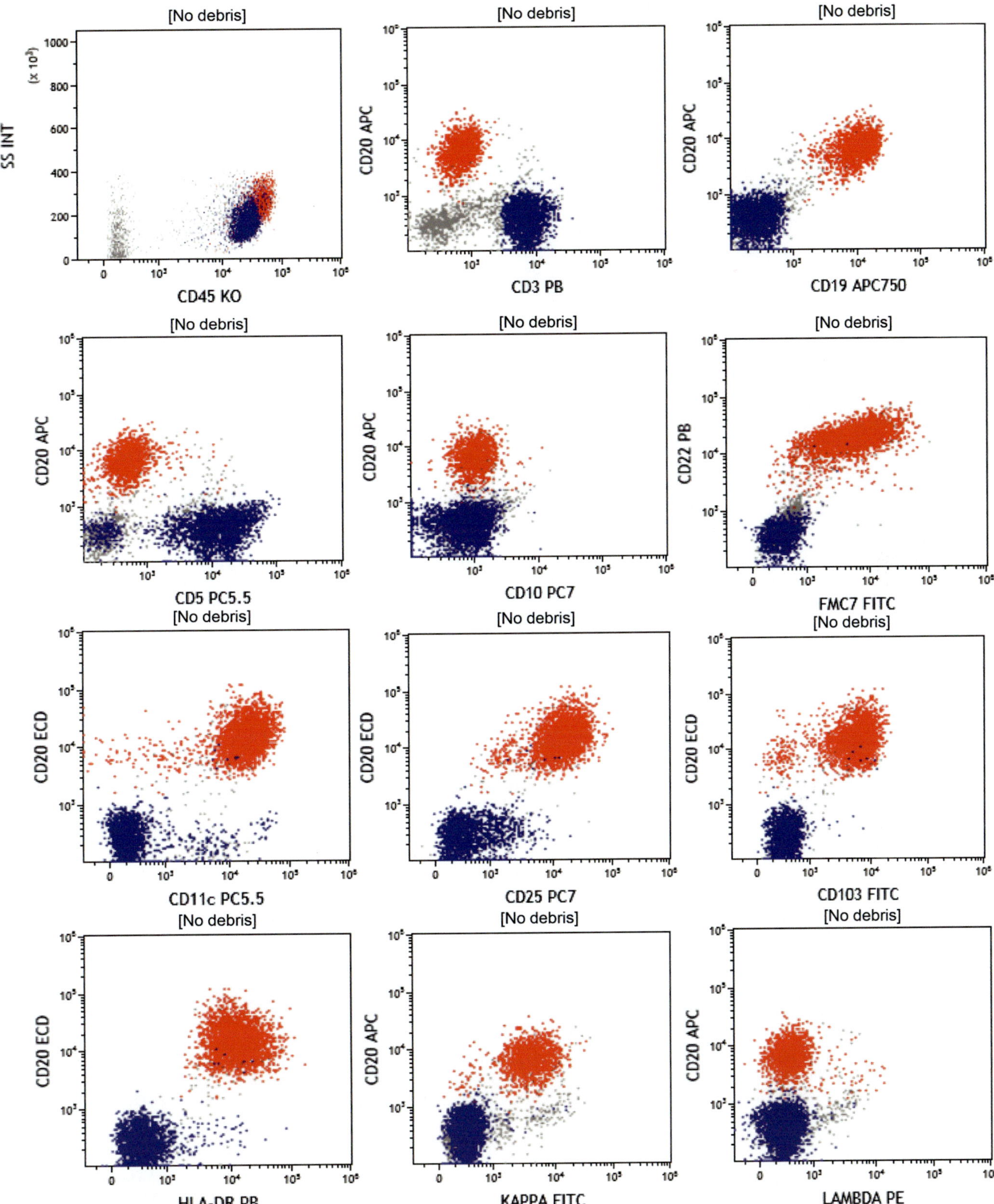

Fig. 4.7 Flow cytometric histogram of classic HCL. Leukemic cells are clonal, with mature B-cell phenotype (CD19, CD20, CD22), and coexpress CD25, CD11c, CD103, FMC7, and HLA-DR with surface kappa light chain restriction. The tumor cells usually lack expression of CD5 and CD10

Splenic Marginal Zone Lymphoma (SMZL)

Both SMZL and HCL can present with splenomegaly and circulating lymphocytes with cytoplasmic projections. However, SMZL cells usually have short bipolar projections compared to HCL. SMZL is a primarily white pulp disease

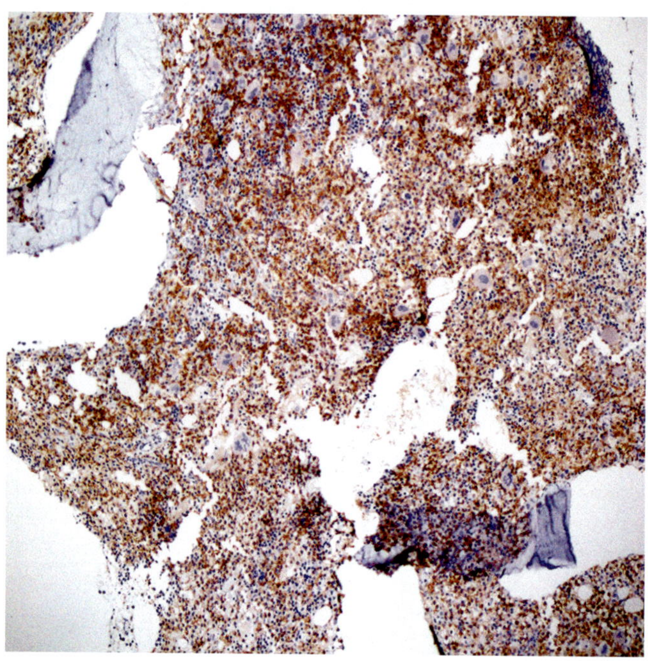

Fig. 4.8 Immunohistochemical stain (Ventana anti-BRAF V600E (VE1) Cat. No 790–5095) for mutated *BRAF*, a surrogate marker for *BRAF* V600E mutation

Table 4.1 Prototypic features of HCL

Parameter	Comments
Clinical	Usually onset in male patients in their sixth decades, with general weakness, fatigue, infections of variable degree, hemorrhagic events, and splenomegaly
CBC findings	Pancytopenia, profound monocytopenia, and neutropenia
Peripheral blood smear	Round to oval nuclei with "spongy" chromatin and inconspicuous nucleoli. Abundant pale cytoplasm with circumferential hairy projections
Bone marrow	Inaspirable (dry tap) in most cases due to diffuse reticulin fibrosis directly associated with hairy cell infiltrates. Subtle, patchy infiltrates on core biopsy (may be inconspicuous). The leukemic cells have abundant cytoplasm, producing a perinuclear halo or "fried egg" appearance in core biopsy
Flow cytometry	Monoclonal B-cells with bright CD20, bright CD22, bright CD11c, bright CD103, bright surface Ig, and CD25
Immunohistochemical stains	Positive immunoreactivity to CD20, annexin 1, CD123, DBA.44 (strong, diffuse), and cyclin D1 (weak and subset)
Cytochemical findings	Stained positive for TRAP
Cytogenetic features	No cytogenetic abnormalities are specific for HCL. Numerical abnormality of chromosome 5 or 7 is occasionally reported
Molecular features	*BRAF* V600E
Normal counterpart	A late, activated memory B-cells

Table 4.2 Histomorphology, immunophenotyping, and molecular characteristics of CLL/SLL, MCL, HCL, HCL-V, and SDRPL

	CLL/SLL	MCL	HCL	HCL-V	SDRPL	SMZL
Cytology	Small, round to oval nuclei, clumped chromatin, inconspicuous nucleoli	Small, round to oval nuclei, condense chromatin, prominent nucleoli	Small to medium, kidney-bean/indented nuclei, inconspicuous nucleoli, radiated cytoplasmic hairy projection	Similar to HCL with polar villous cytoplasmic projection	Small, round to oval nuclei, villous cytoplasmic projection similar to SMZL	Small mature lymphoid cells, plasmacytoid lymphocytes and plasma cells
Splenic infiltrating pattern	Nodular pattern found in white and red pulps	White pulp expansion	Involving primarily red pulps and forming "blood lake" lined by HCL cells	Diffuse involvement of the red pulp	Diffuse involvement of the red pulp	"Biphase" infiltrating pattern, involving both white and red pulps
Immunophenotyping	CD19+, CD20+ (dim), CD22+, CD5+, CD23+, CD11c(−/+) FMC7−, CD103−	CD19+, CD20+ (bright), CD22+, CD5+, CD11c+, BCl-1+, CD23−, CD103−	CD19+, CD20+ (bright), CD22+, CD11c+, CD25+, CD103+, CD123+, CD200+, Annexin 1+, BCL-1+, FMC7+, TRAP+, CD5−, CD10−/+ (10–20%)	CD19+, CD20+, CD22+, CD11c+, CD103−, CD123−/dim+, FCM7+, Annexin 1−, TRAP−, CD25−	CD19+, CD20+, CD22+, Annexin 1−, TRAP−, CD5−, CD10−, CD11c−, CD23−, CD25−, CD103−, CD123−	CD19+, CD20+, CD22+, CD11c + (50%), CD25+ (25%), CD103+ (25%), FMC7+, Annexin 1−, TRAP−, CD5−, CD10−, CD23−, CD43−
BRAF V600E	Neg	Neg	Pos (70–100%)	Neg (0%)	0–2%	0–2%

CLL/SLL chronic lymphocytic leukemia/small lymphocytic lymphoma, *MCL* mantle cell lymphoma, *HCL* hairy cell leukemia, *HCL-V* hairy cell leukemia - variant, *SDRPL* Splenic diffuse red pulp small B-cell lymphoma, *SMZL* splenic marginal zone lymphoma

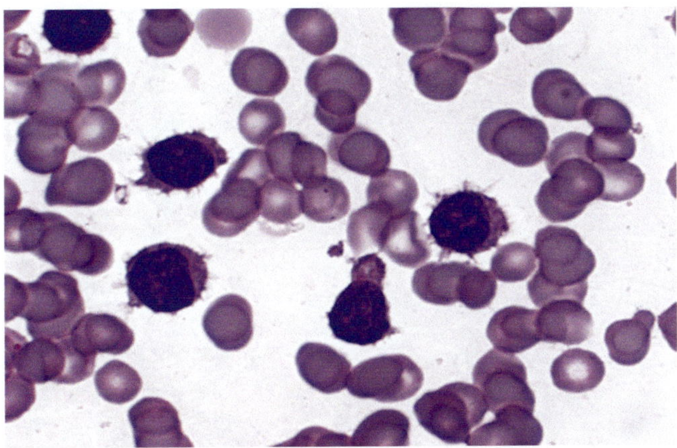

Fig. 4.9 HCL-V involving bone marrow (aspirable). The bone marrow aspirate smears show few lymphoid cells with typical villous projections, round to folded nuclei, and abundant cytoplasm. Nucleoli were inconspicuous to prominent in the case (Wright Giemsa stain, 1000×). Uniformly prominent central nucleoli mimicking prolymphocytic cells are typical findings (not shown here)

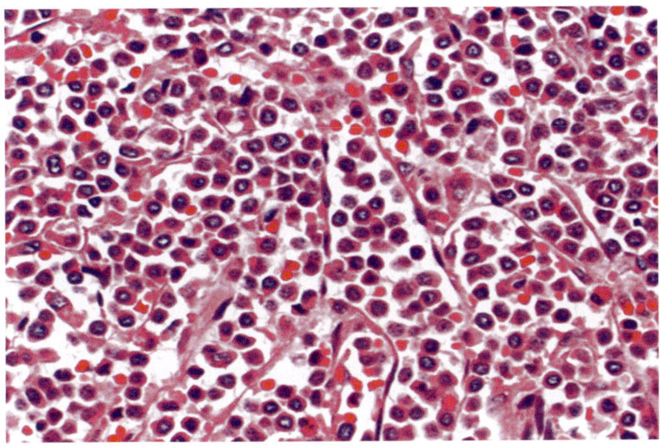

Fig. 4.10 HCL-V involving the spleen shows extensive splenic red pulp infiltrating with monomorphic population of tumor cells filled in sinuses (H&E, magnification 400×)

with nodular infiltrate of small B-cells and is negative for CD11c, CD25, CD103, and annexin A1. *BRAF V600E* mutations are absent or very rare in SMZL.

Mantle Cell Lymphoma

Mantle cell lymphoma can present with splenomegaly and peripheral blood involvement. However, "hairy" cytoplasm is not a feature of mantle cell lymphoma, and it has an immunophenotype that is easily distinguished from HCL. Although both HCL and MCL express cyclin D1 that can be detected by IHC study, FISH study proves *IgH/CCND1* gene rearrangement is only found in MCL. MCL expresses CD5 and has more strong and uniform expression of cyclin D1/BCL-1; it does not express CD25, CD103, or annexin A1.

Chronic Lymphocytic Leukemia (CLL)

CLL can present with splenomegaly and circulating lymphoid cells. However, CLL cells usually have a regular, smooth cytoplasmic outline with dim express of CD20, dim to absent surface light chains, and coexpression of CD5 and lacks expression of CD103. Most cases of splenic involvement in CLL demonstrate diffuse and nodular infiltrates due to involvement of both the red and white pulp.

Splenic Diffuse Red Pulp Small B-Cell Lymphoma (SDRPL)

SDRPL is a rare entity characterized by diffuse infiltration of the bone marrow, peripheral blood, and splenic red pulp by small monomorphous B lymphocytes, usually with villous projections (Fig. 4.11). In contrast to HCL, these tumor cells typically do not express annexin A1, CD25, CD103, CD123, and CD11c phenotypically and lack *BRAF V600E* mutation genetically.

Aplastic Anemia

Patients with advanced HCL may have hypocellular bone marrow that resembles patients with aplastic anemia. In the setting, bone marrow hypocellularity is due to loss of hematopoietic elements, especially the granulocytic lineage. Immunostaining for a B-cell antigen such as CD20 will identify an abnormal B-cell infiltrate. The diagnosis of HCL can then be confirmed using immunohistochemical stains as well as flow cytometry [6].

Prognosis and Treatment

The 10-year median survival of HCL exceeds 90%. Many patients with HCL are asymptomatic and can be observed for months and occasionally years after the diagnosis. The goal of treatment is alleviation of symptoms and cytopenias. For initial treatment, a purine analog, e.g., 2-chloro-2′-deoxyadenosine (2CdA), as first-line therapy is recommended with overall response rates of approximately 96–100% [36]. Although splenectomy does not produce pathologic remissions, peripheral blood counts return to normal in approximately 40–70% of patients [37]. For patients who do not respond to initial therapy, switching to an alternative purine analog, interferon alpha, surgery (splenectomy), or monoclonal antibodies directed against B-cell determinants on the malignant cell are recommended. Available monoclonal antibodies include anti-CD20 antibody (rituximab), anti-CD22 antibody (BL22), anti-CD25 antibody (LMB-2), and, more recently, BRAF inhibition [38].

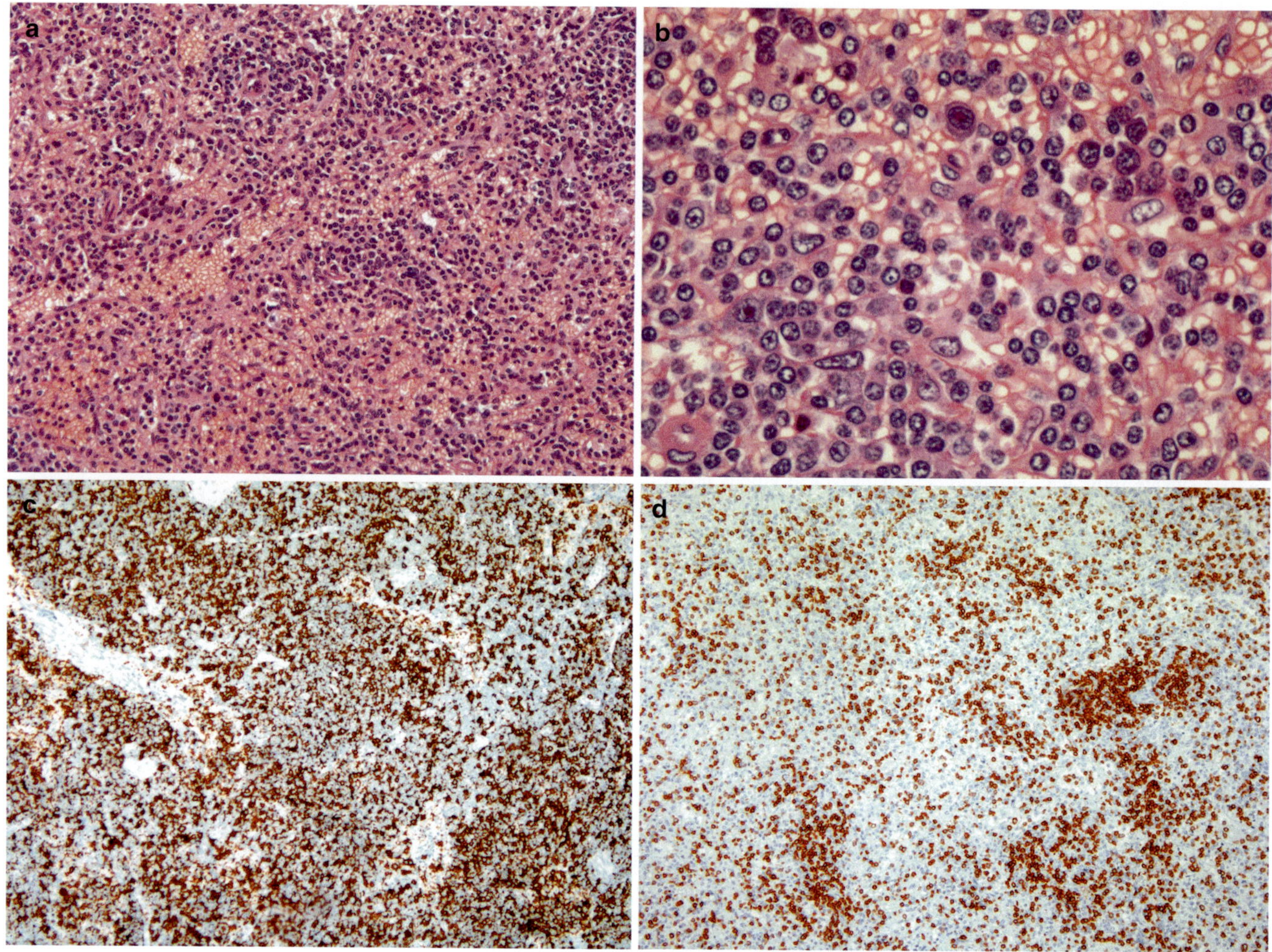

Fig. 4.11 (**a**) The spleen showed predominantly diffuse infiltrate of monomorphic small lymphoid cells in the red pulp in a patient diagnosed with SDRPL (H&E stain, 200x); (**b**) H&E stain, 600x. (**c**) CD20 (immunoperoxidase, 100x). (**d**) CD3 (immunoperoxidase, 100x)

Diagnostic Caveats

- Characteristic features of HCL include circulating atypical mature lymphoid cells with cytoplasmic hairy projection, splenic diffuse red pulp infiltration associated with "blood lake" lined by HCL cells, and bone marrow "fried egg" appearance of HCL arrangements with increased reticulin fibrosis.
- Flow cytometric analysis reveals HCL cells express B-cell markers, CD11c, CD25, and CD103.
- Strong diffuse TRAP positivity is characteristic of HCL, while weak expression may be present in many other disorders.
- Annexin 1 is specific for HCL but also expresses on myeloid cells and T-cells. Interpretation of annexin 1 IHC staining should compare with the expression of B-cell markers.
- Patch infiltrates of hairy cells can be very subtle. A low-level involvement or composite with other neoplasm could be missed without performing additional immunohistochemical study, which may be needed for diagnosis.
- Convoluted, multilobulated, blastic, and spindled variants of hairy cells have been described.

Splenic B-Cell Lymphoma/Leukemia, Unclassifiable

There are a number of variably well-defined entities that represent small B-cell clonal lymphoproliferations involving the spleen, which could not be fit in any of the other types of B-cell lymphoid neoplasms established currently. Hairy cell leukemia variant (HCL-V) and splenic diffuse red pulp small B-cell lymphoma (SDRPL), which are listed under WHO splenic B-cell lymphoma, unclassifiable, will be discussed in the session.

Hairy Cell Leukemia, Variant

The disease known as hairy cell leukemia variant (HCL-V) is rare. This disease was initially identified as a pro-lymphocytic variant of HCL. However, it is no longer considered to be biologically related to HCL due to significant morphologic, immunophenotypic, and genetic differences.

Etiology and Pathogenesis

The cause of HCL-V is still not fully understood. Activated B-cell at late stage of maturation is postulated as the normal counterpart [6]. HCL-V does not harbor *BRAF* V600E mutation. About 40% of HCL-V cases show VH4-34 family usage, which is similar to 10% of classical [39]. More recently, mutations in *MAP2K1*, which encodes MEK1, have been reported in almost half of HCL-V [39]. In 2017, *KMT2C* (*MLL3*) were identified in 25% HCL-V [9]. Moreover, approximately 13% of HCL-V cases harbored predicted activating mutations in *CCND3*, a change-of-function mutation in the splicing factor U2AF1 [15].

Epidemiology

HCL-V constitutes 0.4% of all lymphoid malignancies. In the United States, the estimated incidence rate is 0.03 per million persons per year [38]. It shares a similar male to female ratio with classic HCL. In a recent study, patients with HCL-V were comprised of a male to female ratio of 4.8:1. However, HCL-V tends to involve older patients with an age range from 40 to 98 years (median, 65 years) [24].

Clinical Presentations

Patients with HCL-V tend to have more advanced disease at initial presentation. However, HCL-V and classic HCL are difficult to distinguish based on symptoms and physical examinations only. Splenic discomfort, weakness, and weight loss are the most common clinical complains. Physical findings may include splenomegaly, hepatomegaly, and minimal lymphadenopathy. Instead of the presence of neutropenia, monocytopenia, anemia, and thrombocytopenia that are commonly seen in HCL, patients with HCL-V show marked leukocytosis with a white blood cell count over 30×10^9/L and numerous circulating neoplastic cells. The absolute monocyte count is typically within normal range.

Morphology

The leukemic cells resemble hairy cells in terms of having abundant cytoplasm and surface projections but may also have prominent central nucleoli that are not typically seen in HCL. Nuclear features range from condensed chromatin with prominent central nucleoli of a prolymphocytic cell to dispersed chromatin with highly irregular nuclear contours. Blastic and convoluted subtypes have also been reported. Convoluted HCL was described referring transformation to large cells with convoluted nuclei [37]. The interstitial or patchy involvement pattern in bone marrow is similar to that in classic HCL, although the extent is less severe. The tumor cells may have "fried egg" appearance in biopsy and tissue, which could be subtle and very inconspicuous. Bone marrow fibrosis is usually not seen in HCL-V. Red pulp of the spleen is diffusely involved and expanded in HCL-V. The leukemic cells fill dilated sinusoids and red blood cell lakes may be noted. Liver involvement is characterized by both portal tract and sinusoidal infiltrates and involves less than one third of the patients [40] (Figs. 4.9 and 4.10).

Cytochemical Findings and Immunophenotyping

Tartrate-resistant acid phosphatase (TRAP) is commonly weak to negative in HCL-V. HCL-V shares some similarities with classic HCL in that it expresses CD11c and often CD103, but it usually is negative for CD123, cyclin D1, annexin A1, and CD25.

Cytogenetics and Molecular Findings

For molecular findings, please refer to Etiology and Pathogenesis section. Of importance, *IGHV4-34* immunoglobulin rearrangements are present in 40% of HCL-V [39]. There is no specific cytogenetic abnormality reported, which may be attributed to the lack of complete cytogenetic workup for the rare entity.

Differential Diagnosis

Hairy Cell Leukemia (HCL)

Patients with HCL-V tend to be older than HCL at presentation and have a more aggressive course, which have marked leukocytosis without monocytopenia. The leukemic cells of HCL-V have prominent central nucleoli that are not typically seen in HCL. Bone marrow invasion is less severe and "dry tap" in aspiration is uncommon. The most important difference is frequent presence of *IGHV4-34* immunoglobulin rearrangements and *MAP2K1* mutation without *BRAF* V600E mutation.

Splenic Marginal Zone Lymphoma (SMZL)

SMZL and HCL-V can present with splenomegaly and circulating lymphocytes with cytoplasmic projections. Basically, SMZL is a white pulp disease in the spleen. While the circulating lymphocytes in HCL-V usually have cytoplasmic projections around the entire perimeter of the cell (hairy cells), SMZL cells usually have short bipolar projections. In addition, white blood cell count usually elevates with absolute lymphocytosis. SMZL does not express CD103 and CD11c, all of which are commonly expressed in HCL-V.

Splenic Diffuse Red Pulp Small B-cell Lymphoma (SDRPL)

The abnormal lymphoid cells of SDRPL have a polar distribution of their villi and their nucleolus is small or not visible. The monoclonal B-cells in these subjects express CD11c, have inconsistent CD103 expression, and rarely express CD123 or CD25. However, while there are many overlapping features in clinical and pathologic aspects, the exact relationship between HCL-V and SDRPL remains uncertain.

Treatment

The clinical course of HCL-V is more aggressive than that of HCL, with a median survival of 9 years in one study, significantly shorter than that of HCL. About 50% of patients are resistant to conventional treatment with purine analogues [34]. However, there is no established consensus concerning the treatment of HCL-V. Patients should be treated if they exhibit symptoms, while asymptomatic patients may be managed with a watch-and-wait strategy.

Splenic Diffuse Red Pulp Small B-Cell Lymphoma (SDRPL)

SDRPL is characterized by a diffuse pattern of involvement of the splenic red pulp by small monomorphous B lymphocytes.

Etiology and Pathogenesis

Our knowledge of the molecular mechanisms involved in SDRPL is very limited because the incidence of this lymphoma is low and few splenectomy specimens are available. SDRPL rarely harbors *BRAF V600E* mutations, ranging from 0% to 2% [41]. Most SDRPL cases display a mutated *IGHV* status, with a selective VH gene usage and overrepresentation of VH4-34 [1]. A few *NOTCH2* mutations (4/42 pts., 10%) were described [41]. Recently, increased expression of cyclin D3 was reported in more than 50% of the neoplastic cells in 24/37 splenectomy specimens via next-generation whole-exome sequencing (WES) [42]. Increased expression is sometimes the result of somatic mutations in the proline, glutamic acid, serine, and threonine PEST domain of the *CCND3* gene.

Epidemiology

This indolent but incurable disease is rare and accounts for <1% of non-Hodgkin lymphomas. It represents about 10% of the B-cell lymphomas diagnosed in splenectomy specimens. This disorder is more common in older men with no gender bias [43].

Clinical Presentations

Almost all the patients with SDRPL present in a late stage with splenomegaly and involvement of bone marrow and peripheral blood. Moderate lymphocytosis is also seen. However, fevers, night sweats, and weight losses, which are B symptoms, are usually not associated with SDRPL. A small group of these patients present cutaneous infiltration [43].

Morphology

In peripheral blood smear, the abnormal lymphoid cells have a polar distribution of their villi with small or not visible nucleolus. In the spleen, predominantly red pulp involvement is characteristic, with a monomorphous population of tumor cells resembling marginal zone B-cells and scattered nucleolated blast cells [44]. Some cases have reactive hyperplastic follicles in the white pulp isolated in the middle of a diffuse infiltrate of neoplastic cells. Within the spleen and bone marrow, these cases have a characteristic intrasinusoidal pattern of involvement [45] (Fig. 4.11).

Cytochemical Findings and Immunophenotyping

TRAP is negative in SDRPL. The tumor cells express CD11c (97%), have inconsistent CD103 expression (38%), and rarely express CD123 (16%) or CD25 (3%) [46]. Large majority of cases lack annexin A1 expression [44]. More frequent expression of IgG and DBA.44 has been found in these cases compared with SMZL. Most splenic red pulp small B-cell lymphomas (79%) were IgH mutated, with an overrepresentation of V(H)3 and V(H)4 gene families [46].

Cytogenetics and Molecular Findings

Please refer to Sect. "Etiopathogenesis".

Differential Diagnosis

Hairy Cell Leukemia (HCL)

Patients with SDRPL tend to present at a late stage compared to HCL, with splenomegaly and bone marrow and peripheral blood involvement. Compared to HCL, the tumor cells of SDRPL have a polar distribution of their villi and smaller nuclei. Spleen red pulp is always involved. Most SDRPL cases display a mutated *IgVH* status without *BRAF* mutation. In addition, increased cyclin D3 expression was reported in SDRPL by next-generation whole-exome sequencing (WES), which was rarely observed in HCL [42].

Splenic Marginal Zone Lymphoma (SMZL)

SMZL and SDRPL can present with splenomegaly and circulating lymphocytes with polar cytoplasmic projections. However, SMZL does not express CD103 and CD11c [40], which are commonly expressed in SDRPL. More frequent expression of IgG and DBA.44 has been found in these cases compared with SMZL. In addition, CCND3 expression was reported in more than 50% of the neoplastic cells of SDRPL, which was rarely observed in SMZL [42].

Hairy Cell Leukemia Variant (HCL-V)

Morphologically, SDRPL has abnormal lymphoid cells with a polar distribution of their villi and expresses CD11c (97%), inconsistent CD103 (38%), and rarely CD123 (16%) or CD25 (3%). In contrast to HCL-V, *CCND3* mutations were identified in a much higher rate of SDRPL cases. Approximately 13% of HCL-V cases harbored predicted activating mutations in *CCND3* [15], while in the neoplastic cells of SDRPL, the mutation rate was reported above 50% [42].

Treatment

Treatment of SDRPL has no consensus, but splenectomy with or without chemotherapy should be considered. Given the implication of CCND3 in the pathogenesis of SDRPL, cell cycle inhibitors, such as CDK4/CDK6 inhibitors [47], could be alternative therapeutic option in the near future.

Diagnostic Caveats

- Clinical presentation and morphologic or immunophenotypic characteristics are key elements for diagnosis of HCL-V and SDRPL.
- *BRAF* V600E molecular study is helpful for differential diagnosis of classic HCL.
- Whether or not HCL-V and SDRPL are the same disease with slightly different clinical and pathologic presentation still remains to be determined.

References

1. Traverse-Glehen A, Verney A, Gazzo S, Jallades L, Chabane K, Hayette S, et al. Splenic diffuse red pulp small B-cell lymphoma has a distinct pattern of somatic mutations amongst B-cell malignancies. Leuk Lymphoma. 2017;58(3):666–75.
2. Bouroncle B, Wiseman B, Doan C. Leukemic reticuloendotheliosis. Blood. 1958;13(7):609–30.
3. Foucar K, Catovsky D. Hairy cell leukaemia. In: Jaffe E, Harris N, Stein H, editors. Pathology and genetics of tumours of haematopoietic and lymphoid tissues – World Health Organization classification of tumours. Lyon: IARC Press; 2001. p. 138–41.
4. Foucar K, Falini B, Catovsky D, Stein H. Hairy cell leukaemia. In: Swerdlow S, Campo E, Harris N, editors. World health organization classification of tumours of haematopoietic and lymphoid tissues. Lyon: IARC Press; 2008. p. 188–90.
5. Tiacci E, Liso A, Piris M, Falini B. Evolving concepts in the pathogenesis of hairy-cell leukaemia. Nat Rev Cancer. 2006;6(6):437–48.
6. Foucar K, Falini B, Stein H. Hairy cell leukaemia. In: Swerdlow S, Campo E, Harris N, editors. World Health Organization classification of tumours of haematopoietic and lymphoid tissues. Lyon: IARC Press; 2016. p. 226–8.
7. Morton LM, Wang SS, Devesa SS, Hartge P, Weisenburger DD, Linet MS. Lymphoma incidence patterns by WHO subtype in the United States, 1992–2001. Blood. 2006;107(1):265–76.
8. Frassoldati A, Lamparelli T, Federico M, Annino L, Capnist G, Pagnucco G, et al. Hairy cell leukemia: a clinical review based on 725 cases of the Italian Cooperative Group (ICGHCL). Italian Cooperative Group for Hairy Cell Leukemia. Leuk Lymphoma. 1994;13(3–4):307–16.
9. Quest GR, Johnston JB. Clinical features and diagnosis of hairy cell leukemia. Best Pract Res Clin Haematol. 2015;28(4):180–92.
10. Dores GM, Matsuno RK, Weisenburger DD, Rosenberg PS, Anderson WF. Hairy cell leukaemia: a heterogeneous disease? Br J Haematol. 2008;142(1):45–51.
11. Tiacci E, Trifonov V, Schiavoni G, Holmes A, Kern W, Martelli MP, et al. BRAF mutations in hairy-cell leukemia. N Engl J Med. 2011;364(24):2305–15.
12. Tiacci E, Schiavoni G, Forconi F, Santi A, Trentin L, Ambrosetti A, et al. Simple genetic diagnosis of hairy cell leukemia by sensitive detection of the BRAF-V600E mutation. Blood. 2012;119(1):192–5.
13. Boyd EM, Bench AJ, van't Veer MB, Wright P, Bloxham DM, Follows GA, et al. High resolution melting analysis for detection of BRAF exon 15 mutations in hairy cell leukaemia and other lymphoid malignancies. Br J Haematol. 2011;155(5):609–12.
14. Chilosi M, Chiarle R, Lestani M, Menestrina F, Montagna L, Ambrosetti A, et al. Low expression of p27 and low proliferation index do not correlate in hairy cell leukaemia. Br J Haematol. 2000;111(1):263–71.
15. Durham BH, Getta B, Dietrich S, Taylor J, Won H, Bogenberger JM, et al. Genomic analysis of hairy cell leukemia identifies novel recurrent genetic alterations. Blood. 2017;130(14):1644–8.
16. Monnereau A, Slager SL, Hughes AM, Smith A, Glimelius B, Habermann TM, et al. Medical history, lifestyle, and occupational risk factors for hairy cell leukemia: the InterLymph Non-Hodgkin Lymphoma Subtypes Project. J Natl Cancer Inst Monogr. 2014;2014(48):115–24.

17. Orsi L, Delabre L, Monnereau A, Delval P, Berthou C, Fenaux P, et al. Occupational exposure to pesticides and lymphoid neoplasms among men: results of a French case-control study. Occup Environ Med. 2009;66(5):291–8.

18. Colovic MD, Jankovic GM, Wiernik PH. Hairy cell leukemia in first cousins and review of the literature. Eur J Haematol. 2001;67(3):185–8.

19. Hoffman MA. Clinical presentations and complications of hairy cell leukemia. Hematol Oncol Clin North Am. 2006;20(5):1065–73.

20. Golomb HM, Braylan R, Polliack A. 'Hairy' cell leukaemia (leukaemic reticuloendotheliosis): a scanning electron microscopic study of eight cases. Br J Haematol. 1975;29(3):455–60.

21. Lee WM, Beckstead JH. Hairy cell leukemia with bone marrow hypoplasia. Cancer. 1982;50(10):2207–10.

22. Burke JS, Rappaport H. The diagnosis and differential diagnosis of hairy cell leukemia in bone marrow and spleen. Semin Oncol. 1984;11(4):334–46.

23. Yam LT, Li CY, Lam KW. Tartrate-resistant acid phosphatase isoenzyme in the reticulum cells of leukemic reticuloendotheliosis. N Engl J Med. 1971;284(7):357–60.

24. Shao H, Calvo KR, Grönborg M, Tembhare PR, Kreitman RJ, Stetler-Stevenson M, et al. Distinguishing hairy cell leukemia variant from hairy cell leukemia: development and validation of diagnostic criteria. Leuk Res. 2013;37(4):401–9.

25. Robbins BA, Ellison DJ, Spinosa JC, Carey CA, Lukes RJ, Poppema S, et al. Diagnostic application of two-color flow cytometry in 161 cases of hairy cell leukemia. Blood. 1993;82(4):1277–87.

26. Barak V, Ginzburg M, Kalickman I, Polliack A. Serum soluble interleukin-2 receptor levels are associated with clinical disease status and histopathological grade in non-Hodgkin's lymphoma and chronic lymphocytic leukemia. Leuk Lymphoma. 1992;7(5–6):431–8.

27. Möller P, Mielke B, Moldenhauer G. Monoclonal antibody HML-1, a marker for intraepithelial T cells and lymphomas derived thereof, also recognizes hairy cell leukemia and some B-cell lymphomas. Am J Pathol. 1990;136(3):509–12.

28. Cornfield DB, Mitchell Nelson DM, Rimsza LM, Moller-Patti D, Braylan RC. The diagnosis of hairy cell leukemia can be established by flow cytometric analysis of peripheral blood, even in patients with low levels of circulating malignant cells. Am J Hematol. 2001;67(4):223–6.

29. Pillai V, Pozdnyakova O, Charest K, Li B, Shahsafaei A, Dorfman DM. CD200 flow cytometric assessment and semiquantitative immunohistochemical staining distinguishes hairy cell leukemia from hairy cell leukemia-variant and other B-cell lymphoproliferative disorders. Am J Clin Pathol. 2013;140(4):536–43.

30. Carulli G, Cannizzo E, Zucca A, Buda G, Orciuolo E, Marini A, et al. CD45 expression in low-grade B-cell non-Hodgkin's lymphomas. Leuk Res. 2008;32(2):263–7.

31. Schiller AL, Strauchen JA. Foucar K: chronic lymphoid leukemias and lymphoproliferative disorders. Mod Pathol. 1999;12:990.

32. Haglund U, Juliusson G, Stellan B, Gahrton G. Hairy cell leukemia is characterized by clonal chromosome abnormalities clustered to specific regions. Blood. 1994;83(9):2637–45.

33. Swerdlow SH, Campo E, Pileri SA, Harris NL, Stein H, Siebert R, et al. The 2016 revision of the World Health Organization classification of lymphoid neoplasms. Blood. 2016;127(20):2375–90.

34. Troussard X, Cornet E. Hairy cell leukemia 2018: update on diagnosis, risk-stratification, and treatment. Am J Hematol. 2017;92(12):1382–90.

35. Haroche J, Charlotte F, Arnaud L, von Deimling A, Hélias-Rodzewicz Z, Hervier B, et al. High prevalence of BRAF V600E mutations in Erdheim-Chester disease but not in other non-Langerhans cell histiocytoses. Blood. 2012;120(13):2700–3.

36. Else M, Dearden CE, Matutes E, Garcia-Talavera J, Rohatiner AZ, Johnson SA, et al. Long-term follow-up of 233 patients with hairy cell leukaemia, treated initially with pentostatin or cladribine, at a median of 16 years from diagnosis. Br J Haematol. 2009;145(6):733–40.

37. Golomb HM, Vardiman JW. Response to splenectomy in 65 patients with hairy cell leukemia: an evaluation of spleen weight and bone marrow involvement. Blood. 1983;61(2):349–52.

38. Robak T. Current treatment options in hairy cell leukemia and hairy cell leukemia variant. Cancer Treat Rev. 2006;32(5):365–76.

39. Waterfall JJ, Arons E, Walker RL, Pineda M, Roth L, Killian JK, et al. High prevalence of MAP2K1 mutations in variant and IGHV4-34-expressing hairy-cell leukemias. Nat Genet. 2014;46(1):8–10.

40. Piris MA, Foucar K, Mollejo M, Matutes E. Splenic B-cell lymphoma/leukaemia, unclassifiable. In: Swerdlow S, Campo E, Harris N, editors. World health organization classification of tumours of haematopoietic and lymphoid tissues. Lyon: IARC Press; 2017. p. 230–1.

41. Jallades L, Baseggio L, Sujobert P, Huet S, Chabane K, Callet-Bauchu E, et al. Exome sequencing identifies recurrent BCOR alterations and the absence of KLF2, TNFAIP3 and MYD88 mutations in Splenic diffuse red pulp small B-cell lymphoma. Haematologica. 2017;102(10):1758–66.

42. Curiel-Olmo S, Mondéjar R, Almaraz C, Mollejo M, Cereceda L, Marès R, et al. Splenic diffuse red pulp small B-cell lymphoma displays increased expression of cyclin D3 and recurrent CCND3 mutations. Blood. 2017;129(8):1042–5.

43. Swerdlow S, Campo E, Harris N, Jaffe E, Pileri S, Stein H, et al. WHO classification of tumours of haematopoietic and lymphoid tissues. Lyon: IARC Press; 2008.

44. Traverse-Glehen A, Baseggio L, Salles G, Coiffier B, Felman P, Berger F. Splenic diffuse red pulp small-B cell lymphoma: toward the emergence of a new lymphoma entity. Discov Med. 2012;13(71):253–65.

45. Jaffe E, Arber DA, Campo E, Harris N, Quintanilla-Fend L. Hematopathology. Philidophia, US: Elsevier; 2016.

46. Traverse-Glehen A, Baseggio L, Bauchu EC, Morel D, Gazzo S, Ffrench M, et al. Splenic red pulp lymphoma with numerous basophilic villous lymphocytes: a distinct clinicopathologic and molecular entity? Blood. 2008;111(4):2253–60.

47. Schmitz R, Young RM, Ceribelli M, Jhavar S, Xiao W, Zhang M, et al. Burkitt lymphoma pathogenesis and therapeutic targets from structural and functional genomics. Nature. 2012;490(7418):116–20.

Haipeng Shao

Introduction

As a secondary lymphoid tissue, the spleen is commonly involved by small B-cell non-Hodgkin lymphomas, including chronic lymphocytic leukemia/small lymphocytic lymphoma (CLL/SLL), follicular lymphoma (FL), mantle cell lymphoma (MCL), and lymphoplasmacytic lymphoma (LPL). Most splenic small B-cell lymphomas represent secondary involvement by systemic lymphomas. Primary splenic small B-cell lymphomas, as strictly defined by lymphoma confined to the spleen and hilar lymph nodes and without evidence of involvement of other tissues, are rare. Splenic marginal zone lymphoma (SMZL) is a well-characterized low-grade B-cell lymphoma with primary location in the spleen but also invariably involving the bone marrow. Patients with SMZL present with splenomegaly, anemia, or thrombocytopenia and variable villous lymphocytes in the peripheral blood. Histologically, SMZL is characterized by white pulp expansion with lymphoid nodules showing a biphasic pattern and red pulp infiltrate. The bone marrow involvement by SMZL cells is characterized by intrasinusoidal/intravascular infiltrate. SMZL lacks recurrent chromosomal changes, and the most frequent mutated genes are *NOTCH2* and *KLF2*. The other small B-cell lymphomas in the spleen show similar morphologic and phenotypic features as their corresponding nodal/systemic diseases. While CLL/SLL, FL, and MCL show predominant white pulp involvement with variable red pulp infiltrate, LPL primarily involves the red pulp. Similar to the spleen, the liver is also commonly involved by small B-cell lymphomas, and primary hepatic small B-cell lymphomas are very rare. SMZL infiltrates the liver in a nodular pattern in the portal tracts along with intrasinusoidal infiltrate, and a nodular pattern in the portal tracts is the prominent histo-

logic feature in CLL/SLL, MCL, and FL involving the liver. The differential diagnosis of these small B-cell lymphomas and others such as hairy cell leukemia (HCL), hairy cell leukemia variant (HCL-v), and splenic diffuse red pulp small B-cell lymphoma (SDRPBCL) is based on the integration of clinical presentation, morphology, immunophenotype, and genetic findings (also refer to chapter 4).

Splenic Marginal Zone Lymphoma

Definition

Splenic marginal zone lymphoma (SMZL) is a low-grade B-cell lymphoma involving the spleen, bone marrow, and frequently peripheral blood and with distinctive clinicopathologic features. It is defined by the World Health Organization (WHO) Classification of Tumors of Haematopoietic and Lymphoid Tissues as "a B-cell neoplasm composed of small lymphocytes that surround and replace the splenic white pulp germinal centres, efface the follicle mantle, and merge with a peripheral (marginal) zone of large cells, including scattered transformed blasts; both small and larger cells infiltrate the red pulp" [1].

Epidemiology and Etiology

Though SMZL is the most common primary splenic lymphoma, it is rare, accounting for <2% of all lymphomas and approximately 20% of all nodal and extranodal marginal zone lymphomas [1, 2]. In the United States, SMZL accounts for 0.6% of non-Hodgkin lymphomas in the registries of the Surveillance, Epidemiology, and End Results (SEER) [3]. The overall age-adjusted annual incidence is 0.13 per 100,000 persons per year. There is an increasing trend in the incidence of SMZL, and the annual percent change in age-adjusted incidence is 4.81% with increasing trends in patients who are

H. Shao (✉)
Department of Pathology, H. Lee Moffitt Cancer Center and Research Institute, Tampa, FL, USA
e-mail: Haipeng.shao@moffitt.org

© Springer Nature Switzerland AG 2020
L. Zhang et al. (eds.), *Diagnostic Pathology of Hematopoietic Disorders of Spleen and Liver*,
https://doi.org/10.1007/978-3-030-37708-3_5

white, male, or over 70 years old [3]. The incidence of SMZL in whites is approximately twice that of non-whites [3]. Most patients are over the age of 50 years with a median age of 69 years (ranging 30 to 90 years) and no gender predilection.

There is an association of SMZL with B-cell activating autoimmune conditions, asthma without other atopy, and permanent hair dye use [4, 5]. The association of SMZL with chronic hepatitis C virus (HCV) infection is common in Southern Europe (Italy) [6–8].

Clinical Presentation

The most common sign is splenomegaly, which is identified in 75% of patients. Most patients are asymptomatic at the time of diagnosis, but splenomegaly is invariably present. Unlike other non-Hodgkin lymphomas, peripheral lymphadenopathy is rarely seen (in <20% of patients). Abdominal lymph node involvement is relatively frequent and documented in approximately ¼ of patients. Many patients present with lymphocytosis, anemia, and/or thrombocytopenia that are more often due to hypersplenism and less frequently to autoimmune cytopenia or bone marrow infiltrate [9–13]. B symptoms (fatigue, night sweats, weight loss) and elevation of lactate dehydrogenase (LDH) are rare. A small number of patients present with symptoms related to marked splenomegaly such as abdominal discomfort and early satiety. Approximately ½ of patients had an involvement of SMZL in peripheral blood (>5% of neoplastic cells or absolute lymphocytosis). Some patients could present with isolated clonal B-cell lymphocytosis without splenomegaly, and the atypical lymphoid cells in the peripheral blood have the immunophenotypic features consistent with SMZL [14]. Only a minority of these cases represents SMZL as patients eventually developed splenomegaly, while most cases remained stable and may represent monoclonal B-cell lymphocytosis of non-CLL phenotype. Approximately 20% of patients with SMZL present with autoimmune disorders (autoimmune hemolytic anemia, autoimmune thrombocytopenia, acquired coagulation disorders, positive Coombs test, lupus anticoagulant and thrombosis, and acquired C1 inhibitor deficiency) [15–17]. Serum monoclonal paraprotein (most commonly IgM) and/or Bence Jones proteinuria can be detected in approximately 20–30% of patients with SMZL [18]. The M-spike is less than 30 g/L with predominance of IgM followed by IgG and IgA. The clinical course of SMZL is chronic, and approximately 10% of SMZL eventually transform to diffuse large B-cell lymphoma [19]. The median survival is about 10 years [9, 10, 13, 18, 20,

21]. Solid secondary primary cancers, especially urinary tract and lung cancers, occur in about 10% patients with SMZL [22].

Pathologic Features

The diagnosis is traditionally made on splenectomy specimen, but it can also be based on pathologic features of lymphoma cells in the bone marrow and peripheral blood.

Morphology

Gross Features

The spleen, post splenectomy, is enlarged with weight ranging from 270 to 5500 grams (median, 1750 grams) and numerous small- to moderate-sized gray-tan nodules throughout parenchyma on the cut surfaces [23] (Fig. 5.1).

Microscopic Features

Microscopically, the SMZL typically shows white pulp expansion with variable degree of red pulp infiltrate by atypical lymphoid cells in contrast to normal spleen (Fig. 5.2). In the white pulps, there are nodular lymphoid infiltrate composed of reactive germinal centers surrounded or more frequently replaced by expanded SMZL cells [24, 25]. The mantle zones of the germinal centers are effaced. The SMZL cells display a biphasic pattern with two zones surrounding the reactive germinal centers (Fig. 5.3). The inner zone cells

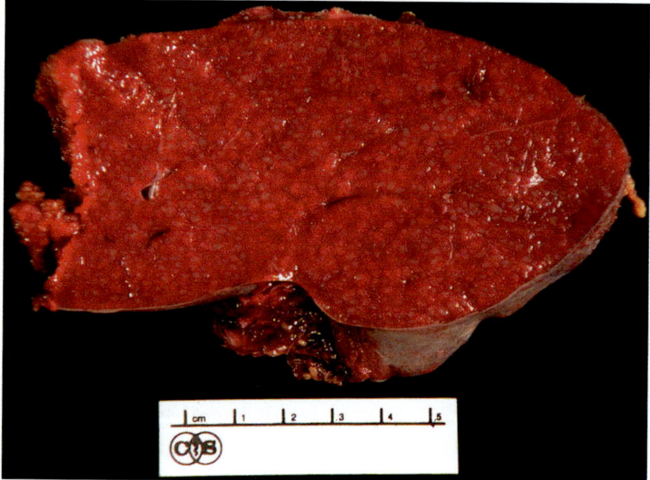

Fig. 5.1 SMZL (gross image). Gross image of splenic marginal zone lymphoma diffusely involving in splenic parenchyma with numerous pink-tan, evenly distributed nodules

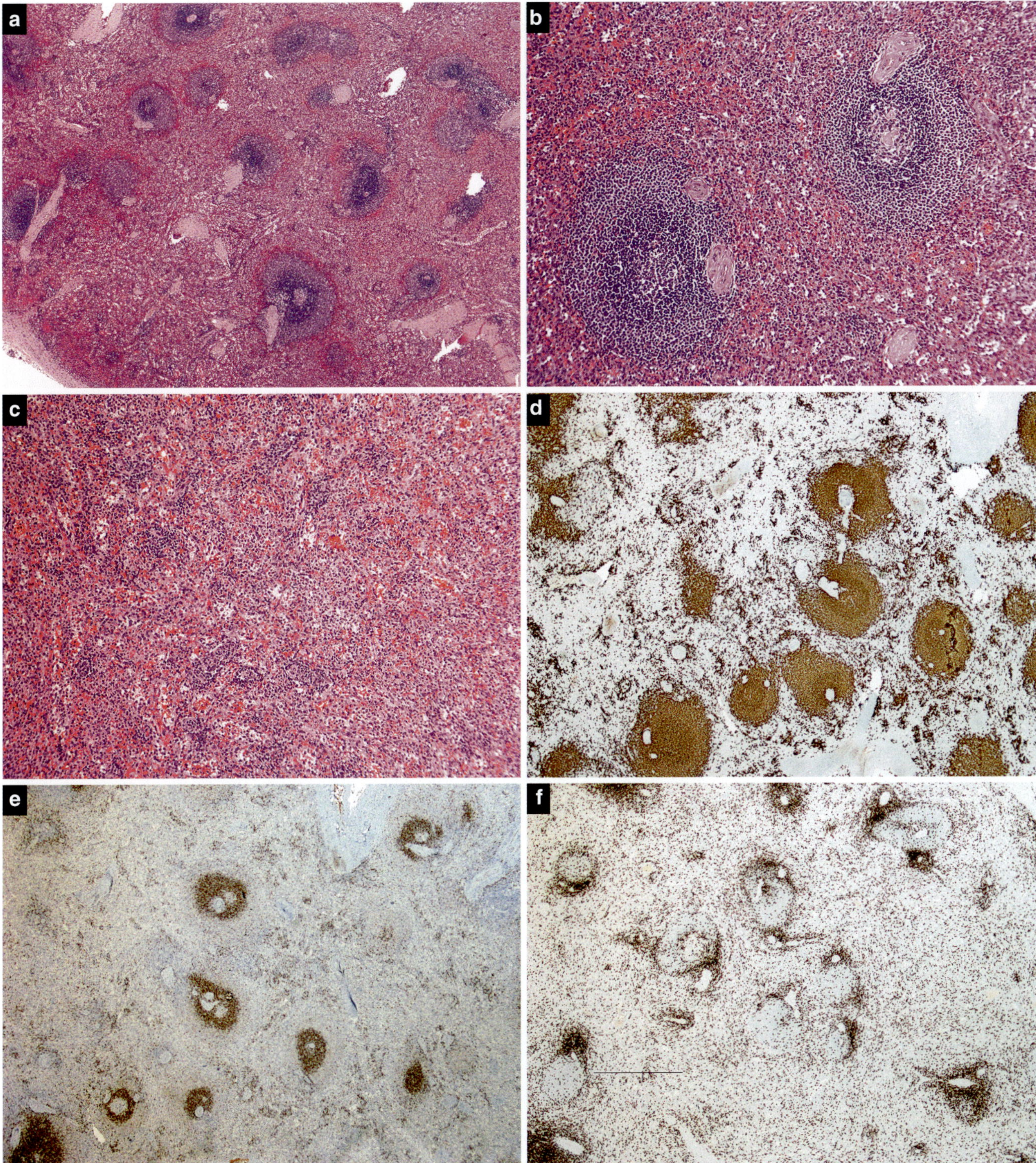

Fig. 5.2 Normal spleen (microscopic image). The normal spleen shows well-separated lymphoid follicles in the white pulps (**a**, H&E). The benign lymphoid follicles show a central germinal center, a dark stained mantle zone, and an exterior marginal zone (**b**, H&E). The marginal zones are distinct but without significant expansion. Except for perivascular lymphocytes, there is no significant increase of lymphocytes in the red pulp areas (**c**, H&E). CD20 highlights the lymphoid follicles and no significant B-cell infiltrate in the red pulp other than variable numbers of perivascular B-cells (**d**). IgD shows the mantle zones of the follicles and the perivascular naïve B-cells (**e**). CD3 shows T-cells surrounding the follicles and scattered T-cells in the red pulp (**f**)

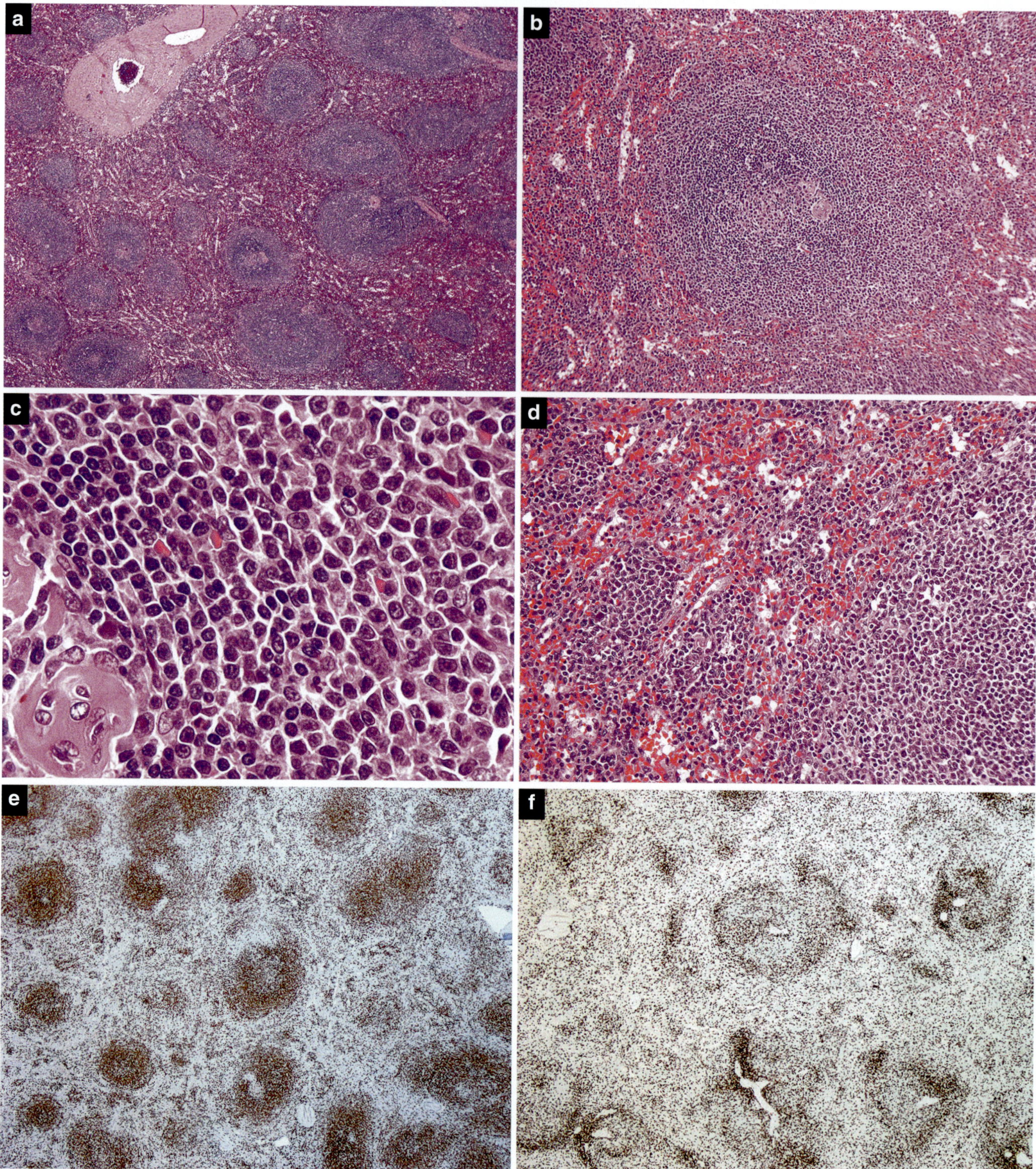

Fig. 5.3 Splenic marginal zone lymphoma in the spleen, biphasic pattern. The spleen shows increased density of atypical lymphoid follicles (**a**, H&E). The follicles in SMZL show biphasic cytology with pale staining exterior marginal zone cells and darker interior cells surrounding a pale central residual germinal center (**b** and **c**, H&E). The red pulp shows many clusters of SMZ cells (**d**, H&E). CD20 shows the lymphoid follicles and increased B-cells in the red pulp in clusters (**e**). CD3 highlight the background T-cells (**f**). The SMZL cells are positive for IgD (**g**) and BCL2 (**h**). Ki-67 shows a targetoid pattern with increased proliferation rate in the central residual germinal center and exterior marginal zone (**i**). In follicles without residual germinal centers, the exterior marginal zones are highlighted by Ki-67 with higher proliferation rate

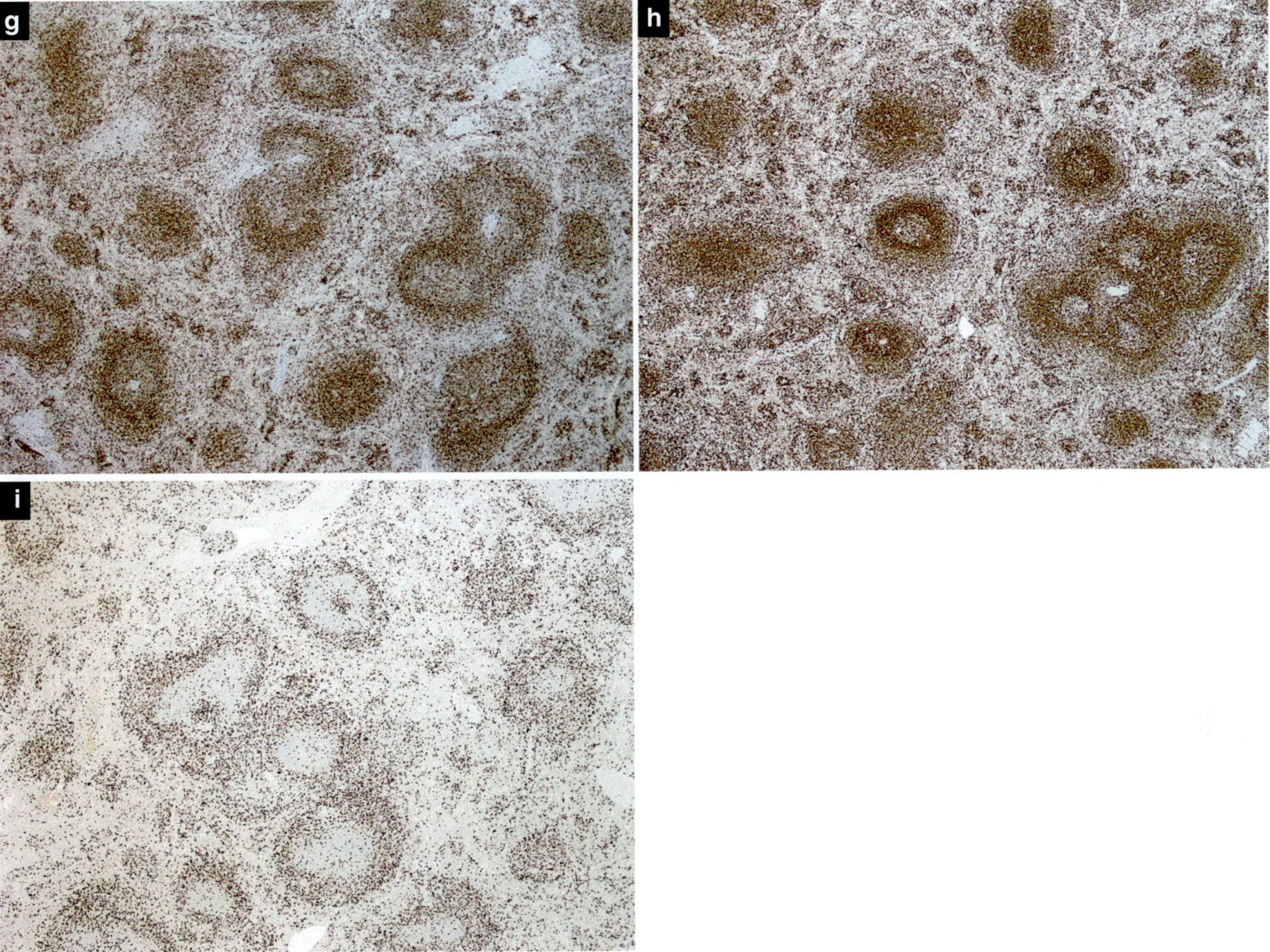

Fig. 5.3 (continued)

are small to medium sized with round nuclei, coarse chromatin, and scant cytoplasm. The SMZL cells in the external zone show cytological features of marginal zone B-cells with mildly irregular nuclei, more dispersed chromatin, and moderately abundant pale cytoplasm, admixed with scattered large transformed centroblasts or immunoblasts. The relative proportion of inner zone and external marginal zone SMZL cells varies from case to case [26]. The red pulp is invariably infiltrated by small clusters of the marginal zone cells and/or sheets of small lymphoid cells, typically with infiltrate of splenic sinuses and splenic cords. The SMZL cells in the sinuses have the cytological features of marginal zone cells. At the early stage of the disease, the marginal zone expansion by SMZL cells may be indistinguishable from reactive marginal hyperplasia. With disease progression, the reactive germinal centers are effaced by SMZL cells (Fig. 5.4). In advanced phases, the splenic architecture can be completely effaced by sheets of SMZL cells. A variable degree of plasmacytic differentiation may be present in up to approximately 40% cases (Fig. 5.5) [27–29]. Clusters of epithelioid histiocytes, sometimes numerous, can be seen [29]. The splenic hilar lymph nodes are invariably involved by SMZL [29]. An aggressive variant of SMZL with aggressive clinical course shows typical morphology with biphasic pattern and marginal zone differentiation but is characterized by a conspicuous component of large lymphoid cells in the marginal zone ring, occasionally overrunning it [30].

Immunophenotyping

The SMZL cells display a nonspecific immunophenotype by immunohistochemistry and flow cytometry. They are consistently positive for B-cell markers such as CD19, CD20, CD22, CD79a, CD79b, FMC7 and PAX5, IgM, and BCL2; variably positive for IgD, CD23, and DBA.44; and negative

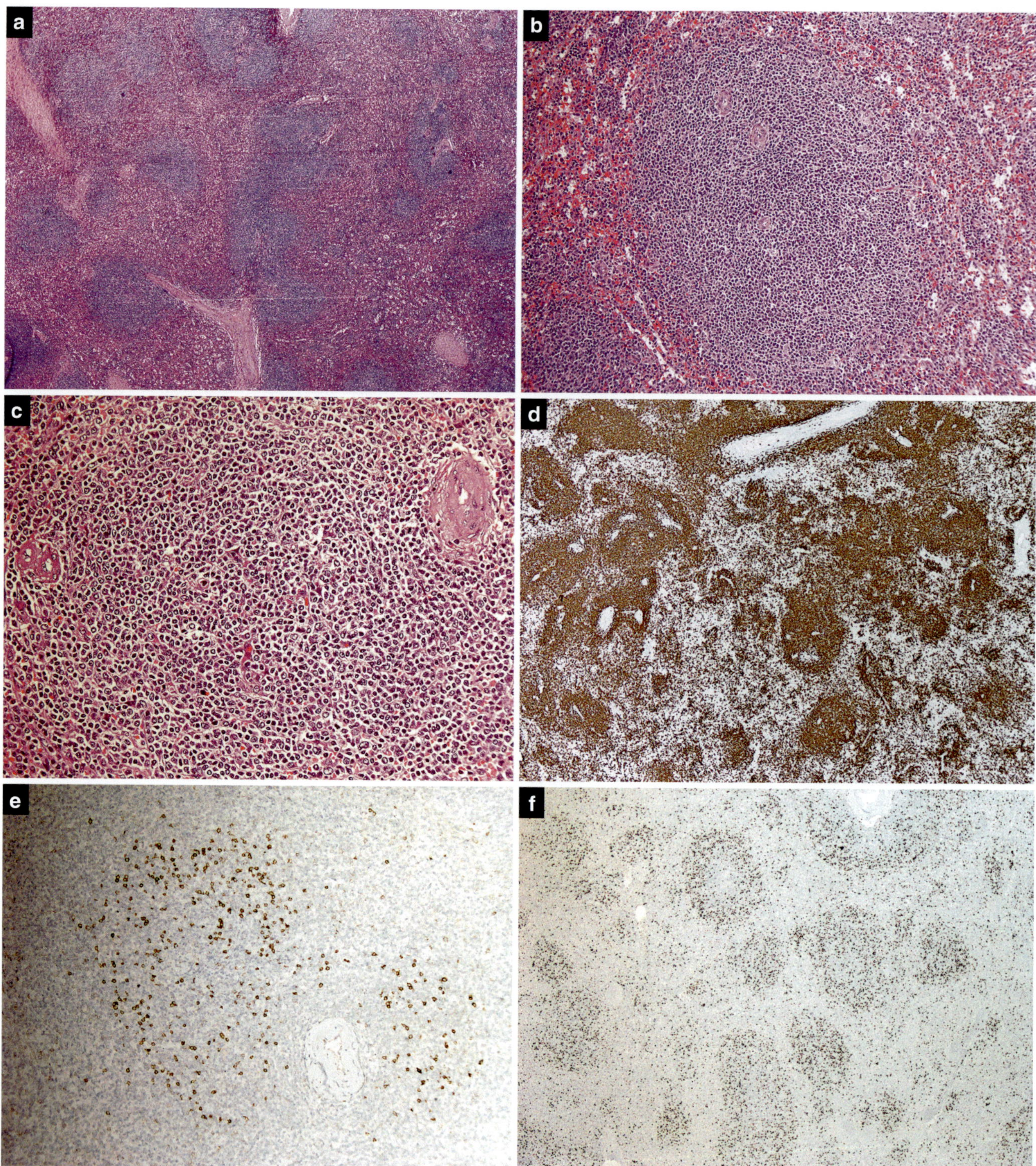

Fig. 5.4 Splenic marginal zone lymphoma in the spleen, monomorphic pattern. Some cases of SMZL do not show the typical biphasic pattern in many follicles, due to replacement of residual germinal centers by mixture of small- and medium-sized marginal zone cells (**a–c**, H&E). The SMZL cells are highlighted by CD20 in the follicles and red pulp (**d**) and are negative for IgD (**e**). Ki-67 (**f**) shows no targetoid pattern in many follicles and highlights the exterior marginal zones in other follicles

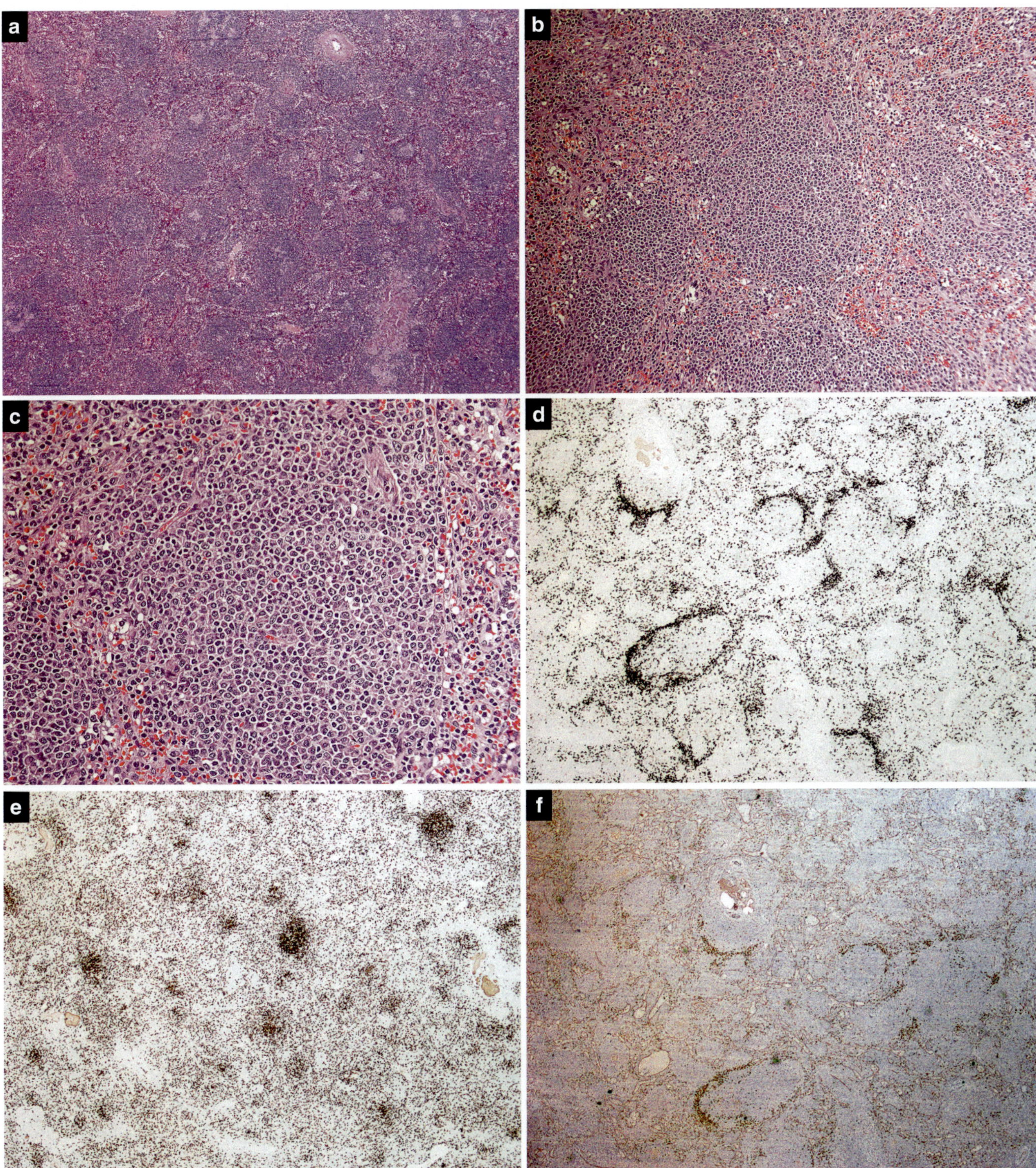

Fig. 5.5 Splenic marginal zone lymphoma with extensive plasmacytic differentiation in the spleen. The spleen shows a nodular infiltrate pattern (**a**, H&E). The nodules are more monomorphic without biphasic pattern (**b**, H&E). The nodules are composed predominantly of plasma cells with few admixed lymphocytes (**c**, H&E). The nodules show thin layers of residual SMZL cells at the periphery that are positive for CD20 (**d**), PAX5 (**f**), and IgD (**g**). The majority of small lymphocytes inside the nodules are CD3-positive T-cells (**e**). Most of the cells in the nodules are plasma cells that are positive for CD79a (**h**) and CD138 (**i**) and show kappa light chain restriction by in situ hybridization for kappa (**j**) and lambda (**k**) light chains. Ki-67 shows low proliferation rate (**l**)

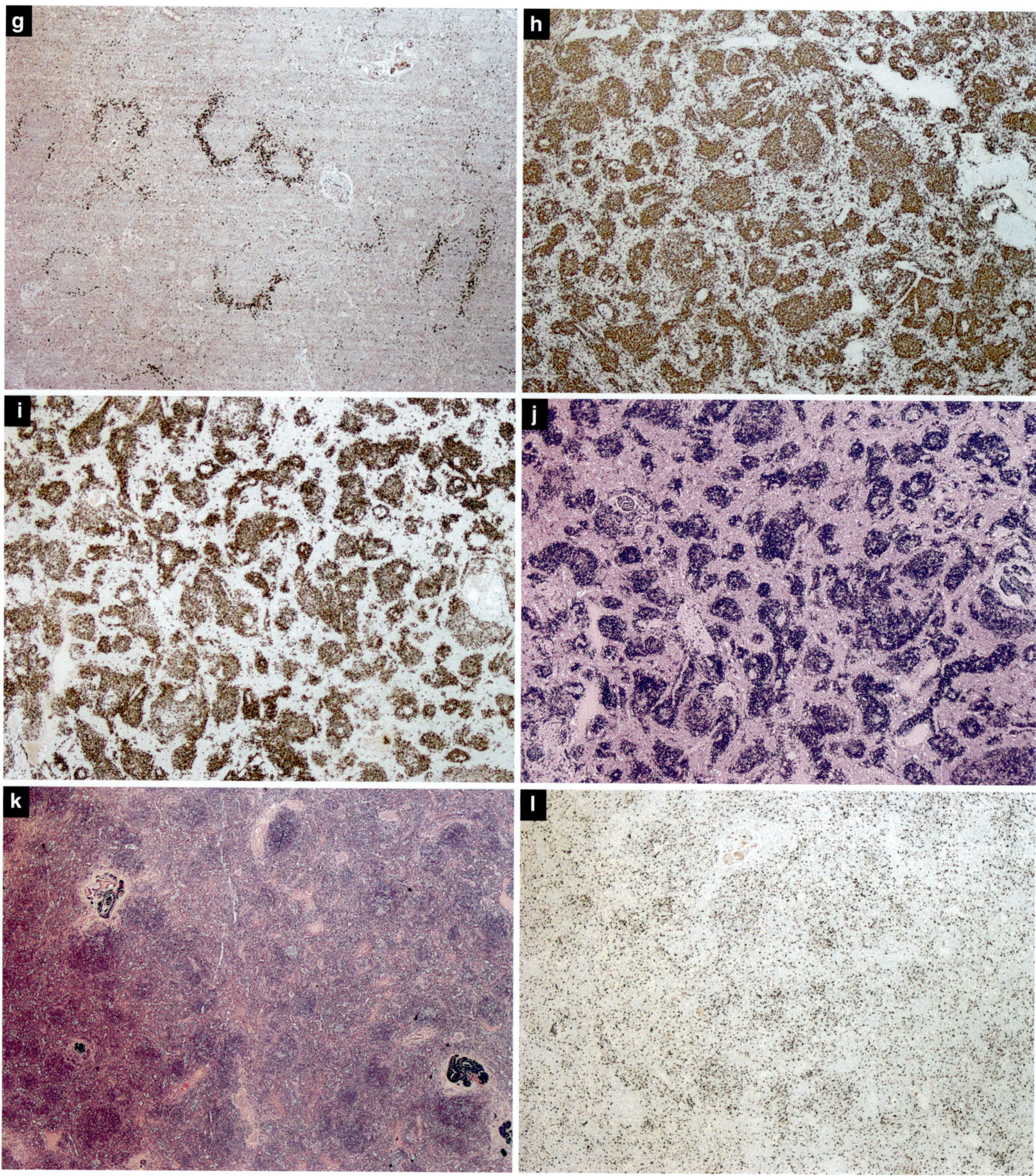

Fig. 5.5 (continued)

for CD10, BCL6, CD43, cyclin D1, CD103, CD123, annexin A1, LEF1, and SOX11 [24, 26, 31–33]. Aberrant expression of CD5 is seen in <20% cases of SMZL and are not uncommon with expression of CD23 and CD11c as well [9, 12, 20, 34, 35]. The CD5$^+$ SMZL tends to show higher lymphocy-tosis at diagnosis and more frequent diffuse bone marrow infiltrate but shows no significant difference in clinical course from CD5$^-$ SMZL [36]. The SMZL cells show dim to nega-tive CD200 by flow cytometry [37, 38]. SMZL has modified Matutes score of <3 points by flow cytometry based on the immunophenotypic analysis of five markers (CD79b, CD5, CD23, FMC7, and surface immunoglobulin) (Table 5.1) [39]. Immunostaining with Ki-67 shows a distinctive targetoid pattern due to increased proliferation rate in the central residual germinal center and exterior marginal zone.

In the absence of splenectomy, the diagnosis of SMZL can be made based on the clinical presentation of splenomegaly and the morphologic findings of peripheral blood and bone marrow biopsy. SMZL cells almost invariably infiltrate bone marrow and are frequently present in peripheral blood (approximately 70% cases) [10, 11, 26, 27, 40–42]. The SMZL cells in the peripheral blood smears show various degree of heterogeneous cytology ranging from unremarkable small mature lymphoid cells to medium-sized plasmacytoid lymphoid cells. A subset of SMZL cells has round nuclei, coarse chromatin, and basophilic cytoplasm with short villi, often at the poles of the cells, which are called "villous lymphocytes" (Fig. 5.6). Large lymphoid cells are rare. SMZLs show various patterns of infiltrate in the bone marrow, most frequently intravascular/intrasinusoidal and nodular patterns (Fig. 5.7) and rarely interstitial, massive, or extensive plasmacytic patterns [43, 44]. The intravascular infiltrate is present in nearly all cases and may be the only pattern, especially in early stage of the disease [43, 45–48]. In the intravascular/intrasinusoidal pattern, the SMZL cells form linear chains in capillaries and/or small clusters in venous sinuses with frequent distention. These SMZL cells are small to intermediate sized with round to oval nuclei, coarse chromatin, and often more abundant cytoplasm. The intravascular infiltrate is very difficult to identify on H&E sections and frequently can only be recognized by immunohistochemistry with anti-CD20 antibody. The intravascular infiltrate is most frequently associated with nodular lymphoid infiltrate. The lymphoid nodules are often homogeneous and may show marginal zone at the periphery. These lymphoid nodules are more commonly intertrabecular but can also be paratrabecular. The interstitial infiltrate is often localized and consists of SMZL cells mixed with hematopoietic cells. The massive infiltrate by sheets of lymphoid cells and plasmacytic infiltrate by monoclonal plasma cells and lymphoplasmacytic cells are rare. The intravascular infiltrate pattern is characteristic, but not specific, of SMZL. The diagnosis of SMZL can be based on the intravascular infiltrate pattern in bone marrow, often associated lymphoid nodules with germinal centers and/or marginal zone, and nonspecific immunophenotype.

The hilar lymph nodes are frequently involved, and peripheral lymph nodes are less frequently involved [32]. The lymph nodes show preserved sinuses mostly in the hilar lymph nodes and nodular lymphoid infiltrate partially or completely effacing the nodal architecture (Fig. 5.8). The lymph nodules generally lack the biphasic pattern and are composed of mixture of the two SMZL cell types: small lymphoid cells and medium marginal zone cells. Residual central germinal centers can be present in some nodules. Focal biphasic pattern may be seen in some cases but is much less prominent than that in the spleen. Scattered large lymphoid cells with nucleoli are present largely at the periphery of the nodules. The SMZL cells are positive for IgD, which allows distinction from most nodal marginal zone lymphomas (NMZL) that are IgD negative. However, a small subset of primary nodal marginal zone lymphomas is of SMZL type with expression of IgD but without splenomegaly [49].

The liver is involved in up to approximately 80% of cases [26, 50, 51]. SMZL shows nodular lymphoid infiltrate in the portal tracts along with sinusoidal infiltrate by SMZL cells (Fig. 5.9). SMZL involvement in nonhematopoietic sites is rare (approximately 6.6%) and is characterized by infiltrate of typical SMZL cells [10].

Approximately 5–19% of SMZL transform to diffuse large B-cell lymphoma during disease progression [10, 18, 19, 52–55]. The transformation can occur within a year to over 10 years after the diagnosis of SMZL. At the time of transformation, the patient usually presents with development of B symptoms, elevated serum lactate dehydrogenase, poor performance status, bulky lymphadenopathy, and dis-

Table 5.1 Modified Matutes scoring system for B-cell lymphoproliferative disorders

Membrane marker	Points	
	0	1
CD79b	Moderate/strong	Weak/negative
CD5	Negative	Positive
CD23	Negative	Positive
FMC7	Positive	Negative
Surface immunoglobulin	Moderate/strong	Weak

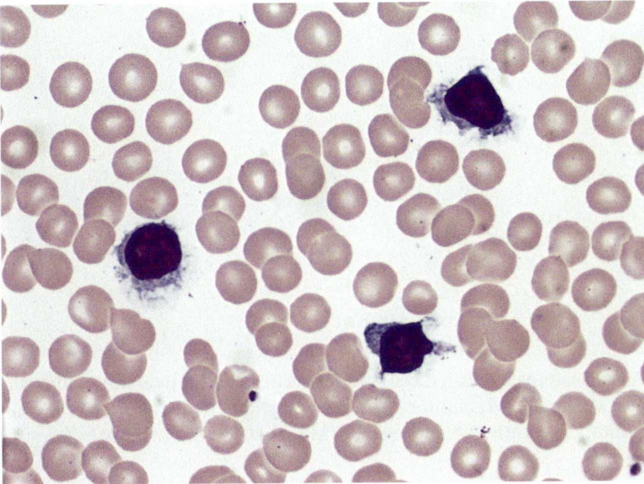

Fig. 5.6 Splenic marginal zone lymphoma in peripheral blood. Circulating SMZL cells as villous lymphocytes show round nuclei, coarse chromatin, and pale basophilic cytoplasm with short villi (Giemsa, ×1000)

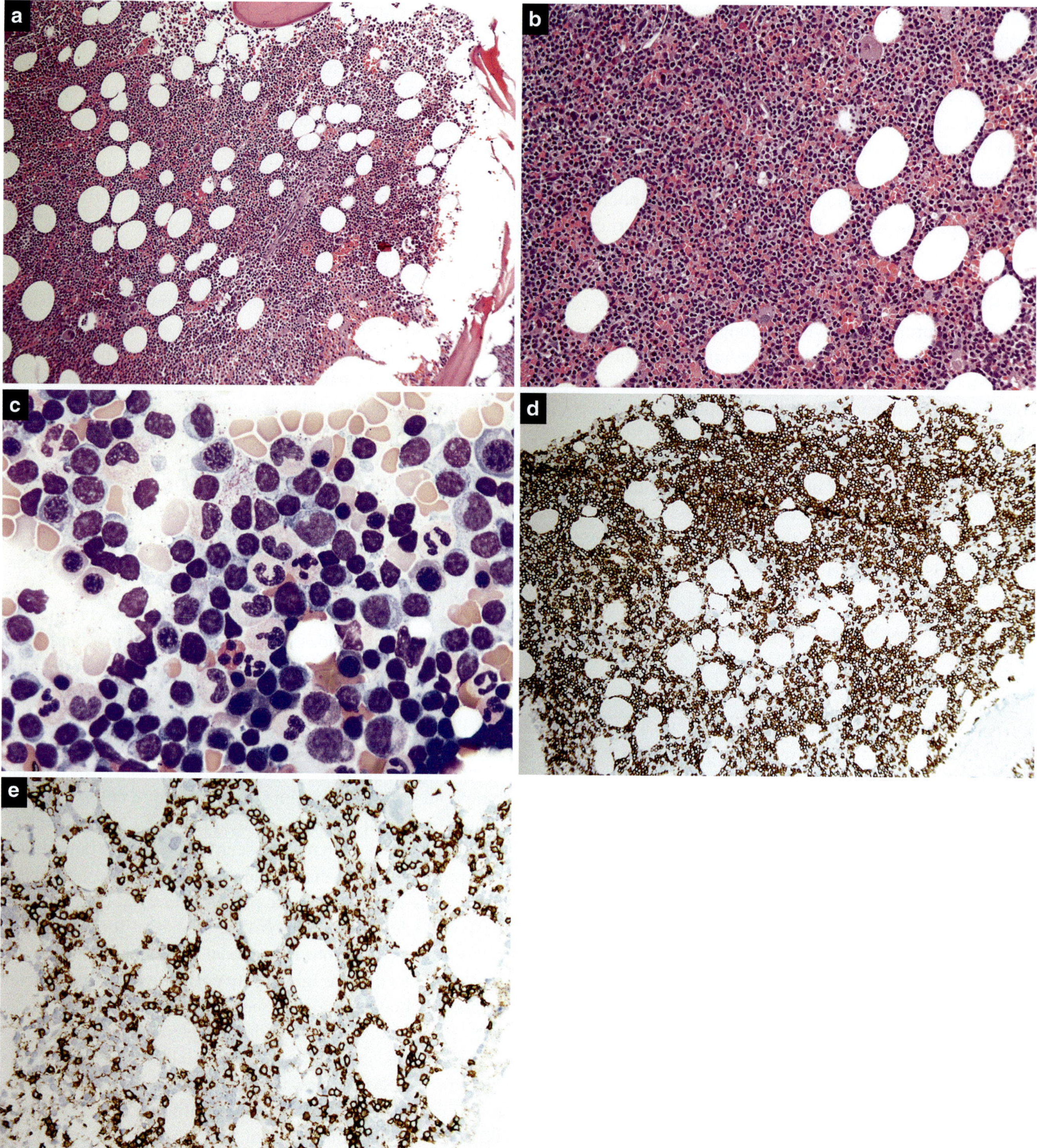

Fig. 5.7 Splenic marginal zone lymphoma in bone marrow. SMZL shows diffuse infiltrate in the bone marrow (**a**, H&E) by small mature lymphoid cells (**b**, H&E). Aspirate smear shows small lymphoid cells with round nuclei, mature chromatin, and variable cytoplasm (**c**, Wright-Giemsa Stain). CD20 highlights diffuse and interstitial infiltrate by SMZL cells (**d**) and focally characteristic intravascular/intrasinusoidal infiltrate with linear arrays of SMZL cells in the capillaries (**e**)

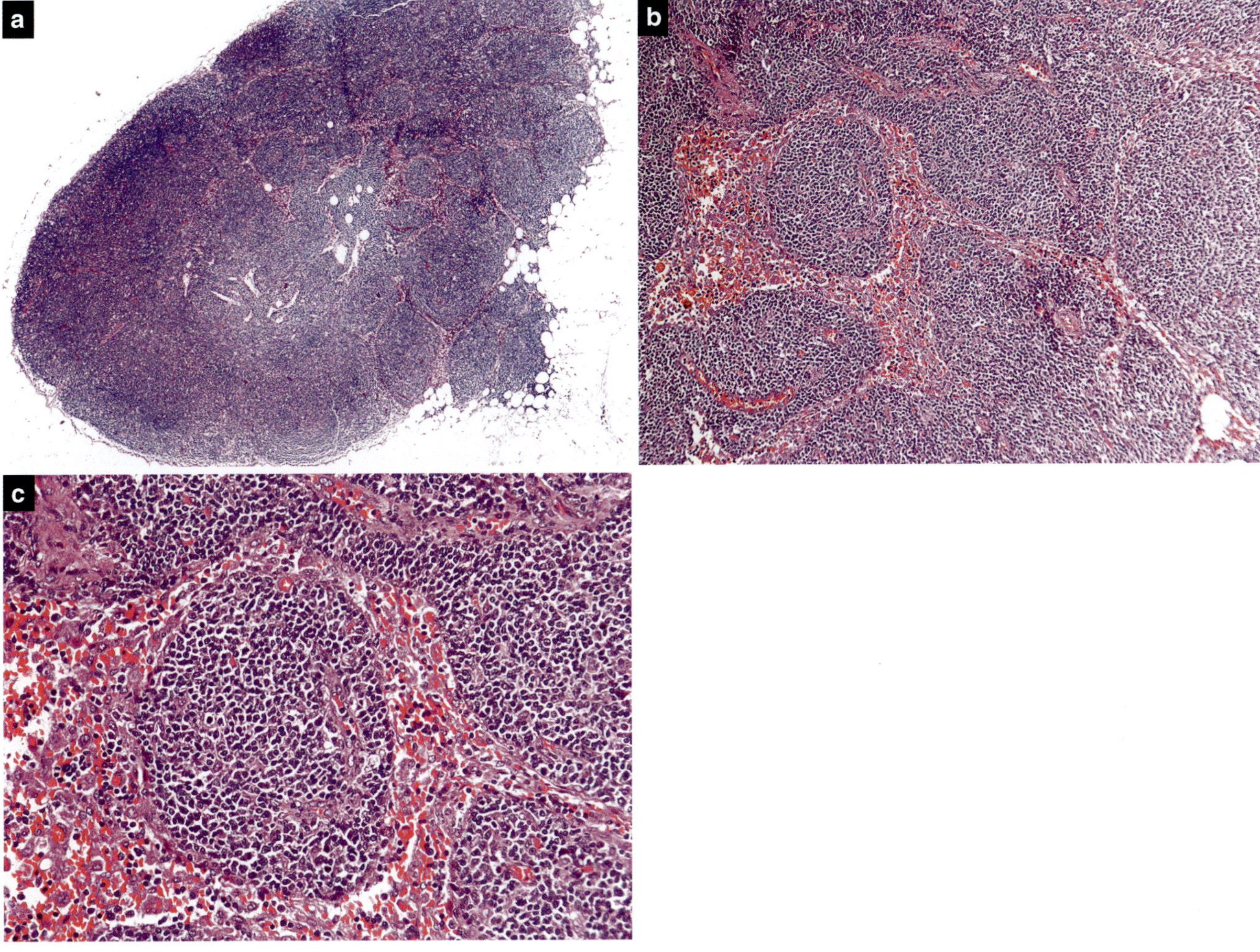

Fig. 5.8 Splenic marginal zone lymphoma in hilar lymph nodes. The hilar lymph node involved by SMZL shows a micronodular pattern (**a**, H&E). The lymphoid nodules lack biphasic pattern with preservation or dilation of sinuses (**b**, H&E). The SMZL cells in the hilar lymph node are more monomorphic and composed of small, round nuclei, coarse chromatin, and scant cytoplasm and no significant marginal zone differentiation (**c**)

seminated disease in extranodal sites. The most frequent sites of transformation are peripheral lymph nodes and bone marrow. Diffuse large B-cell lymphoma can also develop in the spleen and the central nervous system [56]. Blastic transformation with leukemic infiltrate of peripheral blood and bone marrow by blastoid lymphoid cells is reported in rare cases [57, 58]. Transformation to classic Hodgkin lymphoma occurs in occasional cases of SMZL [54].

Cytogenetics and Molecular Studies

SMZL is genetically heterogeneous. Cytogenetic abnormalities are present in approximately 70–80% cases, in which single cytogenetic aberration, two cytogenetic aberrations, and complex karyotypes are seen in approximately 30%, 20%, and 50% cases, respectively [12, 59]. The chromosomes most frequently involved in order of frequency are 7, 3, 1, 8, 6, 12, and 14. Chromosomal gains are more common than losses. The most frequent numerical aberrations are gains of chromosome 3/3q (approximately 20–30%), trisomy 18 (approximately 10%), and trisomy 12 (approximately 15–20%). The most frequent structural aberration is deletion 7q (about 40% of cases). The deletion breakpoints at 7q are heterogeneous with 7q22 as the most recurrent breakpoint followed by 7q32 [59–65]. Comparative genomic hybridization (CGH) shows additional chromosomal aberrations: gains involved 5q, 12q, 20q, 9q (21%),

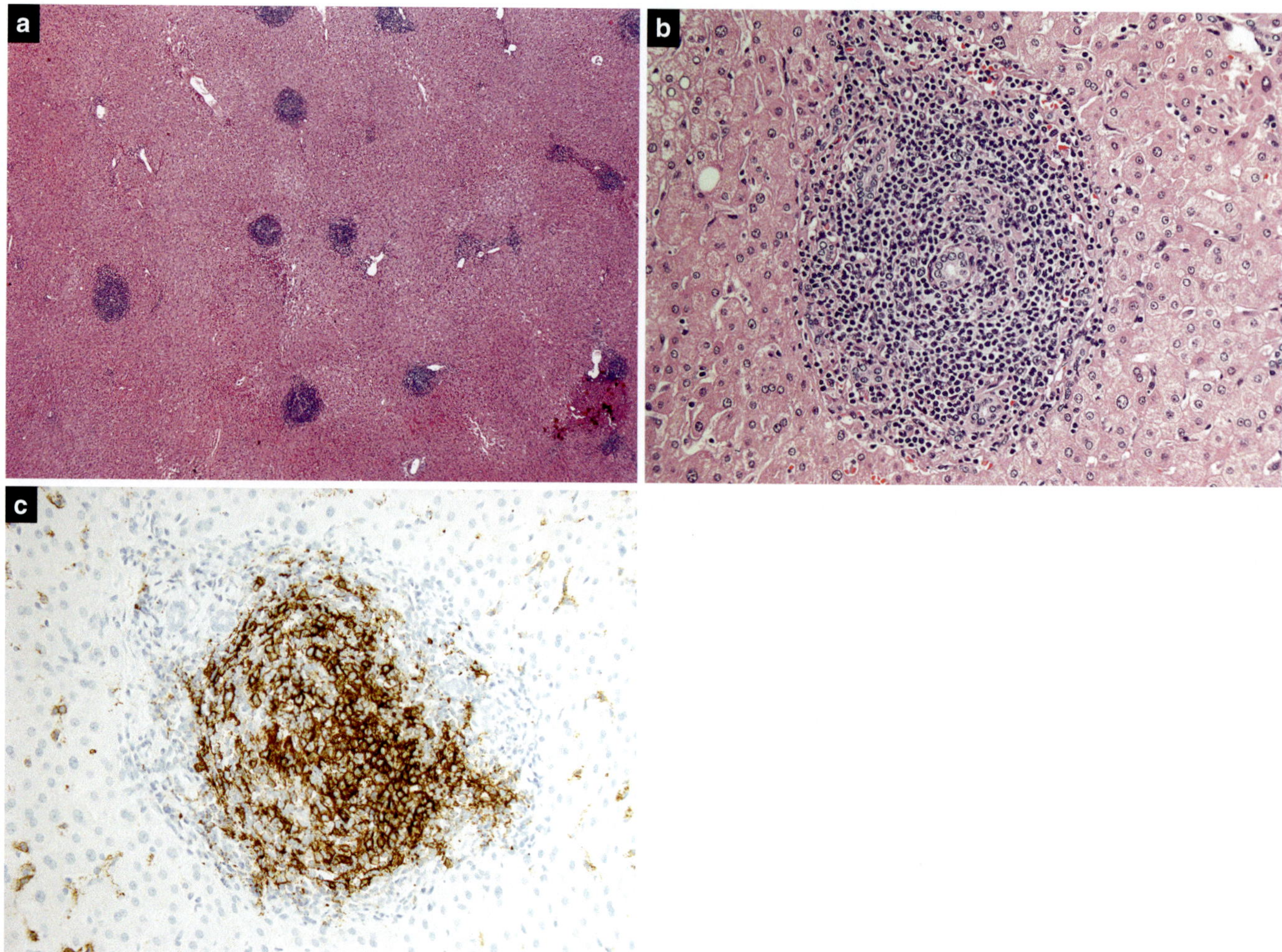

Fig. 5.9 Splenic marginal zone lymphoma in the liver. SMZL shows nodular lymphoid infiltrate in the liver (**a**, H&E). The lymphoid nodules are localized in the portal tracts and are composed of small mature lymphoid cells (**b**). CD20 highlights SMZL cells in the portal tracts and only few SMZL cells in the sinusoids in this case (**c**)

and 4q and losses 17p (10%) in addition to the common ones identified by karyotyping [62, 66, 67]. There are no recurrent chromosomal translocations in SMZL. t(11;14) (q13;q32) of mantle cell lymphoma, t(14;18)(q32;q21) of follicular lymphoma, and translocations associated with marginal zone lymphoma of mucosa-associated lymphoid tissue (MALT lymphoma) such as t(11;18)(q21;q21), t(1;14)(p22;q32), t(14;18)(q32;q21), and t(3;14)(p14;q32) are absent in SMZL. Approximately 7–15% of SMZL has immunoglobulin (*IG*) translocations, with the vast majority involving immunoglobulin heavy chain gene locus (*IGH*) at chromosome 14q and a small minority involving immunoglobulin kappa (*IGK*) or lambda (*IGL*) light chain gene loci at chromosomes 2p and 22q [59, 68]. Most of these translocations occur in complex karyotypes with the majority showing 3–5 aberrations. In approximately half of the cases, the *IG* translocation partner cannot be identified. A number of the translocations partners have been identified including *PAX5*, *BCL6*, *BCL3*, *CDK6*, *CCND3*, and *IRF4/ MUM1* in t(9;14)(p13;q32), t(3;14)(q27;q32), t(14;19) (q32;q13), t(2;7)(p11–p12;q22), t(6;14)(p21;q32), and t(6;14)(p25;q32) [59, 61, 69–77]. Small numbers of SMZL cases show other breakpoints including 1p22, 1p34, 1q21, 1q32, 3p13, 3q13, 4p13, 6p12, 9p11, 9p13, 10q24, 11q21, 11q23, 12q24, 13p11, and 19p13 [19, 59, 61, 64, 69, 73, 78–81].

SMZL shows clonal *IG* heavy and light chain gene rearrangements. The most frequent *IGHV* gene is *IGHV1-2* (approximately 30%), followed by *IGHV4-34* and *IGHV3-23* (approximately 10% each). Cases with *IGHV1–2* show significantly more frequent 7q deletions, alterations at 14q, and abnormal karyotypes. *IGHV* genes are mutated in approximately 60% of the cases, and there are no significant differences in the clinical features between cases with mutated and unmutated *IGHV* genes [59, 82, 83]. SMZL displays a largely homogeneous gene expression signature with deregulated genes involved in B-cell receptor (BCR) signaling, tumor necrosis factor (TNF) signaling and nuclear factor-kappa B (NF-κB) activation, and upregulation of genes involved in marginal zone differentiation, such as *Notch2* [84–86]. The miRNA expression profile of SMZL reflects normal marginal zone and memory B-cells, and the microRNAs target genes involved in B-cell pathways such as NF-κB and CD40 signaling pathways, interleukins, inflammatory pathways, and memory B-cell-related pathways [86].

Whole genome/exome sequencing studies identified recurrent mutations in genes required for marginal zone B-cell development, such as NOTCH, NF-κB, B-cell receptor, and Toll-like receptor signaling, and chromatin remodeling and transcriptional regulation in ~60% cases of SMZL. Recurrent gain-of-function mutations in *NOTCH2* are identified in approximately 10–25% cases of SMZL [87–91]. The mutations in *NOTCH2* lead to elimination or truncation of the C-terminal PEST domain, which is required for proteasomal recruitment, and impaired degradation of the NOTCH2 protein. *NOTCH2* mutations are essentially restricted to SMZL and not present in other B-cell lymphomas, such as CLL/SLL, mantle cell lymphoma, follicular lymphoma, and hairy cell leukemia, and only rarely in extranodal marginal zone lymphoma and diffuse large B-cell lymphomas [87, 89, 92]. Therefore, *NOTCH2* mutations can be helpful to confirm the diagnosis of SMZL in challenging cases.

Recurrent inactivating mutations in Krüppel-like factor 2 (*KLF2*) zinc-finger gene are identified in approximately 20–40% cases of SMZL [91, 93, 94]. The mutations inactivate the suppression of NF-κB activation by KLF2. *NOTCH2* and *KLF2* mutations are not mutually exclusive. IGHV1–2 rearrangement and del(7q) are present mostly in SMZL with *KLF2* mutation. *MYD88* and *TP53* mutations are nearly exclusively seen in SMZL without *KLF2* mutation. Recurrent *KLF2* mutations are not specific for SMZL and are also present infrequently (3–16%) in other low-grade B-cell lymphomas, including nodal and extranodal marginal zone lymphomas. *MYD88* L265P mutation, which is highly specific for lymphoplasmacytic lymphoma, is identified in up to 15% cases of SMZL [88, 90, 95–97].

Cell of Origin/Normal Counterpart

SMZL is considered to arise from marginal zone B-cells in secondary lymphoid follicles [1]. There are two types of SMZLs based on cell or origin. Approximately two thirds of SMZLs originate from post-germinal center marginal zone memory B-cells that show somatic mutation in immunoglobulin heavy chain variable (V$_H$) genes, while about one third of cases originate from naïve marginal zone B-cells without antigen stimulation and with unmutated V$_H$

gene [98]. The expression of both IgD and IgM in most cases of SMZL, low frequency of somatic mutation in cases with mutated V$_H$ genes, and very low frequency of *BCL6* mutations suggest that SMZLs originate from marginal zone B-cell subset involved in T-cell-independent antigen response distinct from classic germinal center-derived memory B-cells [99, 100].

Differential Diagnoses

The diagnosis of SMZL requires integration of clinical, histologic, immunophenotypic, and genetic findings and exclusion of some reactive lymphoid hyperplasia and other small B-cell lymphomas involving the spleen primarily or secondarily.

Splenic Marginal Zone Hyperplasia

Splenic marginal zone hyperplasia may be associated with autoimmune disorders such as systemic lupus erythematosus, immune thrombocytopenic purpura, or other chronic autoimmune disorders [101]. In splenic marginal zone hyperplasia, the spleen shows no or only mild splenomegaly, and the white pulp lymphoid nodules show no or minimal expansion. Unlike in most lymph nodes, the normal lymphoid follicles in the spleen typically show distinct marginal zones. In splenic marginal zone hyperplasia, the marginal zones are expanded, and its hyperplasia has been arbitrarily defined as marginal zone layers over 12 cells in thickness [102–104]. There is no increase of B-cells in the red pulp, and the marginal zone B-cells are negative for IgD. The presence of clusters of B-cells in the red pulp, IgD$^+$, and presence of clonal plasma cells by immunohistochemistry are consistent with SMZL. Splenic marginal zone hyperplasia can be indistinguishable from early SMZL by morphology [105, 106]. These rare cases of early SMZL are often found incidentally and without splenomegaly. The diagnosis of these early SMZLs is only possible through flow cytometric analysis or polymerase chain reaction (PCR) study for clonal B-cell gene rearrangement.

Persistent Polyclonal B-Cell Lymphocytosis (PPBL)

Persistent polyclonal B-cell lymphocytosis (PPBL), also called "polyclonal B-cell lymphocytosis with binucleated lymphocytes," is a rare hematological disorder of uncertain cause predominantly in young to middle-aged female smokers [107]. PPBL is characterized by persistent mild to moderate polyclonal B-cell lymphocytosis and elevated polyclonal serum IgM. Mild splenomegaly is the most common clinical finding and present in approximately 10% of patients [108], but massive splenomegaly is occasionally seen [109, 110]. The hallmark feature of PPBL is the presence of variable numbers of binucleated small mature lymphocytes with two round or ovoid nuclei and moderately abundant basophilic cytoplasm on peripheral blood smears. Patients with PPBL have an indolent clinical course, but PPBL resembles lymphoma in many aspects, including morphology in the spleen and bone marrow and frequent cytogenetic and molecular abnormalities. PPBL shows genetic predisposition with close association with HLA-DR7 allele [111]. Multiple t(14;18) translocations are detected by PCR in all patients with PPBL and an isochromosome 3q+, i[3](q10), is present in a variable proportion of the B-cells [112–114]. The involved spleen shows histologic features resembling SMZL, including white pulp expansion by lymphoid follicles, enlargement of the marginal zone areas of the follicles, biphasic pattern, and infiltrate of the red pulp sinuses [115]. Some cases show white pulp expansion by lymphoid nodules without apparent marginal zones but with massive red pulp infiltrate, simulating low-grade B-cell lymphoma other than SMZL [110]. The hilar lymph nodes show follicular hyperplasia with reactive germinal centers and sinus histiocytosis. The bone marrow shows intrasinusoidal infiltrate by B-cells in chains or small clusters [115, 116]. The B-cells are positive for CD20 and BCL2 and negative for CD5, CD10, CD23, and cyclin D1. The B-cells are CD27$^+$, IgM$^+$, and IgD $^+$ memory B-cells. So the histologic features in the spleen and bone marrow closely resemble SMZL. However, the B-cells do not show monotypic surface light chain restriction by flow cytometry or clonal immunoglobulin gene rearrangement by molecular analysis. Therefore, close attention to the clinical presentation, evaluation of the peripheral blood smear for the characteristic binucleated lymphocytes, and flow cytometric and/or molecular analysis for B-cell clonality are essential to differentiate between PPBL and SMZL in difficult cases.

Other Small B-Cell Lymphomas

The malignant lymphomas in the differential diagnosis of SMZL include hairy cell leukemia (HCL), hairy cell leukemia variant (HCL-v), splenic diffuse red pulp small B-cell lymphoma (SDRPBCL), chronic lymphocytic leukemia/small lymphocytic lymphoma (CLL/SLL), mantle cell lymphoma (MCL), follicular lymphoma (FL), lymphoplasmacytic lymphoma (LPL), and nodal marginal zone lymphoma (NMZL) and MALT lymphoma. A micronodular pattern and marginal zone differentiation are frequently present in FL and MCL and lesser frequency in CLL/SLL and LPL [117]. Occasional lymphoid cells of these small B-cell lymphomas may have hairy cytoplasmic projections in the peripheral blood.

Like SMZL, both CLL/SLL and MCL show expansion of white pulp by nodular lymphoid infiltrate and red pulp infiltrate in the spleen. MCL may show intrasinusoidal/intravascular infiltrate in the bone marrow biopsy [118]. CLL/SLL and MCL are especially important to differenti-ate from CD5$^+$ SMZL. In splenectomy specimen, the pattern of lymphoid nodules and cellular composition are different. SMZL shows biphasic pattern with expansion of marginal zones, and the SMZL cells include small mature lymphocytes, marginal zones, and admixed large transformed lymphoid cells. CLL/SLL shows lymphoid nodules composed of monotonous small mature lymphoid cells with dense chromatin and scattered prolymphocytes and paraimmunoblasts. Proliferation centers may be seen. MCL shows lymphoid follicles with either expanded mantle zones or homogeneous lymphoid nodules composed of monotonous population of MCL cells. Immunohistochemistry is required for the differential diagnosis. CD5$^+$ SMZL is often positive for CD23, but they are negative for LEF1, while CLL/SLL cells are positive for LEF1 [27, 119]. The differential diagnosis of CLL and CD5$^+$ SMZL can be easily resolved by flow cytometry analysis. In modified Matutes scoring system based on expression of CD5, CD23, FMC7, CD79a, and surface IgM, a score of 4 or 5 is consistent with CLL/SLL, while SMZL is associated with a score of <3 points [39]. In the new CLL flow scoring system based on expression of CD5, CD23, FMC7, CD79a, and CD200, a CLL flow score is calculated as %CD200$^+$ + %CD5/CD23$^+$ − %CD79b$^+$ − %FMC7$^+$. A score higher than zero correlates with the diagnosis of CLL, and SMZL is associated with a score of zero or below [120]. MCL is usually excluded by negative cyclin D1 and SOX11 and absence of t(11;14) by fluorescence in situ hybridization (FISH) analysis.

Unlike SMZL, FL shows fairly restricted white pulp infiltrate in the spleen [121]. The FL cells may be present in the red pulp in small numbers. The white pulp may show closely packed neoplastic follicles or scattered neoplastic follicles. The FL follicles show mixture of centrocytes and centroblasts in various numbers depending on the grade. Reactive germinal centers are absent. The SMZL cells may show irregular nuclei resembling FL cells, and the SMZL lymphoid nodules may appear more homogeneous. The absence of expression of germinal center markers (CD10 and BCL6) and/or absence of t(14;18)(q32;q21) or *IGH@-BCL2* rearrangement by FISH analysis exclude the diagnosis of FL. The intrasinusoidal infiltrate by SMZL cells can be easily distinguished from the characteristic paratrabecular lymphoid nodules in bone marrow infiltrated by FL.

LPL is a major differential diagnosis of SMZL with plasmacytic differentiation. Like SMZL, the LPL cells also show nonspecific phenotype. In contrast to SMZL, LPL is characterized by predominantly red pulp infiltrate with relative sparing of the white pulp. LPL shows more prominent plasmacytic differentiation and many plasma cells compared with SMZL. The bone marrow involvement by LPL is characterized by nodular, diffuse, and/or interstitial lymphoid infiltrate, which is distinct from the intravascular infiltrate by SMZL cells. Clinically, LPL shows higher level of IgM paraproteinemia and milder splenomegaly. The *MYD88* L265P somatic point mutation is present in >90% of LPL and rarely seen in SMZL. The diagnosis is often straightforward based on evaluation of the clinical and morphologic features in the spleen and bone marrow. Molecular study for *MYD88* L265P is reserved for challenging cases.

While the presence of hairy bipolar cells and massive splenomegaly in SMZL resemble HCL and HCL-v, the differential diagnosis is usually straightforward based on histology in the spleen and difference in immunophenotype. Unlike SMZL, HCL demonstrates diffuse infiltrate in the red pulp and frequently associated red cell lakes composed of extravasated red blood cells. The white pulps are atrophic. The bone marrow involvement by HCL is characterized by interstitial and patchy infiltrate with relative preservation of the fat and hematopoietic cells and increased reticulin fibrosis. The HCL cells in both spleen and bone marrow sections show fried egg appearance due to abundant cytoplasm. On peripheral blood and bone marrow aspirate smears, the HCL cells display abundant cytoplasm with circumferential hairy projections and often dumbbell-shaped nuclei with ground glass-appearing chromatin, in contrast to the more common bipolar villi and more condensed chromatin of SMZL cells. The HCL cells are positive for CD103, CD25, strong CD11c, and CD123 by flow cytometry and positive for tartrate-resistant acid phosphatase (TRAP), DBA.44, and annexin A1 by immunohistochemistry. SMZL cells are consistently negative for CD103, TRAP, and annexin A1. *BRAF* V600E mutation is characteristically present in HCL and absent in HCL-v and SMZL. HCL-v shows the same morphologic features in the spleen as HCL with diffuse red pulp infiltrate and atrophic white pulp. HCL-v display intrasinusoidal infiltrate in the bone marrow, similar to SMZL. But HCL-v cells are positive for CD103 and negative for CD25 by flow cytometry.

SDRPBCL may be indistinguishable from SMZL without evaluation of splenectomy specimen due to overlapping cytologic, histologic, and immunophenotypic features [44]. SDRPBCL is characterized clinically by massive splenomegaly and relative low atypical lymphocytosis. Similar to SMZL, the peripheral blood shows the presence of villous lymphocytes, and SDRPBCL cells infiltrate the bone marrow invariably in intrasinusoidal pattern, often accompanied by interstitial and nodular infiltrate. The SDRPBCL cells are monomorphic small to medium sized with round to mildly irregular nuclei, coarse chromatin, inconspicuous nucleoli, and scant to moderate pale cytoplasm. The immunophenotypic profile of SDRPBCL and SMZL is nearly identical and nonspecific. The SDRPBCL cells are mostly positive for DBA.44 and negative for HCL markers such as CD103, CD25, CD11c, and annexin A1. Most cases are negative for IgD, so expression of IgD would favor IgD⁺ SMZL. The definitive differential diagnosis of SDRPBCL and SMZL can only be made on histologic evaluation of the spleen. In contrast to SMZL, SDRPBCL shows a diffuse pattern in the red pulp with both cord and sinusoidal infiltrate and atrophic white pulp. The proliferation rate by Ki-67 immunostain is uniformly low. The distinction is not essential as the treatment approaches are not different between SMZL and SDRPBCL [122].

Nodal marginal zone lymphoma (NMZL) and extranodal marginal zone lymphoma of mucosa-associated lymphoid tissue (MALT) may rarely involve the spleen with nodular infiltrate in the white pulp and expansion of marginal zones. In contrast to SMZL, MALT lymphoma is typically negative for IgD, but a subset of NMZL is splenic type with expression of IgD. The t(11;18)(q21;q21) in MALT lymphoma, IgD expression in SMZL, 7q abnormalities in SMZL, and expression of IRTA1 in NMZL [123] are useful features for the differential diagnosis. Ultimately, correlation of clinical and pathologic features is essential for the correct diagnosis.

Clinical Course and Prognostic Factors

The majority of patients with SMZL show an indolent clinical course with median overall survival (OS) of approximately 10 years and >60% patients alive at 5 years [3, 9, 10, 13, 18, 20, 21, 122, 124]. For the conventional type, a "watch-and-wait" approach is enough. Approximately one third of patients have an aggressive course with a median survival of 1.4 years [10], and treatments such as splenectomy or chemotherapy and/or rituximab are required. As most cases of SMZL have bone marrow and/or peripheral blood involvement, the international prognostic index (IPI) designed for diffuse large B-cell lymphoma, and Ann Arbor staging system cannot be used to stratify patients with SMZL for appropriate management.

A number of clinical features are associated with shorter survival including advanced age, anemia, leukocytosis, lymphopenia, lymphocytosis, thrombocytopenia, high lactate dehydrogenase level, performance status >2, monoclonal component, high β2-microglobulin level, extrahilar lymphadenopathy, use of chemotherapy, lack of response to therapy, diffuse bone marrow involvement, and histologic transformation [9, 15, 18, 52, 125]. Genetic and molecular features, such as del(7q), unmutated *IgVH*, *NOTCH2*, and *TP53* gene mutations, and expression of NF-κB pathway genes, including *TRAF5*, *REL*, and *PKCA*, are also associated with worse survival [59, 82, 84, 91, 126, 127]. The presence of high proliferation index and del(7q) may be associated with disease progression.

Currently, there are two prognostic indices specific for patients with SMZL: the Integruppo Italiano Linfomi (IIL) prognostic index and Hemoglobin-Platelet-LDH-extrahilar-Lymphadenopathy (HPLL) score. In the IIL prognostic index, three factors (hemoglobin <12 g/dL, elevated serum lactate dehydrogenase (LDH) level, and albumin <3.5 g/dL) are predictive of shorter cause-specific survival (CSS) [21]. With these three factors, patients with SMZL are grouped into three prognostic categories: low risk, intermediate risk, and high risk with 0, 1, and 2–3 factors, respectively. Patients of low-risk, intermediate-risk, and high-risk groups have five-year CSS rate of 88%, 73%, and 50%, respectively. Approximately half of the lymphoma-related deaths occur in the high-risk group. The validity of the IIL prognostic index has been confirmed in a number of studies [122, 125, 128].

In the HPLL score developed by the SMZL Study Group (SMZLSG), four factors (hemoglobin<9.5 g/dL, platelets <80 × 10⁹/L, LDH > normal, extrahilar lymphadenopathy) are independently associated with lymphoma-specific survival (LSS) [125]. With these four factors, a prognostic index (PI) is calculated as 0.02 × hemoglobin (g/L) + 0.006 × platelet count (10⁹/L) – 1 × LDH (1 when high, 0 when normal) – 1 × extrahilar lymphadenopathy (1 when present, 0 when absent). Patients with SMZL are stratified into three, risk groups: group A (low risk) with PI ≥2.6, group B (intermediate risk) with PI ≥0.9 and <2.6, and group C (high risk) with PI <0.9. Patients with HPLLA, HPLLB, and HPLLC have five-year CSS of 94–96%, 78–88%, and 69–44%, respectively. Compared with the IIL index, the HPLL score shows better discriminative power in patients with low and intermediate risks and appears to be the most appropriate score for SMZL.

Other Small B-Cell Lymphomas

Introduction

The spleen is a common site of involvement by small B-cell lymphomas. This section focuses on chronic lymphocytic leukemia/small lymphocytic lymphoma (CLL/SLL), mantle cell lymphoma (MCL), follicular lymphoma (FL), lymphoplasmacytic lymphoma (LPL), and non-splenic marginal zone lymphomas. Hairy cell leukemia, hairy cell leukemia variant, and splenic diffuse red pulp small B-cell lymphoma are discussed separately in Chap. 4 in this book. These small B-cell lymphomas most frequently involve the spleen secondarily as part of systemic disease [129, 130]. The spleen is typically enlarged, but approximately one third of involved spleens are non-palpable [131]. In contrast, primary splenic small B-cell lymphomas confined to the spleen and hilar lymph nodes are rare, accounting for <1% of lymphomas [117, 132–140]. The primary splenic small B-cell lympho-

mas present with prominent splenomegaly clinically. There are essentially no differences in the gross and histologic findings of primary and secondary splenic small B-cell lymphomas. With the exception of LPL, the small B-cell lymphomas typically show nodular growth pattern in the white pulp with variable red pulp infiltrate. The morphologic features in the white pulp nodules of the spleen are often similar to those in the lymph nodes involved by the same type of lymphoma. In diagnostic challenging cases due to ambiguous morphology in the spleen, evaluation of the hilar lymph node is important for the diagnosis, as the characteristic morphologic features are more often seen in the hilar lymph nodes.

Chronic Lymphocytic Leukemia/Small Lymphocytic Lymphoma

CLL/SLL is a small mature B-cell lymphoma that coexpresses CD5 and CD23 and affects mostly elderly patients (>70 years). It is the most common leukemia/lymphoma in the western countries. Clinically, it shows peripheral absolute lymphocytosis (monoclonal B-cell >5 × 10⁹/L) or generalized lymphadenopathy or both. It frequently involves the spleen.

Morphology

The spleen shows prominent white pulp nodules in a miliary pattern grossly [137]. Histologically, CLL/SLL show white pulp expansion and invariably red pulp infiltrate (Fig. 5.10). The white pulp areas are expanded by small mature lymphoid cells with round nuclei, densely clumped chromatin, and scant cytoplasm, admixed with prolymphocytes and/or paraimmunoblasts with central nucleoli. Proliferation centers composed of clusters of prolymphocytes and paraimmunoblasts are uncommon. The nuclear contours of CLL/SLL cells can be irregular in some cases. The red pulps are infiltrated by the same types of lymphoid cells in nodular, nodular and diffuse, or diffuse patterns. Reactive germinal centers are rarely seen in the lymphoid infiltrate, and marginal zones are generally absent. The CLL/SLL cells may show prominent infiltrate of trabecular vessels.

Immunophenotyping

Phenotypically, the CLL/SLL cells are characteristically positive for CD5 and CD23 and show expression of CD200, dim expression of CD20 and CD22, and dim to negative expression of FMC7 by flow cytometry. The modified Matutes score of 4 or CLL flow score >0 is highly specific for the diagnosis of CLL/SLL by flow cytometric analysis with a panel of markers including CD19, CD79b, CD5,

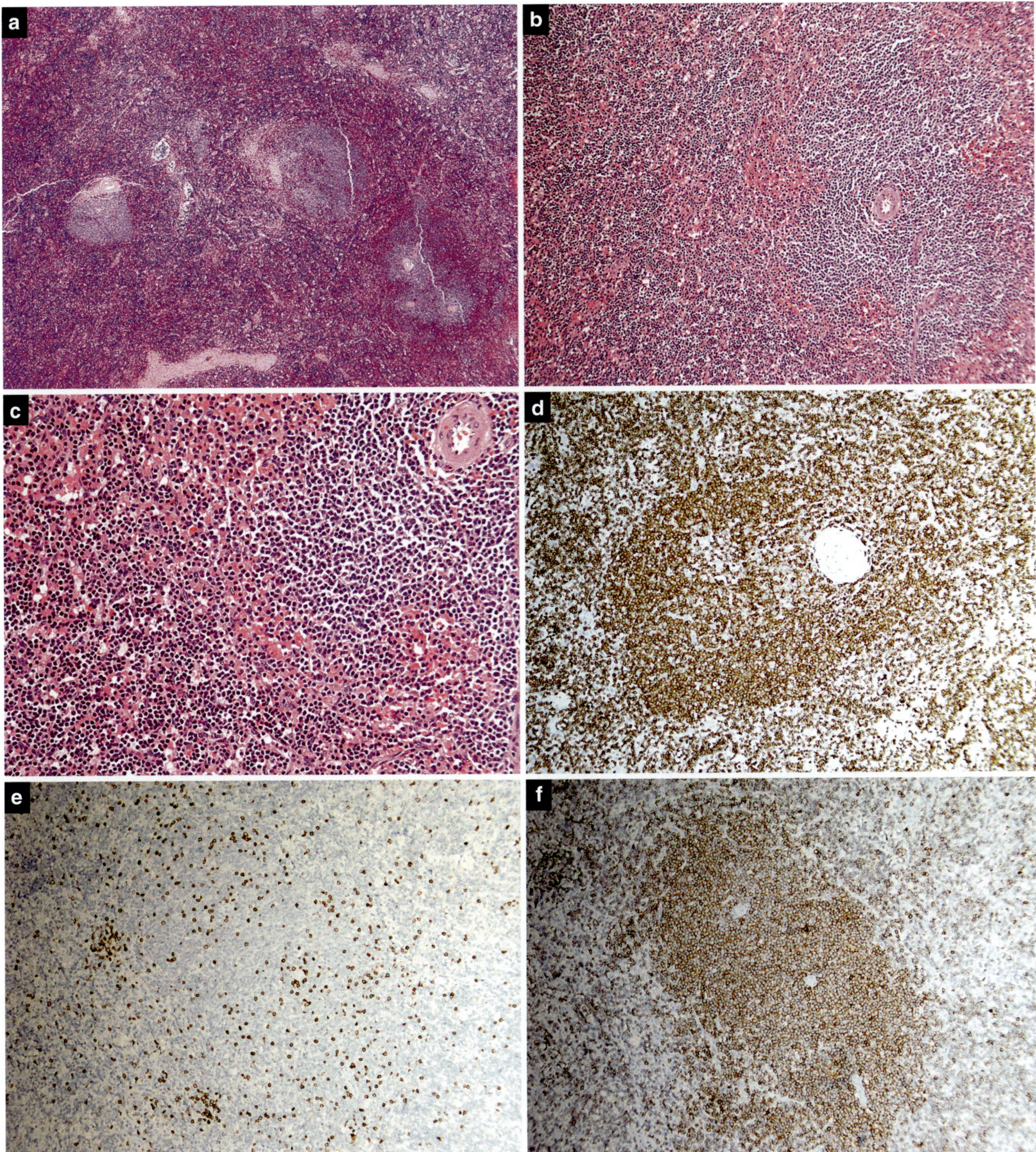

Fig. 5.10 Chronic lymphocytic leukemia/small lymphocytic lymphoma in the spleen. CLL/SLL in the spleen shows lymphoid nodules in the white pulp (**a**, H&E) and also marked diffuse infiltrate of the red pulp (**b**, H&E). The CLL/SLL cells are monotonous and composed of small mature lymphoid cells with round nuclei, coarse chromatin, and scant cytoplasm (**c**, H&E). The CLL/SLL cells are positive for B-cell markers CD79a (**d**), CD5 (**f**), CD23 (**g**), and LEF1 (**h**). CD3 shows background T-cells (**e**)

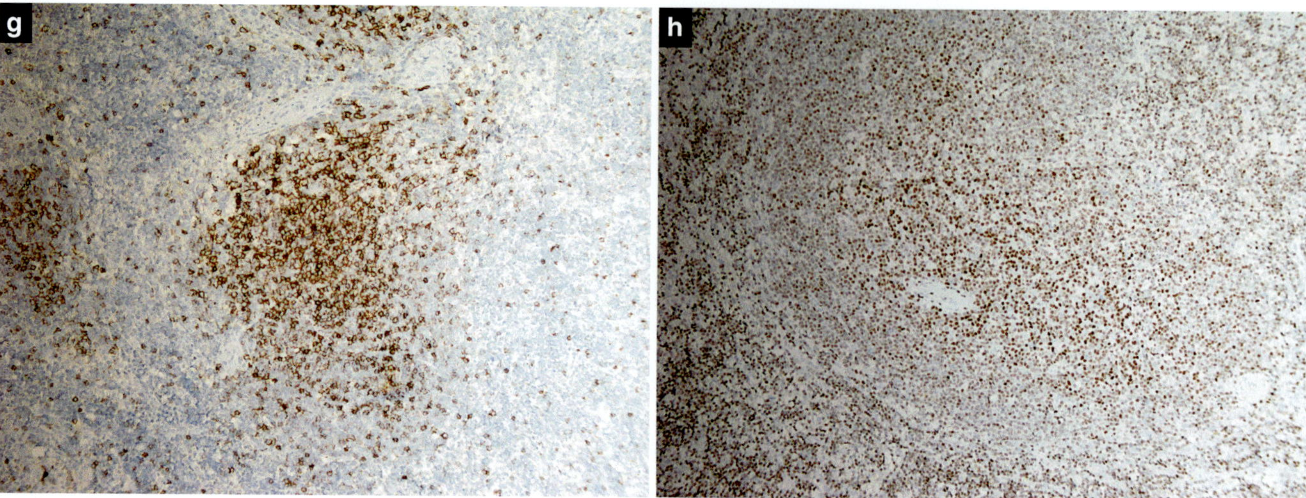

Fig. 5.10 (continued)

CD23, and FMC7 without/with CD200 [120]. Early involvement of the spleen by CLL/SLL may show lymphoid nodules in the white pulp that are indistinguishable from benign primary lymphoid nodules. The presence of significant red pulp infiltrate by B-cells, scattered admixed prolymphocytes and paraimmunoblasts, and abnormal immunophenotype by immunohistochemistry or flow cytometry would support the diagnosis of CLL/SLL.

CLL/SLL in the Liver

CLL/SLL also frequently involves liver (up to approximately 70% cases), and abnormal liver function tests (LFTs) and radiographic abnormalities are the most common indications for a biopsy [141]. The most common histologic finding in liver biopsy is the infiltrate of portal tracts by CLL/SLL cells. A minor subset of cases shows lobular or sinusoidal infiltrate by CLL/SLL cells. Proliferation centers are uncommon.

Mantle Cell Lymphoma

Mantle cell lymphoma (MCL) is a mature B-cell lymphoma with its hallmark of characteristic chromosomal translocation, t(11;14)(q13;q32)/*CCND1-IgH*. It occurs predominantly in middle-aged to old patients. The incidence rate is around 6.5% of non-Hodgkin lymphoma. MCL frequently involves the spleen with prominent splenomegaly [135, 138, 139, 142]. An indolent variant of MCL has been recognized and is characterized by a leukemic presentation with splenomegaly and no lymphadenopathy [143, 144].

Morphology

Grossly, the spleen displays numerous nodules composed of prominent white pulps.

Microscopically, MCL shows predominantly white pulp expansion associated with red pulp infiltrate (Fig. 5.11). The white pulp shows lymphoid follicles with expanded mantle zones surrounding atrophic reactive germinal centers. An external marginal zone is not uncommon giving rise to a triphasic pattern. The MCL may completely replace the residual germinal centers with the formation of monomorphic lymphoid nodules. The coalescence of these lymphoid follicles can generate massive nodules. MCL cells infiltrate the red pulp in small nodules, and occasionally diffusely. The typical MCL cells are small with variably irregular nuclei, coarse chromatin, indistinct nucleoli, and scant cytoplasm. Scattered or clusters of pale histiocytes are often present. The blastoid variant of MCL composed of larger cells with fine chromatin associated with frequent mitotic figures has been reported in the spleen as well. The hilar lymph nodes show at least partial preservation of the sinuses and lymphoid follicles with expanded mantle zones or nodules composed of MCL cells. The lymphoid nodules in the hilar lymph nodes do not show marginal zone differentiation.

Immunophenotyping

Immunophenotypically, the MCL cells are positive for CD5, cyclin D1, SOX11, and CD43 and negative for CD23. The MCL cells of indolent MCL are typically negative for SOX11 [145].

In the liver, MCL shows a dense portal infiltrate pattern [146].

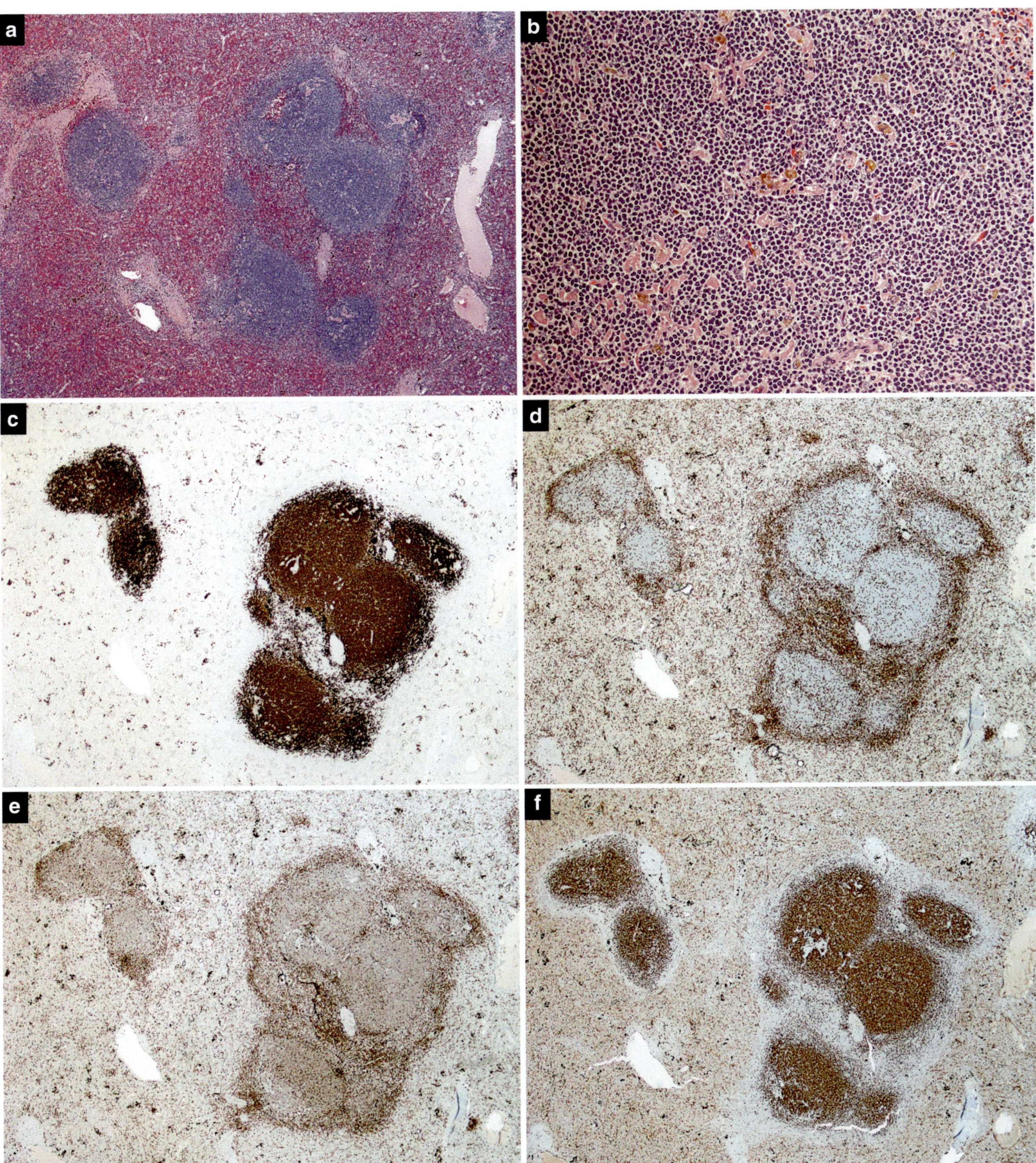

Fig. 5.11 Mantle cell lymphoma in the spleen. MCL shows predominant nodular lymphoid infiltrate in the white pulp (**a**). The MCL cells are monotonous and composed of small mature lymphoid cells with mildly irregular nuclei, coarse chromatin, and scant cytoplasm (**b**, H&E). The MCL cells are positive for B-cell markers CD20 (**c**), dim CD5 (**e**), and cyclin D1 (**f**). CD20 shows no significant red pulp infiltrate in this case (**c**). CD3 shows background T-cells (**d**)

Follicular Lymphoma

Follicular lymphoma is also a common type of non-Hodgkin lymphoma and accounts approximately 20% of all non-Hodgkin lymphoma diagnosed in the United States. It often builds up in lymph node but also occurs in other parts of the body. FL shows frequent involvement of the spleen at the time of diagnosis or during disease progression. Primary splenic FL is very rare [147].

Morphology

Grossly, the spleen shows a micronodular pattern due to expanded white pulps. Large masses from coalesced nodules can occasionally be seen. Microscopically, FL shows prominent white pulp areas with neoplastic follicles as well as red pulp infiltrate in most cases [137]. The splenic FL shows morphologic, immunophenotypic, and cytogenetic features resembling typical nodal FL. The lymphoid follicles are often enlarged and closely packed with disruption of underlying structure (Fig. 5.12). The neoplastic follicles frequently show marginal zones at the periphery [137, 148]. Extracellular hyaline deposit is frequently seen within the neoplastic follicles. Like nodal FL, the neoplastic follicles lack polarization or tingible body macrophages and are composed of centrocytes and variable numbers of centroblasts.

Immunophenotyping

The neoplastic follicles are positive for CD10, BCL6, and BCL2. Immunostains show increased interfollicular neoplastic B-cells that are often CD10 positive. A subset of the spleen FL is characterized by lack of BCL2 and CD10

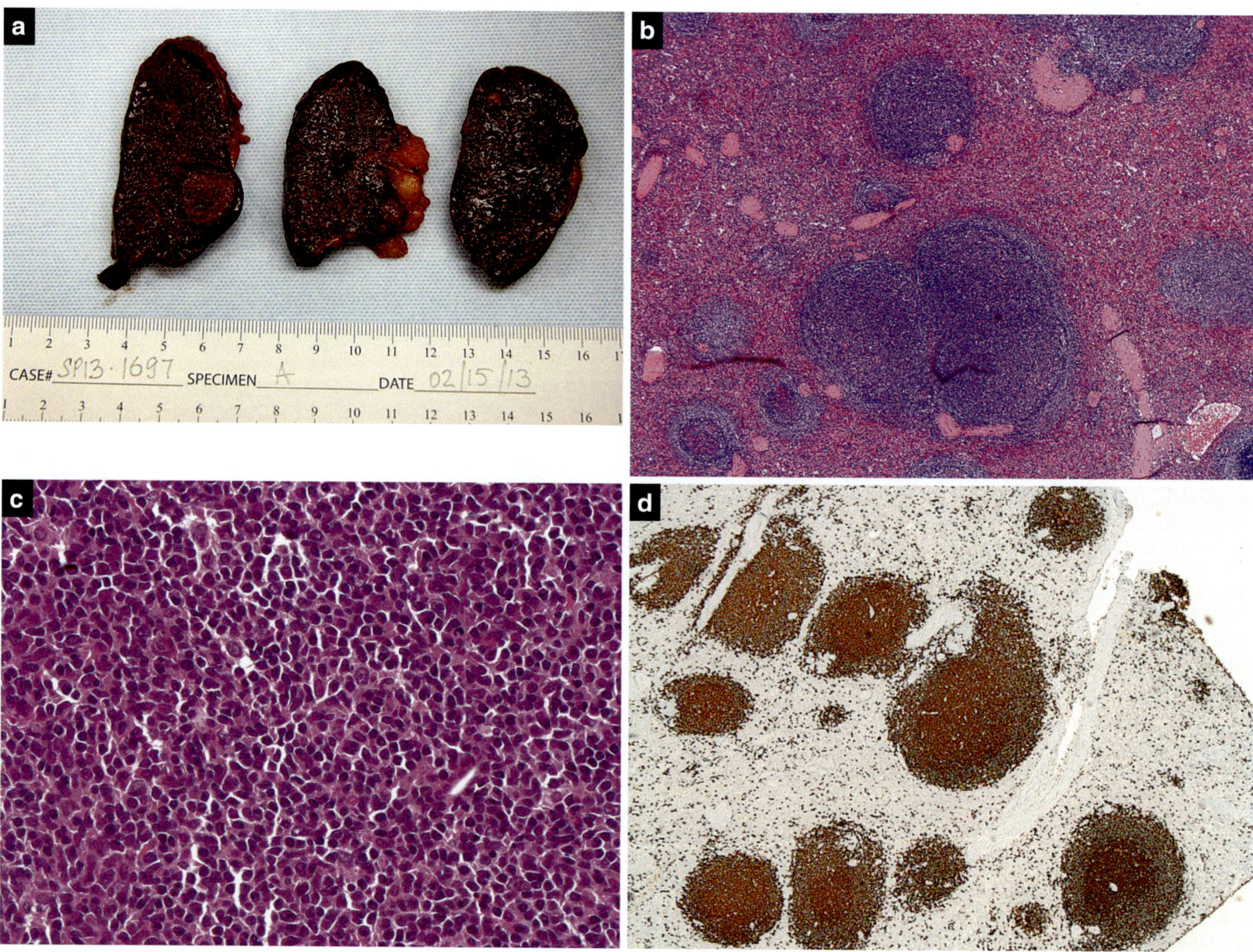

Fig. 5.12 Follicular lymphoma in the spleen. FL in the spleen shows numerous micronodules grossly and a focal large nodule (**a**). H&E sections show nodular lymphoid infiltrate in the white pulp (**b**, H&E). The lymphoid follicles show some degree of marginal zone differentiation (**b**). The atypical lymphoid follicles are composed predominantly of centrocytes and few centroblasts (**c**). The atypical lymphoid follicles are positive for CD20 (**d**), CD10 (data not shown), BCL6 (**e**), and BCL2 (**f**) and show low proliferate rate by Ki-67 (**h**). CD20 shows no significant red pulp infiltrate by FL cells (**d**). The follicular dendritic meshworks of the follicles are highlighted by CD21 stain (**g**)

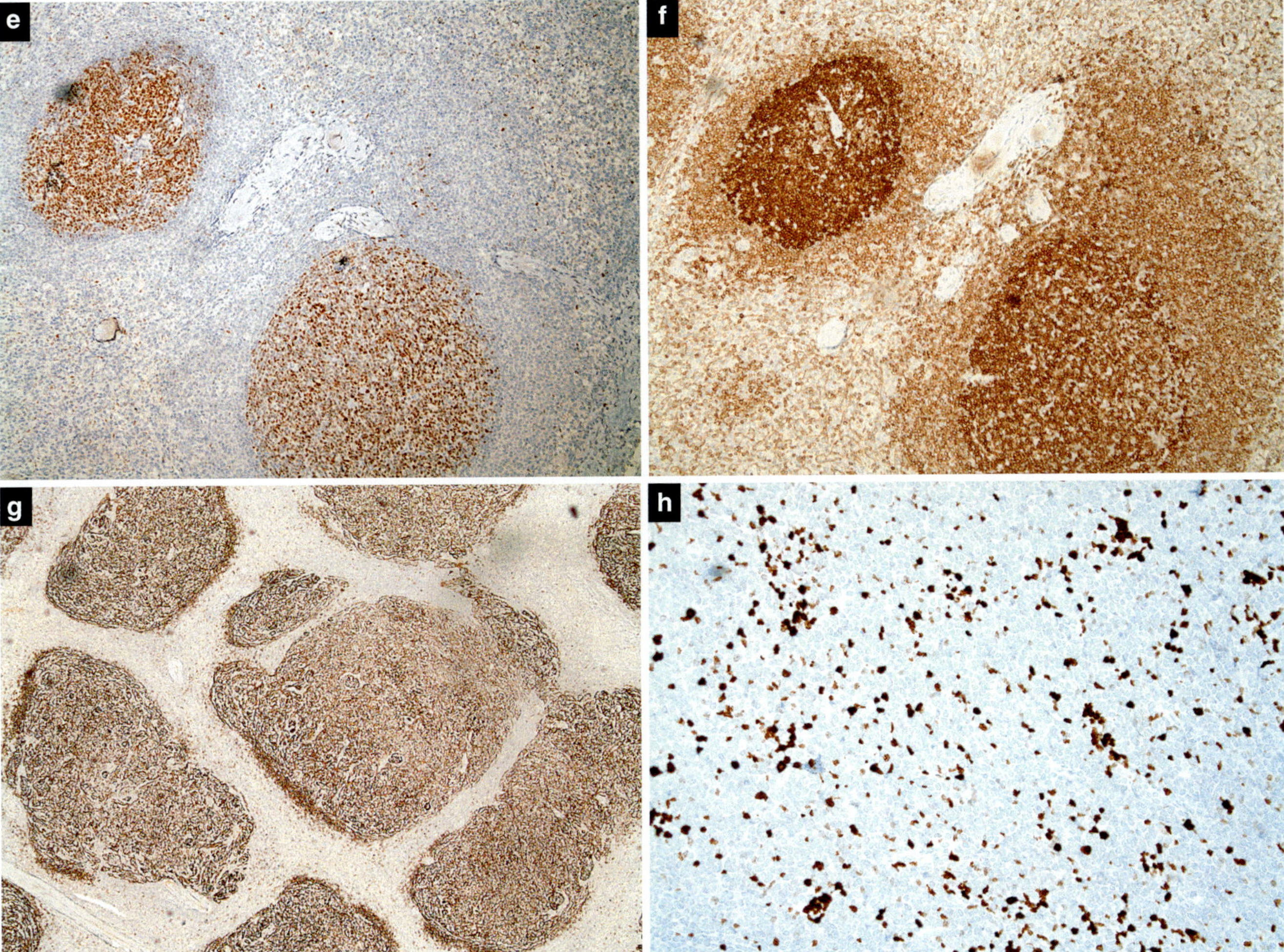

Fig. 5.12 (continued)

expression, higher histologic grade, and proliferation index, and these cases are frequently restricted to the spleen [148]. There are no significant differences in survival between the BCL2-positive and BCL2-negative FL in the spleen. The red pulp infiltrate is most frequently in the form of small lymphoid nodules but can be diffuse in occasional cases. Cases of "in situ" FL or intrafollicular lymphoid hyperplasia of undetermined significance with or without extrasplenic FL have also been reported [121]. In these cases, the spleen shows preserved splenic architecture and scattered lymphoid follicles with prominent marginal zones in the white pulp. The lymphoid follicles show germinal centers with FL grade 1 morphologic features and expression of CD10, BCL6, and BCL2. There are no increased interfollicular B-cells. These "in situ" FLs are difficult to distinguish from reactive lymphoid hyperplasia without the use of immunohistochemistry. The spleen may be the site of transformation to diffuse large B-cell lymphoma in systemic FL.

Cytogenetics

Similar to FL in lymph node, splenic FL also shows *IGH/BCL2* fusion or *BCL6* rearrangement by cytogenetics and FISH analysis.

FL in the Liver

As in the spleen, the liver is not uncommonly involved by systemic/nodal FL, but primary hepatic FL is rare. FL in the liver shows a dense portal infiltration pattern without sinusoidal infiltrate [146, 149]. The FL cells show typical immunophenotype in the liver with expression of CD10, BCL6, and BCL2.

Lymphoplasmacytic Lymphoma

LPL is a B-cell non-Hodgkin lymphoma composed of small B lymphocytes, plasmacytoid lymphocytes, and plasma cells, usually involving bone marrow. Involvement of lymph nodes or other body sites can occur. Approximately one third of patients with LPL present with splenomegaly or hepatomegaly and lymphadenopathy [150].

Clinical Presentation

Patients usually present with Waldenstrom macroglobulinemia with anemia, IgM paraproteinemia, and hyperviscosity.

Morphology

The most common pattern of involvement by LPL in the spleen is red pulp infiltrate by clusters and/or sheets of small mature lymphoid cells, plasmacytoid lymphoid cells, and plasma cells [151, 152]. Dutcher bodies and Russell bodies may be numerous. Large transformed lymphoid cells are rarely seen. A mixed pattern of white and red pulp infiltrate similar to the infiltrate pattern of CLL/SLL and SMZL can be seen [117]. A marginal zone differentiation is less frequently seen. A primary diagnosis of LPL in the spleen is rarely required.

The diagnosis of LPL is typically made on bone marrow biopsies. In cases that require differentiation from CLL/SLL and SMZL, the diagnosis of LPL in the spleen is facilitated by the cellular composition of many plasmacytoid lymphoid cells and plasma cells, absence of large transformed cells, and presence of *MYD88* mutation. Transformation of LPL to diffuse large cell lymphoma also occurs in the spleen [153].

LPL can involve the liver, rarely as a primary disease. The infiltrate by LPL in the liver is usually located to portal tracts [154, 155].

Non-splenic Marginal Zone Lymphomas

Secondary involvement in the spleen and liver by established nodal marginal zone lymphoma (NMZL) or extranodal marginal zone lymphoma of mucosa-associated lymphoid tissue (MALT lymphoma) diagnosed based on the most up-to-date WHO classification is exceptionally rare and may be seen in advanced diseases.

Primary hepatic MALT lymphoma is very rare and can be associated with primary biliary cirrhosis and hepatitis C infection [156–160]. The hepatic infiltrate is characterized by dense nodular lymphoid infiltrate in the portal tracts as well as lymphoepithelial lesions of the bile ducts, which may mimic hepatitis or an inflammatory bile duct disorder. Some of the lymphoid nodules show atrophic reactive germinal centers with expanded marginal zones. The MALT lymphoma cells are small centrocyte-like cells with moderate to abundant cytoplasm. The phenotype is nonspecific without expression of CD5, CD10, or BCL6.

t(14;18)(q32;q21) involving *IGH* and *MALT1* has been reported in primary hepatic MALT lymphoma [161].

References

1. Swerdlow SH, Campo E, Harris NL, Jaffe ES, Pileri SA, Stein H, Thiele J, Arber DA, Hasserjian RP, Le Beau MM, Orazi A, Siebert R. WHO classification of tumours of haematopoietic and lymphoid tissues. Lyon: IARC; 2017.
2. Armitage JO, Weisenburger DD. New approach to classifying non-Hodgkin's lymphomas: clinical features of the major histologic subtypes. Non-Hodgkin's Lymphoma Classification Project. J Clin Oncol. 1998;16:2780–95.
3. Liu L, Wang H, Chen Y, Rustveld L, Liu G, Du XL. Splenic marginal zone lymphoma: a population-based study on the 2001–2008 incidence and survival in the United States. Leuk Lymphoma. 2013;54:1380–6.
4. Morton LM, Slager SL, Cerhan JR, Wang SS, Vajdic CM, Skibola CF, Bracci PM, de Sanjose S, Smedby KE, Chiu BC, et al. Etiologic heterogeneity among non-Hodgkin lymphoma subtypes: the InterLymph Non-Hodgkin Lymphoma Subtypes Project. J Natl Cancer Inst Monogr. 2014;2014:130–44.
5. Bracci PM, Benavente Y, Turner JJ, Paltiel O, Slager SL, Vajdic CM, Norman AD, Cerhan JR, Chiu BC, Becker N, et al. Medical history, lifestyle, family history, and occupational risk factors for marginal zone lymphoma: the InterLymph Non-Hodgkin Lymphoma Subtypes Project. J Natl Cancer Inst Monogr. 2014;2014:52–65.
6. Arcaini L, Merli M, Volpetti S, Rattotti S, Gotti M, Zaja F. Indolent B-cell lymphomas associated with HCV infection: clinical and virological features and role of antiviral therapy. Clin Dev Immunol. 2012;2012:638185.
7. Tasleem S, Sood GK. Hepatitis C associated B-cell non-Hodgkin lymphoma: clinical features and the role of antiviral therapy. J Clin Transl Hepatol. 2015;3:134–9.
8. Arcaini L, Paulli M, Boveri E, Vallisa D, Bernuzzi P, Orlandi E, Incardona P, Brusamolino E, Passamonti F, Burcheri S, et al. Splenic and nodal marginal zone lymphomas are indolent disorders at high hepatitis C virus seroprevalence with distinct presenting features but similar morphologic and phenotypic profiles. Cancer. 2004;100:107–15.
9. Troussard X, Valensi F, Duchayne E, Garand R, Felman P, Tulliez M, Henry-Amar M, Bryon PA, Flandrin G. Splenic lymphoma with villous lymphocytes: clinical presentation, biology and prognostic factors in a series of 100 patients. Groupe Francais d'Hematologie Cellulaire (GFHC). Br J Haematol. 1996;93:731–6.
10. Chacon JI, Mollejo M, Munoz E, Algara P, Mateo M, Lopez L, Andrade J, Carbonero IG, Martinez B, Piris MA, et al. Splenic marginal zone lymphoma: clinical characteristics and prognostic factors in a series of 60 patients. Blood. 2002;100:1648–54.
11. Berger F, Felman P, Thieblemont C, Pradier T, Baseggio L, Bryon PA, Salles G, Callet-Bauchu E, Coiffier B. Non-MALT marginal zone B-cell lymphomas: a description of clinical presentation and outcome in 124 patients. Blood. 2000;95:1950–6.
12. Matutes E, Oscier D, Montalban C, Berger F, Callet-Bauchu E, Dogan A, Felman P, Franco V, Iannitto E, Mollejo M, et al. Splenic marginal zone lymphoma proposals for a revision of diagnostic, staging and therapeutic criteria. Leukemia. 2008;22:487–95.
13. Iannitto E, Ambrosetti A, Ammatuna E, Colosio M, Florena AM, Tripodo C, Minardi V, Calvaruso G, Mitra ME, Pizzolo G, et al. Splenic marginal zone lymphoma with or without villous lymphocytes. Hematologic findings and outcomes in a series of 57 patients. Cancer. 2004;101:2050–7.

14. Xochelli A, Kalpadakis C, Gardiner A, Baliakas P, Vassilakopoulos TP, Mould S, Davis Z, Stalika E, Kanellis G, Angelopoulou MK, et al. Clonal B-cell lymphocytosis exhibiting immunophenotypic features consistent with a marginal-zone origin: is this a distinct entity? Blood. 2014;123:1199–206.

15. Thieblemont C, Felman P, Berger F, Dumontet C, Arnaud P, Hequet O, Arcache J, Callet-Bauchu E, Salles G, Coiffier B. Treatment of splenic marginal zone B-cell lymphoma: an analysis of 81 patients. Clin Lymphoma. 2002;3:41–7.

16. Gebhart J, Lechner K, Skrabs C, Sliwa T, Muldur E, Ludwig H, Nosslinger T, Vanura K, Stamatopoulos K, Simonitsch-Klupp I, et al. Lupus anticoagulant and thrombosis in splenic marginal zone lymphoma. Thromb Res. 2014;134:980–4.

17. Castelli R, Wu MA, Arquati M, Zanichelli A, Suffritti C, Rossi D, Cicardi M. High prevalence of splenic marginal zone lymphoma among patients with acquired C1 inhibitor deficiency. Br J Haematol. 2016;172:902–8.

18. Parry-Jones N, Matutes E, Gruszka-Westwood AM, Swansbury GJ, Wotherspoon AC, Catovsky D. Prognostic features of splenic lymphoma with villous lymphocytes: a report on 129 patients. Br J Haematol. 2003;120:759–64.

19. Camacho FI, Mollejo M, Mateo MS, Algara P, Navas C, Hernandez JM, Santoja C, Sole F, Sanchez-Beato M, Piris MA. Progression to large B-cell lymphoma in splenic marginal zone lymphoma: a description of a series of 12 cases. Am J Surg Pathol. 2001;25:1268–76.

20. Thieblemont C, Felman P, Callet-Bauchu E, Traverse-Glehen A, Salles G, Berger F, Coiffier B. Splenic marginal-zone lymphoma: a distinct clinical and pathological entity. Lancet Oncol. 2003;4:95–103.

21. Arcaini L, Lazzarino M, Colombo N, Burcheri S, Boveri E, Paulli M, Morra E, Gambacorta M, Cortelazzo S, Tucci A, et al. Splenic marginal zone lymphoma: a prognostic model for clinical use. Blood. 2006;107:4643–9.

22. Iannitto E, Minardi V, Callea V, Stelitano C, Calvaruso G, Tripodo C, Quintini G, De Cantis S, Ambrosetti A, Pizzolo G, et al. Assessment of the frequency of additional cancers in patients with splenic marginal zone lymphoma. Eur J Haematol. 2006;76:134–40.

23. Franco V, Florena AM, Iannitto E. Splenic marginal zone lymphoma. Blood. 2003;101:2464–72.

24. Isaacson PG, Matutes E, Burke M, Catovsky D. The histopathology of splenic lymphoma with villous lymphocytes. Blood. 1994;84:3828–34.

25. Mollejo M, Menarguez J, Lloret E, Sanchez A, Campo E, Algara P, Cristobal E, Sanchez E, Piris MA. Splenic marginal zone lymphoma: a distinctive type of low-grade B-cell lymphoma. A clinicopathological study of 13 cases. Am J Surg Pathol. 1995;19: 1146–57.

26. Hammer RD, Glick AD, Greer JP, Collins RD, Cousar JB. Splenic marginal zone lymphoma. A distinct B-cell neoplasm. Am J Surg Pathol. 1996;20:613–26.

27. Arcaini L, Rossi D, Paulli M. Splenic marginal zone lymphoma: from genetics to management. Blood. 2016;127:2072–81.

28. Molina TJ, Lin P, Swerdlow SH, Cook JR. Marginal zone lymphomas with plasmacytic differentiation and related disorders. Am J Clin Pathol. 2011;136:211–25.

29. Dufresne SD, Felgar RE, Sargent RL, Surti U, Gollin SM, McPhail ED, Cook JR, Swerdlow SH. Defining the borders of splenic marginal zone lymphoma: a multiparameter study. Hum Pathol. 2010;41:540–51.

30. Lloret E, Mollejo M, Mateo MS, Villuendas R, Algara P, Martinez P, Piris MA. Splenic marginal zone lymphoma with increased number of blasts: an aggressive variant? Hum Pathol. 1999;30:1153–60.

31. Matutes E, Morilla R, Owusu-Ankomah K, Houlihan A, Catovsky D. The immunophenotype of splenic lymphoma with villous lymphocytes and its relevance to the differential diagnosis with other B-cell disorders. Blood. 1994;83:1558–62.

32. Mollejo M, Lloret E, Menarguez J, Piris MA, Isaacson PG. Lymph node involvement by splenic marginal zone lymphoma: morphological and immunohistochemical features. Am J Surg Pathol. 1997;21:772–80.

33. Menter T, Trivedi P, Ahmad R, Flora R, Dirnhofer S, Tzankov A, Naresh KN. Diagnostic utility of lymphoid enhancer binding factor 1 immunohistochemistry in small B-cell lymphomas. Am J Clin Pathol. 2017;147:292–300.

34. Gimeno E, Salido M, Sole F, Florensa L, Granada I, Domingo A, Woessner S. CD5 negative and CD5 positive splenic marginal B-cell lymphomas have differential cytogenetic patterns. Leuk Res. 2005;29:981–2.

35. Kojima M, Sato E, Oshimi K, Murase T, Koike T, Tsunoda S, Matsumoto T, Marutsuka K, Ogiya D, Moriuchi M, et al. Characteristics of CD5-positive splenic marginal zone lymphoma with leukemic manifestation; clinical, flow cytometry, and histopathological findings of 11 cases. J Clin Exp Hematop. 2010;50: 107–12.

36. Baseggio L, Traverse-Glehen A, Petinataud F, Callet-Bauchu E, Berger F, Ffrench M, Couris CM, Thieblemont C, Morel D, Coiffier B, et al. CD5 expression identifies a subset of splenic marginal zone lymphomas with higher lymphocytosis: a clinico-pathological, cytogenetic and molecular study of 24 cases. Haematologica. 2010;95:604–12.

37. El Desoukey NA, Afify RA, Amin DG, Mohammed RF. CD200 expression in B-cell chronic lymphoproliferative disorders. J Investig Med. 2012;60:56–61.

38. Challagundla P, Medeiros LJ, Kanagal-Shamanna R, Miranda RN, Jorgensen JL. Differential expression of CD200 in B-cell neoplasms by flow cytometry can assist in diagnosis, subclassification, and bone marrow staging. Am J Clin Pathol. 2014;142:837–44.

39. Moreau EJ, Matutes E, A'Hern RP, Morilla AM, Morilla RM, Owusu-Ankomah KA, Seon BK, Catovsky D. Improvement of the chronic lymphocytic leukemia scoring system with the monoclonal antibody SN8 (CD79b). Am J Clin Pathol. 1997;108:378–82.

40. Santos TSD, Tavares RS, Farias DLC. Splenic marginal zone lymphoma: a literature review of diagnostic and therapeutic challenges. Rev Bras Hematol Hemoter. 2017;39:146–54.

41. Behdad A, Bailey NG. Diagnosis of splenic B-cell lymphomas in the bone marrow: a review of histopathologic, immunophenotypic, and genetic findings. Arch Pathol Lab Med. 2014;138:1295–301.

42. Melo JV, Hegde U, Parreira A, Thompson I, Lampert IA, Catovsky D. Splenic B cell lymphoma with circulating villous lymphocytes: differential diagnosis of B cell leukaemias with large spleens. J Clin Pathol. 1987;40:642–51.

43. Audouin J, Le Tourneau A, Molina T, Camilleri-Broet S, Adida C, Comperat E, Benattar L, Delmer A, Devidas A, Rio B, et al. Patterns of bone marrow involvement in 58 patients presenting primary splenic marginal zone lymphoma with or without circulating villous lymphocytes. Br J Haematol. 2003;122:404–12.

44. Ponzoni M, Kanellis G, Pouliou E, Baliakas P, Scarfo L, Ferreri AJ, Doglioni C, Bikos V, Dagklis A, Anagnostopoulos A, et al. Bone marrow histopathology in the diagnostic evaluation of splenic marginal-zone and splenic diffuse red pulp small B-cell lymphoma: a reliable substitute for spleen histopathology? Am J Surg Pathol. 2012;36:1609–18.

45. Franco V, Florena AM, Campesi G. Intrasinusoidal bone marrow infiltration: a possible hallmark of splenic lymphoma. Histopathology. 1996;29:571–5.

46. Labouyrie E, Marit G, Vial JP, Lacombe F, Fialon P, Bernard P, de Mascarel A, Merlio JP. Intrasinusoidal bone marrow involvement by splenic lymphoma with villous lymphocytes: a helpful immunohistologic feature. Mod Pathol. 1997;10:1015–20.

47. Kent SA, Variakojis D, Peterson LC. Comparative study of marginal zone lymphoma involving bone marrow. Am J Clin Pathol. 2002;117:698–708.

48. Catovsky D, Matutes E. Splenic lymphoma with circulating villous lymphocytes/splenic marginal-zone lymphoma. Semin Hematol. 1999;36:148–54.

49. Campo E, Miquel R, Krenacs L, Sorbara L, Raffeld M, Jaffe ES. Primary nodal marginal zone lymphomas of splenic and MALT type. Am J Surg Pathol. 1999;23:59–68.

50. Schmid C, Kirkham N, Diss T, Isaacson PG. Splenic marginal zone cell lymphoma. Am J Surg Pathol. 1992;16:455–66.

51. Domingo-Domenech E, Romagosa V, González-Barca E, Rodriguez-Aliberas M, Oliveira A, de la Banda E, Santiago Mercadal JS, Petit J, de Sevilla AF. Liver infiltration in splenic marginal zone lymphoma: prevalence and prognostic implication. Blood. 2010;116:4137.

52. Lenglet J, Traulle C, Mounier N, Benet C, Munoz-Bongrand N, Amorin S, Noguera ME, Traverse-Glehen A, Ffrench M, Baseggio L, et al. Long-term follow-up analysis of 100 patients with splenic marginal zone lymphoma treated with splenectomy as first-line treatment. Leuk Lymphoma. 2014;55:1854–60.

53. Xing KH, Kahlon A, Skinnider BF, Connors JM, Gascoyne RD, Sehn LH, Savage KJ, Slack GW, Shenkier TN, Klasa R, et al. Outcomes in splenic marginal zone lymphoma: analysis of 107 patients treated in British Columbia. Br J Haematol. 2015;169:520–7.

54. Conconi A, Franceschetti S, Aprile von Hohenstaufen K, Margiotta-Casaluci G, Stathis A, Moccia AA, Bertoni F, Ramponi A, Mazzucchelli L, Cavalli F, et al. Histologic transformation in marginal zone lymphomas. Ann Oncol. 2015;26:2329–35.

55. Dungarwalla M, Appiah-Cubi S, Kulkarni S, Saso R, Wotherspoon A, Osuji N, Swansbury J, Cunningham DC, Catovsky D, Dearden CE, et al. High-grade transformation in splenic marginal zone lymphoma with circulating villous lymphocytes: the site of transformation influences response to therapy and prognosis. Br J Haematol. 2008;143:71–4.

56. Thoennissen NH, Keyvani K, Voelker HU, Bremer J, Krug U, Muller-Tidow C, Koch P, Muller-Hermelink HK, Berdel WE. Splenic marginal zone lymphoma: transformation to diffuse large B-cell lymphoma with isolated cerebral manifestation. J Clin Oncol. 2008;26:4509–11.

57. Cualing H, Steele P, Zellner D. Blastic transformation of splenic marginal zone B-cell lymphoma. Arch Pathol Lab Med. 2000;124:748–52.

58. Kakinoki Y, Kubota H, Sakurai H, Sato T, Tokusashi Y. Blastic transformation after splenectomy in a patient with nonvillous splenic marginal zone lymphoma with p53 overexpression: a case report. Int J Hematol. 2005;81:417–20.

59. Salido M, Baro C, Oscier D, Stamatopoulos K, Dierlamm J, Matutes E, Traverse-Glehen A, Berger F, Felman P, Thieblemont C, et al. Cytogenetic aberrations and their prognostic value in a series of 330 splenic marginal zone B-cell lymphomas: a multicenter study of the Splenic B-Cell Lymphoma Group. Blood. 2010;116:1479–88.

60. Callet-Bauchu E, Baseggio L, Felman P, Traverse-Glehen A, Berger F, Morel D, Gazzo S, Poncet C, Thieblemont C, Coiffier B, et al. Cytogenetic analysis delineates a spectrum of chromosomal changes that can distinguish non-MALT marginal zone B-cell lymphomas among mature B-cell entities: a description of 103 cases. Leukemia. 2005;19:1818–23.

61. Gazzo S, Baseggio L, Coignet L, Poncet C, Morel D, Coiffier B, Felman P, Berger F, Salles G, Callet-Bauchu E. Cytogenetic and molecular delineation of a region of chromosome 3q commonly gained in marginal zone B-cell lymphoma. Haematologica. 2003;88:31–8.

62. Hernandez JM, Garcia JL, Gutierrez NC, Mollejo M, Martinez-Climent JA, Flores T, Gonzalez MB, Piris MA, San Miguel JF. Novel genomic imbalances in B-cell splenic marginal zone lymphomas revealed by comparative genomic hybridization and cytogenetics. Am J Pathol. 2001;158:1843–50.

63. Oscier DG, Matutes E, Gardiner A, Glide S, Mould S, Brito-Babapulle V, Ellis J, Catovsky D. Cytogenetic studies in splenic lymphoma with villous lymphocytes. Br J Haematol. 1993;85:487–91.

64. Sole F, Salido M, Espinet B, Garcia JL, Martinez Climent JA, Granada I, Hernandez JM, Benet I, Piris MA, Mollejo M, et al. Splenic marginal zone B-cell lymphomas: two cytogenetic subtypes, one with gain of 3q and the other with loss of 7q. Haematologica. 2001;86:71–7.

65. Troussard X, Mauvieux L, Radford-Weiss I, Rack K, Valensi F, Garand R, Vekemans M, Flandrin G, Macintyre EA. Genetic analysis of splenic lymphoma with villous lymphocytes: a Groupe Francais d'Hematologie Cellulaire (GFHC) study. Br J Haematol. 1998;101:712–21.

66. Andersen CL, Gruszka-Westwood A, Atkinson S, Matutes E, Catovsky D, Pedersen RK, Pedersen BB, Pulczynski S, Hokland P, Jacobsen E, et al. Recurrent genomic imbalances in B-cell splenic marginal-zone lymphoma revealed by comparative genomic hybridization. Cancer Genet Cytogenet. 2005;156:122–8.

67. Boonstra R, Bosga-Bouwer A, van Imhoff GW, Krause V, Palmer M, Coupland RW, Dabbagh L, van den Berg E, van den Berg A, Poppema S. Splenic marginal zone lymphomas presenting with splenomegaly and typical immunophenotype are characterized by allelic loss in 7q31-32. Mod Pathol. 2003;16:1210–7.

68. Remstein ED, Law M, Mollejo M, Piris MA, Kurtin PJ, Dogan A. The prevalence of IG translocations and 7q32 deletions in splenic marginal zone lymphoma. Leukemia. 2008;22:1268–72.

69. Morrison AM, Jager U, Chott A, Schebesta M, Haas OA, Busslinger M. Deregulated PAX-5 transcription from a translocated IgH promoter in marginal zone lymphoma. Blood. 1998;92:3865–78.

70. Andrieux J, Fert-Ferrer S, Copin MC, Huyghe P, Pocachard P, Lespinasse J, Bauters F, Lai JL, Quesnel B. Three new cases of non-Hodgkin lymphoma with t(9;14)(p13;q32). Cancer Genet Cytogenet. 2003;145:65–9.

71. Daibata M, Taguchi T, Nemoto Y, Iwasaki S, Ohtsuki Y, Taguchi H. In vitro Epstein-Barr virus-immortalized lymphoma cell line carrying t(9;14)(p13;q32) chromosome abnormality, derived from splenic lymphoma with villous lymphocytes. Int J Cancer. 2006;118:513–7.

72. Dierlamm J, Pittaluga S, Stul M, Wlodarska I, Michaux L, Thomas J, Verhoef G, Verhest A, Depardieu C, Cassiman JJ, et al. BCL6 gene rearrangements also occur in marginal zone B-cell lymphoma. Br J Haematol. 1997;98:719–25.

73. Aamot HV, Micci F, Holte H, Delabie J, Heim S. G-banding and molecular cytogenetic analyses of marginal zone lymphoma. Br J Haematol. 2005;130:890–901.

74. Soma LA, Gollin SM, Remstein ED, Ketterling RP, Flynn HC, Rajasenan KK, Swerdlow SH. Splenic small B-cell lymphoma with IGH/BCL3 translocation. Hum Pathol. 2006;37:218–30.

75. Brito-Babapulle V, Gruszka-Westwood AM, Platt G, Andersen CL, Elnenaei MO, Matutes E, Wotherspoon AC, Weston-Smith SG, Catovsky D. Translocation t(2;7)(p12;q21-22) with dysregulation of the CDK6 gene mapping to 7q21-22 in a non-Hodgkin's lymphoma with leukemia. Haematologica. 2002;87:357–62.

76. Corcoran MM, Mould SJ, Orchard JA, Ibbotson RE, Chapman RM, Boright AP, Platt C, Tsui LC, Scherer SW, Oscier DG. Dysregulation of cyclin dependent kinase 6 expression in splenic marginal zone lymphoma through chromosome 7q translocations. Oncogene. 1999;18:6271–7.

77. Sonoki T, Harder L, Horsman DE, Karran L, Taniguchi I, Willis TG, Gesk S, Steinemann D, Zucca E, Schlegelberger B, et al. Cyclin D3 is a target gene of t(6;14)(p21.1;q32.3) of mature B-cell malignancies. Blood. 2001;98:2837–44.

78. Dierlamm J, Pittaluga S, Wlodarska I, Stul M, Thomas J, Boogaerts M, Michaux L, Driessen A, Mecucci C, Cassiman JJ, et al. Marginal

zone B-cell lymphomas of different sites share similar cytogenetic and morphologic features. Blood. 1996;87:299–307.

79. Gruszka-Westwood AM, Hamoudi R, Osborne L, Matutes E, Catovsky D. Deletion mapping on the long arm of chromosome 7 in splenic lymphoma with villous lymphocytes. Genes Chromosomes Cancer. 2003;36:57–69.

80. Martinez-Climent JA, Sanchez-Izquierdo D, Sarsotti E, Blesa D, Benet I, Climent J, Vizcarra E, Marugan I, Terol MJ, Sole F, et al. Genomic abnormalities acquired in the blastic transformation of splenic marginal zone B-cell lymphoma. Leuk Lymphoma. 2003;44: 459–64.

81. Jadayel D, Matutes E, Dyer MJ, Brito-Babapulle V, Khohkar MT, Oscier D, Catovsky D. Splenic lymphoma with villous lymphocytes: analysis of BCL-1 rearrangements and expression of the cyclin D1 gene. Blood. 1994;83:3664–71.

82. Algara P, Mateo MS, Sanchez-Beato M, Mollejo M, Navas IC, Romero L, Sole F, Salido M, Florensa L, Martinez P, et al. Analysis of the IgV(H) somatic mutations in splenic marginal zone lymphoma defines a group of unmutated cases with frequent 7q deletion and adverse clinical course. Blood. 2002;99:1299–304.

83. Bikos V, Darzentas N, Hadzidimitriou A, Davis Z, Hockley S, Traverse-Glehen A, Algara P, Santoro A, Gonzalez D, Mollejo M, et al. Over 30% of patients with splenic marginal zone lymphoma express the same immunoglobulin heavy variable gene: ontogenetic implications. Leukemia. 2012;26:1638–46.

84. Ruiz-Ballesteros E, Mollejo M, Rodriguez A, Camacho FI, Algara P, Martinez N, Pollan M, Sanchez-Aguilera A, Menarguez J, Campo E, et al. Splenic marginal zone lymphoma: proposal of new diagnostic and prognostic markers identified after tissue and cDNA microarray analysis. Blood. 2005;106:1831–8.

85. Troen G, Nygaard V, Jenssen TK, Ikonomou IM, Tierens A, Matutes E, Gruszka-Westwood A, Catovsky D, Myklebost O, Lauritzsen G, et al. Constitutive expression of the AP-1 transcription factors c-jun, junD, junB, and c-fos and the marginal zone B-cell transcription factor Notch2 in splenic marginal zone lymphoma. J Mol Diagn. 2004;6:297–307.

86. Arribas AJ, Gomez-Abad C, Sanchez-Beato M, Martinez N, Dilisio L, Casado F, Cruz MA, Algara P, Piris MA, Mollejo M. Splenic marginal zone lymphoma: comprehensive analysis of gene expression and miRNA profiling. Mod Pathol. 2013;26:889–901.

87. Kiel MJ, Velusamy T, Betz BL, Zhao L, Weigelin HG, Chiang MY, Huebner-Chan DR, Bailey NG, Yang DT, Bhagat G, et al. Whole-genome sequencing identifies recurrent somatic NOTCH2 mutations in splenic marginal zone lymphoma. J Exp Med. 2012;209:1553–65.

88. Martinez N, Almaraz C, Vaque JP, Varela I, Derdak S, Beltran S, Mollejo M, Campos-Martin Y, Agueda L, Rinaldi A, et al. Whole-exome sequencing in splenic marginal zone lymphoma reveals mutations in genes involved in marginal zone differentiation. Leukemia. 2014;28:1334–40.

89. Rossi D, Trifonov V, Fangazio M, Bruscaggin A, Rasi S, Spina V, Monti S, Vaisitti T, Arruga F, Fama R, et al. The coding genome of splenic marginal zone lymphoma: activation of NOTCH2 and other pathways regulating marginal zone development. J Exp Med. 2012;209:1537–51.

90. Peveling-Oberhag J, Wolters F, Doring C, Walter D, Sellmann L, Scholtysik R, Lucioni M, Schubach M, Paulli M, Biskup S, et al. Whole exome sequencing of microdissected splenic marginal zone lymphoma: a study to discover novel tumor-specific mutations. BMC Cancer. 2015;15:773.

91. Parry M, Rose-Zerilli MJ, Ljungstrom V, Gibson J, Wang J, Walewska R, Parker H, Parker A, Davis Z, Gardiner A, et al. Genetics and prognostication in splenic marginal zone lymphoma: revelations from deep sequencing. Clin Cancer Res. 2015;21: 4174–83.

92. Lee SY, Kumano K, Nakazaki K, Sanada M, Matsumoto A, Yamamoto G, Nannya Y, Suzuki R, Ota S, Ota Y, et al. Gain-of-function mutations and copy number increases of Notch2 in diffuse large B-cell lymphoma. Cancer Sci. 2009;100:920–6.

93. Clipson A, Wang M, de Leval L, Ashton-Key M, Wotherspoon A, Vassiliou G, Bolli N, Grove C, Moody S, Escudero-Ibarz L, et al. KLF2 mutation is the most frequent somatic change in splenic marginal zone lymphoma and identifies a subset with distinct genotype. Leukemia. 2015;29:1177–85.

94. Piva R, Deaglio S, Fama R, Buonincontri R, Scarfo I, Bruscaggin A, Mereu E, Serra S, Spina V, Brusa D, et al. The Kruppel-like factor 2 transcription factor gene is recurrently mutated in splenic marginal zone lymphoma. Leukemia. 2015;29:503–7.

95. Troen G, Warsame A, Delabie J. CD79B and MYD88 mutations in splenic marginal zone lymphoma. ISRN Oncol. 2013;2013:252318.

96. Yan Q, Huang Y, Watkins AJ, Kocialkowski S, Zeng N, Hamoudi RA, Isaacson PG, de Leval L, Wotherspoon A, Du MQ. BCR and TLR signaling pathways are recurrently targeted by genetic changes in splenic marginal zone lymphomas. Haematologica. 2012;97:595–8.

97. Varettoni M, Arcaini L, Zibellini S, Boveri E, Rattotti S, Riboni R, Corso A, Orlandi E, Bonfichi M, Gotti M, et al. Prevalence and clinical significance of the MYD88 (L265P) somatic mutation in Waldenstrom's macroglobulinemia and related lymphoid neoplasms. Blood. 2013;121:2522–8.

98. Bahler DW, Pindzola JA, Swerdlow SH. Splenic marginal zone lymphomas appear to originate from different B cell types. Am J Pathol. 2002;161:81–8.

99. Traverse-Glehen A, Davi F, Ben Simon E, Callet-Bauchu E, Felman P, Baseggio L, Gazzo S, Thieblemont C, Charlot C, Coiffier B, et al. Analysis of VH genes in marginal zone lymphoma reveals marked heterogeneity between splenic and nodal tumors and suggests the existence of clonal selection. Haematologica. 2005;90:470–8.

100. Traverse-Glehen A, Verney A, Baseggio L, Felman P, Callet-Bauchu E, Thieblemont C, Ffrench M, Magaud JP, Coiffier B, Berger F, et al. Analysis of BCL-6, CD95, PIM1, RHO/TTF and PAX5 mutations in splenic and nodal marginal zone B-cell lymphomas suggests a particular B-cell origin. Leukemia. 2007;21:1821–4.

101. Jiang DY, Li CY. Immunohistochemical study of the spleen in chronic immune thrombocytopenic purpura. With special reference to hyperplastic follicles and foamy macrophages. Arch Pathol Lab Med. 1995;119:533–7.

102. Farhi DC, Ashfaq R. Splenic pathology after traumatic injury. Am J Clin Pathol. 1996;105:474–8.

103. Harris S, Wilkins BS, Jones DB. Splenic marginal zone expansion in B-cell lymphomas of gastrointestinal mucosa-associated lymphoid tissue (MALT) is reactive and does not represent homing of neoplastic lymphocytes. J Pathol. 1996;179:49–53.

104. Kroft SH, Singleton TP, Dahiya M, Ross CW, Schnitzer B, Hsi ED. Ruptured spleens with expanded marginal zones do not reveal occult B-cell clones. Mod Pathol. 1997;10:1214–20.

105. Dunphy CH, Bee C, McDonald JW, Grosso LE. Incidental early detection of a splenic marginal zone lymphoma by polymerase chain reaction analysis of paraffin-embedded tissue. Arch Pathol Lab Med. 1998;122:84–6.

106. Rosso R, Neiman RS, Paulli M, Boveri E, Kindl S, Magrini U, Barosi G. Splenic marginal zone cell lymphoma: report of an indolent variant without massive splenomegaly presumably representing an early phase of the disease. Hum Pathol. 1995;26:39–46.

107. Gordon DS, Jones BM, Browning SW, Spira TJ, Lawrence DN. Persistent polyclonal lymphocytosis of B lymphocytes. N Engl J Med. 1982;307:232–6.

108. Cornet E, Lesesve JF, Mossafa H, Sebahoun G, Levy V, Davi F, Troussard X, Groupe Francais d'Hematologie C. Long-term follow-up of 111 patients with persistent polyclonal B-cell lymphocytosis with binucleated lymphocytes. Leukemia. 2009;23:419–22.

109. Bhagwandin SB, Weisenberg ES, Ozer H, Maker AV. Symptomatic massive splenomegaly in persistent polyclonal B-cell lymphocytosis requiring splenectomy. Open J Clin Med Case Rep. 2015;1:1017.

110. Sun P, Juskevicius R. Histological and immunohistochemical features of the spleen in persistent polyclonal B-cell lymphocytosis closely mimic splenic B-cell lymphoma. Diagn Pathol. 2012;7:107.

111. Troussard X, Valensi F, Debert C, Maynadie M, Schillinger F, Bonnet P, Macintyre EA, Flandrin G. Persistent polyclonal lymphocytosis with binucleated B lymphocytes: a genetic predisposition. Br J Haematol. 1994;88:275–80.

112. Delage R, Roy J, Jacques L, Bernier V, Delage JM, Darveau A. Multiple bcl-2/Ig gene rearrangements in persistent polyclonal B-cell lymphocytosis. Br J Haematol. 1997;97:589–95.

113. Delage R, Roy J, Jacques L, Darveau A. All patients with persistent polyclonal B cell lymphocytosis present Bcl-2/Ig gene rearrangements. Leuk Lymphoma. 1998;31:567–74.

114. Callet-Bauchu E, Renard N, Gazzo S, Poncet C, Morel D, Pages J, Salles G, Coeur P, Felman P. Distribution of the cytogenetic abnormality +i(3)(q10) in persistent polyclonal B-cell lymphocytosis: a FICTION study in three cases. Br J Haematol. 1997;99:531–6.

115. Del Giudice I, Pileri SA, Rossi M, Sabattini E, Campidelli C, Starza ID, De Propris MS, Mancini F, Perrone MP, Gesuiti P, et al. Histopathological and molecular features of persistent polyclonal B-cell lymphocytosis (PPBL) with progressive splenomegaly. Br J Haematol. 2009;144:726–31.

116. Feugier P, De March AK, Lesesve JF, Monhoven N, Dorvaux V, Braun F, Gregoire MJ, Jonveaux P, Lederlin P, Bene MC, et al. Intravascular bone marrow accumulation in persistent polyclonal lymphocytosis: a misleading feature for B-cell neoplasm. Mod Pathol. 2004;17:1087–96.

117. Piris MA, Mollejo M, Campo E, Menarguez J, Flores T, Isaacson PG. A marginal zone pattern may be found in different varieties of non-Hodgkin's lymphoma: the morphology and immunohistology of splenic involvement by B-cell lymphomas simulating splenic marginal zone lymphoma. Histopathology. 1998;33:230–9.

118. Schenka AA, Gascoyne RD, Duchayne E, Delsol G, Brousset P. Prominent intrasinusoidal infiltration of the bone marrow by mantle cell lymphoma. Hum Pathol. 2003;34:789–91.

119. Tandon B, Peterson L, Gao J, Nelson B, Ma S, Rosen S, Chen YH. Nuclear overexpression of lymphoid-enhancer-binding factor 1 identifies chronic lymphocytic leukemia/small lymphocytic lymphoma in small B-cell lymphomas. Mod Pathol. 2011;24:1433–43.

120. Kohnke T, Wittmann VK, Bucklein VL, Lichtenegger F, Pasalic Z, Hiddemann W, Spiekermann K, Subklewe M. Diagnosis of CLL revisited: increased specificity by a modified five-marker scoring system including CD200. Br J Haematol. 2017;179:480–7.

121. Howard MT, Dufresne S, Swerdlow SH, Cook JR. Follicular lymphoma of the spleen: multiparameter analysis of 16 cases. Am J Clin Pathol. 2009;131:656–62.

122. Perrone S, D'Elia GM, Annechini G, Ferretti A, Tosti ME, Foa R, Pulsoni A. Splenic marginal zone lymphoma: prognostic factors, role of watch and wait policy, and other therapeutic approaches in the rituximab era. Leuk Res. 2016;44:53–60.

123. Falini B, Agostinelli C, Bigerna B, Pucciarini A, Pacini R, Tabarrini A, Falcinelli F, Piccioli M, Paulli M, Gambacorta M, et al. IRTA1 is selectively expressed in nodal and extranodal marginal zone lymphomas. Histopathology. 2012;61:930–41.

124. Olszewski AJ, Castillo JJ. Survival of patients with marginal zone lymphoma: analysis of the surveillance, epidemiology, and end results database. Cancer. 2013;119:629–38.

125. Montalban C, Abraira V, Arcaini L, Domingo-Domenech E, Guisado-Vasco P, Iannitto E, Mollejo M, Matutes E, Ferreri A, Salar A, et al. Risk stratification for Splenic Marginal Zone Lymphoma based on haemoglobin concentration, platelet count, high lactate dehydrogenase level and extrahilar lymphadenopathy: development and validation on 593 cases. Br J Haematol. 2012;159:164–71.

126. Hockley SL, Else M, Morilla A, Wotherspoon A, Dearden C, Catovsky D, Gonzalez D, Matutes E. The prognostic impact of clinical and molecular features in hairy cell leukaemia variant and splenic marginal zone lymphoma. Br J Haematol. 2012;158:347–54.

127. Gruszka-Westwood AM, Hamoudi RA, Matutes E, Tuset E, Catovsky D. p53 abnormalities in splenic lymphoma with villous lymphocytes. Blood. 2001;97:3552–8.

128. Cervetti G, Ghio F, Cecconi N, Morganti R, Galimberti S, Petrini M. How to treat splenic marginal zone lymphoma (SMZL) in patients unfit for surgery or more aggressive therapies: experience in 30 cases. J Chemother. 2017;29:126–9.

129. Kim H, Dorfman RF. Morphological studies of 84 untreated patients subjected to laparotomy for the staging of non-Hodgkin's lymphomas. Cancer. 1974;33:657–74.

130. Warnke RA, Weiss LM, Chan JKC, Cleary ML, Dorfman RF. Tumors of the lymph nodes and spleen. Atlas of tumor pathology, 3rd Series, Fascicle 14. Washington, D.C.: Armed Forces Institute of Pathology; 1995.

131. Goffinet DR, Warnke R, Dunnick NR, Castellino R, Glatstein E, Nelsen TS, Dorfman RF, Rosenberg SA, Kaplan HS. Clinical and surgical (laparotomy) evaluation of patients with non-Hodgkin's lymphomas. Cancer Treat Rep. 1977;61:981–92.

132. Ahmann DL, Kiely JM, Harrison EG Jr, Payne WS. Malignant lymphoma of the spleen. A review of 49 cases in which the diagnosis was made at splenectomy. Cancer. 1966;19:461–9.

133. Brox A, Bishinsky JI, Berry G. Primary non-Hodgkin lymphoma of the spleen. Am J Hematol. 1991;38:95–100.

134. Kraemer BB, Osborne BM, Butler JJ. Primary splenic presentation of malignant lymphoma and related disorders. A study of 49 cases. Cancer. 1984;54:1606–19.

135. Narang S, Wolf BC, Neiman RS. Malignant lymphoma presenting with prominent splenomegaly. A clinicopathologic study with special reference to intermediate cell lymphoma. Cancer. 1985;55:1948–57.

136. Spier CM, Kjeldsberg CR, Eyre HJ, Behm FG. Malignant lymphoma with primary presentation in the spleen. A study of 20 patients. Arch Pathol Lab Med. 1985;109:1076–80.

137. Kansal R, Ross CW, Singleton TP, Finn WG, Schnitzer B. Histopathologic features of splenic small B-cell lymphomas. A study of 42 cases with a definitive diagnosis by the World Health Organization classification. Am J Clin Pathol. 2003;120:335–47.

138. Pittaluga S, Verhoef G, Criel A, Wlodarska I, Dierlamm J, Mecucci C, Van den Berghe H, De Wolf-Peeters C. "Small" B-cell non-Hodgkin's lymphomas with splenomegaly at presentation are either mantle cell lymphoma or marginal zone cell lymphoma. A study based on histology, cytology, immunohistochemistry, and cytogenetic analysis. Am J Surg Pathol. 1996;20:211–23.

139. Arber DA, Rappaport H, Weiss LM. Non-Hodgkin's lymphoproliferative disorders involving the spleen. Mod Pathol. 1997;10:18–32.

140. Kraus MD, Fleming MD, Vonderheide RH. The spleen as a diagnostic specimen: a review of 10 years' experience at two tertiary care institutions. Cancer. 2001;91:2001–9.

141. Hampel PJ, King RL, Hanson CA, Simonetto D, Chaffee KG, Call TG, Ding W, Kenderian SS, Slager SL, Kay NE, and others. Liver biopsy in patients with chronic lymphocytic leukemia: indications and pathological findings. Blood. 2016;128:5592.

142. Ruchlemer R, Wotherspoon AC, Thompson JN, Swansbury JG, Matutes E, Catovsky D. Splenectomy in mantle cell lymphoma

with leukaemia: a comparison with chronic lymphocytic leukaemia. Br J Haematol. 2002;118:952–8.

143. Hsi ED, Martin P. Indolent mantle cell lymphoma. Leuk Lymphoma. 2014;55:761–7.

144. Furtado M, Rule S. Indolent mantle cell lymphoma. Haematologica. 2011;96:1086–8.

145. Ondrejka SL, Lai R, Smith SD, Hsi ED. Indolent mantle cell leukemia: a clinicopathological variant characterized by isolated lymphocytosis, interstitial bone marrow involvement, kappa light chain restriction, and good prognosis. Haematologica. 2011;96:1121–7.

146. Loddenkemper C, Longerich T, Hummel M, Ernestus K, Anagnostopoulos I, Dienes HP, Schirmacher P, Stein H. Frequency and diagnostic patterns of lymphomas in liver biopsies with respect to the WHO classification. Virchows Arch. 2007;450: 493–502.

147. Shimono J, Miyoshi H, Kamimura T, Eto T, Miyagishima T, Sasaki Y, Kurita D, Kawamoto K, Nagafuji K, Seto M, et al. Clinicopathological features of primary splenic follicular lymphoma. Ann Hematol. 2017;96:2063–70.

148. Mollejo M, Rodriguez-Pinilla MS, Montes-Moreno S, Algara P, Dogan A, Cigudosa JC, Juarez R, Flores T, Forteza J, Arribas A, et al. Splenic follicular lymphoma: clinicopathologic characteristics of a series of 32 cases. Am J Surg Pathol. 2009;33:730–8.

149. Lei KI. Primary non-Hodgkin's lymphoma of the liver. Leuk Lymphoma. 1998;29:293–9.

150. Dimopoulos MA, Panayiotidis P, Moulopoulos LA, Sfikakis P, Dalakas M. Waldenstrom's macroglobulinemia: clinical features, complications, and management. J Clin Oncol. 2000;18:214–26.

151. Hamadeh F, MacNamara SP, Aguilera NS, Swerdlow SH, Cook JR. MYD88 L265P mutation analysis helps define nodal lymphoplasmacytic lymphoma. Mod Pathol. 2015;28:564–74.

152. Lin P, Bueso-Ramos C, Wilson CS, Mansoor A, Medeiros LJ. Waldenstrom macroglobulinemia involving extramedullary sites: morphologic and immunophenotypic findings in 44 patients. Am J Surg Pathol. 2003;27:1104–13.

153. Pescarmona E, Pignoloni P, Orazi A, Lo Coco F, Lavinia AM, Martelli M, Baroni CD. "Composite" lymphoma, lymphoplasmacytoid and diffuse large B-cell lymphoma of the spleen: molecular-genetic evidence of a common clonal origin. Virchows Arch. 1999;435:442–6.

154. Borgonovo G, d'Oiron R, Amato A, Leger-Ravet MB, Iseni MC, Smadja C, Lemaigre G, Franco D. Primary lymphoplasmacytic lymphoma of the liver associated with a serum monoclonal peak of IgG kappa. Am J Gastroenterol. 1995;90:137–40.

155. Polprasert C, Wongchitrat C, Assanasen T, Prayongratana K. Lymphoplasmacytic lymphoma with IgA hypergammaglobulinemia and liver involvement. J Med Assoc Thail. 2009;92(Suppl 3):S65–8.

156. Isaacson PG, Banks PM, Best PV, McLure SP, Muller-Hermelink HK, Wyatt JI. Primary low-grade hepatic B-cell lymphoma of mucosa-associated lymphoid tissue (MALT)-type. Am J Surg Pathol. 1995;19:571–5.

157. Maes M, Depardieu C, Dargent JL, Hermans M, Verhaeghe JL, Delabie J, Pittaluga S, Troufleau P, Verhest A, De Wolf-Peeters C. Primary low-grade B-cell lymphoma of MALT-type occurring in the liver: a study of two cases. J Hepatol. 1997;27:922–7.

158. Prabhu RM, Medeiros LJ, Kumar D, Drachenberg CI, Papadimitriou JC, Appelman HD, Johnson LB, Laurin J, Heyman M, Abruzzo LV. Primary hepatic low-grade B-cell lymphoma of mucosa-associated lymphoid tissue (MALT) associated with primary biliary cirrhosis. Mod Pathol. 1998;11:404–10.

159. Kirk CM, Lewin D, Lazarchick J. Primary hepatic B-cell lymphoma of mucosa-associated lymphoid tissue. Arch Pathol Lab Med. 1999;123:716–9.

160. Nagata S, Harimoto N, Kajiyama K. Primary hepatic mucosa-associated lymphoid tissue lymphoma: a case report and literature review. Surg Case Rep. 2015;1:87.

161. Streubel B, Lamprecht A, Dierlamm J, Cerroni L, Stolte M, Ott G, Raderer M, Chott A. T(14;18)(q32;q21) involving IGH and MALT1 is a frequent chromosomal aberration in MALT lymphoma. Blood. 2003;101:2335–9.

Madhu P. Menon, Min Shi, and Karthik Ganapathi

Introduction

The diagnosis of diffuse large B-cell lymphoma (DLBCL) in the current era is complex and involves a subclassification scheme that incorporates morphologic, immunophenotypic, and genetic features. In addition, there are large B-cell lymphomas that have a unique biology or site predilection, which justifies separate diagnostic entities (e.g., Epstein-Barr virus (EBV) + DLBCL, not otherwise specified (NOS); primary DLBCL of the CNS; primary cutaneous DLBCL, leg type; DLBCL associated with chronic inflammation; plasmablastic lymphoma). This chapter covers large B-cell lymphomas that are known to involve the spleen, primary or secondary. The most common lymphoma of the spleen is DLBCL, NOS, and most of these are secondary in nature. We discuss both the common macronodular manifestation and the less common diffuse red pulp variant of DLBCLs. T-cell-/histiocyte-rich large B-cell lymphoma (TCRBL) has morphologic features (micronodular) unique to the spleen as compared to the typical morphology observed in nodal TCRBL. EBV+ DLBCL, NOS, of the spleen has morphology similar to that observed in other sites, however, with important differential diagnoses that need to be considered. Lastly, we discuss the recently introduced high-grade B-cell lymphomas (HGBL), which include double-/triple-hit lymphomas (involving *MYC*, *BCL2*, and/or *BCL6* translocations) and high-grade B-cell lymphoma, NOS.

M. P. Menon (✉)
Department of Pathology and Laboratory Medicine, Henry Ford Hospital, Detroit, MI, USA
e-mail: MMENON2@hfhs.org

M. Shi
Department of Laboratory Medicine and Pathology, Mayo Clinic, Rochester, MN, USA

K. Ganapathi
Department of Laboratory Medicine, University of California, San Francisco, CA, USA

Diffuse Large B-Cell Lymphoma (DLBCL), Not Otherwise Specified (NOS)

Definition

As per the World Health Organization (WHO) classification of tumors of hematopoietic and lymphoid tissue, diffuse large B-cell lymphoma is defined as an aggressive mature B-cell lymphoma with diffuse proliferation of medium to large cells whose nuclei are the same size or larger than that of macrophages or twice that of normal lymphocytes [1].

Diagnosis of DLBCL in the modern era is complex and requires further subclassification based on morphologic, molecular, and immunohistochemical attributes, EBV status, and specific organ sites [1]. Several studies have pointed toward the prognostic relevance of subclassification based on cell of origin (COO) into an activated B-cell subtype (ABC) or a germinal center B-cell subtype (GCB) subtype as defined by gene expression profiling studies [2–4]. Patients with ABC subtypes treated with rituximab + cyclophosphamide, hydroxydaunorubicin, oncovin, and prednisone (R-CHOP) tend to have worse prognosis than those with GCB subtype and benefit from the addition of drugs such as bortezomib, lenalidomide, and ibrutinib to R-CHOP [1]. Recent studies by Schmitz et al. have further defined the genetic landscape of DLBCLs and identified four distinct subtypes: MCD (*MYD88* and *CD79B* mutations), BN2 (*BCL6* rearrangements and *NOTCH2* mutations), N1 (*NOTCH1* mutation), and EZB (*BCL2* translocations and *EZH2* mutations) [5]. Interestingly, these subtypes have prognostic differences, favorable in BN2 and EZB subtypes, while inferior in MCD and N1 subtypes [5]. Several immunohistochemical surrogate schemes were developed to distinguish DLBCL ABC from DLBCL GCB subtype; the most commonly used algorithm is the Hans classifier, which uses CD10, BCL6, and MUM1 [6]. Other immunohistochemical algorithms in existence include Colomo (MUM1, CD10, and BCL6), Muris (BCL2, CD10, and MUM1), Choi (GCET1, MUM1, CD10, FOXP1,

© Springer Nature Switzerland AG 2020
L. Zhang et al. (eds.), *Diagnostic Pathology of Hematopoietic Disorders of Spleen and Liver*,
https://doi.org/10.1007/978-3-030-37708-3_6

and BCL6), and Tally (CD10, GCET1, MUM1, FOXP1, and LMO2) [7–10]. Recent studies have also demonstrated the importance of genetic studies, primarily the identification of double-hit (*MYC* + *BCL2* or *BCL6* translocations) or triple-hit (*MYC* + *BCL2* + *BCL6* translocations) lymphomas with a highly aggressive clinical course. In addition, the use of MYC and BCL2 immunohistochemistry (IHC) identifies a specific subtype with inferior prognosis, the so-called double expressers, with expression of MYC (more than 40% of cells) and BCL2 (more than 50% of cells) [11, 12].

The most common lymphoma involving the spleen is DLBCL that constitutes approximately 30–50% of splenic lymphomas [13, 14]. While there is no precise definition, it is generally accepted that splenic manifestation with possible involvement of regional lymph nodes and/or adjacent organs/tissues but without generalized lymphadenopathy would define a primary splenic DLBCL [15].

Epidemiology

The bulk of the DLBCLs in the spleen are secondary in nature, and primary splenic DLBCLs appear to be less common (ranging from approximately 11–30%) [13–15]. Three major macroscopic patterns are recognized: macronodular; micronodular, and diffuse red pulp infiltration [15, 16]. The macronodular pattern is most common, while the diffuse red pulp pattern is least common. Both macronodular and micronodular patterns have a roughly equal sex distribution and a mean age of 64 years (range of 32–84 years) and 55.1 years (range of 32–80 years). The diffuse red pulp infiltration pattern (R-DLBCL) has a median age of 64 years (range of 40–81 years) with a male predominance (18:6) [15–24]. Association of hepatitis C virus with DLBCL has been reported albeit with different rates in different countries: 44% in Taiwan, 51% in Japan, 64% in Italy, and 9% in Israel [25–28].

Clinical Features

Patients with the typical macronodular pattern of DLBCL generally tend to be in clinical stage I with primary presentation of abdominal pain and splenomegaly [15]. In contrast, most patients with micronodular pattern frequently present in stage IV [15]. Patients with diffuse red pulp DLBCL (R-DLBCL) usually have an aggressive presentation with cytopenia, B symptoms, and splenomegaly [15–23]. Most patients also have elevated lactate dehydrogenase (LDH) and soluble interleukin-2 receptor, CD25, hypoalbuminemia, and moderately elevated C-reactive protein. Patients with R-DLBCL are usually in stage IV and, unlike the macronodular DLBCL, tend to have more bone marrow, liver, and peripheral blood involvement [15–23]. A subset of R-DLBCL cases is positive for CD5 [16]. Similar to the *de novo* CD5+ large B-cell lymphoma, the CD5+ R-DLBCL particularly tends to behave more aggressively with high clinical stage, international prognostic index (IPI) score, and LDH levels [16]. Lymph node involvement is generally limited to the perisplenic or abdominal lymph nodes in all morphologic patterns. Regardless of the morphologic patterns, a generalized lymphadenopathy at the time of diagnosis is not a feature and, in most cases, would be considered exclusionary for a diagnosis of primary splenic large B-cell lymphoma. The macronodular DLBCL seems to have a better prognosis and a higher survival rate as compared to that of the micronodular or diffuse red pulp DLBCL [15]. The recommended treatment approach is generally similar to that of typical nodal DLBCLs [29].

Pathologic Features

As mentioned above, there are three major morphologic patterns of splenic involvement by large B-cell lymphoma: macronodular, micronodular, and diffuse red pulp infiltration.

Morphology

Gross Features

Macronodular DLBCL This is the most common type of DLBCL manifestation in the spleen. Grossly, the spleens are enlarged, and the cut surface demonstrates a visible large mass or multiple nodules of variable sizes that sometimes coalesce (Fig. 6.1a). The mean reported splenic weight is 1015 grams (range of 150–2089 grams) [15]. Broad areas of necrosis might be seen (Fig. 6.1a).

Micronodular DLBCL Spleens are enlarged with a median weight of 1880 grams (range of 800–4000 grams). Unlike the macronodular DLBCL, large nodules or masses are not seen. Instead, the cut surface demonstrates a uniform miliary pattern with numerous small, discrete, and uniform nodules [15].

Diffuse Red Pulp Infiltration DLBCL Spleens are enlarged with a median weight of 1300 grams (range of 220–2600 grams). The cut surface either appears normal or beefy red in color (Fig. 6.2a). Discrete masses or nodules are generally not seen [15–23].

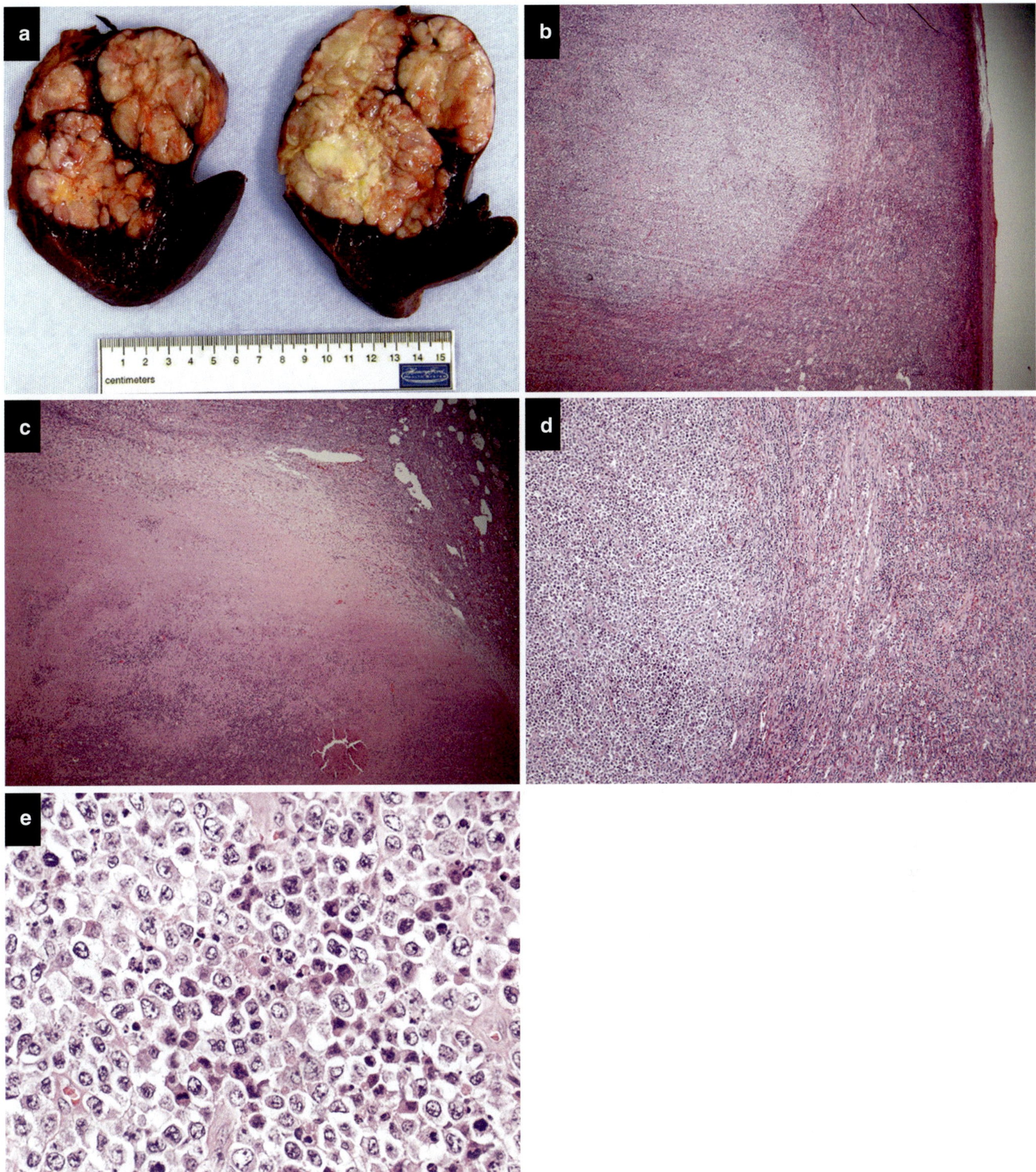

Fig. 6.1 Diffuse large B-cell lymphoma, macronodular: (**a**) Gross photograph demonstrates discrete large masses within the spleen with areas of necrosis. (**b**) Low power microscopy demonstrates distinction between the mass on the left and non-neoplastic splenic tissue on the right (Hematoxylin and eosin (H&E), magnification ×40). (**c**) Broad areas of necrosis are noted; note normal splenic tissue with sinusoids at the top (H&E, magnification ×40). (**d**) The mass is composed of sheets of large atypical lymphocytes (H&E, magnification ×100). (**e**) Diffuse proliferation of centroblasts (multiple membrane bound nucleoli) is seen. Frequent mitoses and apoptosis are also noted (H&E, magnification ×400)

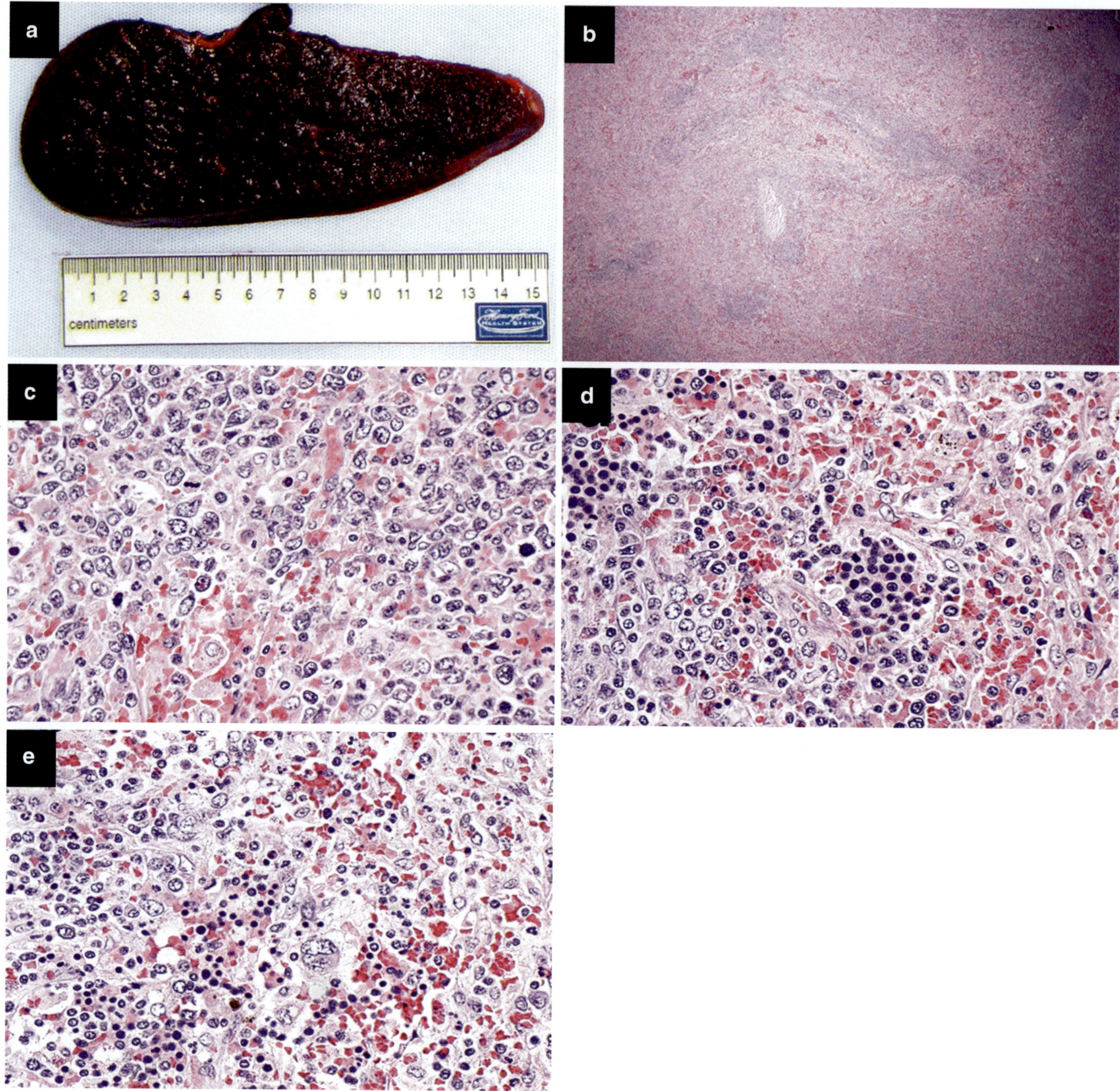

Fig. 6.2 Diffuse large B-cell lymphoma, diffuse red pulp variant: (**a**) Gross photograph does not demonstrate any discrete masses, instead, the cut surface appears to be beefy red with areas of nodularity (**b**) Low power microscopy demonstrates expanded red pulp with retained, albeit attenuated white pulp (H&E. magnification ×40). (**c**) The red pulp cords and sinuses are infiltrated by centroblasts (H&E, with multiple membrane bound nucleoli). Frequent mitotic figures are seen (H&E, magnification ×400). (**d**) Exuberant extramedullary hematopoiesis is noted (H&E, magnification ×400). (**e**) Frequent areas of extramedullary hematopoiesis with presence of megakaryocytes noted (H&E, magnification ×400)

Microscopic Features

Macronodular DLBCL Microscopically, there are discrete discernible tumor areas (replacing normal splenic architecture) separated in a circumscribed fashion from the normal splenic parenchyma (Fig. 6.1b, d). Areas of necrosis and sclerosis can be seen quite frequently within the tumor nodules (Fig. 6.1c). The tumor nodules are composed of sheets of medium to large atypical lymphoid cells, which most commonly are centroblastic (large atypical cells with vesicular nuclei and multiple peripheralized nucleoli) (Fig. 6.1e) but can also appear to be immunoblastic (large atypical cells with vesicular nuclei and prominent single nucleolus) or polylobated. Increased macrophages are noted in several cases; nevertheless, sheeting of the large neoplastic lymphoid cells is obvious. The residual spleen demonstrates an intact architecture with retained white and red pulp. Regional and abdominal lymph nodes, when involved, demonstrate effacement of the architecture by sheets of large atypical lymphoid cells. Bone marrow involvement is rare with the macronodular DLBCL. However, when the bone marrow is involved, both concordant involvement (large lymphoid cell infiltration in the bone marrow) and discordant involvement (small B-cell lymphoma in the bone marrow) can be identified.

Micronodular DLBCL Numerous small nodules centered in the white pulp with some infiltration of the red pulp are seen. Most cases demonstrate clustering and sheeting of predominantly large atypical lymphoid cells with fewer non-neoplastic T-cells forming nodules in the background. The cases with nodular morphology, abundant histiocytes, and scattered large cells of B-cell phenotype (not clustering, coalescing, or sheeting) are best diagnosed as micronodular T-cell-/histiocyte-rich large B-cell lymphoma (discussed later in this chapter). When regional lymph nodes are involved, they are either replaced by sheets of large lymphoid cells or demonstrate similar nodular morphology.

Diffuse Red Pulp Infiltration DLBCL The splenic red pulp demonstrates expansion and infiltration of the cords and sinuses by non-cohesive large lymphoma cells (Fig. 6.2b). Cells appear either centroblastic, pleomorphic, or polylobated (Fig. 6.2c) [15]. Areas with extramedullary hematopoiesis are frequently noted (Fig. 6.2d and e). Hemophagocytosis in the spleen and bone marrow is also a frequent phenomenon. Involvement of the bone marrow is common and is manifested in the form of characteristic intrasinusoidal and interstitial infiltrates of large lymphoid cells. In addition, involvement of the liver is also seen commonly in the form of intrasinusoidal and portal infiltrates. Lymph node involvement is less common and is seen in the form of diffuse as well as intravascular infiltration.

Immunohistochemistry

Macronodular DLBCL The large lymphoid cells are consistently positive for pan B-cell markers including CD20

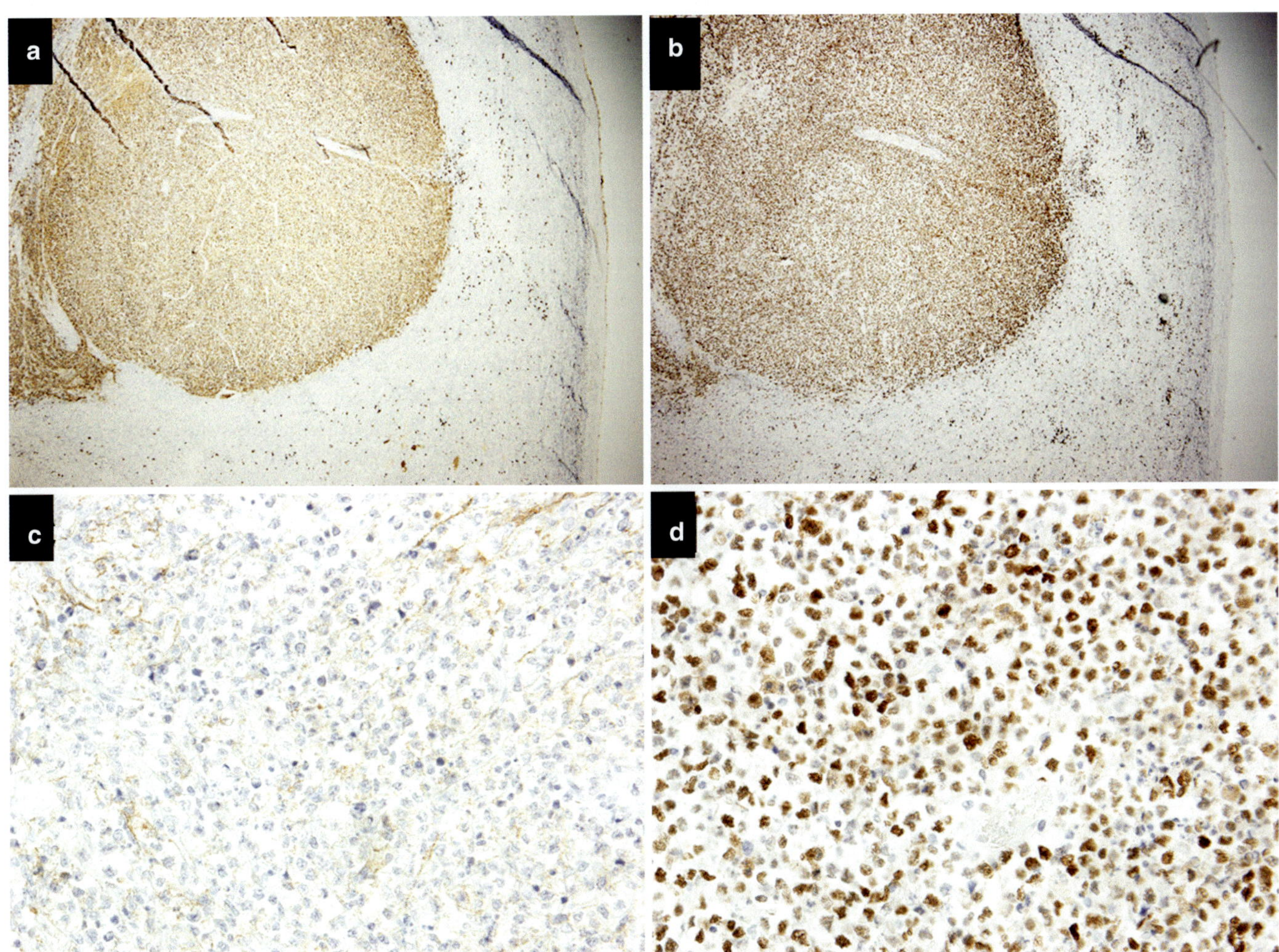

Fig. 6.3 Diffuse large B-cell lymphoma, macronodular: The neoplastic lymphocytes are positive for CD20 (**a**) and demonstrate a high MIB1 proliferation index (**b**) (immunoperoxidase, magnification ×40). In addition, these cells are negative for CD10 (**c**), positive for BCL6 (**d**) and negative for MUM1 (**e**) immunoperoxidase, magnification ×400). (**f**) MYC immunostain demonstrates greater than 40% positivity (immunoperoxidase, magnification ×400)

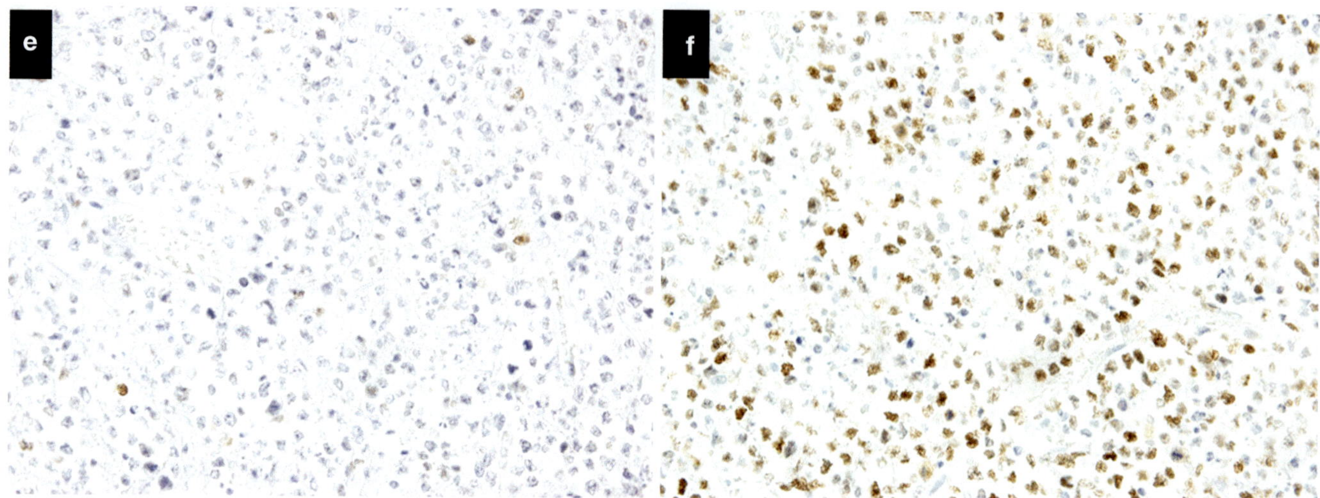

Fig. 6.3 (continued)

(Fig. 6.3a). They are often positive for BCL6 (Fig. 6.3d), while CD10 seems to be more frequently negative (Fig. 6.3c). BCL2 is positive in approximately half the cases. IgD expression is seen in approximately one-fourth of the cases, while cyclin D1, DBA.44, and CD5 are usually negative. CD21, CD23, or CD35 do not highlight any follicular dendritic cell meshworks. P53 expression and loss of P16 expression are seen in a minor subset of cases. MIB1 or Ki-67 proliferation index is high (Fig. 6.3b) and more than 70% in majority of the cases. Most cases are EBV negative by Epstein-Barr virus-encoded RNA (EBER) in situ hybridization (ISH). MYC positivity can also be observed in these cases (Fig. 6.3f).

Micronodular DLBCL Cases that are best diagnosed as micronodular T-cell-/histiocyte-rich large B-cell lymphoma are discussed later. Otherwise, cases with micronodular pattern are CD20 and BCL6 positive and negative for CD10, CD5, and BCL1. There is variable positivity for BCL2 and IgD. Expression of DBA.44, CD43, or CD38 is rare. MIB1 or Ki-67 proliferation index is moderate to high (>50% in all cases and >75% in a subset). Most cases are EBV negative by EBER-ISH.

Diffuse Red Pulp Infiltration DLBCL The lymphoma cells are consistently positive for pan B-cell markers including CD20 (Fig. 6.4a, c) and negative for CD3 (Fig. 6.4b). These cases demonstrate variable positivity for CD10, BCL6, MUM1, and BCL2. Most cases are IgM$^+$, while a minor subset can be IgD$^+$. Aberrant CD5 expression is seen in a subset of cases (Fig. 6.4d). The intrasinusoidal nature of the infiltrate can be demonstrated by PAS stain or Factor VIII immunostain. Occasionally, these cases can also be CD38 or DBA.44 positive. They are consistently negative for cyclin D1. P53 overexpression is seen in a minor subset of cases. MIB1 or Ki-67 proliferation index is variable, ranging from 10% to 80% in the majority of the cases (Fig. 6.4f). Most cases are EBV negative by EBER-ISH.

Flow Cytometry

Flow cytometry can be used for immunophenotypic analysis of the lymphoma cells, especially for the detection of dim CD5 expression in the diffuse red pulp infiltration type. However, in general, flow cytometry can be negative in approximately 25% of large B-cell lymphoma cases for various reasons including non-viability of cells, cell fragility, necrosis, apoptosis, and routine gating strategies missing out on gating the large cells [30].

Molecular Studies

Polymerase chain reaction (PCR) for immunoglobulin heavy chain (IgH) and T-cell receptor (TCR) gamma rearrangement usually demonstrates monoclonality of B-cells and polyclonal nature of background T-cells. In addition, CD5$^+$ diffuse red pulp infiltrate DLBCL demonstrates complex cytogenetic abnormalities including 3q27 and 11q13 abnormalities, which have been previously reported in de novo DLBCL [16, 31].

Differential Diagnoses

The diagnosis of macronodular DLBCL is usually straightforward. However, the diffuse red pulp infiltration DLBCL might

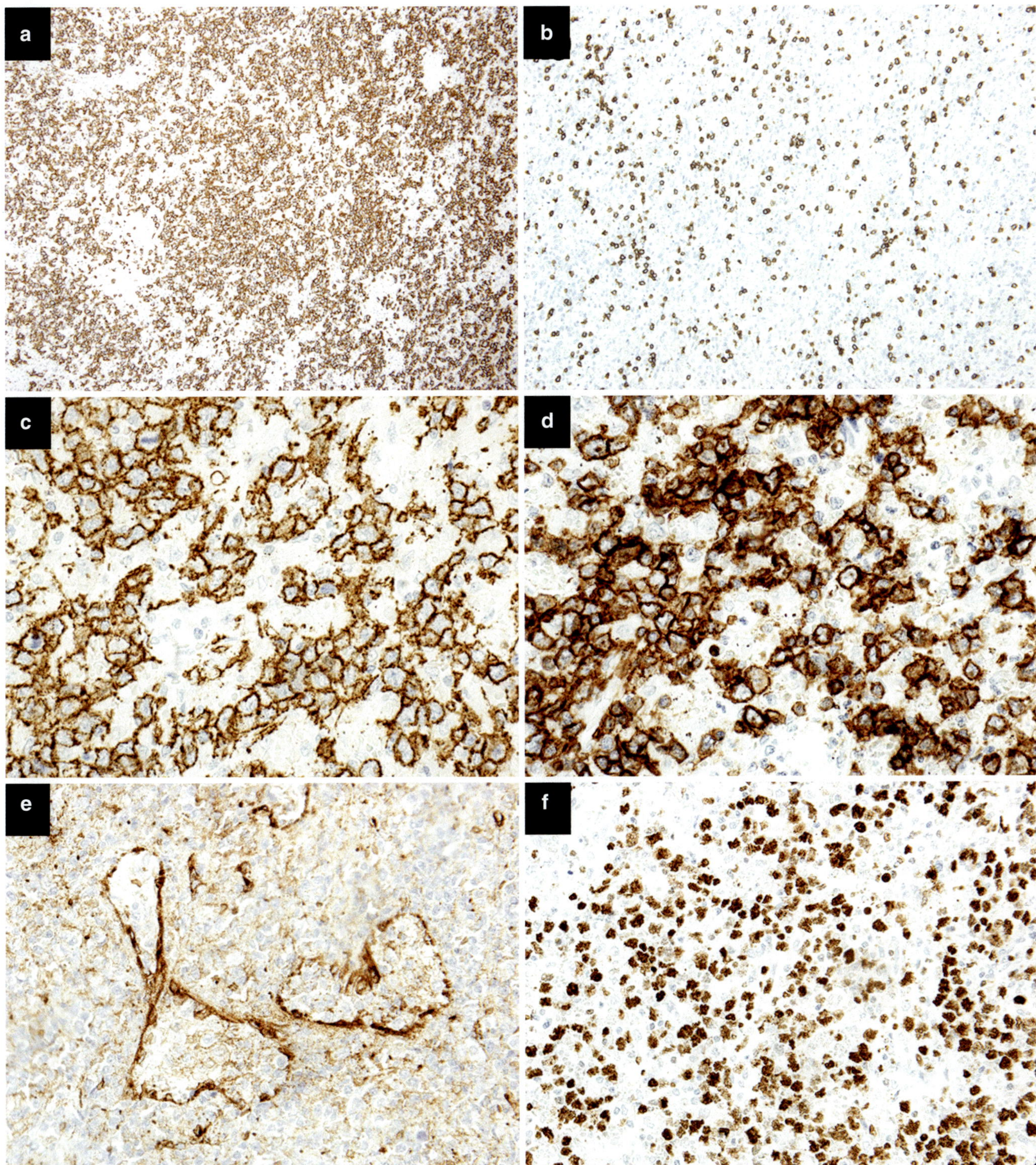

Fig. 6.4 Diffuse large B-cell lymphoma, diffuse red pulp variant: The neoplastic lymphocytes are positive for CD20 (**a**) and negative for CD3 (**b**) (immunoperoxidase, magnification ×40). CD20 demonstrates infiltration of splenic cords (**c**) and sinuses by neoplastic lymphocytes, which are also positive for CD5 (**d**) (immunoperoxidase, magnification ×400). (**e**) Factor VIII staining demonstrates the sinusoidal infiltration by the neoplastic B lymphocytes. The surrounding splenic cords are also infiltrated by lymphoma cells (immunoperoxidase, magnification ×400). (**f**) Ki-67 demonstrates a high proliferation index (immunoperoxidase, magnification ×400)

Table 6.1 Differential diagnoses of diffuse red pulp variant of diffuse large B-cell lymphoma

	Gross findings of the spleen	Morphology	IHC and ISH	Genetic and molecular studies	Miscellaneous
Diffuse red pulp variant of diffuse large B-cell lymphoma (R-DLBCL)	Enlarged Normal cut surface or beefy red	Expansion of red pulp Infiltration of cords and sinuses by large cells with centroblastic, pleomorphic, or polylobated cells Extramedullary hematopoiesis Hemophagocytosis Bone marrow: intrasinusoidal and interstitial infiltrates	B-cell markers Variable expression of CD10, BCL6, MUM1, and BCL2 Subset of cases are CD5+ Surface IgM+ in most cases EBER-ISH negative	Positive Ig gene rearrangement Negative TCRγ rearrangement Complex cytogenetics	Regional lymph node involvement can be seen Aggressive clinical presentation
Intravascular large B-cell lymphoma (Asian variant)	Enlarged or normal Normal cut surface	Spleen and BM: predominantly intrasinusoidal infiltrate of large cells Hemophagocytosis Interstitial infiltrate of BM generally *not* seen	Similar to R-DLBCL	Positive Ig gene rearrangement Negative TCRγ rearrangement	Lymph node involvement generally *not* seen
B-cell prolymphocytic leukemia	Enlarged Prominent nodules can be seen	Prolymphocytes noted in peripheral blood (PB) and BM Spleen: expanded white pulp and red pulp by prolymphocytes	Similar to R-DLBCL CD5+ in a subset of cases	Positive Ig gene rearrangement Negative TCRγ rearrangement	Involvement of lymph node is rare High WBC counts and prolymphocytic cytology in PB
Hairy cell leukemia (HCL)	Enlarged with presence of "blood lakes"	Expansion of red pulp with proliferation of small- to medium-sized lymphocytes with abundant pale cytoplasm PB: hairy lymphoid cells BM: interstitial infiltrate	Pan B-cell markers Positive for CD103, CD123, DBA.44, TRAP, and annexin A1 Low MIB1 or Ki-67 proliferation	Positive Ig gene rearrangement Negative TCRγ rearrangement Positive *BRAF*-V600E mutation	Indolent clinical course
Hairy cell leukemia variant (HCLv)	Enlarged spleen Normal-appearing cut surface or presence of "blood lakes"	Expansion of red pulp with proliferation of small- to medium-sized lymphoid cells with abundant pale cytoplasm albeit with prominent nucleoli, blastic, or convoluted nuclei PB: hybrid features of prolymphocyte and hairy cells BM: generally intrasinusoidal infiltrates	Pan B-cell markers DBA.44+, CD11c+, bright monotypic immunoglobulin+, and CD103+ Negative for CD25, annexin A1, TRAP, CD123	Positive Ig gene rearrangement Negative TCRγ rearrangement Negative *BRAF*-V600E mutation	Variant clinical, morphologic, and immunophenotypic features as compared to HCL
Splenic marginal zone lymphoma (SMZL) transforming to large B-cell lymphoma	Enlarged with presence of prominent nodules	Areas of SMZL seen with prominent white pulp nodules and targetoid appearance of proliferation of small to medium lymphoid cells Areas with sheets of large cells can be seen replacing the white and red pulp	Pan B-cell marker Surface IgD+ Can be CD5+	Positive Ig gene rearrangement Negative TCRγ rearrangement Can have loss of 7q21–32 or trisomy 3	

Ig immunoglobulin, *TCRγ* T-cell receptor gamma, *IHC* immunohistochemistry, *ISH* in situ hybridization, *EBER* EBV-encoded small RNA, *BM* bone marrow, *PB* peripheral blood

pose diagnostic challenges, and certain differential diagnoses need to be considered (Table 6.1). On pure morphologic grounds, various T/NK cell lymphomas, which involve the red pulp like hepatosplenic T-cell lymphoma, T-large granular lymphocytic leukemia, T-prolymphocytic leukemia, and intravascular NK/T-cell lymphoma, might be considered. However, the B-cell phenotype of the lymphoid cells would easily exclude these T-cell lymphomas except for rare cases with aberrant CD20 expression. There are some aggressive B-cell lymphomas, which need to be considered in the differential diagnoses because of overlapping morphologic features and/or immunophenotype. The focus would be on those B-cell lymphomas, which characteristically involve the red pulp (Table 6.1).

Intravascular Large B-Cell Lymphoma (IVBL)

Intravascular large B-cell lymphomas are either the classic type seen in the Western population (predominantly neurologic and cutaneous involvement) or the Asian variant (hepatosplenomegaly, cytopenias, multi-organ failure, and hemophagocytosis) [1]. The Asian type particularly can involve the spleen and bone marrow in an intrasinusoidal fashion, which mimics the R-DLBCL. An intrasinusoidal large B-cell lymphoma has also been described in the Asian population with characteristic splenic histiocytic proliferation and prominent hemophagocytosis [20]. This variant is perhaps best classified as an IVBL. While the morphologic features and immunophenotype of both IVBL and R-DLBCL can be similar (including CD5 positivity in a subset of both entities), the involvement of lymph nodes would generally exclude IVBL [1]. Also, the characteristic interstitial and intrasinusoidal involvement of the bone marrow is a feature of R-DLBCL, while WHO definition limits IVBL to only intrasinusoidal involvement in addition to capillaries [1, 16].

B-Prolymphocytic Leukemia (B-PLL)

B-prolymphocytic leukemia is an aggressive leukemia with characteristically high WBC counts and greater than 55% prolymphocytes in the peripheral blood [1]. Prolymphocytes are defined as medium to large cells with moderately condensed nuclei and prominent central nucleoli. They generally involve the bone marrow, peripheral blood, and spleen. Splenic involvement is in the form of expanded white pulp nodules and red pulp infiltrate by medium to large size cells with moderate to abundant cytoplasm and mature-appearing nuclei with prominent central eosinophilic nucleolus [1]. The cytology and immunophenotype of B-PLL can be similar to that of R-DLBCL. However, high WBC counts, characteristic morphology of the prolymphocytes in the peripheral blood, and the white pulp involvement in the spleen would favor B-PLL over R-DLBCL. In addition, involvement of lymph nodes by B-PLL is rare.

Hairy Cell Leukemia (HCL)

Hairy cell leukemia is a low-grade B-cell lymphoma, which characteristically involves the peripheral blood, bone marrow, and splenic red pulp. These cells characteristically are small to medium sized with oval to indented mature-appearing nuclei and moderate to abundant clear cytoplasm. Nucleoli are generally not seen. They characteristically involve the red pulp cords of the spleen and form pools of red blood cells, the so-called blood lakes. In general, the low-grade cytomorphology and the characteristic hairy cytoplasmic projections of the cells in the peripheral blood would distinguish hairy cell leukemia from R-DLBCL. Also, involvement of the bone marrow in HCL is in the form of interstitial infiltrates. Intrasinusoidal bone marrow infiltrates seen in R-DLBCL are generally not seen in HCL. There are some key immunophenotypic attributes of HCL, which distinguish them from R-DLBCL; in addition to B-cell markers, HCL cells are also positive for CD11c, CD25, CD103, CD123, DBA.44, tartrate resistant acid phosphatase (TRAP), cyclin

D1 (subset), and annexin A1. Classic HCL cells characteristically demonstrate *BRAF*-V600E mutation.

Hairy Cell Leukemia Variant (HCLv)

Hairy cell leukemia variant shares some morphologic and immunophenotypic features with HCL. However, it also demonstrates variant clinical (i.e., presence of leukocytosis and monocytosis), morphologic (i.e., presence of cells with prominent nucleoli, blastic or convoluted nuclei, and/or variable degree of hairy projections), or immunophenotypic features (i.e., negativity for CD25, CD123, annexin A1, and TRAP). HCLv can occasionally demonstrate variable nuclear features including prolymphocytic morphology and the so-called convoluted appearance [1, 32, 33]; some of these cases mimic R-DLBCL. Key differentiating features of HCLv (especially the transformed "convoluted" cases) from R-DLBCL would be the identification of the variable hairy projections in peripheral blood and the characteristic HCLv immunophenotype: DBA.44+, CD11c+, bright monotypic immunoglobulin+, and CD103+.

Splenic Marginal Zone Lymphoma (SMZL) Transforming to Large B-Cell Lymphoma

Splenic marginal zone lymphoma can occasionally undergo a large cell transformation, sometimes with a CD5+ phenotype [34, 35]. These cases need to be distinguished from R-DLBCL. The transformed SMZLs tend to retain proliferative areas of small- to medium-sized cells with some areas demonstrating the classic targetoid white pulp nodules (see chapter on SMZL). In addition, most R-DLBCL cases are surface IgM+, while transformed SMZLs are positive for surface IgD [16]. R-DLBCL cases tend to demonstrate complex cytogenetic abnormalities but usually lack trisomy 3 or allelic loss of 7q21–32, a characteristic finding in SMZL [16].

Micronodular T-Cell-/Histiocyte-Rich Large B-Cell Lymphoma (mTCRBL)

Definition

T-cell-/histiocyte-rich large B-cell lymphoma (TCRBL) is considered to be a subtype of large B-cell lymphoma, which is characterized morphologically by limited number of scattered large B-cells in a T-cell- and histiocyte-rich background [1, 36]. The term "T-cell-rich large B-cell lymphoma" was coined initially by Ramsay et al. to describe this peculiar subset of large B-cell lymphomas, which accounts for less than 10% of all DLBCLs [37]. TCRBL is primarily a nodal disease; however, other organs such as the bone marrow, liver, and spleen can be frequently involved [1]. While lymph nodes generally exhibit effacement of the architecture, a peculiar micronodular appearance in the spleen was initially described in cases of predominantly nodal TCRBL that secondarily involved the spleen [36, 38, 39]. Subsequently, Dogan et al. described the largest series of 17 patients with primarily splenic micronodular TCRBL (mTCRBL) (without a predominant nodal component), which demonstrated a similar micronodular appearance [40]. Other studies have also described similar micronodular morphology of TCRBL involving the spleen [15, 41]. In rare instances, mTCRBL can represent transformation from underlying low-grade B-cell lymphomas [42, 43]. mTCRBL is an aggressive disease with poor prognosis and should be treated as a variant of large B-cell lymphoma [29, 40].

Epidemiology

In the series by Mollejo et al., 3/33 (9%) of all primary splenic large B-cell lymphomas were mTCRBL [15]. Secondary involvement of the spleen by a "systemic" nodal TCRBL is much more common. It predominantly affects males with an age range of 35–70 (median age of 56 years) [40].

Clinical Features

Patients usually present with cytopenias, B-symptoms, and splenomegaly. While a generalized lymphadenopathy is not frequently seen in this entity, involvement of the regional lymph nodes, bone marrow, lungs, and liver has been reported [15, 40].

Pathologic Features

Primary or secondary involvement of the spleen by TCRBL demonstrates similar micronodular features. Diffuse effacement of the spleen in either context is not seen.

Morphology

Gross Features

The spleen is grossly enlarged and the weight usually ranges from 850 to 2500 grams [15, 40]. The cut surface either appears normal or miliary with presence of many small nodules (micronodular). Macroscopically identifiable tumor masses are not a feature of this entity.

Microscopic Features

Microscopically, the spleen demonstrates an intact architecture with retained normal-appearing red pulps. However, the white pulps are almost entirely replaced by atypical pale "histiocytic" nodules (Fig. 6.5a). The nodules exhibit varia-

tion in size, and in some cases, they coalesce to form larger nodules. At higher magnification, these nodules are composed of non-epithelioid histiocytes, small lymphocytes, and admixed large atypical lymphoid cells (Fig. 6.5b), which exhibited a spectrum of morphology ranging from Reed-Sternberg-like cells (as seen in classic Hodgkin lymphoma, cHL) (Fig. 6.5c), to centroblasts (large atypical cells with vesicular nuclei and multiple peripheralized nucleoli) (Fig. 6.5d), to immunoblasts or "pop-corn" lymphocyte/histiocyte (L&H/LP) cells that are seen in nodular lymphocyte predominant Hodgkin lymphoma (NLPHL). Areas of necrosis, extramedullary hematopoiesis, and some degree of fibrosis can be seen [40, 41]. The nodules can also demonstrate central sclerosis/hyalinization and either abut or surround the arterioles [41]. Plasma cells, eosinophils, or neutrophils are generally not a prominent feature of this entity. When it involves the liver, it causes expansion of the portal triads and presence of large lymphoid cells. Involvement of the bone marrow is in the form of numerous well-defined nodules, which are either inter- or occasionally paratrabecular in location [40]. These nodules have a similar histology as seen in the spleen with presence of numerous histiocytes, small lymphocytes, and scattered large lymphoid cells [40]. Other organs such as the lymph node and lung demonstrate similar nodular morphology as seen in the spleen [40].

Immunohistochemistry

By immunohistochemistry [40], the nodules are composed of small numbers of large B-cells as demonstrated by CD20 (Fig. 6.6a, c, d) and exhibit a predominance of T-cells (Fig. 6.6b). The large atypical lymphoid cells are positive for CD79a, OCT2 (Fig. 6.6e), PAX-5, BCL6, BCL2, and CD45 and negative for CD10, CD5, CD3, and CD138 [15, 40, 41]. EMA and CD30 are usually negative or variably positive, while CD15 is uniformly negative. Strong and diffuse CD30 expression is not a feature of this entity. Kappa and lambda immunostains may demonstrate kappa or lambda light chain restriction (Fig. 6.6f). The follicular dendritic cell markers (CD21, CD23, or CD35) do not demonstrate any follicular dendritic cell meshworks within the nodules. The background small cells are uniformly positive for CD3 (Fig. 6.6b) demonstrating their T-cell lineage and also demonstrating a cytotoxic T-cell phenotype [41]. The ratio of background T-cells to histiocytes can vary from case to case. CD57- or PD1(CD279)-positive T-cells are usually not increased in the background. MIB1 or Ki-67 proliferation index is usually high (>80%) in the large cell component (Fig. 6.6g). EBV-LMP immunohistochemical studies and in situ hybridization for EBV (EBER-ISH) are negative [40, 41].

Flow Cytometry

Flow cytometry is not a reliable methodology to confirm light chain restriction because of the paucity of the large lymphoid cells [41].

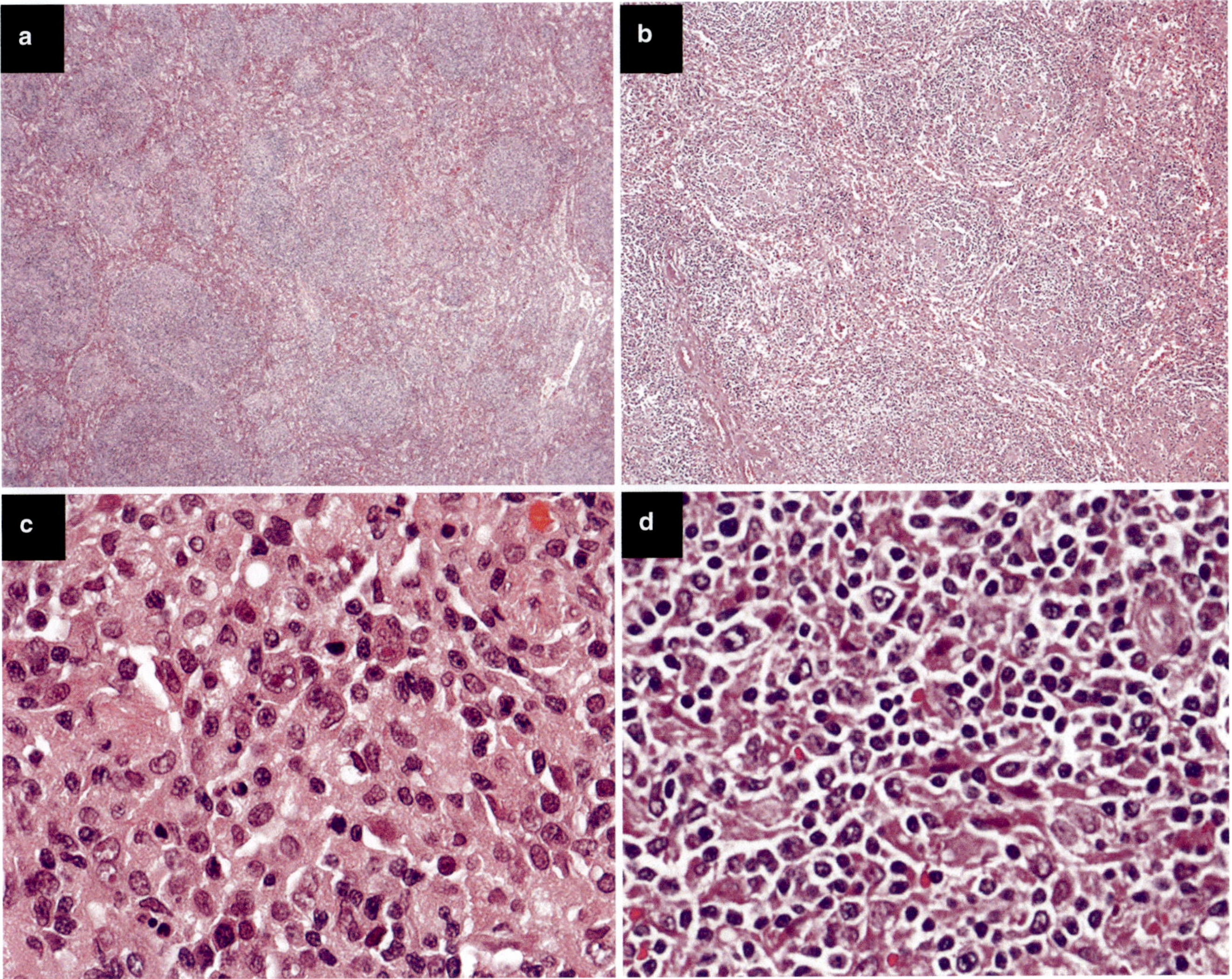

Fig. 6.5 Micronodular T-cell/histiocyte-rich large B-cell lymphoma: (**a**) Low power microscopy demonstrates nodular pale proliferations with intact red pulp (H&E, magnification ×40). (**b**) Higher magnification demonstrates that these nodules are composed of mostly histiocytes, small lymphocytes and large scattered atypical lymphocytes (H&E, magnification ×100). (**c**) Nodules demonstrate abundant histiocytes, small lymphocytes and large atypical cells with Reed-Sternberg cell like morphology (H&E, magnification ×400). (**d**) The large atypical lymphocytes can also have centroblast-like morphology (with multiple membrane bound nucleoli) (H&E, magnification ×400). Courtesy of Dr. Ahmet Dogan (Memorial Sloan Kettering Cancer Center) and Drs. Stefania Pittaluga and Gaurav Gupta (National institutes of Health)

Molecular Studies

PCR for immunoglobulin heavy chain (IgH) and TCR gamma gene rearrangement usually demonstrates monoclonality of B-cells and the polyclonal nature of background T-cells [41].

Differential Diagnoses

The differential diagnoses mainly include benign granulomatous inflammation, follicular lymphoma, cHL, NLPHL, EBV+ large B-cell lymphoma, and peripheral T-cell lymphoma (Table 6.2) [40]. Grossly, these entities might look like mTCRBL, i.e., miliary appearance or even a normal appearance; an exception could be cHL, which generally has prominent nodules or large masses.

Benign Granulomatous Inflammation

The presence of nodular lesions in mTCRBL with a predominance of histiocytes might initially give an impression of well-formed granulomas. However, the key features in support of the neoplastic nature of mTCRBL are the presence of large atypical lymphoid cells with a B-cell phenotype and absence of any residual follicles with intact FDC meshworks. In challenging cases, light chain restriction by IHC or ISH can be demonstrated. An alternative method to establish clonality would be IgH polymerase chain reaction (PCR) analysis.

Follicular Lymphoma

The appearance of nodular lesions in mTCRBL might sometimes simulate a follicular lymphoma. However, the absence of centrocytes and centroblasts, predominance of T-cells (as highlighted by CD3 immunohistochemistry) and histiocytes (as highlighted by CD68), and absence of FDC meshworks would support the diagnosis of mTCRBL over follicular lymphoma. Also, CD20 staining in follicular lymphoma would demonstrate a predominance of B-cells, which are CD10 positive unlike mTCRBL. Flow cytometric or immunohistochemistry studies would reveal a clonal CD20$^+$ and CD10$^+$ B-cell population in follicular lymphoma, while as mentioned above, flow cytometric studies are generally negative in mTCRBL.

Classic Hodgkin Lymphoma

The presence of large Reed-Sternberg-/Hodgkin-like cells in mTCRBL could easily be mistaken for a classic Hodgkin lymphoma. However, the key differentiating morphologic factor would be the absence of the characteristic inflammatory milieu of classic Hodgkin lymphoma, i.e., eosinophils, neutrophils, and plasma cells. In addition, immunohistochemistry demonstrates that the large lymphoma cells in TCRBL have a completely retained B-cell phenotype (i.e., CD20$^+$, CD79a$^+$, OCT2$^+$, PAX5 strong$^+$) along with positivity for CD45. In addition, unlike cHL, the large cells in mTCRBL would be either negative or weakly positive for CD30 accompanied by CD15 negativity.

Nodular Lymphocyte Predominant Hodgkin Lymphoma (NLPHL)

Nodular lymphocyte predominant Hodgkin lymphoma is primarily a nodal disease with very rare involvement of the spleen [42]. While the large cells in mTCRBL can be morphologically and immunophenotypically identical to that of

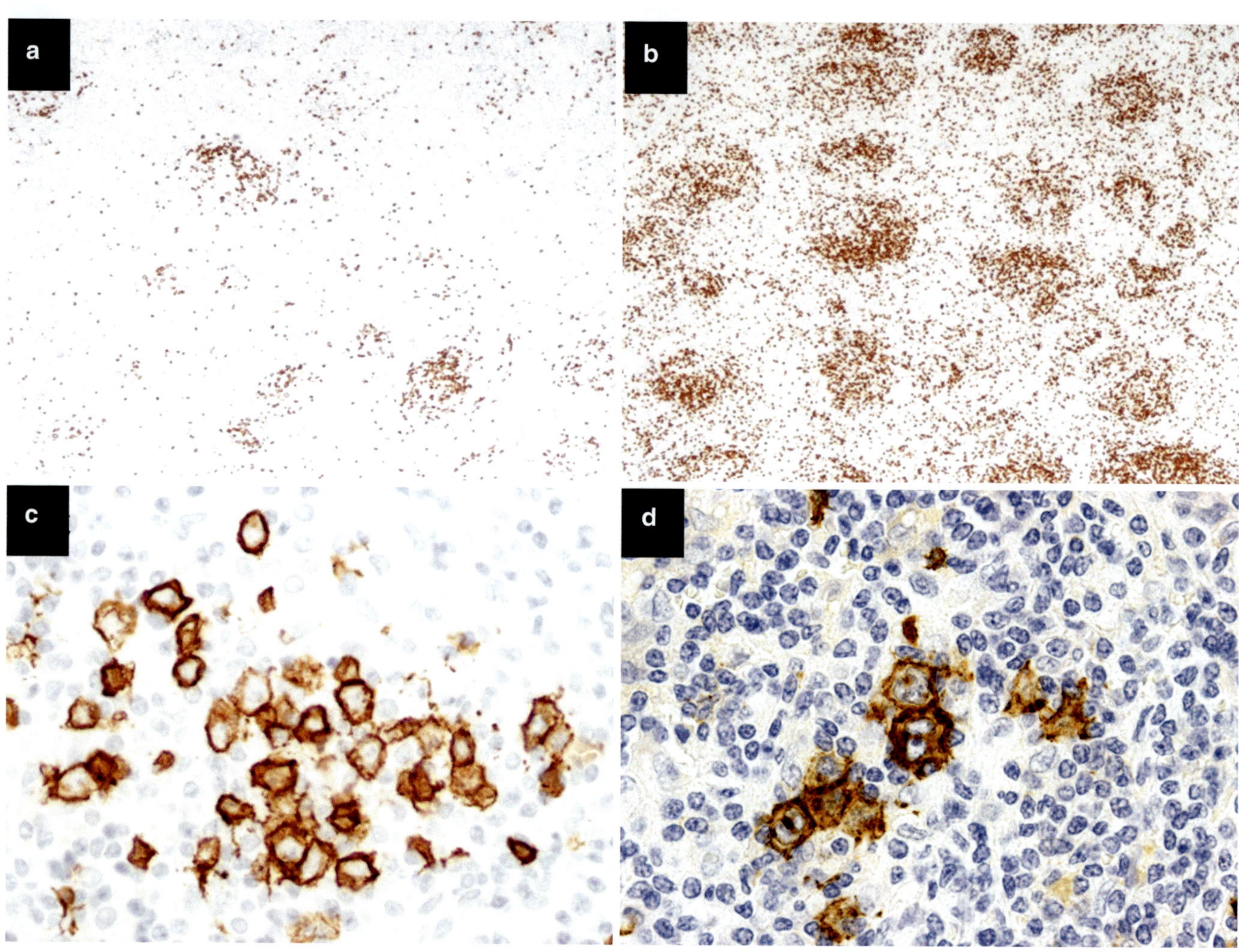

Fig. 6.6 Micronodular T-cell/histiocyte-rich large B-cell lymphoma: The nodules are composed of scattered large CD20 positive B-cells (**a**) and a predominant CD3 positive T-cell population (**b**) (immunoperoxidase, magnification ×40). (**c**, **d**) CD20 demonstrates scattered large neoplastic B-cells, which constitutes a minor population within the nodules (immunoperoxidase, magnification ×400). These cells are also positive for OCT2 (**e**), kappa light chain restricted (**f**) and demonstrate high proliferation index (**g**) (immunoperoxidase, magnification ×400). Courtesy of Dr. Ahmet Dogan (Memorial Sloan Kettering Cancer Center) and Drs. Stefania Pittaluga and Gaurav Gupta (National institutes of Health)

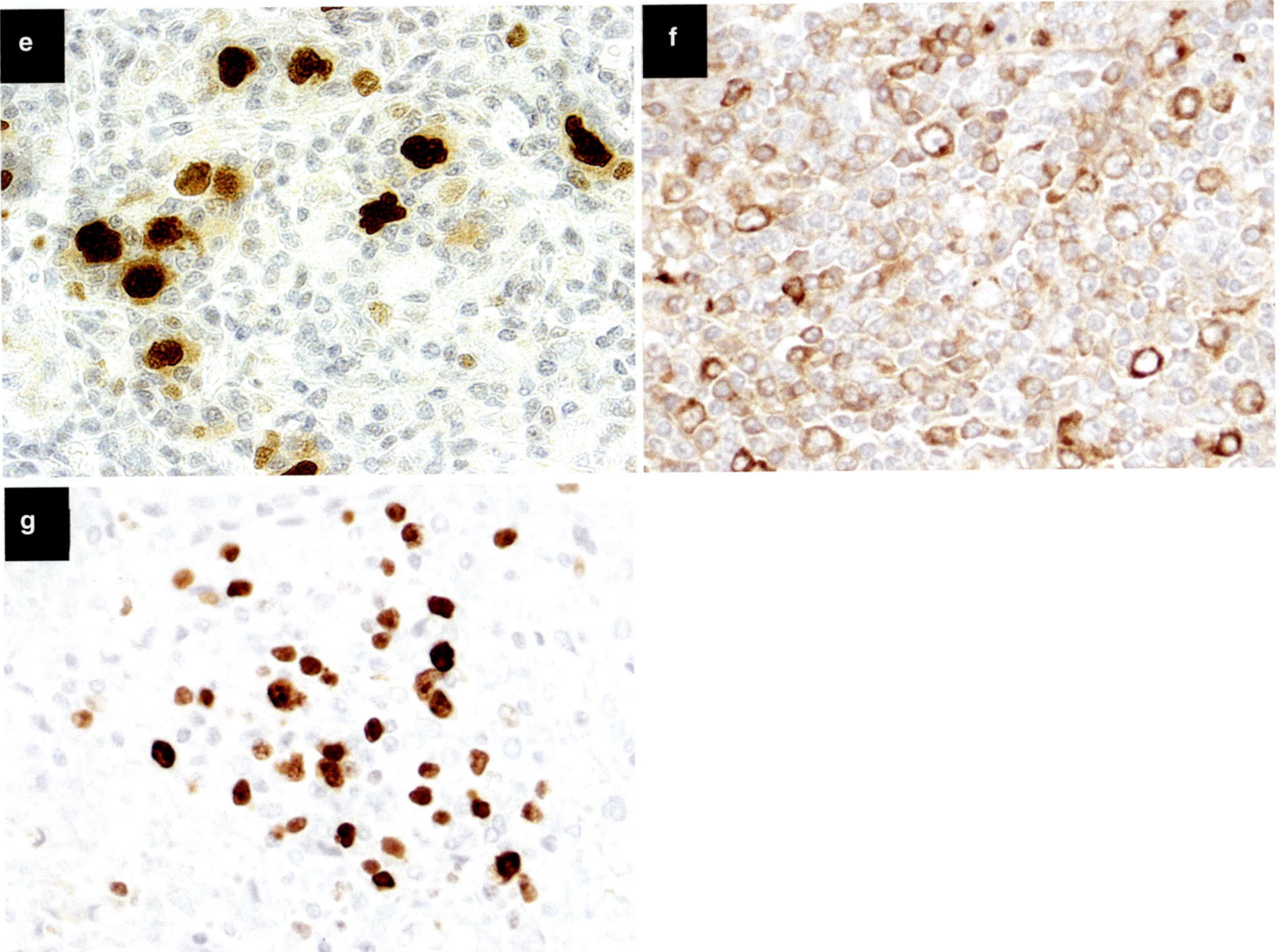

Fig. 6.6 (continued)

NLPHL, there are some distinguishing features; the small lymphocytes within the nodules are usually predominantly B-cells (IgD[+]) in NLPHL (with the exception of the rare T-cell-rich variant) unlike mTCRBL, which houses mostly T-cells. In addition, NLPHL nodules would demonstrate expanded FDC meshworks, which are absent in mTCRBL [42]. Unlike TCRBL, which demonstrates a predominance of cytotoxic CD8[+] T-cells, NLPHL demonstrates CD4[+], CD57[+], and PD1[+] T-cell rosettes around L&H/LP cells [44, 45].

EBV[+] Large B-Cell Lymphoma

Sometimes, the neoplastic cells in EBV[+] large B-cell lymphoma might mimic lymphocyte predominant cells (LP-cells) or immunoblasts, in a T-cell-/histiocyte-rich background (Fig. 6.8 D). These EBV[+] large B-cell lymphomas usually have a retained B-cell phenotype like mTCRBL; however, CD20 or CD45 can be downregulated along with expression of MUM1. EBER-ISH is strongly recommended in all cases of large B-cell lymphomas involving the spleen including mTCRBL. The presence of EBV in the scattered large B-cells would favor a diagnosis of EBV[+] large B-cell lymphoma over mTCRBL.

Mature T-Cell Lymphoma

Finally, the abundance of background T-cells in mTCRBL would raise the possibility of a T-cell lymphoma. T-large granular lymphocytic leukemia (T-LGL) and hepatosplenic T-cell lymphoma are the two main mature T-cell lymphomas involving the spleen, and both demonstrate diffuse red pulp involvement as opposed to the nodular appearance in mTCRBL [29]; this should not raise any diagnostic conundrums. However, while rare T-cell lymphomas, similar to mTCRBL, might appear nodular, especially the follicular type of peripheral T-cell lymphoma [23, 46], these lymphomas generally exhibit cytologic atypia in T-cells along with T-cell immunophenotypic aberrancies and a clonal T-cell gene rearrangement distinguishing them from mTCRBL.

Table 6.2 Differential diagnoses of micronodular T-cell-/histiocyte-rich large B-cell lymphoma

	Gross findings	Morphology	IHC and ISH	Genetic and molecular studies
Micronodular T-cell-/histiocyte-rich large B-cell lymphoma	Enlarged Normal cut surface or many small nodules	Intact architecture White pulp replaced by nodular pale lesions Composed of histiocytes, small lymphocytes, and few admixed large atypical lymphoid cells	Large atypical lymphoid cells: CD20$^+$, CD79a$^+$, OCT2$^+$, BCL6$^+$, PAX5$^+$, BCL2$^+$, CD45$^+$, CD10 negative, and CD138 negative Majority of the small lymphocytes are CD3$^+$ T-cells CD30 and EMA are negative or variably positive CD21, CD23, and CD35 are negative for FDC meshworks EBER-ISH and LMP-1 are negative	Positive IgH rearrangement Negative TCRγ rearrangement
Benign granulomatous inflammation	Normal or scattered nodular areas (with or without necrosis)	Granulomas with histiocytic proliferation (with or without necrosis) No large atypical cells seen	CD68$^+$ histiocytes GMS, AFB stains might reveal fungal or mycobacterial organism	Negative IgH rearrangement Negative TCRγ rearrangement
Follicular lymphoma	Many nodules	White pulp replaced by atypical follicles Centrocytes and centroblasts Prominent histiocytic component generally absent	Majority of the lymphoid cells: CD20$^+$, CD10$^+$, CD79a$^+$, PAX5$^+$, BCL6$^+$, BCL2$^+$ CD21, CD23, and CD35 demonstrate FDC meshworks	Positive IgH rearrangement Negative TCRγ rearrangement
Classic Hodgkin lymphoma	Prominent large nodules with or without necrosis	Reed-Sternberg cells and variants in background of small lymphocytes, eosinophils, and plasma cells	Hodgkin cells: CD30$^+$, CD15$^+$, PAX5 dim$^+$, CD20$^{+/-}$, CD79$^{-/+}$, CD45 negative EBER-ISH$^{+/-}$	Negative IgH rearrangement Negative TCRγ rearrangement
Nodular lymphocyte predominant Hodgkin lymphoma	Prominent small nodules or unremarkable cut surface	LP cells in a background of small lymphocytes	Large atypical lymphoid cells: CD20$^+$, CD79a$^+$, OCT2$^+$, BCL6$^+$, PAX5$^+$, CD45$^+$, CD10$^-$, CD30$^-$ and CD138$^-$ Majority of the small lymphocytes are CD20$^+$ B-cells CD3$^+$, CD57$^+$, PD1$^+$ rosettes CD21, CD23, and CD35 demonstrate expanded FDC meshworks EBER-ISH and LMP-1 are negative	Negative IgH rearrangement Negative TCRγ rearrangement
Mature T-cell lymphoma	Enlarged with generally unremarkable cut surface	Alteration of architecture Atypical small, medium, or large lymphoid cells	Lymphoma cells exhibit a T-cell phenotype Might exhibit immunophenotypic aberrancies including loss of T-cell markers	Clonal TCRγ rearrangement Negative IgH rearrangement

IgH immunoglobulin heavy chain, *TCRγ* T-cell receptor gamma, *IHC* immunohistochemistry, *ISH* in situ hybridization, *EBER* EBV-encoded small RNA, *FDC* follicular dendritic cell, *LMP-1* latent membrane protein-1, *GMS* Gomori Methenamine-Silver stain, *AFB* acid-fast bacilli stain

EBV-Positive Diffuse Large B-Cell Lymphoma (DLBCL), Not Otherwise Specified (NOS)

Definition

EBV-positive diffuse large B-cell lymphoma, NOS, is an EBV-positive clonal large B-cell proliferation, affecting both nodal and extranodal sites. Based on the spleen involvement, it can be further subclassified into primary and secondary EBV-positive DLBCL, NOS, of the spleen. Primary EBV-positive DLBCL, NOS, of the spleen is limited primarily to the spleen or splenic hilar lymph nodes without diffuse lymphadenopathy or widespread systemic involvement

[47]. The diagnosis of EBV-positive DLBCL, NOS, of the spleen should not be made when the spleen is involved by other EBV-associated specific entities, such as plasmablastic lymphoma, classic Hodgkin lymphoma, Burkitt lymphoma (BL), post-transplant lymphoproliferative disorder, DLBCL associated with chronic inflammation, or extracavitary primary effusion lymphoma.

Epidemiology

The spleen is not a common extranodal site to be involved by EBV-positive DLBCL, NOS [48]. When compared with primary splenic DLBCL, NOS [13, 14], primary EBV-positive DLBCL, NOS, of the spleen is even rarer, accounting for <5% of primary splenic DLBCL, NOS [15, 26, 49]. Less than 10% of patients with EBV-positive DLBCL, NOS, primarily present with spleen involvement [50–53]. The vast majority of primary EBV-positive DLBCL, NOS, of the spleen occurs in patients aged over 50 years without underlying immunodeficiency or prior lymphoma [15, 50–53]. Only one patient less than 50 years has been reported to have primary EBV-positive DLBCL, NOS, of the spleen [49].

Etiology and Pathogenesis

The increased incidence of EBV-positive DLBCL, NOS, in the elderly is thought to be associated with immunosenescence, an age-dependent dysfunction of the immune system characterized by dysregulation of adaptive immunity, decreased generation of immune cells, and decreased function of cytotoxic T-cells [54, 55]. Immunosenescence leads to impaired immune surveillance of latent EBV infection as well as activation of oncogenic pathway predominantly via latent membrane protein-1 (LMP-1) [56, 57]. Alternatively, local tolerogenic immune milieu may play a role in tumorogenesis, supported by the finding that PD-L1 is overexpressed on tumor cells in patients with EBV-positive DLBCL, NOS [58, 59]. Although hepatitis C virus infection has been associated with primary splenic DLBCL, NOS [26, 28], it usually does not induce EBV-positive DLBCL, NOS, of the spleen [26].

Clinical Features

Clinical presentations are variable, including fever, fatigue, weight loss, and left-sided abdominal pain. Rarely, spontaneous splenic rupture may occur due to massive splenomegaly. Physical and radiological examinations normally reveal splenomegaly without lymphadenopathy. Cytopenia(s) (especially thrombocytopenia) can be present, likely due to hypersplenism. Patients may have high level of lactate dehydrogenase (LDH) and detectable EBV DNA in the serum.

Pathologic Features

Primary EBV-positive DLBCL, NOS, of the spleen shows similar pathologic features as those seen in secondary splenic involvement by systemic EBV-positive DLBCL, NOS.

Morphology

The spleen is generally enlarged. Most cases grossly show a solitary mass that is clearly demarcated from the normal spleen tissue. The mass lesion is tan-whitish and firm, with areas of yellowish necrosis frequently observed (Fig. 6.7a). In some cases, the gross finding of the splenic cut surface could

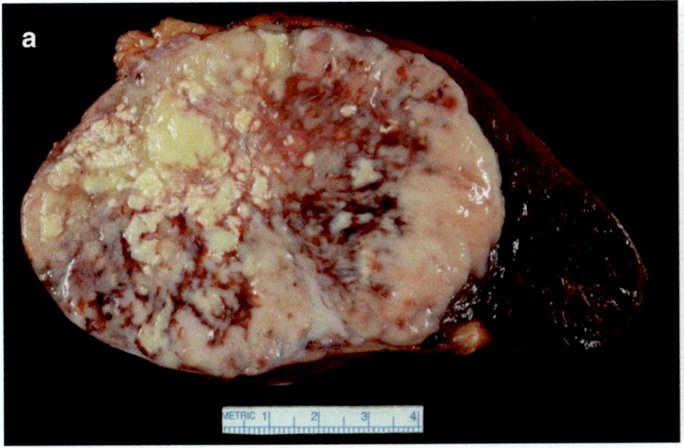
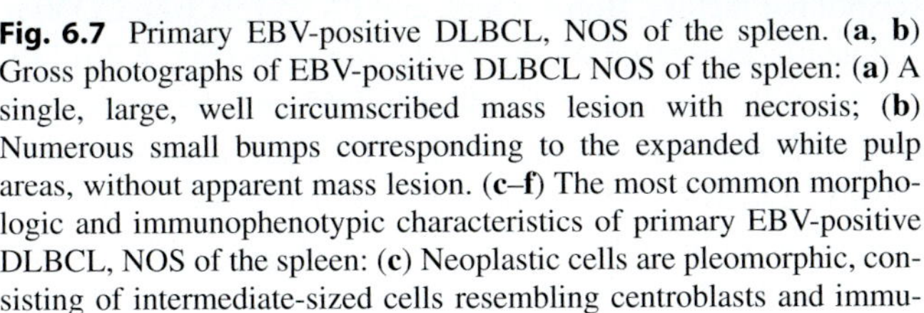
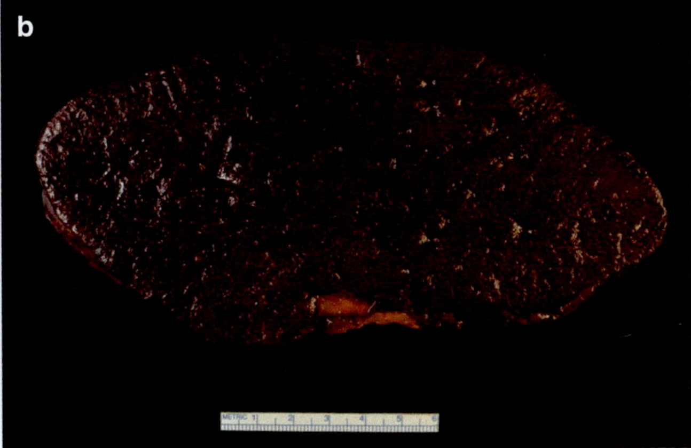

Fig. 6.7 Primary EBV-positive DLBCL, NOS of the spleen. (**a**, **b**) Gross photographs of EBV-positive DLBCL NOS of the spleen: (**a**) A single, large, well circumscribed mass lesion with necrosis; (**b**) Numerous small bumps corresponding to the expanded white pulp areas, without apparent mass lesion. (**c**–**f**) The most common morphologic and immunophenotypic characteristics of primary EBV-positive DLBCL, NOS of the spleen: (**c**) Neoplastic cells are pleomorphic, consisting of intermediate-sized cells resembling centroblasts and immunoblasts, and large-sized cells mimicking Hodgkin-Reed-Sternberg cells. Background small reactive T-lymphocytes and histiocytes are present; (**c**, H&E, magnification ×400); **d**) Immunohistochemical studies show the neoplastic cells are uniformly and strongly positive for CD20; (**e**) the neoplastic cells are partially positive for CD30; (**d**–**e**. immunoperoxidase, magnification ×400); **f**) In situ hybridization detects EBER expression in most neoplastic cells. (**f**, ISH, magnification ×400)

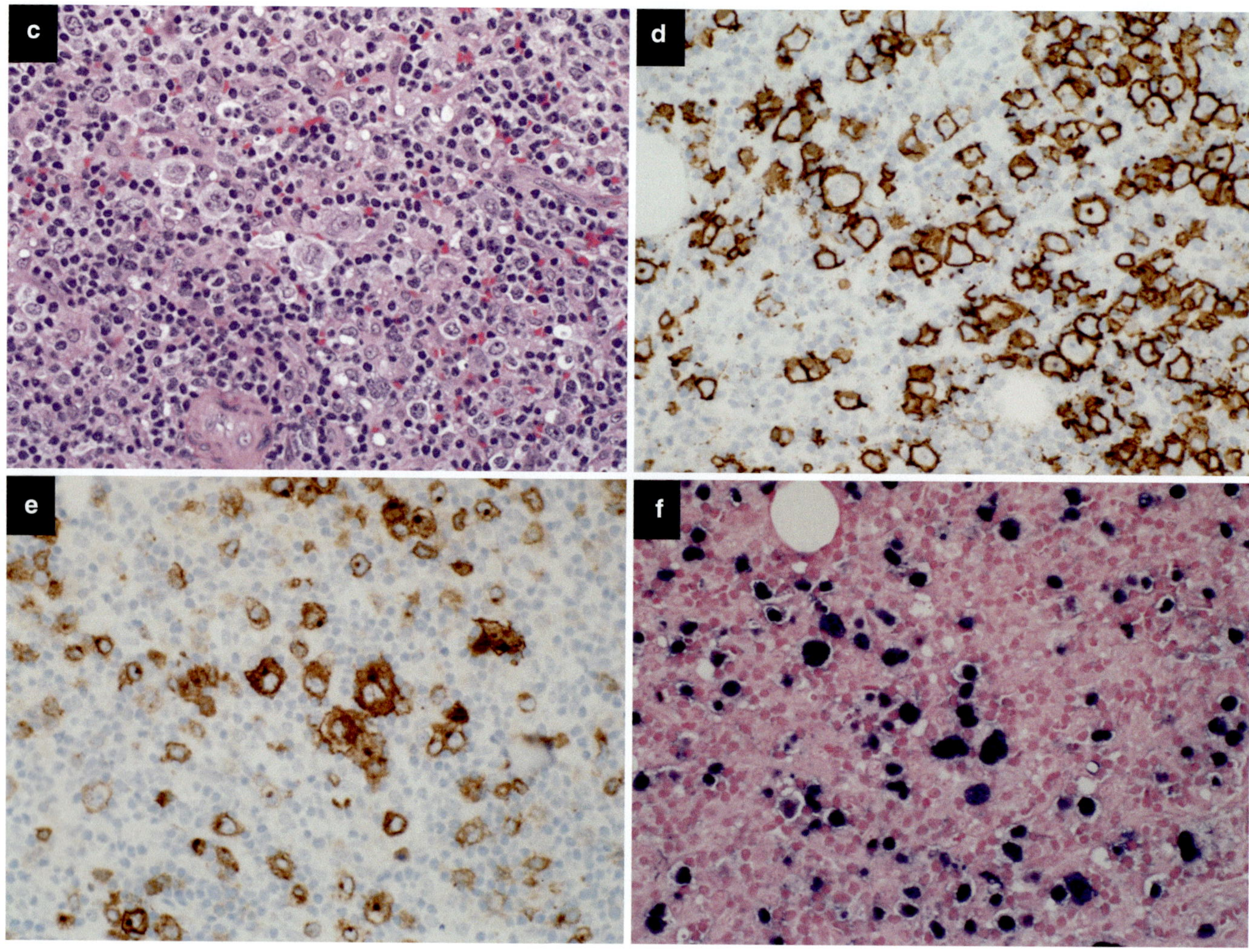

Fig. 6.7 (continued)

be very subtle: other than a "bumpy" appearance representing numerous enlarged white pulps, there is no dominant mass (Fig. 6.7b).

Histologic sections show splenic architecture effacement by a predominantly white pulp or dual white and red pulp expansion consisting of large atypical lymphoid cells, in a nodular or diffuse pattern, often accompanied by necrosis. Exclusive red pulp involvement has not been reported in primary EBV-positive DLBCL, NOS, of the spleen [15, 16, 60]. EBV-positive DLBCL, NOS, of the spleen display a wide range of morphologic variations. A marked pleomorphism is present in most cases, containing Hodgkin-Reed-Sternberg-like, immunoblast-like, or centroblast-like cells (Figs. 6.7c and 6.8a, d). Although pleomorphic, the neoplastic cells are all large and lack the small B lymphoid cells seen in EBV-positive polymorphic lymphoproliferative disorder. A monomorphic appearance with centroblastic or immunoblastic lymphoma cells can be seen in some cases, resembling "conventional" DLBCL, NOS (Fig. 6.8a). Rarely, the morpho-

logic features may simulate those in T-cell-/histiocyte-rich large B-cell lymphoma, with neoplastic cells mimicking lymphocyte predominant cells (LP cells) or immunoblasts, in a T-cell-/histiocyte-rich background (Fig. 6.8d).

Immunophenotype

The neoplastic cells normally express pan B-cell markers, such as CD19, CD20 (Figs. 6.7d and 6.8b, e), CD22, CD79a, Bob.1, Oct2, and PAX5. While EBV-transformed B-cells may demonstrate partial loss of CD20 or CD45 expression, they typically maintain the strong expression of B-lineage transcriptional factors, Bob.1, Oct2, and PAX5 [59, 61]. CD30 is frequently expressed on the neoplastic cells (Fig. 6.7e) [49, 51, 61, 62]. The loss of CD20 or CD45 and the expression of CD30 may cause diagnostic challenges between EBV-positive DLBCL, NOS, and EBV-positive classic Hodgkin lymphoma of the spleen. EBV-positive DLBCL, NOS, of the spleen lacks the typical inflammatory background of classic Hodgkin lymphoma. In addition, the neoplastic cells in

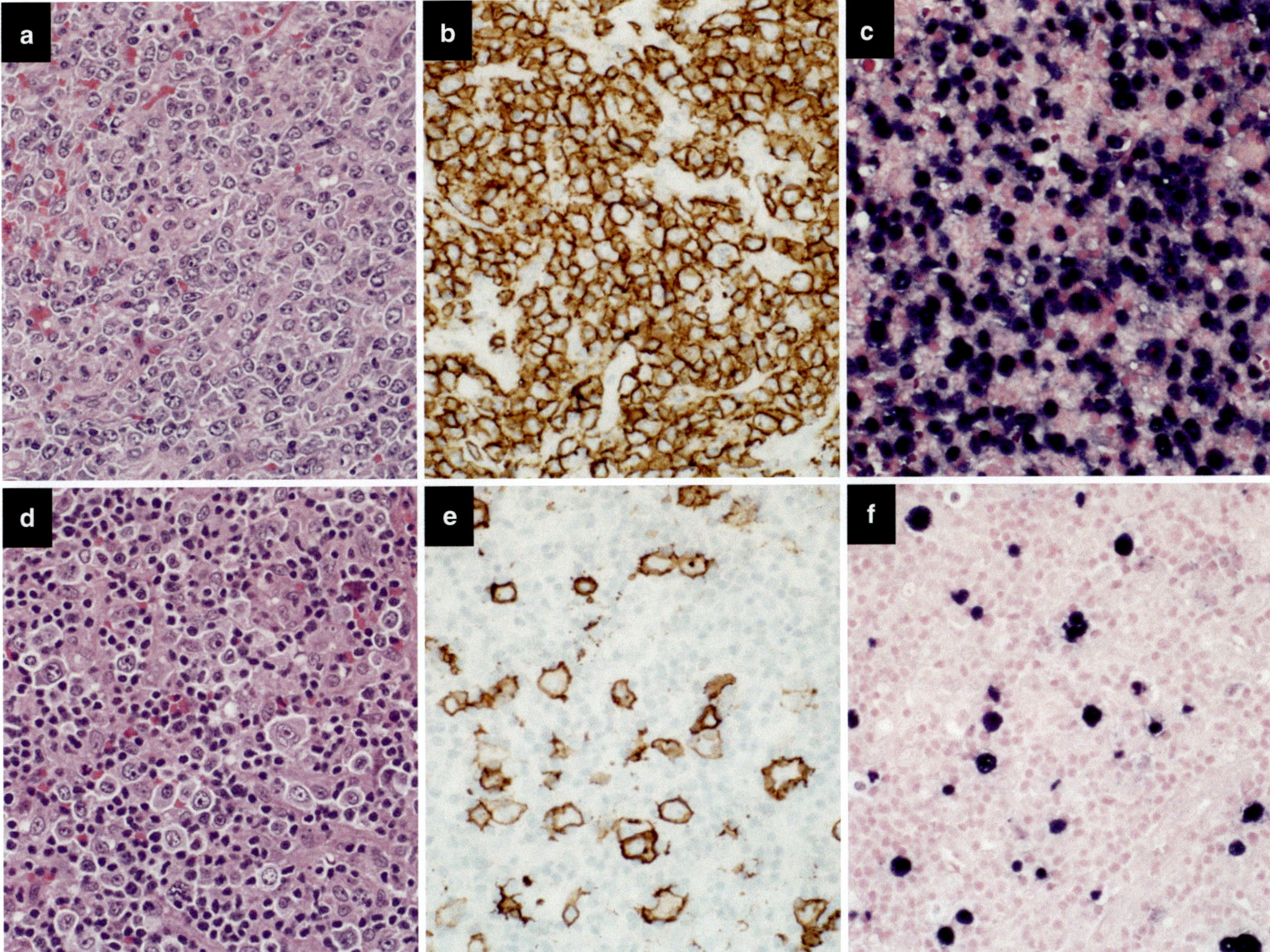

Fig. 6.8 The less common morphologic and immunophenotypic characteristics of primary EBV-positive DLBCL, NOS of the spleen. (**a–c**) Some cases show monomorphic appearance: (**a**) A monotonous proliferation of centroblasts with multiple small nucleoli bound to the nuclear membrane; (H&E, magnification ×400); (**b**) Neoplastic cells are uniformly positive for CD20 by an immunohistochemical study (immunoperoxidase, magnification ×400); (**c**) The vast majority of neoplastic cells are positive for EBER by in situ hybridization (ISH, magnification ×400). (**d–f**) Rare cases reveal a T-cell/histiocyte-rich large B-cell lymphoma-like pattern: (**d**) The singly distributed large atypical cells resembling immunoblasts or LP cells (H&E, magnification ×400); (**e**) They are positive for CD20 (immunoperoxidase, magnification ×400); (**f**) Most of neoplastic cells are positive for EBER (ISH, magnification ×400)

EBV-positive DLBCL, NOS, demonstrate a broad morphologic spectrum including immunoblastic, centroblastic, and Hodgkin-cell like features, and exhibit a strong B-cell program as per CD79a, Bob.1, Oct2, and PAX-5.

The neoplastic cells in EBV-positive DLBCL, NOS, of the spleen are commonly negative for CD10 and positive for IRF4/MUM1 with variable BCL6 expression, consistent with an active B-cell (ABC) subtype [26, 50–52]. Infrequently, they show a germinal center B-cell (GCB) subtype [51].

The majority of tumor cells are positive for EBV-encoded small RNA (EBER) using ISH assay. If only a small subset of tumor cells is positive for EBER, EBV infection may not be the driver of tumorigenesis, and whether those cases belong to this category is debatable. Based on the different expression patterns of latent proteins LMP-1 and EBV nuclear antigen 2 (EBNA2), latency can be classified as type I (LMP-1$^-$EBNA2$^-$), type II (LMP-1$^+$ EBNA2$^-$), and type III (LMP-1$^+$ EBNA2$^+$). Primary EBV-positive DLBCL, NOS, of the spleen exhibits both type II and type III EBV latency [51–53], similar to EBV-positive DLBCL, NOS, involving other sites [59, 61–67].

Genetic and Molecular Features

Clonality is confirmed by a clonal immunoglobulin gene rearrangement or a clonal EBV genome using molecular assays [49, 51]. *IGH*@/14q32 translocation is identified in around 15% of cases, but *MYC/IGH* translocation is rare [61]. Although EBV-positive DLBCL, NOS, of the spleen commonly displays the ABC subtype immunophenotypically, it carries the genetic features of both ABC and GCB subtypes of DLBCL, NOS. Similar to the ABC subtype of conventional DLBCL, EBV-positive DLBCL, NOS, of the spleen reveals enhanced activation of nuclear factor kappa B (*NF-kB*) pathway, and it rarely carries *EZH2* mutations [51, 68–70]. Akin to the GCB subtype, it demonstrates increased activation of the Janus kinase-signal transducer and activator of transcription (*JAK-STAT*) pathway and no *CD79B* and *MYD88* mutations [68–70]. Array comparative genomic hybridization (CGH) analyses in cases of EBV-positive DLBCL, NOS, have shown a high frequency in chromosome gains at 9p24.1 [71], a chromosomal gain characteristic of primary mediastinal large B-cell lymphoma, but rarely detected in DLBCL, NOS. These findings indicate that EBV-positive DLBCL, NOS, of the spleen is a molecularly distinct variant of DLBCL, NOS.

Prognosis

EBV-positive DLBCL, NOS, is an aggressive disease and carries unfavorable clinical outcomes, especially in patients older than 70 years [62], with B symptoms [51, 62], positive for CD30 [69], positive for EBNA2 [72], or having gains of chromosome at 9p24.1 [71]. The prognosis of primary EBV-positive DLBCL, NOS, in the spleen is hard to predict given the rarity of the entity. The overexpression of CD30 and the activation of *NF-kB* and *JAK-STAT* pathways are potential therapeutic targets for this lymphoma.

Differential Diagnosis

Differential diagnosis mainly includes EBV-associated reactive lymphoid hyperplasia, EBV-associated polymorphic lymphoproliferative disorder of the spleen, fibrin-associated EBV-positive large B-cell lymphoma of the spleen, inflammatory pseudotumor of the spleen, and post-transplant lymphoproliferative disorder (PTLD). Other differential diagnoses, which may demonstrate EBER-ISH positivity, include plasmablastic lymphoma, classic Hodgkin lymphoma, Burkitt lymphoma, and aggressive NK-cell leukemia.

The key features are summarized in Table 6.3.

Table 6.3 Differential diagnosis of EBV-positive DLBCL, NOS, of the spleen

	Splenic architecture	Morphology	Immunophenotype	EBER positivity	Hallmark cytogenetics	Critical clinical history
EBV-positive DLBCL, NOS, of the spleen	Effaced	Large lymphoid cells	CD19$^+$ CD20$^{+/-}$, CD79a$^+$, BOB.1$^+$, OCT2$^+$, PAX5$^+$, MUM1$^+$, CD10$^-$, BCL6$^{+/-}$, CD30$^{+/-}$, CD15$^-$	In the vast majority of large lymphoid cells	N/A	N/A
EBV-associated reactive lymphoid hyperplasia of the spleen	Preserved, with white pulp hyperplasia including B-cell and T-cell zones	A mixed population of small lymphocytes, plasma cells, and immunoblasts	Immunoblasts positive for CD30	In many small lymphocytes and immunoblasts	N/A	Current EBV infection
EBV-associated polymorphic lymphoproliferative disorder of the spleen	Partially or totally effaced	A spectrum of B-cell maturation from immunoblasts to plasma cells	CD19$^+$ CD20$^+$, CD79a$^+$, BOB.1$^+$, OCT2$^+$, PAX5$^+$, CD10$^-$, BCL6$^{+/-}$, MUM1$^+$ CD30$^{+/-}$, CD15$^-$	In a range of cell sizes including small-, intermediate, and large-sized cells	N/A	N/A
Fibrin-associated EBV-positive large B-cell lymphoma of the spleen	Pseudocyst containing amorphous eosinophilic materials	Large lymphoid cells	CD19$^+$, CD20$^+$, CD79a$^+$, BOB.1$^+$, OCT2$^+$, PAX5$^+$, CD10$^-$,BCL6$^{+/-}$,MUM1$^{+/-}$	In the vast majority of large lymphoid cells	N/A	N/A
Inflammatory pseudotumor of the spleen	Effaced	Spindle-shaped cells and bland looking	CD21$^+$, CD35$^+$, CXCL13$^+$, clusterin$^+$, smooth muscle actin$^+$	In the spindle-shaped cells, not lymphocytes	N/A	N/A

Table 6.3 (continued)

	Splenic architecture	Morphology	Immunophenotype	EBER positivity	Hallmark cytogenetics	Critical clinical history
Post-transplant lymphoproliferative disorder, monomorphic type	Effaced	Large lymphoid cells	CD19$^+$, CD20$^+$, CD79a$^+$, BOB.1$^+$, OCT2$^+$, PAX5$^+$, CD10$^-$, BCL6$^{+/-}$, MUM1$^+$, CD30$^-$, CD15$^-$	In the vast majority of large lymphoid cells	N/A	History of a solid organ or allogeneic stem cell transplant
Plasmablastic lymphoma	Effaced	Large lymphoid cells with plasmablastic morphology	CD38$^+$, CD138$^+$, MUM1$^+$, CD30$^{+/-}$, CD79a$^{-/+}$, CD19$^-$, CD20$^-$, CD45$^-$, CD56$^-$, PAX5$^-$, with light chain restriction	In large lymphoid cells	*MYC/IG* translocation in 50% of cases	Immunodeficiency
Classic Hodgkin lymphoma	Effaced	Reed-Sternberg cells in the background of lymphocytes, eosinophils, histiocytes, and plasma cells	CD30$^+$, CD15$^+$, PAX5$^+$, CD19$^-$, CD20$^-$, CD45$^-$	In Reed-Sternberg cells	N/A	N/A
Burkitt lymphoma	Effaced	Intermediated-sized lymphoid cells	CD19$^+$, CD20$^+$, CD79a$^+$, BOB.1$^+$, OCT2$^+$, PAX5$^+$, CD10$^+$, BCL6$^+$, BCL2$^-$	Variable	*MYC/IGH* or *IHK/MYC* or *MYC/IGL* translocation	N/A
Aggressive NK-cell leukemia	Effaced, with a splenic cord expansion	Intermediate- to large-sized lymphoid cells	CD2$^+$, CD3$^+$, CD7$^+$, CD56$^+$, granzyme B$^+$, TIA1$^+$, CD4$^-$, CD5$^-$, CD8$^-$,TCR$\alpha\beta^-$,andTCR$\gamma\delta^-$	In the vast majority of large lymphoid cells	N/A	N/A

EBV Epstein-Barr Virus, *EBER* Epstein Barr-Virus-Encoded RNA

EBV-Associated Reactive Lymphoid Hyperplasia of the Spleen (Infectious Mononucleosis in the Spleen)

Approximately half of patients with infectious mononucleosis have detectable splenomegaly, and some of them may experience splenic rupture secondary to trauma. In contrast to EBV-positive DLBCL, NOS, of the spleen, the splenic architecture is retained in EBV-associated reactive lymphoid hyperplasia. There is a prominence of splenic white pulp, composed of expanded T-cell zones and reactive germinal centers. T-cell zones (corresponds to the periarteriolar lymphoid sheath) are expanded by a mixed population of small lymphocytes, plasma cells, and immunoblasts. Sometimes, the mixed cell population also infiltrates the splenic cords. Many EBER-positive small lymphocytes and immunoblasts are present in the T-cell zones and splenic cords. Correlation with clinical and laboratory findings is necessary.

EBV-Associated Polymorphic Lymphoproliferative Disorder of the Spleen

The architecture of the spleen is partially or completely effaced by a spectrum of B-cell maturation with plasmacytic differentiation (Fig. 6.9a). B-cells show a spectrum of size, including small-, intermediate-, and large-sized cells, contrary to EBV-positive DLBCL, NOS, where the neoplastic B-cells are all large in size (Fig. 6.9b). Plasma cells, plasmacytoid cells, and prominent immunoblasts accompanied by numerous mitotic figures are frequently present (Fig. 6.9b).

Fibrin-Associated EBV-Positive Large B-Cell Lymphoma of the Spleen

This is an unusual form of DLBCL of chronic inflammation, occurring in the setting of local immunodeficiency because of chronic inflammation associated with EBV infection and carrying highly favorable prognosis [73, 74]. It usually forms a pseudocyst in the spleen, rather than a mass lesion. Histologic examination shows a thickened pseudocyst wall containing clusters of large atypical lymphoid cells in a background of fibrous/amorphous materials (Fig. 6.9c and d). These large atypical cells are positive for CD20, CD79a, PAX-5, and EBER.

Inflammatory Pseudotumor of the Spleen

It may mimic primary EBV-positive DLBCL, NOS, in the spleen clinically, radiologically, grossly, and histologically.

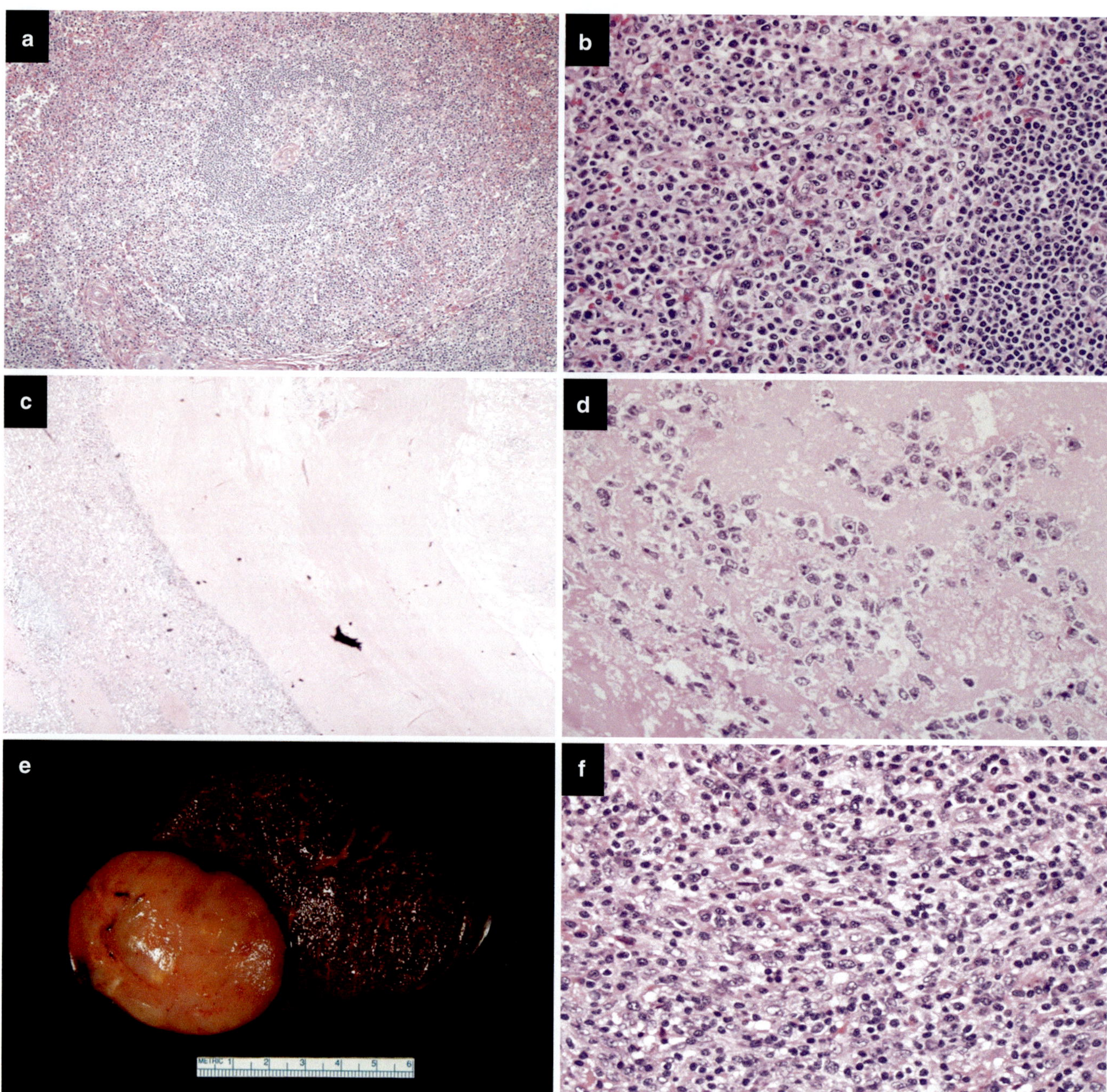

Fig. 6.9 Mimickers of primary EBV-positive DLBCL NOS of the spleen. (**a**, **b**) EBV-positive polymorphic lymphoproliferative disorder of the spleen: (**a**) The architecture of the spleen is partially effaced by a perifollicular expansion of a mixed population of cells (H&E, magnification ×100); (**b**) This mixed population is consisting of small plasmacytoid lymphocytes, immunoblasts, plasma cells, and histiocytes (H&E, magnification ×400). (**c**, **d**) Fibrin-associated DLBCL of the spleen: (**c**) The perisplenic cyst has a thickened capsule and contains scattered foci of atypical cells accompanied by extensive fibrin. The adjacent splenic tissue is morphologically unremarkable (H&E, magni-

fication ×40); (**d**) On a higher magnification power, the atypical cells have intermediate-to-large nuclei, vesicular chromatin, distinct nucleoli and moderate cytoplasm (H&E, magnification ×400). (**e–h**) Inflammatory pseudotumor of the spleen: (**e**) Gross photograph shows a single, solid, well-demarcated mass lesion with bulging appearance; (**f**) A proliferation of spindle cells with elongated nuclei and bland-looking, intermingled with small reactive lymphocytes and histiocytes (**e**, **f**. H&E, magnification ×400); (**g**) The spindle cells are positive for clusterin (Immunoperoxidase, magnification ×400); (**h**) EBER is detected on the spindle cells (ISH, magnification ×400)

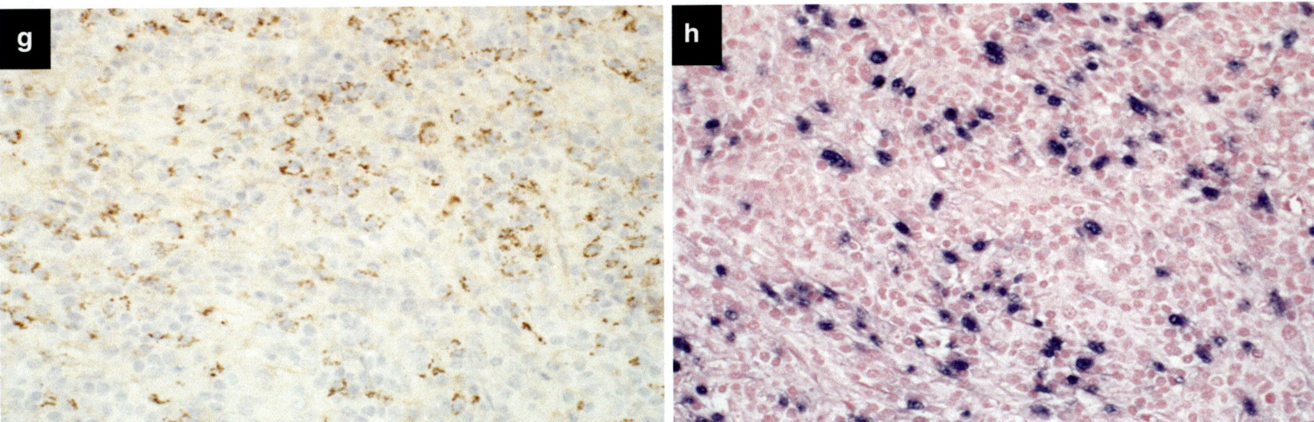

Fig. 6.9 (continued)

Patients frequently have fever, abdominal pain, and weight loss. Radiological examination reveals solitary or multiple splenic solid lesions. The mass is usually tan-white, well-demarcated, and bulging on cut surface (Fig. 6.9e). Histologic sections show a proliferation of bland-looking spindle cells, admixed with abundant chronic inflammatory cells including lymphocytes, plasma cells, and histiocytes (Fig. 6.9f). It is not uncommon to misdiagnose inflammatory pseudotumor of the spleen as B- or T-cell lymphoma. The spindle cells are follicular/fibroblastic dendritic cell origin and may be positive for CD21, CD35, clusterin (Fig. 6.9g), CXCL13, or smooth muscle actin. Importantly, it is the spindle cell population, not lymphocytic population, that is positive for EBER (Fig. 6.9h). It is a curable disease with splenectomy.

Post-transplant Lymphoproliferative Disorder (PTLD)

Post-transplant lymphoproliferative disorder is frequently associated with EBV infection and has a wide range of morphology: nondestructive, polymorphic, monomorphic, and classic Hodgkin lymphoma PTLD. Monomorphic B-cell PTLD of DLBCL subtype could be identical to EBV-positive DLBCL, NOS, of the spleen, both morphologically and immunophenotypically. The key point is that patients with PTLD have history of a solid organ or allogeneic stem cell transplant.

Burkitt Lymphoma of the Spleen

Definition

Burkitt lymphoma is a highly aggressive mature B-cell lymphoma, composed of monomorphic intermediate-sized B-cells with germinal center B-cell phenotype. It has a very high proliferative rate and a frequently detectable *MYC* gene translocation to an *IG* (heavy or light chain) locus. There are three variants of Burkitt lymphoma: endemic, sporadic, and immunodeficiency associated. These variants display considerable differences in epidemiology, clinical presentation, anatomic location, and etiology (Table 6.4).

Epidemiology

While all three variants of Burkitt lymphoma (BL) can involve the abdomen, they often spare the spleen. Only one case of primary BL of the spleen has been reported after examining 1280 patients who underwent splenectomy, and it represents <1% of primary splenic lymphoma [13]. The secondary splenic involvement at the diagnosis of BL is also rare, even at the advanced stage. Several radiological studies using position emission tomography (PET)/computed tomography (CT) scans for Burkitt lymphoma staging have not shown splenic involvement, except in cases with direct extension from adjacent peritoneal masses [75–77]. These findings suggest that the spleen is characteristically not affected by BL. However, when BL is widely disseminated, the spleen can be involved among multiple other organs [78, 79].

Pathologic Features

Morphology

When BL involves the spleen, it effaces the splenic architecture and often infiltrates both white pulp and red pulp. Occasionally, selective white pulp involvement is noted [78].

Table 6.4 Clinical variants of Burkitt lymphoma

	Endemic	Sporadic	Immunodeficiency associated
Epidemiology	Equatorial Africa and Papua New Guinea (malaria-endemic areas)	Throughout the word	Throughout the word
Age of the patients	Young children (peaked at 4–7 years)	Children; young individuals (median age, 30)	Adults (median age, 44)
Anatomic locations	Most commonly involves jaws and other facial bones, followed by the abdomen (gastrointestinal tract)	Predominantly involves the abdomen: ileocecal region, gastrointestinal tract, mesentery, retroperitoneum, genitourinary tract	More lymph node and bone marrow involvement than the other two variants; the abdomen (gastrointestinal tract) can be involved
EBER positivity	>95%	A wide range (10–87%)	25–40%
Etiology	EBV and *Plasmodium falciparum* malaria infections cooperate *MYC*-driven tumorigenesis	EBV infection cooperates *MYC*-driven tumorigenesis	EBV infection cooperates *MYC*-driven tumorigenesis

All three variants of BL share similar morphology [78]. Low magnification power examination reveals a "starry-sky" appearance, as a result of numerous evenly spaced tingible body macrophages intermingled with a diffuse proliferation of neoplastic cells (Fig. 6.10a). The monotonous neoplastic cells are intermediate in size, with round nuclear contours, finely clumped chromatin and several distinct, paracentrally located nucleoli. The basophilic cytoplasm usually shows cytoplasmic molding and cytoplasmic vacuoles. Immunodeficiency-associated BL sometimes displays plasmacytoid appearance.

Immunohistochemistry

The neoplastic cells are positive for pan B-cell markers, such as CD19, CD20 (Fig. 6.10b), CD22, CD79a, and PAX-5. They usually express membrane IgM immunoglobulin heavy chain with surface light chain restriction. They are positive for germinal center B-cell markers, CD10 (Fig. 6.10c) and BCL6 (Fig. 6.10d), and usually negative for BCL2 (Fig. 6.10e). In some cases, the neoplastic cells can weakly/partially express BCL2. The neoplastic cells also show a diffuse expression of MYC protein (Fig. 6.10f) and a very high Ki-67 proliferative index (Ki-67 > 95%) (Fig. 6.10g). In contrast to B-lymphoblastic leukemia/lymphoma, the neoplastic cells in BL are typically negative for nuclear terminal deoxynucleotidyl transferase (TdT).

EBER (Epstein-Barr virus (EBV)-encoded RNA) is variably detected in different variants of BL that involve the spleen (Fig. 6.10h). EBER is identified in nearly all endemic BL [80], 10–87% of sporadic type [81–84] and 25–40% of immunodeficiency-associated type [85]. Different from most EBV-associated lymphomas, all three BL variants are mainly negative for LMP-1 (latent membrane protein) and EBNA2 (Epstein-Barr virus nuclear antigen 2), reflexing EBV latency type I [83, 84, 86–88].

Genetic and Molecular Features

Regardless of the subtypes and EBV infection status, almost all BLs harbor a reciprocal chromosomal translo-cation involving the *MYC* gene on chromosome 8 and one of the immunoglobulin chain loci on chromosome 14, 2, or 22, resulting in *MYC/IGH*, *IGK/MYC*, or *MYC/IGL* fusion, respectively [89]. t(8;14) (q24;q32) is the most frequent cytogenetic abnormality, seen in approximately 80% of cases, followed by t(8;22)(q24;q11) in 5–10% and t(2;8) (p11;q24) in 5% of cases. These chromosomal translocations bring the *MYC* oncogene under the transcriptional control of an immunoglobulin locus, resulting in the overexpression of MYC protein that promotes the high proliferation of neoplastic cells [90]. The breakpoints of *MYC* translocation can substantially vary in their locations among the three variants, suggesting that there might be distinct pathogenetic mechanisms at play among the epidemiologic variants [81, 89, 91, 92].

MYC gene rearrangement is the biological hallmark, but not specific for BL. Other lymphomas can carry *MYC* gene rearrangement as a secondary event, such as large B-cell lymphoma, plasmablastic lymphoma, mantle cell lymphoma, follicular lymphoma, chronic lymphocytic leukemia/small lymphocytic lymphoma, and marginal zone lymphoma [93]. Although *MYC* gene rearrangement in BL is most commonly associated with simple karyotype, additional aberrations have been observed, such as copy number gains involving 1q, 7q, 9q, 12q, 13q, and 20q and losses involving 4q, 6q, 11q, 13q, and 17p [94–96]. There are usually less than two secondary cytogenetic alternations and complex cytogenetics is unusual in BL [94].

Gene expression profile demonstrates that BL is genetically different from diffuse large B-cell lymphoma [97, 98]. Interestingly, a molecular genetic signature is largely shared among the three variants of BL, regardless of the EBV status, indicating the biological homogeneity of BL [99, 100]. Although BL is characterized by deregulation of *MYC* gene, other recurrent genetic mutations are present in BL, including *ID3*, *GNA13*, *RET*, *PIK3R1*, and the SWI/SNF genes *ARID1A* and *SMARCA4*, implicating new pathogenetic factors in BL [101, 102].

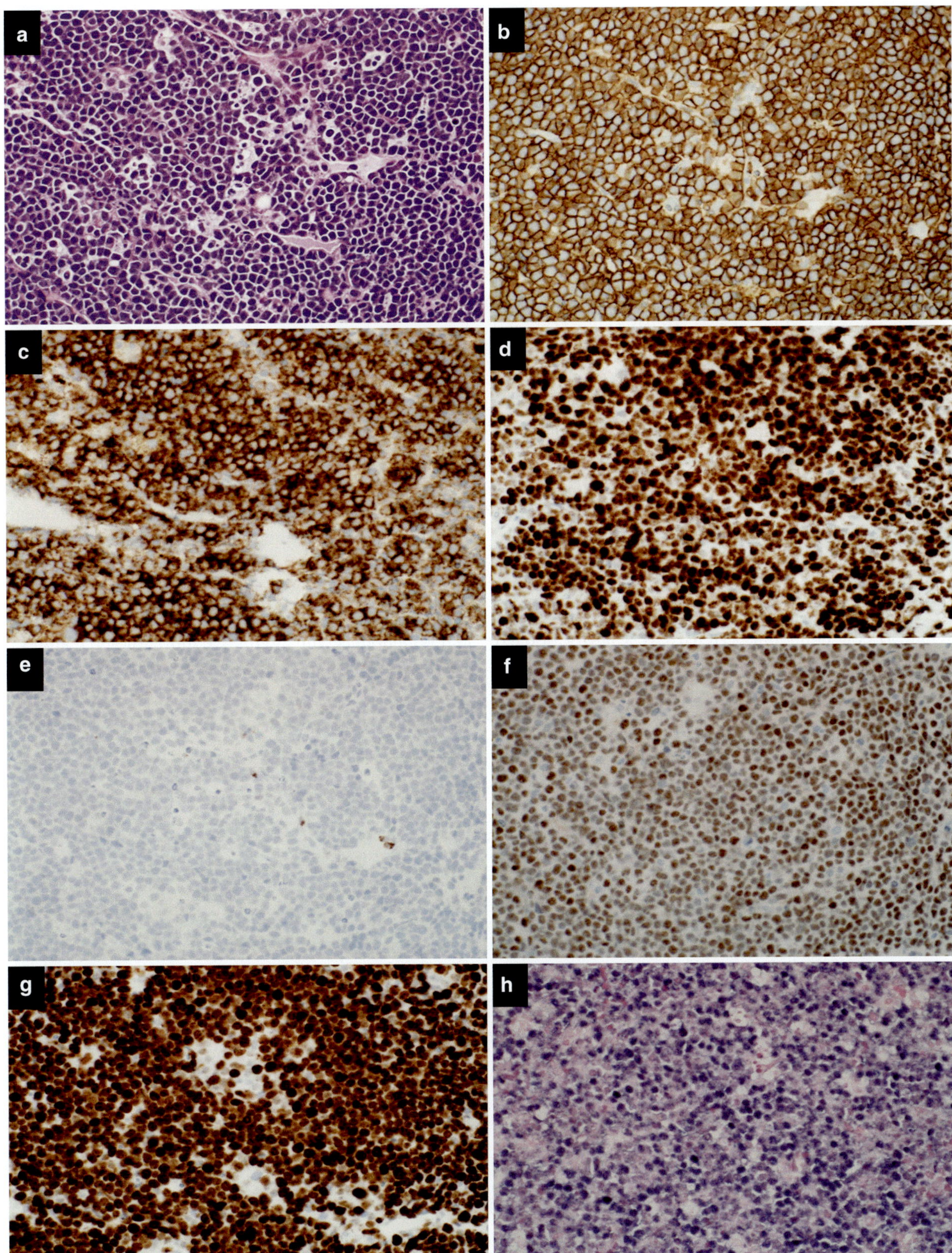

Fig. 6.10 Burkitt lymphoma of the spleen. (**a**) Hematoxylin and eosin stain reveals the classic "starry-sky" pattern, due to scattered phagocytic macrophages intermingled with a monotonous proliferation of neoplastic cells (magnification ×400). Immunohistochemical studies show the neoplastic cells are positive for CD20 (**b**), CD10 (**c**), BCL6 (**d**), and negative for BCL2 (**e**). Neoplastic cells have high expression of MYC protein (**f**), and a very high Ki-67 proliferative index (**g**) (**b**–**g**. immunoperoxidase, magnification ×400). The tumor cells in this case are diffusely positive for EBER by in situ hybridization (magnification ×400) (**h**)

Prognosis

BL is a potential curable disease with the modern intensive chemotherapy and central neural system chemoprophylaxis. However, when disseminated disease with spleen involvement occurs, the more intensive and prolonged chemotherapy is required, and the mortality rate is higher [79].

Differential Diagnosis

Differential diagnosis includes other large B-cell lymphomas, such as high-grade B-cell lymphoma (HGBL) with *MYC* and *BCL2* and/or *BCL6* rearrangements; HGBL, NOS; diffuse large B-cell lymphoma, NOS; and mantle cell lymphoma, blastoid type (Table 6.5). Occasionally, it can be very challenging to distinguish BL from B-lymphoblastic leukemia/lymphoma. The critical diagnostic features are listed in Table 6.5.

High-Grade B-Cell Lymphoma

Definition

High-grade B-cell lymphoma (HGBL) is a newly defined entity in the revised fourth edition of the WHO classifica-

tion of hematopoietic neoplasms [1]. HGBL are mature, aggressive B-cell neoplasms that should not be diagnosed as DLBCL or Burkitt lymphoma as they have a unique biology, which impacts management and prognosis. HGBL are subdivided into two categories, HGBL with *MYC*, *BCL2*, and/or *BCL6* rearrangements ("double-/triple-hit lymphoma") and HGBL, not otherwise specified (HGBL, NOS).

High-Grade B-Cell Lymphoma, with *MYC*, *BCL2*, and/or *BCL6* Rearrangements ("Double-/Triple-Hit Lymphoma")

Definition

High-grade B-cell lymphomas (HGBL) with *MYC*, *BCL2*, and/or *BCL6* rearrangements, also referred to as "double-/triple-hit lymphoma," are defined strictly by the presence of *MYC* rearrangements in addition to *BCL2* and/or *BCL6* rearrangement(s). Lymphomas with concurrent rearrangements of other oncogenes without *MYC* rearrangements and lymphomas with concurrent rearrangements of *MYC* and genes other than *BCL2* and *BCL6* are not included in this category. For example, lymphomas with concurrent rearrangements of *MYC* and *CCND1* are best classified as mantle cell lymphomas with aggressive morphologic features [103–105]. Aggressive B-cell lymphomas may show rearrange-

Table 6.5 Differential diagnosis for Burkitt lymphoma

	Burkitt lymphoma	HGBL with *MYC* and *BCL2* and/or *BCL6*	HGBL, NOS	DLBCL, NOS	Mantle cell lymphoma, blastoid type	B-lymphoblastic leukemia/lymphoma
Starry-sky pattern	Frequent	Less frequent	Less frequent	Less frequent	Less frequent	Less frequent
Cytoplasmic molding	Y	N	N	N	N	N
Nucleoli	Multiple small, paracentrally located	More prominent nucleoli	More prominent nucleoli	More prominent nucleoli	Indistinct nucleoli	Indistinct nucleoli
CD20	+	+	+	+	+	−
CD5	−	−	−	−	+	−
CD10	+	+/−	Variable	Variable	−/+	+
BCL2	−	+/−	+/−	Variable	+	−
BCL6	+	+/−	+/−	Variable	−	−
IRF4/MUM1	−	−/+	−/+	Variable	−/+	−
Cyclin D1	−	−	−	−	+	−
TdT	−	−	−	−	−	+
Ki-67	>95%	<90%	Variable	<90%	<90%	<90%
MYC gene rearrangement	>90%	100%	20–35%	10–15%	Rare	Rare
Primary cytogenetic abnormalities	*MYC/IGH* or *IGK/MYC* or *MYC/IGL*	*MYC* and *BCL2* and/or *BCL6* rearrangement	*MYC* or *BCL2* gene rearrangement	Variable	*CCND1/IGH*	Chromosome numeric alternations or recurrent genetic mutations

Y yes, *N* no, *HGBL* high-grade B-cell lymphoma, *NOS* not otherwise specified

ments of one of *MYC*, *BCL2*, or *BCL6* genes in addition to gains/amplifications of the other two, secondary to aneuploidy [106]. Currently, these lymphomas are not included in this category. Similarly, aggressive B-cell lymphomas with isolated *MYC* rearrangements, not fulfilling morphologic or immunophenotypic criteria for Burkitt lymphoma, and those with *MYC*, *BCL2, or BCL6* gains are excluded from this category [107–110]. Conversely, follicular lymphomas and B-lymphoblastic lymphomas with double/triple hits are classified as such based on their morphologic and immunophenotypic features and are excluded from this category [111–113].

The majority of double-/triple-hit lymphomas show *MYC*, *BCL2*, and/or *BCL6* rearrangements in the background of a complex karyotype. It is postulated that the *MYC* rearrangement follows *BCL2* and/or *BCL6* rearrangements, but this has been demonstrated only in cases of follicular lymphoma with *BCL2* rearrangement that transforms into double-hit lymphomas. These cases represent only a subset of double-hit lymphomas, suggesting that de novo double-/triple-hit lymphomas of spleen may exist.

Epidemiology

Double-/triple-hit lymphomas are predominantly diseases of adults with a median age of diagnosis in the sixth or seventh decades of life. More than half of the patients present with advanced disease (stage III/IV, Ann Arbor classification), with frequent involvement of the bone marrow and central nervous system (CNS). Splenic involvement can present as diffuse infiltration of the red pulp or a mass lesion in the white pulp [114, 115].

Pathologic Features

Morphology

Double-/triple-hit lymphomas show variable morphologic features. Nearly half of these cases have the morphology of a DLBCL, NOS [116–118]. This is consistent with the observation that DLBCL, NOS, is the most frequent subtype of lymphoma, and approximately 8% of all DLBCL are double-/triple-hit lymphoma [119]. The cells are seen in diffuse sheets and are large with irregular nuclei, coarse to vesicular chromatin, and variably sized nucleoli. They have moderate to abundant cytoplasm imparting a more eosinophilic appearance. Mitotic activity can be variable, and apoptotic bodies or necrosis may or may not be identified. Starry-sky macrophages can be focally identified.

A significant subset of these tumors also has morphologic features mimicking BL or with features intermedi-ate between BL and DLBCL. The cells grow in a diffuse pattern and are predominantly intermediate sized with interspersed large cells, but foci of monotonous cells reminiscent of BL are noted. They have round or irregular nuclei with coarse chromatin, small or inconspicuous nucleoli, and minimal to moderate basophilic cytoplasm. Mitotic figures and apoptotic bodies are readily identified, and starry-sky macrophages are prominent. This morphologic pattern has been previously named atypical BL and B-cell lymphoma, unclassifiable with features intermediate between Burkitt lymphoma and diffuse large B-cell lymphoma (BCL-U), but these terms are eliminated from 2016 revised WHO classification and no longer recommended for use in the setting of double-/triple-hit lymphoma [114, 116].

Some cases have blastoid morphology, resembling lymphoblasts and composed of sheets of intermediate-sized cells with irregular nuclei, fine chromatin, small nucleoli, and minimal cytoplasm. Mitotic figures are readily noted, but starry-sky macrophages may or may not be identified [115]. Detailed immunohistochemical analysis should be performed in these cases to exclude B-lymphoblastic lymphoma and blastoid variant of mantle cell lymphoma.

Double-/triple-hit lymphomas are defined by their shared genetic aberrations, regardless of morphology; however, a recent study has shown that double-/triple-hit lymphomas with blastoid morphology have a significantly worse prognosis compared to non-blastoid double-/triple-hit lymphomas [120], and it is recommended to describe the morphologic features in a diagnostic comment.

Immunohistochemistry

Double-/triple-hit lymphomas are mature B-cell neoplasms and express pan B-cell markers, including CD19, CD20, PAX-5, and CD79a. However, a subset of cases may show features of immaturity such as weak CD45 expression, weak/absent CD20 expression, and lack of surface immunoglobulin [121]. CD10 and BCL6 expression is present in greater than 75% of cases, and IRF4/MUM1 expression is seen in approximately 25% of cases [122]. EBV-encoded small RNA (EBER) is negative. Using the Hans algorithm [6], essentially 100% of *MYC/BCL2* and *MYC/BCL2/BCL6* rearranged lymphomas are of germinal center B-cell phenotype (GCB), while greater than half of *MYC/BCL6* rearranged tumors are of GCB phenotype. BCL2 is uniformly expressed in almost all cases with *BCL2* rearrangements but is variably expressed in *BCL6* rearranged cases [117, 119, 123]. Unlike BL, which shows strong MYC expression in the majority of cells and a Ki-67 proliferative index approaching 100%, double-/triple-hit lymphomas can have variable MYC expression [119, 124, 125] and proliferative rates [126]. In cases with blastoid morphology, cyclin D1 and TdT stains should be performed to rule out blastoid variant of mantle cell lymphoma and B-lymphoblastic lymphoma, respectively.

Cytogenetics/Fluorescence In Situ Hybridization (FISH)

A definitive diagnosis of double-/triple-hit lymphoma is based on the detection of *MYC*, *BCL2*, and/or *BCL6* rearrangements by cytogenetic techniques. Conventional karyotyping techniques require fresh tissue and do not have the highest sensitivity for these gene rearrangements due to the presence of cryptic rearrangements (*MYC*) [127] or translocation of other genes in the same locus (*BCL2* and *MALT1* at 18q21). Fluorescence in situ hybridization (FISH) cytogenetic studies using labeled probes offer the highest sensitivity and specificity and are currently the preferred diagnostic method of detecting these gene rearrangements [128]. While it is agreed that all mature B-cell lymphomas with high-grade morphologic features (BL, BL/DLBCL, and blastoid lymphoma) need routine FISH evaluation for *MYC*, *BCL2*, and *BCL6* rearrangements, this strategy will only identify half of all double-/triple-hit lymphomas. Since DLBCL are encountered more often than high-grade B-cell lymphomas, it is impractical and cost-ineffective to perform comprehensive FISH analysis in every case. Hence, numerous immunohistochemical (IHC) and FISH screening strategies have been suggested to facilitate accurate diagnosis of double-/triple-hit lymphomas with morphologic features of DLBCL, NOS [122]. Currently, the most sensitive strategy is to perform *MYC* rearrangement testing in all DLBCL cases, regardless of cell of origin (COO) subtype, MYC expression levels by IHC, and proliferative rates; this is followed by testing for *BCL6* and *BCL2* rearrangements in cases positive for *MYC* rearrangement [119, 129]. The results of FISH testing are included in an addendum report and the clinician notified of the results, to facilitate appropriate management.

High-Grade B-Cell Lymphoma, Not Otherwise Specified (HGBL, NOS)

Definition

High-grade B-cell lymphoma, not otherwise specified (HGBL, NOS), is a category of aggressive mature B-cell lymphoma that does not meet morphologic and/or genetic criteria for BL, DLBCL, and double-/triple-hit lymphoma. These lymphomas are rare, and this diagnosis should be rendered carefully, only after exclusion of the abovementioned entities.

Epidemiology

No definitive epidemiologic information is available for this entity, but it appears to be a disease of older adults. Unlike in some cases of double-/triple-hit lymphoma, it is not known if these lymphomas are preceded by a low-grade B-cell lymphoma. Many patients present with advanced disease, and splenic involvement can present as red pulp or white pulp involvement [114, 115].

Pathologic Features

Morphology

Morphologically, the majority of HGBL, NOS, cases have features reminiscent of BL. The cells are intermediate sized with round or irregular nuclei and minimal basophilic cytoplasm. Some cases have monotonous features resembling BL, while others show more variability. Mitotic figures and apoptotic bodies are frequent and starry-sky macrophages are readily identified. Cases with blastoid morphology that do not fulfill criteria for blastoid variant of mantle cell lymphoma and B-lymphoblastic lymphoma are also included in this category.

Immunohistochemistry

HGBL, NOS, are positive for pan B-cell markers, including CD19, CD20, PAX-5, and CD79a. They are usually positive for CD10, BCL6, and BCL2 with rare cases expressing MUM1. EBER is negative. MYC expression is variable, depending on the presence or absence of *MYC* rearrangements. Ki-67 proliferative rates are variable. Cases morphologically resembling BL but with BCL2 expression are included in this category [115, 130, 131].

Genetics and Fluorescence In Situ Hybridization (FISH)

A subset of HGBL, NOS, cases show *MYC* rearrangements or gains. These are usually seen in the background of a complex karyotype associated with *BCL2* and *BCL6* copy number aberrations, but cases with *BCL2* and/or *BCL6* rearrangements in combination with *MYC* rearrangements are excluded from this category. Additionally, cases with morphologic features of DLBCL and with a *MYC* rearrangement or high proliferative rates do not fulfill diagnostic criteria for HGBL, NOS, and must be diagnosed as DLBCL. The differential diagnosis of HGBL is summarized in Table 6.6.

Differential Diagnosis

See Table 6.6.

Table 6.6 Differential diagnoses of high-grade B-cell lymphoma

	Morphology	Immunophenotype	FISH cytogenetics

High-grade B-cell lymphoma with *MYC*, *BCL2*, and/or *BCL6* rearrangements ("double-/triple-hit" lymphoma)	1. Diffuse large B-cell lymphoma-like morphology
	  (a) Sheets of large atypical lymphoid cells with irregular nuclei, mature chromatin, nucleoli, and moderate to abundant cytoplasm
	2. Burkitt lymphoma-like morphology
	  (a) Sheets of medium-sized atypical lymphoid cells with round to irregular nuclei, mature chromatin, small nucleoli, minimal basophilic cytoplasm
	3. Blastoid morphology
	  (a) Sheets of medium-sized atypical lymphoid cells with round to irregular nuclei, fine/open chromatin, small nucleoli, minimal cytoplasm
		Positive: CD45, CD19, CD20, CD79a, PAX5, CD10 (>75%), BCL6 (>75%), BCL2 (100% in *BCL2* rearranged cases, variable in *BCL6* rearranged cases), IRF4/MUM1 (~ 25%), Ki-67 (variable)
		Negative: cyclin D1, TdT, EBER-ISH
			Usually complex karyotype
			Positive for *MYC*, *BCL2*, and/or *BCL6* rearrangements
			Negative for *CCND1* rearrangement

High-grade B-cell lymphoma with, not otherwise specified (HGBL, NOS)	1. Burkitt lymphoma-like morphology
	  (a) Sheets of medium-sized atypical lymphoid cells with round to irregular nuclei, mature chromatin, small nucleoli, minimal basophilic cytoplasm
	2. Blastoid morphology
	  (a) Sheets of medium-sized atypical lymphoid cells with round to irregular nuclei, fine/open chromatin, small nucleoli, minimal cytoplasm
		Positive: CD45, CD19, CD20, CD79a, PAX5, CD10 (subset), BCL6 (subset), BCL2 (variable), IRF4/MUM1 (variable), Ki-67 (variable)
		Negative: cyclin D1, TdT, EBER-ISH
			Usually complex karyotype
			Can be positive for one of *MYC*, *BCL2*, and/or *BCL6* rearrangements but never two rearrangements including *MYC*
			Negative for *CCND1* rearrangement

Burkitt lymphoma	Sheets of monomorphic intermediate-sized atypical lymphoid cells with "squared off" nuclei, coarse chromatin with small nucleoli, and minimal basophilic cytoplasm. Prominent apoptotic debris with "starry-sky" macrophages	Positive: CD45, CD19, CD20, CD79a, PAX5, CD10, BCL6, Ki-67 (~ 100%), EBER-ISH (subset) Negative: BCL2, cyclin D1, TdT	Usually simple karyotype Positive for *MYC* rearrangement
Blastoid variant of mantle cell lymphoma	Sheets of medium-sized atypical lymphoid cells with round to irregular nuclei, fine/open chromatin, small nucleoli, minimal cytoplasm	Positive: CD45, CD19, CD20, CD79a, PAX5, CD5 (majority), CD10 (rarely), BCL2, cyclin D1, SOX11, Ki-67 (variable) Negative: BCL6, IRF4/MUM1, TdT, EBER-ISH	Simple or complex karyotype Positive for *CCND1* rearrangement Some cases may show *MYC* with or without *BCL-2 or BCL-6* rearrangement, but still classified as mantle cell lymphoma, blastoid variant
B-lymphoblastic leukemia/lymphoma	Sheets of medium-sized atypical lymphoid cells with round to irregular nuclei, fine/open chromatin, small nucleoli, minimal cytoplasm	Positive: CD45 (dim), CD19, CD79a, PAX5, CD10, BCL2, TdT Negative: CD20, BCL6, IRF4/MUM1, cyclin D1, EBER-ISH	Variable karyotype May rarely show *MYC*, *BCL6*, and/or *BCL2* rearrangements but still classified as B-lymphoblastic lymphoma due to immature phenotype

References

1. Swerdlow SH, Campo E, Harris NL, Jaffe ES, Pileri S, Stein H, Thiele J, Swiatowa Organizacja Z, International Agency for Research on Cancer. WHO classification of tumours of haematopoietic and lymphoid tissues. Lyon: International Agency for Research on Cancer; 2017.
2. Alizadeh AA, Eisen MB, Davis RE, Ma C, Lossos IS, Rosenwald A, Boldrick JC, Sabet H, Tran T, Yu X, et al. Distinct types of diffuse large B-cell lymphoma identified by gene expression profiling. Nature. 2000;403:503–11.
3. Rosenwald A, Wright G, Leroy K, Yu X, Gaulard P, Gascoyne RD, Chan WC, Zhao T, Haioun C, Greiner TC, et al. Molecular diagnosis of primary mediastinal B cell lymphoma identifies a clinically favorable subgroup of diffuse large B cell lymphoma related to Hodgkin lymphoma. J Exp Med. 2003;198:851–62.
4. Wright G, Tan B, Rosenwald A, Hurt EH, Wiestner A, Staudt LM. A gene expression-based method to diagnose clinically distinct subgroups of diffuse large B cell lymphoma. Proc Natl Acad Sci U S A. 2003;100:9991–6.
5. Schmitz R, Wright GW, Huang DW, Johnson CA, Phelan JD, Wang JQ, Roulland S, Kasbekar M, Young RM, Shaffer AL, et al. Genetics and pathogenesis of diffuse large B-cell lymphoma. N Engl J Med. 2018;378:1396–407.
6. Hans CP, Weisenburger DD, Greiner TC, Gascoyne RD, Delabie J, Ott G, Muller-Hermelink HK, Campo E, Braziel RM, Jaffe ES, et al. Confirmation of the molecular classification of diffuse large B-cell lymphoma by immunohistochemistry using a tissue microarray. Blood. 2004;103:275–82.
7. Muris JJ, Meijer CJ, Vos W, van Krieken JH, Jiwa NM, Ossenkoppele GJ, Oudejans JJ. Immunohistochemical profiling based on Bcl-2, CD10 and MUM1 expression improves risk stratification in patients with primary nodal diffuse large B cell lymphoma. J Pathol. 2006;208:714–23.
8. Choi WW, Weisenburger DD, Greiner TC, Piris MA, Banham AH, Delabie J, Braziel RM, Geng H, Iqbal J, Lenz G, et al. A new immunostain algorithm classifies diffuse large B-cell lymphoma into molecular subtypes with high accuracy. Clin Cancer Res. 2009;15:5494–502.
9. Colomo L, Lopez-Guillermo A, Perales M, Rives S, Martinez A, Bosch F, Colomer D, Falini B, Montserrat E, Campo E. Clinical impact of the differentiation profile assessed by immunophenotyping in patients with diffuse large B-cell lymphoma. Blood. 2003;101:78–84.
10. Meyer PN, Fu K, Greiner TC, Smith LM, Delabie J, Gascoyne RD, Ott G, Rosenwald A, Braziel RM, Campo E, et al. Immunohistochemical methods for predicting cell of origin and survival in patients with diffuse large B-cell lymphoma treated with rituximab. J Clin Oncol. 2011;29:200–7.
11. Johnson NA, Slack GW, Savage KJ, Connors JM, Ben-Neriah S, Rogic S, Scott DW, Tan KL, Steidl C, Sehn LH, et al. Concurrent expression of MYC and BCL2 in diffuse large B-cell lymphoma treated with rituximab plus cyclophosphamide, doxorubicin, vincristine, and prednisone. J Clin Oncol. 2012;30:3452–9.
12. Hu S, Xu-Monette ZY, Tzankov A, Green T, Wu L, Balasubramanyam A, Liu WM, Visco C, Li Y, Miranda RN, et al. MYC/BCL2 protein coexpression contributes to the inferior survival of activated B-cell subtype of diffuse large B-cell lymphoma and demonstrates high-risk gene expression signatures: a report from The International DLBCL Rituximab-CHOP Consortium Program. Blood. 2013;121:4021–31; quiz 4250.
13. Kraus MD, Fleming MD, Vonderheide RH. The spleen as a diagnostic specimen: a review of 10 years' experience at two tertiary care institutions. Cancer. 2001;91:2001–9.
14. Arber DA, Rappaport H, Weiss LM. Non-Hodgkin's lymphoproliferative disorders involving the spleen. Mod Pathol. 1997;10:18–32.
15. Mollejo M, Algara P, Mateo MS, Menarguez J, Pascual E, Fresno MF, Camacho FI, Piris MA. Large B-cell lymphoma presenting in the spleen: identification of different clinicopathologic conditions. Am J Surg Pathol. 2003;27:895–902.
16. Kashimura M, Noro M, Akikusa B, Okuhara A, Momose S, Miura I, Kojima M, Tamaru J. Primary splenic diffuse large B-cell lymphoma manifesting in red pulp. Virchows Arch. 2008;453:501–9.
17. Kuratsune H, Machii T, Aozasa K, Ueda E, Tokumine Y, Morita T, Tagawa S, Taniguchi N, Inoue R, Kitani T. B cell lymphoma showing clinicopathological features of malignant histiocytosis. Acta Haematol. 1988;79:94–8.
18. Betman HF, Vardiman JW, Lau J. T-cell-rich B-cell lymphoma of the spleen. Am J Surg Pathol. 1994;18:323–4.
19. Faravelli A, Gambini S, Perego D, Nobili R, Zoldan MC, Leone BE, Giani L. Splenic lymphoma: unusual case with exclusive red pulp involvement. Pathologica. 1995;87:692–5.
20. Kobrich U, Falk S, Karhoff M, Middeke B, Anselstetter V, Stutte HJ. Primary large cell lymphoma of the splenic sinuses: a variant of angiotropic B-cell lymphoma (neoplastic angioendotheliomatosis)? Hum Pathol. 1992;23:1184–7.
21. Kroft SH, Howard MS, Picker LJ, Ansari MQ, Aquino DB, McKenna RW. De novo CD5+ diffuse large B-cell lymphomas. A heterogeneous group containing an unusual form of splenic lymphoma. Am J Clin Pathol. 2000;114:523–33.
22. Palutke M, Eisenberg L, Narang S, Han LL, Peeples TC, Kukuruga DL, Tabaczka PM. B lymphocytic lymphoma (large cell) of possible splenic marginal zone origin presenting with prominent splenomegaly and unusual cordal red pulp distribution. Cancer. 1988;62:593–600.
23. Stroup RM, Burke JS, Sheibani K, Ben-Ezra J, Brownell M, Winberg CD. Splenic involvement by aggressive malignant lymphomas of B-cell and T-cell types. A morphologic and immunophenotypic study. Cancer. 1992;69:413–20.
24. Salgado C, Feliu E, Montserrat E, Villamor N, Ordi J, Aguilar JL, Vives-Corrons JL, Rozman C. B-type large-cell primary splenic lymphoma with massive involvement of the red pulp. Acta Haematol. 1993;89:46–9.
25. Bairey O, Shvidel L, Perry C, Dann EJ, Ruchlemer R, Tadmor T, Goldschmidt N. Characteristics of primary splenic diffuse large B-cell lymphoma and role of splenectomy in improving survival. Cancer. 2015;121:2909–16.
26. Takeshita M, Sakai H, Okamura S, Oshiro Y, Higaki K, Nakashima O, Uike N, Yamamoto I, Kinjo M, Matsubara F. Splenic large B-cell lymphoma in patients with hepatitis C virus infection. Hum Pathol. 2005;36:878–85.
27. Yu SC, Lin CW. Early-stage splenic diffuse large B-cell lymphoma is highly associated with hepatitis C virus infection. Kaohsiung J Med Sci. 2013;29:150–6.
28. De Renzo A, Perna F, Persico M, Notaro R, Mainolfi C, de Sio I, Ciancia G, Picardi M, Del Vecchio L, Pane F, et al. Excellent prognosis and prevalence of HCV infection of primary hepatic and splenic non-Hodgkin's lymphoma. Eur J Haematol. 2008;81:51–7.
29. Iannitto E, Tripodo C. How I diagnose and treat splenic lymphomas. Blood. 2011;117:2585–95.
30. Bertram HC, Check IJ, Milano MA. Immunophenotyping large B-cell lymphomas. Flow cytometric pitfalls and pathologic correlation. Am J Clin Pathol. 2001;116:191–203.
31. Yoshioka T, Miura I, Kume M, Takahashi N, Okamoto M, Ichinohasama R, Yoshino T, Yamaguchi M, Hirokawa M, Sawada K, et al. Cytogenetic features of de novo CD5-positive diffuse

large B-cell lymphoma: chromosome aberrations affecting 8p21 and 11q13 constitute major subgroups with different overall survival. Genes Chromosomes Cancer. 2005;42:149–57.

32. Matutes E, Wotherspoon A, Catovsky D. The variant form of hairy-cell leukaemia. Best Pract Res Clin Haematol. 2003;16:41–56.

33. Zanelli M, Ragazzi M, Valli R, Piattoni S, Alvarez De Celis MI, Farnetti E, Orcioni GF, Longo R, Ascani S, Falini B, et al. Transformation of IGHV4-34+ hairy cell leukaemia-variant with U2AF1 mutation into a clonally-related high grade B-cell lymphoma responding to immunochemotherapy. Br J Haematol. 2016;173:491–5.

34. Berger F, Felman P, Thieblemont C, Pradier T, Baseggio L, Bryon PA, Salles G, Callet-Bauchu E, Coiffier B. Non-MALT marginal zone B-cell lymphomas: a description of clinical presentation and outcome in 124 patients. Blood. 2000;95:1950–6.

35. Camacho FI, Mollejo M, Mateo MS, Algara P, Navas C, Hernandez JM, Santoja C, Sole F, Sanchez-Beato M, Piris MA. Progression to large B-cell lymphoma in splenic marginal zone lymphoma: a description of a series of 12 cases. Am J Surg Pathol. 2001;25:1268–76.

36. Delabie J, Vandenberghe E, Kennes C, Verhoef G, Foschini MP, Stul M, Cassiman JJ, De Wolf-Peeters C. Histiocyte-rich B-cell lymphoma. A distinct clinicopathologic entity possibly related to lymphocyte predominant Hodgkin's disease, paragranuloma subtype. Am J Surg Pathol. 1992;16:37–48.

37. Ramsay AD, Smith WJ, Isaacson PG. T-cell-rich B-cell lymphoma. Am J Surg Pathol. 1988;12:433–43.

38. Achten R, Verhoef G, Vanuytsel L, De Wolf-Peeters C. Histiocyte-rich, T-cell-rich B-cell lymphoma: a distinct diffuse large B-cell lymphoma subtype showing characteristic morphologic and immunophenotypic features. Histopathology. 2002;40:31–45.

39. Achten R, Verhoef G, Vanuytsel L, De Wolf-Peeters C. T-cell/histiocyte-rich large B-cell lymphoma: a distinct clinicopathologic entity. J Clin Oncol. 2002;20:1269–77.

40. Dogan A, Burke JS, Goteri G, Stitson RN, Wotherspoon AC, Isaacson PG. Micronodular T-cell/histiocyte-rich large B-cell lymphoma of the spleen: histology, immunophenotype, and differential diagnosis. Am J Surg Pathol. 2003;27:903–11.

41. Li S, Mann KP, Holden JT. T-cell-rich B-cell lymphoma presenting in the spleen: a clinicopathologic analysis of 3 cases. Int J Surg Pathol. 2004;12:31–7.

42. Wang SA, Olson N, Zukerberg L, Harris NL. Splenic marginal zone lymphoma with micronodular T-cell rich B-cell lymphoma. Am J Surg Pathol. 2006;30:128–32.

43. Turkoz HK, Polat N, Akin I, Ozcan D. Micronodular T-cell/histiocyte-rich B-cell lymphoma of the spleen in a case of small lymphocytic lymphoma: a Richter's transformation. Ups J Med Sci. 2010;115:217–9.

44. Pittaluga S, Jaffe ES. T-cell/histiocyte-rich large B-cell lymphoma. Haematologica. 2010;95:352–6.

45. Kamel OW, Gelb AB, Shibuya RB, Warnke RA. Leu 7 (CD57) reactivity distinguishes nodular lymphocyte predominance Hodgkin's disease from nodular sclerosing Hodgkin's disease, T-cell-rich B-cell lymphoma and follicular lymphoma. Am J Pathol. 1993;142:541–6.

46. de Leval L, Savilo E, Longtine J, Ferry JA, Harris NL. Peripheral T-cell lymphoma with follicular involvement and a CD4+/bcl-6+ phenotype. Am J Surg Pathol. 2001;25:395–400.

47. Dasgupta T, Coombes B, Brasfield RD. Primary malignant neoplasms of the spleen. Surg Gynecol Obstet. 1965;120:947–60.

48. Shimoyama Y, Asano N, Kojima M, Morishima S, Yamamoto K, Oyama T, Kinoshita T, Nakamura S. Age-related EBV-associated B-cell lymphoproliferative disorders: diagnostic approach to a newly recognized clinicopathological entity. Pathol Int. 2009;59:835–43.

49. Kojima M, Noro M, Nakazato Y, Akikusa B, Tamaru J, Masawa N, Kashimura M. Epstein-Barr virus-associated B-cell lymphoma of the spleen resembling infectious mononucleosis morphologically. Leuk Lymphoma. 2012;53:2504–6.

50. Ozsan N, Cagirgan S, Saydam G, Gunes A, Hekimgil M. Epstein-Barr virus (EBV) positive diffuse large B cell lymphoma of the elderly-experience of a single center from Turkey. Pathol Res Pract. 2013;209:471–8.

51. Montes-Moreno S, Odqvist L, Diaz-Perez JA, Lopez AB, de Villambrosia SG, Mazorra F, Castillo ME, Lopez M, Pajares R, Garcia JF, et al. EBV-positive diffuse large B-cell lymphoma of the elderly is an aggressive post-germinal center B-cell neoplasm characterized by prominent nuclear factor-kB activation. Mod Pathol. 2012;25:968–82.

52. Hofscheier A, Ponciano A, Bonzheim I, Adam P, Lome-Maldonado C, Vela T, Cortes E, Ortiz-Hidalgo C, Fend F, Quintanilla-Martinez L. Geographic variation in the prevalence of Epstein-Barr virus-positive diffuse large B-cell lymphoma of the elderly: a comparative analysis of a Mexican and a German population. Mod Pathol. 2011;24:1046–54.

53. Asano N, Yamamoto K, Tamaru J, Oyama T, Ishida F, Ohshima K, Yoshino T, Nakamura N, Mori S, Yoshie O, et al. Age-related Epstein-Barr virus (EBV)-associated B-cell lymphoproliferative disorders: comparison with EBV-positive classic Hodgkin lymphoma in elderly patients. Blood. 2009;113:2629–36.

54. Aw D, Silva AB, Palmer DB. Immunosenescence: emerging challenges for an ageing population. Immunology. 2007;120:435–46.

55. Hakim FT, Gress RE. Immunosenescence: deficits in adaptive immunity in the elderly. Tissue Antigens. 2007;70:179–89.

56. Kuppers R. B cells under influence: transformation of B cells by Epstein-Barr virus. Nat Rev Immunol. 2003;3:801–12.

57. Ok CY, Papathomas TG, Medeiros LJ, Young KH. EBV-positive diffuse large B-cell lymphoma of the elderly. Blood. 2013;122:328–40.

58. Chen BJ, Chapuy B, Ouyang J, Sun HH, Roemer MG, Xu ML, Yu H, Fletcher CD, Freeman GJ, Shipp MA, et al. PD-L1 expression is characteristic of a subset of aggressive B-cell lymphomas and virus-associated malignancies. Clin Cancer Res. 2013;19:3462–73.

59. Nicolae A, Pittaluga S, Abdullah S, Steinberg SM, Pham TA, Davies-Hill T, Xi L, Raffeld M, Jaffe ES. EBV-positive large B-cell lymphomas in young patients: a nodal lymphoma with evidence for a tolerogenic immune environment. Blood. 2015;126:863–72.

60. Morice WG, Rodriguez FJ, Hoyer JD, Kurtin PJ. Diffuse large B-cell lymphoma with distinctive patterns of splenic and bone marrow involvement: clinicopathologic features of two cases. Mod Pathol. 2005;18:495–502.

61. Dojcinov SD, Venkataraman G, Pittaluga S, Wlodarska I, Schrager JA, Raffeld M, Hills RK, Jaffe ES. Age-related EBV-associated lymphoproliferative disorders in the Western population: a spectrum of reactive lymphoid hyperplasia and lymphoma. Blood. 2011;117:4726–35.

62. Oyama T, Yamamoto K, Asano N, Oshiro A, Suzuki R, Kagami Y, Morishima Y, Takeuchi K, Izumo T, Mori S, et al. Age-related EBV-associated B-cell lymphoproliferative disorders constitute a distinct clinicopathologic group: a study of 96 patients. Clin Cancer Res. 2007;13:5124–32.

63. Oyama T, Ichimura K, Suzuki R, Suzumiya J, Ohshima K, Yatabe Y, Yokoi T, Kojima M, Kamiya Y, Taji H, et al. Senile EBV+ B-cell lymphoproliferative disorders: a clinicopathologic study of 22 patients. Am J Surg Pathol. 2003;27:16–26.

64. Hoeller S, Tzankov A, Pileri SA, Went P, Dirnhofer S. Epstein-Barr virus-positive diffuse large B-cell lymphoma in elderly patients is rare in Western populations. Hum Pathol. 2010;41:352–7.

65. Sato A, Nakamura N, Kojima M, Ohmachi K, Carreras J, Kikuti YY, Numata H, Ohgiya D, Tazume K, Amaki J, et al. Clinical out-

come of Epstein-Barr virus-positive diffuse large B-cell lymphoma of the elderly in the rituximab era. Cancer Sci. 2014;105:1170–5.

66. Ahn JS, Yang DH, Duk Choi Y, Jung SH, Yhim HY, Kwak JY, Sung Park H, Shin MG, Kim YK, Kim HJ, et al. Clinical outcome of elderly patients with Epstein-Barr virus positive diffuse large B-cell lymphoma treated with a combination of rituximab and CHOP chemotherapy. Am J Hematol. 2013;88:774–9.

67. Cohen M, Narbaitz M, Metrebian F, De Matteo E, Preciado MV, Chabay PA. Epstein-Barr virus-positive diffuse large B-cell lymphoma association is not only restricted to elderly patients. Int J Cancer. 2014;135:2816–24.

68. Gebauer N, Gebauer J, Hardel TT, Bernard V, Biersack H, Lehnert H, Rades D, Feller AC, Thorns C. Prevalence of targetable oncogenic mutations and genomic alterations in Epstein-Barr virus-associated diffuse large B-cell lymphoma of the elderly. Leuk Lymphoma. 2015;56:1100–6.

69. Ok CY, Li L, Xu-Monette ZY, Visco C, Tzankov A, Manyam GC, Montes-Moreno S, Dybkaer K, Chiu A, Orazi A, et al. Prevalence and clinical implications of epstein-barr virus infection in de novo diffuse large B-cell lymphoma in Western countries. Clin Cancer Res. 2014;20:2338–49.

70. Kato H, Karube K, Yamamoto K, Takizawa J, Tsuzuki S, Yatabe Y, Kanda T, Katayama M, Ozawa Y, Ishitsuka K, et al. Gene expression profiling of Epstein-Barr virus-positive diffuse large B-cell lymphoma of the elderly reveals alterations of characteristic oncogenetic pathways. Cancer Sci. 2014;105:537–44.

71. Yoon H, Park S, Ju H, Ha SY, Sohn I, Jo J, Do IG, Min S, Kim SJ, Kim WS, et al. Integrated copy number and gene expression profiling analysis of Epstein-Barr virus-positive diffuse large B-cell lymphoma. Genes Chromosomes Cancer. 2015;54:383–96.

72. Stuhlmann-Laeisz C, Borchert A, Quintanilla-Martinez L, Hoeller S, Tzankov A, Oschlies I, Kreuz M, Trappe R, Klapper W. In Europe expression of EBNA2 is associated with poor survival in EBV-positive diffuse large B-cell lymphoma of the elderly. Leuk Lymphoma. 2016;57:39–44.

73. Loong F, Chan AC, Ho BC, Chau YP, Lee HY, Cheuk W, Yuen WK, Ng WS, Cheung HL, Chan JK. Diffuse large B-cell lymphoma associated with chronic inflammation as an incidental finding and new clinical scenarios. Mod Pathol. 2010;23:493–501.

74. Boroumand N, Ly TL, Sonstein J, Medeiros LJ. Microscopic diffuse large B-cell lymphoma (DLBCL) occurring in pseudocysts: do these tumors belong to the category of DLBCL associated with chronic inflammation? Am J Surg Pathol. 2012;36:1074–80.

75. Davidson T, Priel E, Schiby G, Raskin S, Chikman B, Nissan E, Benjamini O, Nissan J, Goshen E, Ben-Haim S, et al. Low rate of spleen involvement in sporadic Burkitt lymphoma at staging on PET-CT. Abdom Radiol (NY). 2018;43(9):2369–74.

76. Zeng W, Lechowicz MJ, Winton E, Cho SM, Galt JR, Halkar R. Spectrum of FDG PET/CT findings in Burkitt lymphoma. Clin Nucl Med. 2009;34:355–8.

77. Karantanis D, Durski JM, Lowe VJ, Nathan MA, Mullan BP, Georgiou E, Johnston PB, Wiseman GA. 18F-FDG PET and PET/CT in Burkitt's lymphoma. Eur J Radiol. 2010;75:e68–73.

78. Banks PM, Arseneau JC, Gralnick HR, Canellos GP, DeVita VT Jr, Berard CW. American Burkitt's lymphoma: a clinicopathologic study of 30 cases. II. Pathologic correlations. Am J Med. 1975;58:322–9.

79. Grogan TM, Warnke RA, Kaplan HS. A comparative study of Burkitt's and non-Burkitt's "undifferentiated" malignant lymphoma: immunologic, cytochemical, ultrastructural, cytologic, histopathologic, clinical and cell culture features. Cancer. 1982;49:1817–28.

80. Burkitt DP. Epidemiology of Burkitt's lymphoma. Proc R Soc Med. 1971;64:909–10.

81. Shiramizu B, Barriga F, Neequaye J, Jafri A, Dalla-Favera R, Neri A, Guttierez M, Levine P, Magrath I. Patterns of chromosomal breakpoint locations in Burkitt's lymphoma: relevance to geography and Epstein-Barr virus association. Blood. 1991;77:1516–26.

82. Gutierrez MI, Bhatia K, Barriga F, Diez B, Muriel FS, de Andreas ML, Epelman S, Risueno C, Magrath IT. Molecular epidemiology of Burkitt's lymphoma from South America: differences in breakpoint location and Epstein-Barr virus association from tumors in other world regions. Blood. 1992;79:3261–6.

83. Anwar N, Kingma DW, Bloch AR, Mourad M, Raffeld M, Franklin J, Magrath I, el Bolkainy N, Jaffe ES. The investigation of Epstein-Barr viral sequences in 41 cases of Burkitt's lymphoma from Egypt: epidemiologic correlations. Cancer. 1995;76:1245–52.

84. Araujo I, Foss HD, Bittencourt A, Hummel M, Demel G, Mendonca N, Herbst H, Stein H. Expression of Epstein-Barr virus-gene products in Burkitt's lymphoma in Northeast Brazil. Blood. 1996;87:5279–86.

85. Hamilton-Dutoit SJ, Raphael M, Audouin J, Diebold J, Lisse I, Pedersen C, Oksenhendler E, Marelle L, Pallesen G. In situ demonstration of Epstein-Barr virus small RNAs (EBER 1) in acquired immunodeficiency syndrome-related lymphomas: correlation with tumor morphology and primary site. Blood. 1993;82:619–24.

86. Rowe M, Rowe DT, Gregory CD, Young LS, Farrell PJ, Rupani H, Rickinson AB. Differences in B cell growth phenotype reflect novel patterns of Epstein-Barr virus latent gene expression in Burkitt's lymphoma cells. EMBO J. 1987;6:2743–51.

87. Hamilton-Dutoit SJ, Rea D, Raphael M, Sandvej K, Delecluse HJ, Gisselbrecht C, Marelle L, van Krieken HJ, Pallesen G. Epstein-Barr virus-latent gene expression and tumor cell phenotype in acquired immunodeficiency syndrome-related non-Hodgkin's lymphoma. Correlation of lymphoma phenotype with three distinct patterns of viral latency. Am J Pathol. 1993;143:1072–85.

88. Niedobitek G, Agathanggelou A, Rowe M, Jones EL, Jones DB, Turyaguma P, Oryema J, Wright DH, Young LS. Heterogeneous expression of Epstein-Barr virus latent proteins in endemic Burkitt's lymphoma. Blood. 1995;86:659–65.

89. Klein G. Specific chromosomal translocations and the genesis of B-cell-derived tumors in mice and men. Cell. 1983;32:311–5.

90. Polack A, Hortnagel K, Pajic A, Christoph B, Baier B, Falk M, Mautner J, Geltinger C, Bornkamm GW. Kempkes B. c-myc activation renders proliferation of Epstein-Barr virus (EBV)-transformed cells independent of EBV nuclear antigen 2 and latent membrane protein 1. Proc Natl Acad Sci U S A. 1996;93:10411–6.

91. Boxer LM, Dang CV. Translocations involving c-myc and c-myc function. Oncogene. 2001;20:5595–610.

92. Ramiro AR, Jankovic M, Eisenreich T, Difilippantonio S, Chen-Kiang S, Muramatsu M, Honjo T, Nussenzweig A, Nussenzweig MC. AID is required for c-myc/IgH chromosome translocations in vivo. Cell. 2004;118:431–8.

93. Nguyen L, Papenhausen P, Shao H. The role of c-MYC in B-cell lymphomas: diagnostic and molecular aspects. Genes (Basel). 2017;8(4):116.

94. Seegmiller AC, Garcia R, Huang R, Maleki A, Karandikar NJ, Chen W. Simple karyotype and bcl-6 expression predict a diagnosis of Burkitt lymphoma and better survival in IG-MYC rearranged high-grade B-cell lymphomas. Mod Pathol. 2010;23:909–20.

95. Aukema SM, Theil L, Rohde M, Bauer B, Bradtke J, Burkhardt B, Bonn BR, Claviez A, Gattenlohner S, Makarova O, et al. Sequential karyotyping in Burkitt lymphoma reveals a linear clonal evolution with increase in karyotype complexity and a high frequency of recurrent secondary aberrations. Br J Haematol. 2015;170:814–25.

96. Havelange V, Ameye G, Theate I, Callet-Bauchu E, Mugneret F, Michaux L, Dastugue N, Penther D, Barin C, Collonge-Rame MA, et al. Patterns of genomic aberrations suggest that Burkitt lymphomas with complex karyotype are distinct from other aggressive B-cell lymphomas with MYC rearrangement. Genes Chromosomes Cancer. 2013;52:81–92.

97. Dave SS, Fu K, Wright GW, Lam LT, Kluin P, Boerma EJ, Greiner TC, Weisenburger DD, Rosenwald A, Ott G, et al. Molecular diagnosis of Burkitt's lymphoma. N Engl J Med. 2006;354:2431–42.

98. Hummel M, Bentink S, Berger H, Klapper W, Wessendorf S, Barth TF, Bernd HW, Cogliatti SB, Dierlamm J, Feller AC, et al. A biologic definition of Burkitt's lymphoma from transcriptional and genomic profiling. N Engl J Med. 2006;354:2419–30.

99. Lenze D, Leoncini L, Hummel M, Volinia S, Liu CG, Amato T, De Falco G, Githanga J, Horn H, Nyagol J, et al. The different epidemiologic subtypes of Burkitt lymphoma share a homogenous micro RNA profile distinct from diffuse large B-cell lymphoma. Leukemia. 2011;25:1869–76.

100. Piccaluga PP, De Falco G, Kustagi M, Gazzola A, Agostinelli C, Tripodo C, Leucci E, Onnis A, Astolfi A, Sapienza MR, et al. Gene expression analysis uncovers similarity and differences among Burkitt lymphoma subtypes. Blood. 2011;117:3596–608.

101. Love C, Sun Z, Jima D, Li G, Zhang J, Miles R, Richards KL, Dunphy CH, Choi WW, Srivastava G, et al. The genetic landscape of mutations in Burkitt lymphoma. Nat Genet. 2012;44:1321–5.

102. Richter J, Schlesner M, Hoffmann S, Kreuz M, Leich E, Burkhardt B, Rosolowski M, Ammerpohl O, Wagener R, Bernhart SH, et al. Recurrent mutation of the ID3 gene in Burkitt lymphoma identified by integrated genome, exome and transcriptome sequencing. Nat Genet. 2012;44:1316–20.

103. Delas A, Sophie D, Brousset P, Laurent C. Unusual concomitant rearrangements of Cyclin D1 and MYC genes in blastoid variant of mantle cell lymphoma: case report and review of literature. Pathol Res Pract. 2013;209:115–9.

104. Choe JY, Yun JY, Na HY, Huh J, Shin SJ, Kim HJ, Paik JH, Kim YA, Nam SJ, Jeon YK, et al. MYC overexpression correlates with MYC amplification or translocation, and is associated with poor prognosis in mantle cell lymphoma. Histopathology. 2016;68:442–9.

105. Hu Z, Medeiros LJ, Chen Z, Chen W, Li S, Konoplev SN, Lu X, Pham LV, Young KH, Wang W, et al. Mantle cell lymphoma with MYC rearrangement: a report of 17 patients. Am J Surg Pathol. 2017;41:216–24.

106. Li S, Seegmiller AC, Lin P, Wang XJ, Miranda RN, Bhagavathi S, Medeiros LJ. B-cell lymphomas with concurrent MYC and BCL2 abnormalities other than translocations behave similarly to MYC/BCL2 double-hit lymphomas. Mod Pathol. 2015;28:208–17.

107. Li S, Weiss VL, Wang XJ, Desai PA, Hu S, Yin CC, Tang G, Reddy NM, Medeiros LJ, Lin P. High-grade B-cell lymphoma with MYC rearrangement and without BCL2 and BCL6 rearrangements is associated with high P53 expression and a poor prognosis. Am J Surg Pathol. 2016;40:253–61.

108. Quesada AE, Medeiros LJ, Desai PA, Lin P, Westin JR, Hawsawi HM, Wei P, Tang G, Seegmiller AC, Reddy NM, et al. Increased MYC copy number is an independent prognostic factor in patients with diffuse large B-cell lymphoma. Mod Pathol. 2017;30:1688–97.

109. Lu TX, Fan L, Wang L, Wu JZ, Miao KR, Liang JH, Gong QX, Wang Z, Young KH, Xu W, et al. MYC or BCL2 copy number aberration is a strong predictor of outcome in patients with diffuse large B-cell lymphoma. Oncotarget. 2015;6:18374–88.

110. Caponetti GC, Dave BJ, Perry AM, Smith LM, Jain S, Meyer PN, Bast M, Bierman PJ, Bociek RG, Vose JM, et al. Isolated MYC cytogenetic abnormalities in diffuse large B-cell lymphoma do not predict an adverse clinical outcome. Leuk Lymphoma. 2015;56:3082–9.

111. Miyaoka M, Kikuti YY, Carreras J, Ikoma H, Hiraiwa S, Ichiki A, Kojima M, Ando K, Yokose T, Sakai R, et al. Clinicopathological and genomic analysis of double-hit follicular lymphoma: comparison with high-grade B-cell lymphoma with MYC and BCL2 and/or BCL6 rearrangements. Mod Pathol. 2018;31:313–26.

112. Geyer JT, Subramaniyam S, Jiang Y, Elemento O, Ferry JA, de Leval L, Nakashima MO, Liu YC, Martin P, Mathew S, et al. Lymphoblastic transformation of follicular lymphoma: a clinicopathologic and molecular analysis of 7 patients. Hum Pathol. 2015;46:260–71.

113. Liu W, Hu S, Konopleva M, Khoury JD, Kalhor N, Tang G, Bueso-Ramos CE, Jorgensen JL, Lin P, Medeiros LJ, et al. De novo MYC and BCL2 double-hit B-cell precursor acute lymphoblastic leukemia (BCP-ALL) in pediatric and young adult patients associated with poor prognosis. Pediatr Hematol Oncol. 2015;32:535–47.

114. Perry AM, Crockett D, Dave BJ, Althof P, Winkler L, Smith LM, Aoun P, Chan WC, Fu K, Greiner TC, et al. B-cell lymphoma, unclassifiable, with features intermediate between diffuse large B-cell lymphoma and burkitt lymphoma: study of 39 cases. Br J Haematol. 2013;162:40–9.

115. Kanagal-Shamanna R, Medeiros LJ, Lu G, Wang SA, Manning JT, Lin P, Penn GM, Young KH, You MJ, Vega F, et al. High-grade B cell lymphoma, unclassifiable, with blastoid features: an unusual morphological subgroup associated frequently with BCL2 and/or MYC gene rearrangements and a poor prognosis. Histopathology. 2012;61:945–54.

116. Li S, Lin P, Fayad LE, Lennon PA, Miranda RN, Yin CC, Lin E, Medeiros LJ. B-cell lymphomas with MYC/8q24 rearrangements and IGH@BCL2/t(14;18)(q32;q21): an aggressive disease with heterogeneous histology, germinal center B-cell immunophenotype and poor outcome. Mod Pathol. 2012;25:145–56.

117. Li S, Desai P, Lin P, Yin CC, Tang G, Wang XJ, Konoplev SN, Khoury JD, Bueso-Ramos CE, Medeiros LJ. MYC/BCL6 double-hit lymphoma (DHL): a tumour associated with an aggressive clinical course and poor prognosis. Histopathology. 2016;68:1090–8.

118. Li S, Huang W, Oki Y, Medeiros LJ. MYC/BCL2/BCL6 triple hit lymphoma: a study of 33 patients who had an aggressive clinical course similar to patients with double hit lymphomas. J Clin Oncol. 2017;35:7559.

119. Scott DW, King RL, Staiger AM, Ben-Neriah S, Jiang A, Horn H, Mottok A, Farinha P, Slack GW, Ennishi D, et al. High-grade B-cell lymphoma with MYC and BCL2 and/or BCL6 rearrangements with diffuse large B-cell lymphoma morphology. Blood. 2018;131:2060–4.

120. Moore EM, Aggarwal N, Surti U, Swerdlow SH. Further exploration of the complexities of large B-cell lymphomas with MYC abnormalities and the importance of a blastoid morphology. Am J Surg Pathol. 2017;41:1155–66.

121. Moench L, Sachs Z, Aasen G, Dolan M, Dayton V, Courville EL. Double- and triple-hit lymphomas can present with features suggestive of immaturity, including TdT expression, and create diagnostic challenges. Leuk Lymphoma. 2016;57:2626–35.

122. Swerdlow SH. Diagnosis of 'double hit' diffuse large B-cell lymphoma and B-cell lymphoma, unclassifiable, with features intermediate between DLBCL and Burkitt lymphoma: when and how, FISH versus IHC. Hematology Am Soc Hematol Educ Program. 2014;2014:90–9.

123. Pillai RK, Sathanoori M, Van Oss SB, Swerdlow SH. Double-hit B-cell lymphomas with BCL6 and MYC translocations are aggressive, frequently extranodal lymphomas distinct from BCL2 double-hit B-cell lymphomas. Am J Surg Pathol. 2013;37:323–32.

124. Kluk MJ, Ho C, Yu H, Chen BJ, Neuberg DS, Dal Cin P, Woda BA, Pinkus GS, Rodig SJ. MYC immunohistochemistry to identify MYC-driven B-cell lymphomas in clinical practice. Am J Clin Pathol. 2016;145:166–79.

125. Horn H, Ziepert M, Becher C, Barth TF, Bernd HW, Feller AC, Klapper W, Hummel M, Stein H, Hansmann ML, et al. MYC status in concert with BCL2 and BCL6 expression predicts outcome in diffuse large B-cell lymphoma. Blood. 2013;121:2253–63.

126. Mationg-Kalaw E, Tan LH, Tay K, Lim ST, Tang T, Lee YY, Tan SY. Does the proliferation fraction help identify mature

B cell lymphomas with double- and triple-hit translocations? Histopathology. 2012;61:1214–8.
127. Landsburg DJ, Nasta SD, Svoboda J, Morrissette JJ, Schuster SJ. 'Double-Hit' cytogenetic status may not be predicted by baseline clinicopathological characteristics and is highly associated with overall survival in B cell lymphoma patients. Br J Haematol. 2014;166:369–74.
128. Foot NJ, Dunn RG, Geoghegan H, Wilkins BS, Neat MJ. Fluorescence in situ hybridisation analysis of formalin-fixed paraffin-embedded tissue sections in the diagnostic work-up of non-Burkitt high grade B-cell non-Hodgkin's lymphoma: a single centre's experience. J Clin Pathol. 2011;64:802–8.
129. Landsburg DJ, Schuster SJ. Who should be tested for double-hit lymphoma? J Oncol Pract. 2016;12:243–4.
130. Chiu A, Frizzera G, Mathew S, Hyjek EM, Chadburn A, Tam W, Knowles DM, Orazi A. Diffuse blastoid B-cell lymphoma: a histologically aggressive variant of t(14;18)-negative follicular lymphoma. Mod Pathol. 2009;22:1507–17.
131. Lin P, Dickason TJ, Fayad LE, Lennon PA, Hu P, Garcia M, Routbort MJ, Miranda R, Wang X, Qiao W, et al. Prognostic value of MYC rearrangement in cases of B-cell lymphoma, unclassifiable, with features intermediate between diffuse large B-cell lymphoma and Burkitt lymphoma. Cancer. 2012;118:1566–73.

Xin Qing and Changjun Yue

Introduction

The liver is an organ that could either be involved by systemic lymphomas or rarely as a primary site of lymphomas. Although secondary involvement of the liver by lymphomas is relatively common, primary hepatic lymphomas (PHL) represent only about 0.016% of all cases of non-Hodgkin lymphomas (NHL) and 0.4% of all primary extranodal non-Hodgkin lymphomas. Most of these cases are B-cell lymphomas. Primary hepatic T-cell lymphomas are extremely rare. There is no national consensus regarding the diagnostic criteria of PHL. In general, it is a lymphoma confined to the liver without evidence of involvement in the spleen, lymph nodes, other lymphoid tissue, or bone marrow at the time of presentation and within the next 6 months. The etiology and pathogenesis of primary hepatic B-cell lymphomas (PHBCLs) are unclear. Most patients with PHBCLs present with right upper quadrant abdominal pain or discomfort, have hepatomegaly on examination, and have elevated liver function tests. Radiologically, PHBCLs may present as a solitary lesion, multiple lesions, or less commonly diffuse infiltrate of the liver. The most common histological type of PHBCL is diffuse large B-cell lymphoma (DLBCL). The prognosis is variable, but patients with PHBCLs may have a more favorable outcome than patients with systemic B-cell lymphomas involving the liver, when treated with early combination chemotherapy.

Definition

There is no consensus regarding the diagnostic criteria of PHL. It was first defined in 1986 by Caccamo et al. as a lymphoma confined to the liver without evidence of involvement in the spleen, lymph nodes, other lymphoid tissue, or bone marrow at the time of presentation and within the next 6 months [1]. However, hepatic lymphomas with extrahepatic involvement at presentation have been accepted by some authors as being PHLs if the extrahepatic involvement was minor and considered as a secondary extension from the liver [2, 3]. In 1998, Lei proposed the following criteria for the diagnosis of PHL: (1) at disease presentation, the clinical symptoms are mainly caused by the lymphomatous involvement in the liver; (2) there is no distant lymphadenopathy by physical examination or radiologic staging studies; and (3) there is no leukemic involvement observed on the peripheral blood film [4].

In this chapter, primary hepatic B-cell lymphomas (PHBCLs) are defined as B-cell lymphomas confined to the liver at presentation with no or minimal involvement of the spleen, lymph node, peripheral blood, bone marrow, or other lymphoid tissues.

Etiology

The exact etiology of PHBCLs is unknown, but their association with viruses such as chronic hepatitis virus B or C, human immunodeficiency virus (HIV), and Epstein-Barr virus (EBV) and other etiologies such as nonviral chronic hepatitis, liver cirrhosis, hemochromatosis, immunosuppression, autoimmune diseases, primary biliary cirrhosis (PBC) and exposure to chemicals have been proposed [5–13]. However, a significant difference in the rate of viral infection between PHBCLs and systemic B-cell lymphomas involving the liver has not been observed. In addition, other chronic inflammatory diseases such as ascariasis and

X. Qing (✉)
Hematopathology and Hematology Laboratory, Department of Pathology, Harbor-UCLA Medical Center, Torrance, CA, USA
e-mail: xqing@dhs.lacounty.gov

C. Yue
Department of Medical Affair, Covance Clinical Trial, Los Angeles, Los Angeles, CA, USA

© Springer Nature Switzerland AG 2020
L. Zhang et al. (eds.), *Diagnostic Pathology of Hematopoietic Disorders of Spleen and Liver*,
https://doi.org/10.1007/978-3-030-37708-3_7

Helicobacter pylori infection were reported to be related to the pathogenesis of primary hepatic extranodal marginal zone lymphoma of mucosa-associated lymphoid tissue (MALT lymphoma) [14].

Epidemiology

PHL are very rare. They account for only 0.1% of malignant liver tumors [15]. These lymphomas constitute about 0.4% of all primary extranodal non-Hodgkin lymphomas and 0.016% of all cases of non-Hodgkin lymphomas [16]. Most of these cases are B-cell lymphomas. Primary hepatic T-cell lymphomas are extremely rare. PHLs typically occur in middle-aged adults, with a median age in the fifth or sixth decade of life, but they can also occur at any age (range, 3–95 years) [4, 17, 18]. They are slightly more common in males than in females, with a male-to-female ratio of about 2:1.

Clinical Presentations

Clinical presentations are generally nonspecific. Patients can be asymptomatic with unexpected lesion at the time of histological diagnosis [19] or present with right upper quadrant pain or discomfort and less commonly fatigue, jaundice, anorexia, nausea, and vomitting [20]. Rare patients may present with acute liver failure [3]. Bililary obstruction is uncommon and often found in late manifestation of hepatic non-Hodgkin lymphoma (NHL), accounting for <2% of patients with NHL [21, 22]. As a local lesion, PHBCLs are less frequently associated with B-symptoms such as fever/chills, weight loss, and night sweats, compared to secondary liver involvement by systemic lymphomas. However, still, 40–85% of these patients were found to have B symptoms [20, 23]. Approximately 57% of patients presented with weight loss [20]. Hepatomegaly is common. Congestive splenomegaly can also be found, possibly due to liver dysfunction and/or portal hypertension. Abnormal liver funtion tests [aspartate aminotransferase (AST), alanine aminotransferase (ALT), alkaline phosphatase (ALK), or bilirubin] are seen in the majority of patients. Lactate dehydrogenase (LDH) and beta-2-microglobulin levels are elevated in approximately a half of patients [4, 24]. However, patients with PHLs overall have lower LDH levels than those who have hepatic involvement by systemic lymphomas [25]. This is likely due to their relatively earlier stage and limited involvement by lymphoma. The α-fetoprotein (AFP), the carbohydrate antigen (CA) 19-9, and the carcinoembryonic antigen (CEA) levels are usually normal [20, 23]. Less commonly, hypercalcemia [23], coagulopathy [7], and a monoclonal spike on serum protein electrophoresis [26] have also been reported. By definition, the bone marrow is not involved, and therefore, blood counts are within the normal range in most patients, except if the patient has marked splenomegaly [8].

Diagnosis

A diagnosis of PHL is based on liver biopsy in conjunction with immunophenotypic findings and no evidence of extensive extrahepatic involvement of the lymphoma [23, 27, 28]. Of note, diffuse large B-cell lymphoma could mimic poorly differentiated carcinoma radiologically and histologically [28]. When biopsy tissue is limited, a small panel of immunohistochemical study or flow cytometry should be applied.

Morphology

Gross or Radiological Findings

PHBCLs may present as a solitary lesion, multiple lesions, or less commonly diffuse infiltrate of the liver [20]. Radiologically, PHLs on ultrasound are hypoechoic relative to normal liver (Fig. 7.1a) and on computed tomography (CT) as hypoattenuating lesions (Fig. 7.1b–d), sometimes with patchy or rim enhancement following intravenous contrast administration [8, 29]. The magnetic resonance imaging (MRI) appearance of these lesions is nonspecific (Fig. 7.1e–f), as lesions have a T1 hypointense and mildly T2 hyperintense signal and enhance less than the adjacent liver parenchyma [30]. When the lymphoma presents as a diffuse infiltrate of the liver, imaging studies may show an enlarged liver without distinct lesions [31].

Histology

The most common histological type of PHBCL is diffuse large B-cell lymphoma (DLBCL). MALT lymphoma is the second most common subtype [32]. Other less common histological types described in the literature include Burkitt lymphoma (BL), follicular lymphoma (FL), small lymphocytic lymphoma (SLL), mantle cell lymphoma (MCL), lymphoplasmacytic lymphoma (LPL), and T-cell/histiocyte-rich large B-cell lymphoma (THRLBCL) [8, 17, 18, 23, 26, 27, 33]. Primary hepatic T-cell lymphomas are extremely rare, representing approximate 3–10% of PHLs [8, 18]. Primary hepatic classical Hodgkin lymphoma (nodular sclerosis type) has also been reported [34].

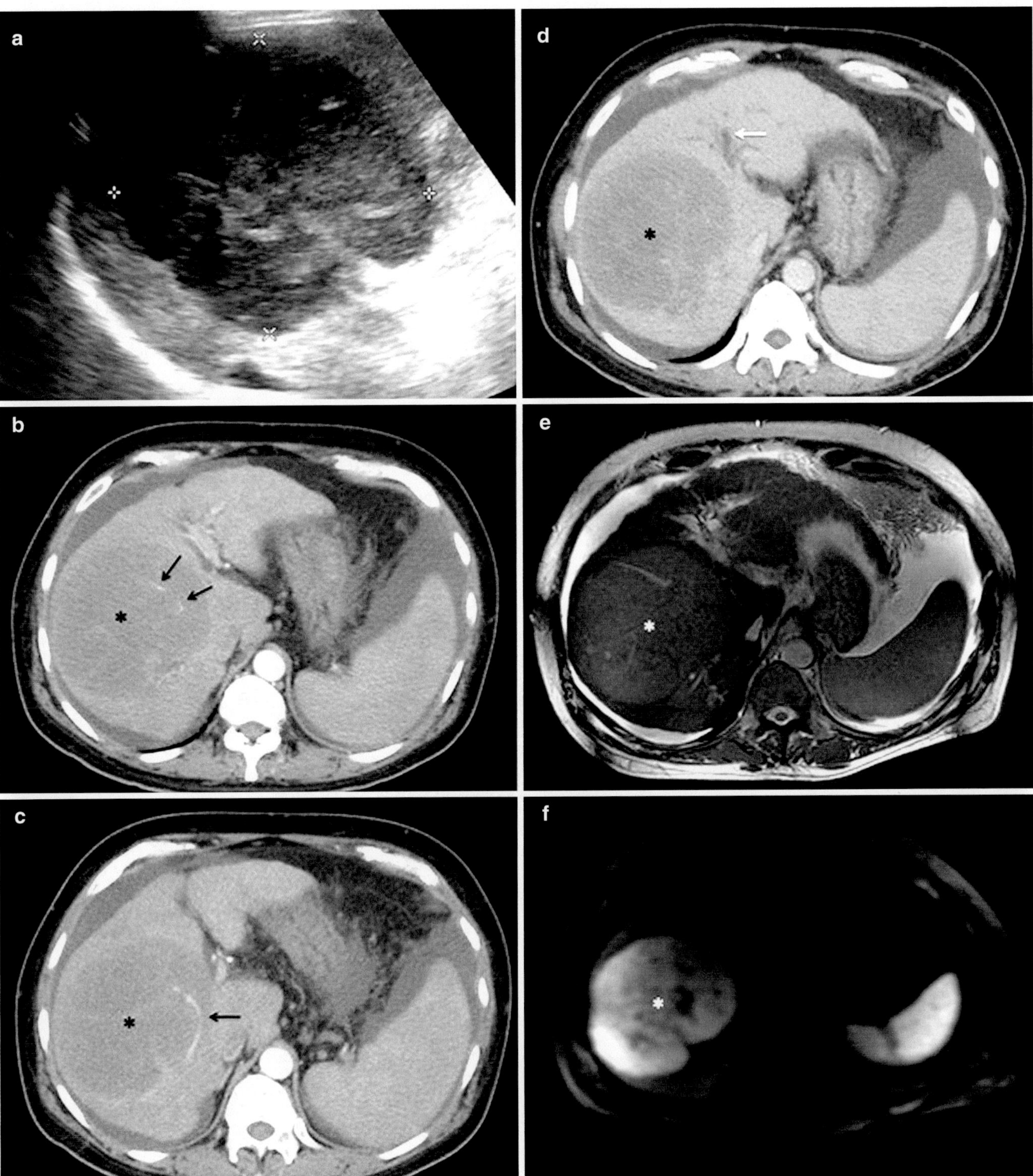

Fig. 7.1 Primary hepatic non-Hodgkin lymphoma. (**a**) Grayscale ultrasound image showing a large, well-defined, markedly hypoechoic lesion in the right lobe of the liver (marked by calipers). Contrast-enhanced computed tomography images (**b**–**d**) demonstrating a hypoenhancing lesion (asterisks) with arterial channels coursing through it (arrows in **b** and **c**). Changes of liver cirrhosis and ascites can also be seen with biliary dilatation (arrow in **d**). The magnetic resonance images reveal a homogeneous, mildly T2 hyperintense, diffusion-restricting lesion (asterisks in **e** and **f**). (Reproduced with permission of the copyright owner [39])

Except for DLBCL, MALT lymphoma, and Burkit lymphoma, the histological characteristics of PHBCLs have not been well described in the literature due to their rarities. Based on the available case reports, the morphological features of PHBCLs do not appear to differ from those of lymphomas of the same histological types seen in other organs. PHLs may infiltrate the liver with one or more of the following patterns: portal infiltrates, nodular growth, sinusoidal growth, loose infiltrate, and dense infiltrate [7, 21].

DLBCL is an aggressive neoplasm composed of intermediate or large lymphoid cells whose nuclei are the same size as, or larger than, those of normal histiocytes or more than twice the size of those of normal small mature lymphocytes, with a diffuse growth pattern. DLBCL, not otherwise specified (NOS), is the most common type of non-Hodgkin lymphoma in the world. They represent 25–35% of all non-Hodgkin lymphomas in developed countries and an even higher incidence in developing countries [35]. Approximately 60–80% of reported PHL cases are diagnosed with DLBCL, NOS (Figs. 7.2, 7.3, and 7.4). DLBCL, NOS, can be subgrouped into germinal center B-cell (GCB) type versus activated B-cell (ABC) type based on gene expression profiling (GEP) and GCB versus non-GCB subtypes by immunohistochemical

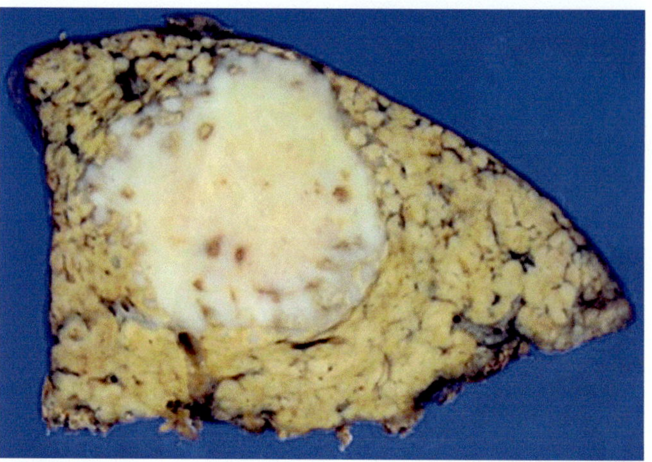

Fig. 7.2 Primary hepatic diffuse large B-cell lymphoma. The liver specimen shows a whitish solid tumor with an irregular margin. (Reproduced with permission of the copyright owner [40])

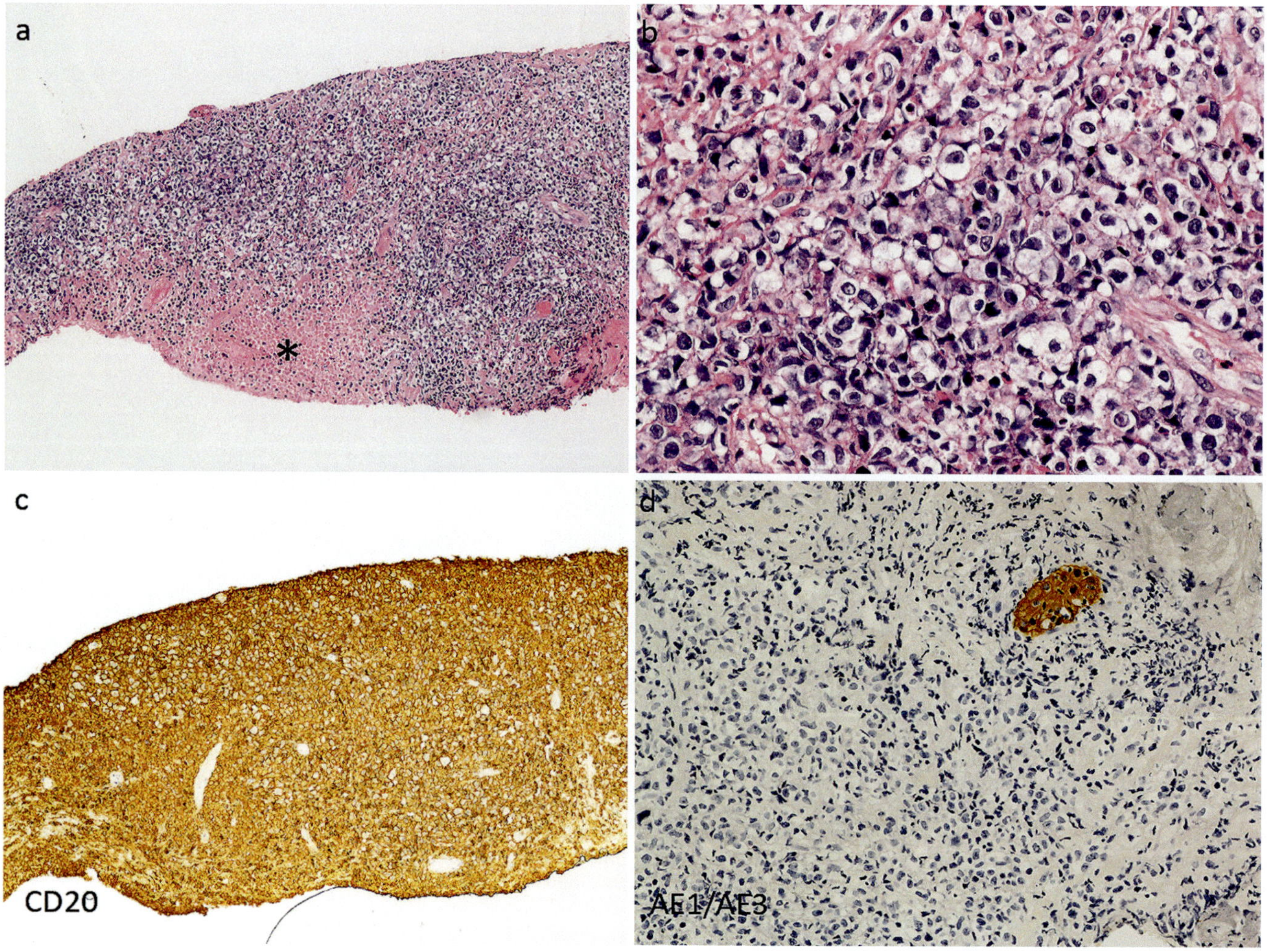

Fig. 7.3 Primary hepatic diffuse large B-cell lymphoma. (**a**, **b**) Normal liver architecture is effaced by sheets of large lymphoma cells with areas of necrosis (asterisk). (**c**) The lymphoma cells are positive for CD20. (**d**) Pancytokeratin AE1/AE3 immunostain highlights an entrapped bile duct

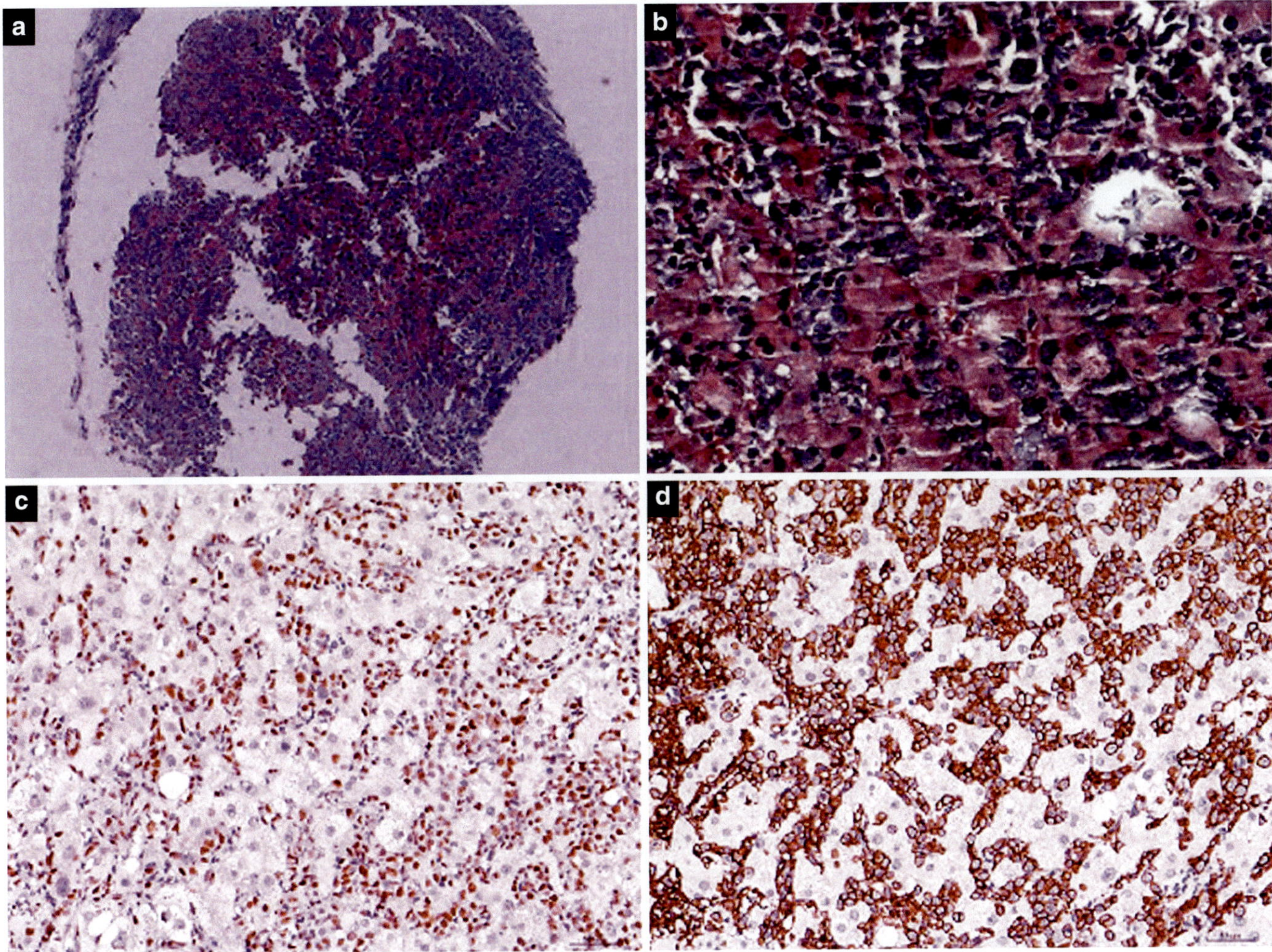

Fig. 7.4 Primary hepatic diffuse large B-cell lymphoma. (**a**, **b**) Lymphoma cells are observed in the hepatic sinusoids and the portal areas. By immunohistochemical stains, the lymphoma cells are positive for BCL-6 (**c**) and CD20 (**d**). (Reproduced with permission of the copyright owner [15])

stains. Both GCB and non-GCB immunophenotypes have been reported in primary hepatic DLBCL.

MALT lymphoma is a low-grade B-cell lymphoma involving extranodal organs. Primary hepatic MALT lymphoma (Fig. 7.5) typically shows lymphoid nodules infiltrating the liver. Normal liver tissue may be entrapped. When underlying chronic necroinflammatory disease or cirrhosis is present, the lymphoma infiltrate may become more confluent and less well defined [36]. The tumor is composed of neoplastic small B-cells with centrocyte-like, monocytoid B-cell-like, or small B lymphocyte-like cytology, admixed with variable numbers of scattered transformed cells that resemble immunoblasts or centroblasts. A plasmacytic differentiation is not uncommon. Lymphoepithelial lesions involving the biliary ducts are seen. The lymphoma cells infiltrate the marginal zones, spread out into the interfollicular areas, and eventually colonize or replace the follicles.

Burkitt lymphoma is a highly aggressive but curable lymphoma characterized by sheets of monomorphic medium-sized B-cells with round nuclei, multiple small nucleoli, and numerous mitotic figures. The cytoplasm is deeply basophilic, often containing lipid vacuoles, best observed in air-dried touch imprints (Fig. 7.6). Many scattered tingible body macrophages are usually present, due to a high rate of apoptosis, and form a so-called starry-sky appearance. *MYC* gene translocation to an immunoglobulin locus can be demonstrated in more than 90% of cases.

FL is a lymphoma composed of germinal center (follicular center) B-cells, i.e., centrocytes and centroblasts. The lymphoma typically shows at least a partially follicular (nodular) growth pattern. However, in liver biopsy specimens, the follicular pattern can be difficult to observe due to the limited size of the needle core biopsy [2]. The relative proportions of centrocytes and centroblasts determine the grade of this lymphoma. Low-grade FL (grade 1–2) is defined as 0–15 centroblasts per high-power (40 x objective, 0.159 mm²) microscopic field (HPF) on average in at least 10 HPFs within 10 representative follicles. Grade 3 FL is defined as >15 centroblasts per HPF, which can be further divided into grade 3A and 3B. Grade 3A is assigned to those

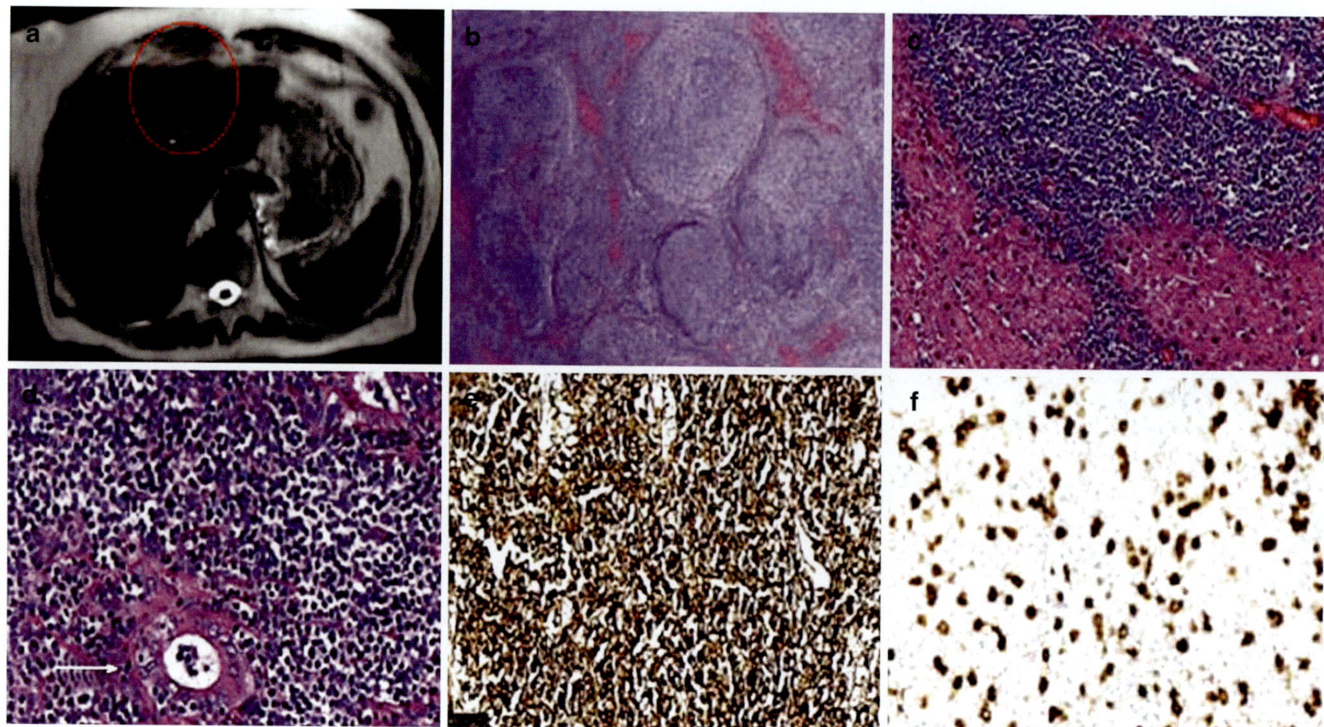

Fig. 7.5 Primary hepatic extranodal marginal zone lymphoma of mucosa-associated lymphoid tissue (MALT lymphoma). (**a**) Computed tomography of the abdomen reveals a large mass, highlighted in red, in the left hepatic lobe. (**b**) Effacement of normal liver architecture by a nodular lymphoid infiltrate. (**c**) Islands of residual hepatocytes surrounded by neoplastic marginal zone cells. (**d**) Lymphoma cells with pale cytoplasm infiltrate into the bile duct epithelium forming lymphoepithelial lesions (arrow). By immunohistochemistry, the lymphoma cells are positive for CD20 (**e**) and negative for CD5 (**f**). (Reproduced with permission of the copyright owner [41])

cases when there is a mixture of centrocytes and centroblasts. When the centroblasts form sheets, the FL is assigned grade 3B. Majority of the reported primary hepatic FL are grade 1–2 [2].

SLL is an indolent small B-cell lymphoma that is morphologically and immunophenotypically indistinguishable from chronic lymphocytic leukemia (CLL) but lacks significant monoclonal lymphocytosis with CLL immunophenotype ($< 5 \times 10^9$/L). It is characterized by a diffuse proliferation of small mature lymphoid cells with usually round nuclei, clumped chromatin, inconspicuous nucleoli, and scant cytoplasm. Scattered paler areas, i.e., proliferation centers (pseudofollicles), are usually present, containing small lymphocytes, prolymphocytes, and paraimmunoblasts, creating a vaguely nodular appearance at low magnification in some cases. In the liver, the proliferation centers can be rare and difficult to identify. However, when there is a heavy infiltration by SLL, proliferation centers may become prominent.

MCL is a neoplasm of mature B-cells. Classic MCL is composed of monomorphic small- to medium-sized lymphoid cells that usually have irregular nuclear contours, conspicuous nucleoli, and scant cytoplasm, with a diffuse, vaguely nodular, mantle zone or rarely follicular growth pattern. Morphological variants of MCL have been recognized, including the aggressive variants (blastoid variant and pleomorphic variant) and other variants (small-cell variant and marginal zone-like variant), mimicking other high-grade and low-grade B-cell lymphomas, respectively. However, centroblasts, paraimmunoblasts, or proliferation centers are not found. In the vast majority of cases, a *CCND1-IGH* translocation can be identified.

LPL is a low-grade small B-cell lymphoma composed of small mature lymphoid cells, plasmacytoid lymphoid cells, and plasma cells. It usually involves bone marrow and sometimes lymph nodes and the spleen. Primary hepatic LPL is extremely rare. Bone marrow biopsy, clinical review, and *MYD88* mutation analysis may be considered for diagnosis of LPL. Moreover, it may be morphologically difficult in distinguishing LPL from MALT lymphoma. Identification of MALT lymphoma-associated cytogenetic abnormalities may contribute to the differential diagnosis.

THRLBCL is another type of aggressive lymphoma of large B-cells, which is rarely reported as PHL. It is a neoplasm with scattered, usually singly dispersed, highly atypical large B-cells in a background of abundant T-cells and histiocytes.

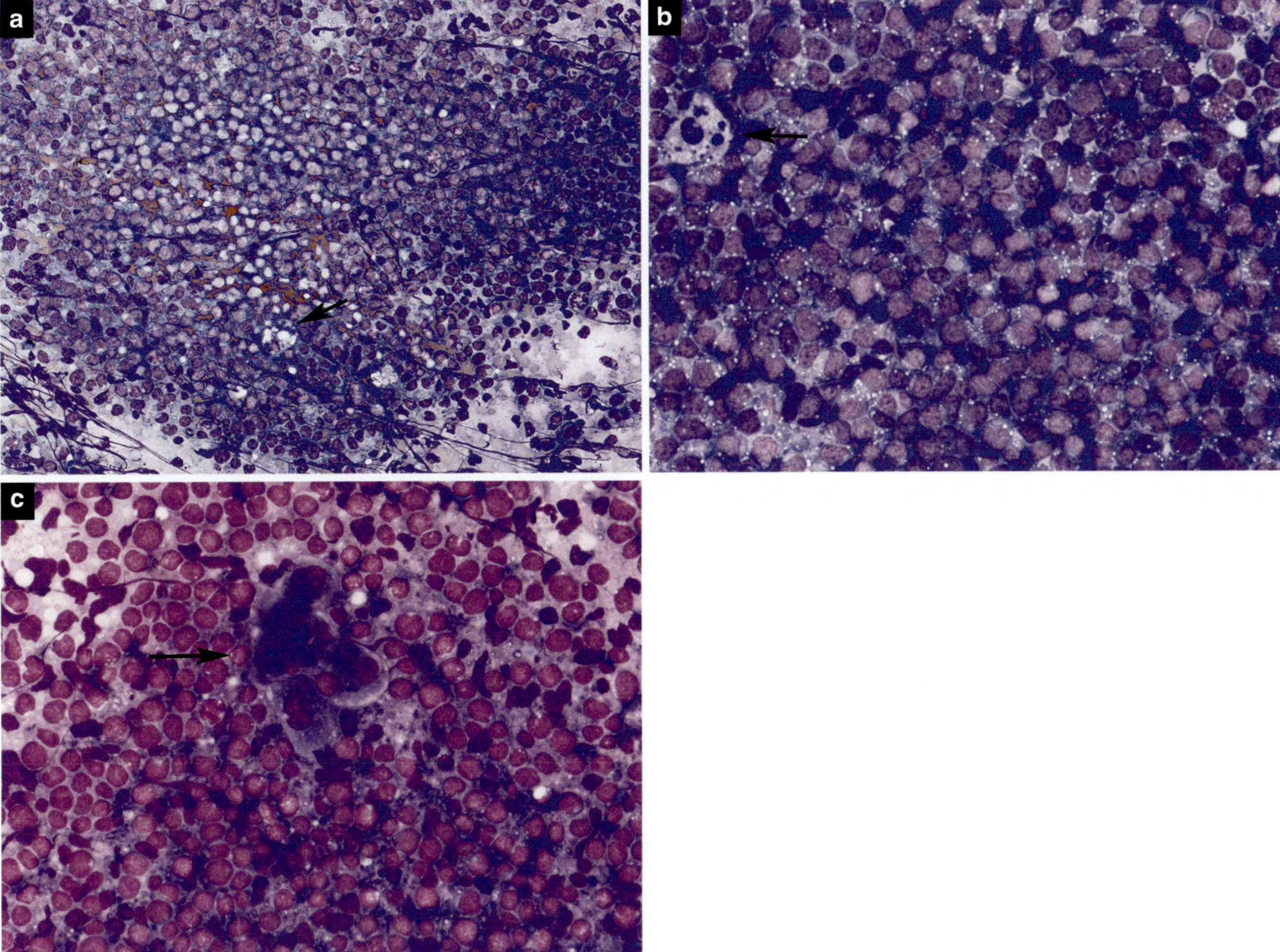

Fig. 7.6 Touch imprints of a case of primary hepatic Burkitt lymphoma. (**a**) Low-power magnification shows sheets of uniform lymphoma cells with interspersed tingible body macrophages (arrow). (**b**) The lymphoma cells are medium sized and have a deeply basophilic cytoplasm containing numerous vacuoles. One tingible body macrophage is shown (arrow). (**c**) Numerous lymphoma cells surround a cluster of hepatocytes (arrow)

Immunophenotype

The immunophenotype of the PHBCLs does not differ from those of lymphomas of similar histological types in the lymph nodes or other extranodal organs. The neoplastic cells typically express pan-B-cell markers such as CD19, CD20, CD22, CD79a, and PAX-5. Surface and cytoplasmic immunoglobulin can be demonstrated in the majority of the cases.

Cytogenetics

Very few PHBCL cases have been studied by cytogenetic analysis. The genotype of these lymphomas does not appear to differ significantly from that of the lymphomas in other organs, with the same histological types. It is noteworthy that,

among the seven cases with primary hepatic MALT lymphoma in which cytogenetic studies were performed, there were two with t(14;18)(q32;q21) and trisomy 3, one with t(14;18)(q32;q21) and trisomy 18, one with t(14;18)(q32;q21), one with t(3;14)(q27;q32), one with trisomy 3 and trisomy 18, and one with neither of these cytogenetic abnormalities [36]. Interestingly, t(11;18)(q21;q21) or t(1;14)(p22;q23) translocations were not detected in any of these cases.

Molecular Findings

Molecular studies show clonally rearranged immunoglobulin genes. Although minimal data are available, PHBCLs are expected to demonstrate the molecular features similar to those of lymphomas of the same histological types in other organs.

Differential Diagnosis

Due to the rarity of these diseases and their relatively non-specific clinical manifestations and laboratory findings, a clinical diagnosis of PHL is difficult. PHLs may be confused with hepatitis, primary hepatic non-lymphoid tumors, metastatic carcinoma, sarcoma, and secondary involvement by systemic lymphomas. In fact, secondary liver involvement by lymphomas is relatively common and can be detected in up to 50% of patients with lymphoma by staging [37, 38]. Imaging studies may provide some clues in differentiating between these possibilities. Radiographically, primary hepatic non-lymphoid tumors appear as hyperechoic lesions on ultrasound, with marked arterial enhancement of the lesion by CT scan, which becomes iso- or hypodense on portovenous and delayed phases. In contrast, PHLs present as a lesion that is hypoechoic on ultrasound and hyoattenuating, non-enhancing, or minimally enhancing on CT scan [8]. Imaging studies may also provide supportive evidence to differentiate primary hepatic tumors/lymphomas from secondary hepatic involvement by a systemic process such as carcinoma or lymphoma. However, a definitive diagnosis of PHL requires liver biopsy. Histologically, reactive lymphoid infiltrate associated with inflammation and autoimmune diseases and in posttransplant setting also has to be excluded. A careful pathologic examination with ancillary studies including flow cytometry, immunohistochmistry, and/or cytogentic and molecular studies would lead to the correct diagnosis. Bone marrow biopsy and other imaging studies must also be performed for staging to confirm the absence of lymphoma outside of the liver.

Reactive lymphoid infiltrate can be seen with virus or autoimmune hepatitis. They are mostly composed of T-cells without aberrant antigen expression, polyclonal B-cells, and occasionally plasma cells. CMV hepatitis can be diagnosed per immunohistochemical staining with anti-CMV antibody.

EBV hepatitis may be difficult to distinguish from PHL, in particular Burkitt lymphoma or classic Hodgkin lymphoma. Of note, the biopsy from EBV hepatitis most commonly shows a lymphohistiocytic infiltrate in sinusoidal pattern, composed of a predominant population of T-cells (CD3 positive) and occasional EBV-positive B-cells per in situ hybridization of Epstein-Barr virus-encoded RNA (EBER) probe [32]. Burkitt lymphoma often present with diffuse proliferation of medium-size atypical lymphoid cells and associated with increased EBER in situ signals. FISH *MYC* translocation can help the diagnosis. Primary hepatic classic Hodgkin lymphoma is extremely rare. If it is systemic involvement by classic Hodgkin lymphoma, identification of the patient's history, histology (EBV commonly positive in mixed cellularity subtype), and inflammatory infiltrating cell background help the differential diagnosis.

Primary and metastatic hepatic carcinoma should be first excluded with laboratory carcinoma markers (AFP, CEA, or CA19.9).

Treatment and Prognosis

PHL conventionally had been considered as an aggressive disease with a poor prognosis [4]. However, Page et al. demonstrated an excellent response rate associated with the use of combination chemotherapy alone with a complete remission rate of 83.3% [23]. Our group found that patients with PHBCLs have a more favorable outcome than patients with systemic B-cell lymphomas involving the liver, when treated with combination chemotherapy [25]. Although HCV is often found to be associated with PHL, the infection does not have impact on the outcome of treatment unless advanced stage of liver disease [23, 27].

Some studies suggested that the poor prognostic factors may include advanced age, constitutional symptoms, bulky disease, unfavorable histological subtypes, diffuse pattern of liver involvement, elevated LDH, and comorbid conditions like cirrhosis, chronic active hepatitis, HIV, and immunosuppression [8]. Multivariate analysis performed by Ugurluer et al. on 41 patients with PHLs showed that the presence of fever, the absence of weight loss, and normal hemoglobin level were the independent factors associated with a more favorable survival [17]. Their study did not show, in univariate analyses, any influence of gender, abdominal pain or discomfort, weight loss, night sweats, preexisting liver disease, multiple or diffuse lesions, elevated liver enzymes, hepatosplenomegaly, or histopathology on the outcome. However, in a multivariable Cox regression analysis performed by El-Fattah et al., the age of ≥80 years, male gender, black race, and T-cell lymphoma histological subtype were found to be unfavorable prognostic factors [18]. Unfortunately, most reports of PHLs published to date have described either single cases or small numbers of patients. Because of the scarcity of this entity, well-defined prognostic factors and standard treatment are difficult to determine. Larger multicenter prospective studies are needed to establish treatment guidelines, outcome, and prognostic factors.

Diagnostic Caveats

Primary hepatic B-cell lymphoma is a rare disease that can be found in a patient with liver mass or liver infiltration but normal CEA and AFP levels.

A needle core biopsy of the liver is the most valuable tool for diagnosis of the clinical cases with high index of suspicion. Imaging findings of PHL are nonspecific.

The treatment guideline is not yet defined. Although surgical treatment, radiotherapy, and chemotherapy alone or in combination are the options, multiple-line chemotherapy remains the main treatment modality and shows a favorable outcome.

The prognosis of patients with primary hepatic lymphoma is better than patients with secondary involvement by systemic B-cell lymphoma.

References

1. Caccamo D, Pervez NK, Marchevsky A. Primary lymphoma of the liver in the acquired immunodeficiency syndrome. Arch Pathol Lab Med. 1986;110(6):553–5.
2. Gomyo H, Kagami Y, Kato H, et al. Primary hepatic follicular lymphoma : a case report and discussion of chemotherapy and favorable outcomes. J Clin Exp Hematop. 2007;47(2):73–7.
3. Haider FS, Smith R, Khan S. Primary hepatic lymphoma presenting as fulminant hepatic failure with hyperferritinemia: a case report. J Med Case Rep. 2008;2:279.
4. Lei KI. Primary non-Hodgkin's lymphoma of the liver. Leuk Lymphoma. 1998;29(3–4):293–9.
5. Honda H, Franken EA Jr, Barloon TJ, Smith JL. Hepatic lymphoma in cyclosporine-treated transplant recipients: sonographic and CT findings. AJR Am J Roentgenol. 1989;152(3):501–3.
6. Lisker-Melman M, Pittaluga S, Pluda JM, et al. Primary lymphoma of the liver in a patient with acquired immune deficiency syndrome and chronic hepatitis B. Am J Gastroenterol. 1989;84(11):1445–8.
7. Santos ES, Raez LE, Salvatierra J, Morgensztern D, Shanmugan N, Neff GW. Primary hepatic non-Hodgkin's lymphomas: case report and review of the literature. Am J Gastroenterol. 2003;98(12):2789–93.
8. Noronha V, Shafi NQ, Obando JA, Kummar S. Primary non-Hodgkin's lymphoma of the liver. Crit Rev Oncol Hematol. 2005;53(3):199–207.
9. Nakayama S, Yokote T, Kobayashi K, et al. Primary hepatic MALT lymphoma associated with primary biliary cirrhosis. Leuk Res. 2010;34(1):e17–20.
10. Kikuma K, Watanabe J, Oshiro Y, et al. Etiological factors in primary hepatic B-cell lymphoma. Virchows Arch. 2012;460(4):379–87.
11. Sekiguchi Y, Yoshikawa H, Shimada A, et al. Primary hepatic circumscribed Burkitt's lymphoma that developed after acute hepatitis B: report of a case with a review of the literature. J Clin Exp Hematop. 2013;53(2):167–73.
12. Mohamed M, Fernando R. Diagnostic and therapeutic quandaries in a patient with primary hepatic lymphoma and concurrent hepatitis C infection. Indian J Hematol Blood Transfus. 2014;30(Suppl 1):394–7.
13. Salmon JS, Thompson MA, Arildsen RC, Greer JP. Non-Hodgkin's lymphoma involving the liver: clinical and therapeutic considerations. Clin Lymphoma Myeloma. 2006;6(4):273–80.
14. Nagata S, Harimoto N, Kajiyama K. Primary hepatic mucosa-associated lymphoid tissue lymphoma: a case report and literature review. Surg Case Rep. 2015;1:87.
15. Liu Y, Jiang J, Wu Q, et al. A case of primary hepatic lymphoma and related literature review. Case Rep Hepatol. 2016;2016:6764121.
16. Freeman C, Berg JW, Cutler SJ. Occurrence and prognosis of extranodal lymphomas. Cancer. 1972;29(1):252–60.
17. Ugurluer G, Miller RC, Li Y, et al. Primary hepatic lymphoma: a retrospective, Multicenter Rare Cancer Network Study. Rare Tumors. 2016;8(3):6502.
18. El-Fattah MA. Non-Hodgkin lymphoma of the liver: a US population-based analysis. J Clin Transl Hepatol. 2017;5(2):83–91.
19. Anthony PP, Sarsfield P, Clarke T. Primary lymphoma of the liver: clinical and pathological features of 10 patients. J Clin Pathol. 1990;43(12):1007–13.
20. Lei KI, Chow JH, Johnson PJ. Aggressive primary hepatic lymphoma in Chinese patients. Presentation, pathologic features, and outcome. Cancer. 1995;76(8):1336–43.
21. Laroia ST, Rastogi A, Panda D, Sarin SK. Primary hepatic non-Hodgkin's lymphoma: an enigma beyond the liver, a case report. World J Oncol. 2015;6(2):338–44.
22. Ravindra KV, Stringer MD, Prasad KR, Kinsey SE, Lodge JP. Non-Hodgkin lymphoma presenting with obstructive jaundice. Br J Surg. 2003;90(7):845–9.
23. Page RD, Romaguera JE, Osborne B, et al. Primary hepatic lymphoma: favorable outcome after combination chemotherapy. Cancer. 2001;92(8):2023–9.
24. Avlonitis VS, Linos D. Primary hepatic lymphoma: a review. Eur J Surg. 1999;165(8):725–9.
25. Peng Y, Qing AC, Cai J, Yue C, French SW, Qing X. Lymphoma of the liver: Clinicopathological features of 19 patients. Exp Mol Pathol. 2016;100(2):276–80.
26. Borgonovo G, d'Oiron R, Amato A, et al. Primary lymphoplasmacytic lymphoma of the liver associated with a serum monoclonal peak of IgG kappa. Am J Gastroenterol. 1995;90(1):137–40.
27. Bronowicki JP, Bineau C, Feugier P, et al. Primary lymphoma of the liver: clinical-pathological features and relationship with HCV infection in French patients. Hepatology. 2003;37(4):781–7.
28. Agmon-Levin N, Berger I, Shtalrid M, Schlanger H, Sthoeger ZM. Primary hepatic lymphoma: a case report and review of the literature. Age Ageing. 2004;33(6):637–40.
29. Maher MM, McDermott SR, Fenlon HM, et al. Imaging of primary non-Hodgkin's lymphoma of the liver. Clin Radiol. 2001;56(4):295–301.
30. Alexander LF, Harri P, Little B, Moreno CC, Mittal PK. Magnetic resonance imaging of primary hepatic malignancies in patients with and without chronic liver disease: a pictorial review. Cureus. 2017;9(8):e1539.
31. Abe H, Kamimura K, Kawai H, et al. Diagnostic imaging of hepatic lymphoma. Clin Res Hepatol Gastroenterol. 2015;39(4):435–42.
32. Choi WT, Gill RM. Hepatic lymphoma diagnosis. Surg Pathol Clin. 2018;11(2):389–402.
33. Cameron AM, Truty J, Truell J, et al. Fulminant hepatic failure from primary hepatic lymphoma: successful treatment with orthotopic liver transplantation and chemotherapy. Transplantation. 2005;80(7):993–6.
34. Colagrande S, Calistri L, Grazzini G, et al. MRI features of primary hepatic lymphoma. Abdom Radiol (NY). 2018;43(9):2277–87.
35. Swerdlow SHCE, Harris NL, Jaffe ES, Pileri SA, Stein H, Thiele J, Arber DA, Hasserjian RP, Le Beau MM, Orazi A, Siebert R. WHO classification of tumours of haematopoietic and lymphoid tissues. Lyon: IARC; 2017.
36. Koubaa Mahjoub W, Chaumette-Planckaert MT, Murga Penas EM, et al. Primary hepatic lymphoma of mucosa-associated lymphoid tissue type: a case report with cytogenetic study. Int J Surg Pathol. 2008;16(3):301–7.
37. Lotz MJ, Chabner B, DeVita VT Jr, Johnson RE, Berard CW. Pathological staging of 100 consecutive untreated patients with non-Hodgkin's lymphomas: extramedullary sites of disease. Cancer. 1976;37(1):266–70.

38. Ferguson DJ, Allen LW, Griem ML, Moran ME, Rappaport H, Ultmann JE. Surgical experience with staging laparotomy in 125 patients with lymphoma. Arch Intern Med. 1973;131(3):356–61.

39. Rajesh S, Bansal K, Sureka B, Patidar Y, Bihari C, Arora A. The imaging conundrum of hepatic lymphoma revisited. Insights Imaging. 2015;6(6):679–92.

40. Takei D, Abe T, Amano H, et al. Methotrexate-associated primary hepatic malignant lymphoma following hepatectomy: a case report. Int J Surg Case Rep. 2017;31:5–9.

41. Obiorah IE, Johnson L, Ozdemirli M. Primary mucosa-associated lymphoid tissue lymphoma of the liver: a report of two cases and review of the literature. World J Hepatol. 2017;9(3):155–60.

Pei Lin

Introduction

Plasma cell neoplasms (PCNs) result from monoclonal expansion of neoplastic plasma cells. They include monoclonal gammopathy of undetermined significance (MGUS) (67%), plasma cell myeloma (PCM) (14%), solitary plasmacytoma of bone or extraosseous tissue (3%), primary amyloidosis (9%) and immunoglobulin (Ig) chain deposition diseases (<1%), POEMS (polyneuropathy, organomegaly, endocrinopathy, M component, and skin changes) syndrome, and TEMPI syndrome (telangiectasias, elevated erythropoietin level and erythrocytosis, monoclonal gammopathy, perinephric fluid collections, and intrapulmonary shunting).

PCNs involving the liver or spleen usually result from localized primary (extraosseous) plasmacytoma or extramedullary dissemination of PCM/plasma cell leukemia (PCL). The latter is far more common and biologically distinct from primary plasmacytoma [1–9]. Primary amyloidosis and less often immunoglobulin (Ig) chain deposition diseases may also involve these organs causing tissue damages. While hepatosplenomegaly (organomegaly) can be observed in POEMS, both PEOMS and TEMPI are paraneoplastic syndromes. MGUS does not usually manifest in the liver and spleen. Thus, this chapter focuses on solitary plasmacytoma, extramedullary involvment of PCM/PCL and primary amyloidosis involving the liver or spleen.

P. Lin (✉)
Department of Hematopathology, University of Texas MD Anderson Cancer Center, Houston, TX, USA
e-mail: peilin@mdanderson.org

Primary (Extraosseous) Plasmacytoma and Extramedullary Myeloma Involving the Liver and Spleen

Definition

Extraosseous plasmacytoma is a localized mass lesion(s) arising *de novo* in the liver or spleen due to monoclonal expansion of plasma cells. More commonly, extramedullary plasmacytoma results from secondary spread of neoplastic cells in patients with established diagnosis of myeloma or PCL [2–4, 10, 11]. Symptomatic (active) myeloma is defined as neoplastic plasma cells ≥10% in the bone marrow with associated M protein and organ damages (hypercalcemia, renal insufficiency, anemia and bone lesions) (CRAB), Table 8.1). PCL is diagnosed when absolute plasmacytosis is more than 2×10^9/L (white blood cell, WBC, count > 10×10^9/L) or plasma cells constitute more than 20% of the total leukocytes (WBC is <10×10^9/L) in the peripheral blood. PCL can be either primary or secondary. Hepatosplenomegaly due to infiltration of neoplastic plasma cells is a common finding in PCL.

Table 8.1 Symptomatic (active) plasma cell myeloma (PCM)

Clonal bone marrow plasma cell percentage ≥10% or biopsy-proven plasmacytoma and ≥1 of the following myeloma-defining events	
End-organ damage attributable to the plasma cell proliferative disorder (*CRAB*): Hypercalcemia: serum calcium >0.25 mmol/L (>1 mg/dL) higher than the upper limit of normal or >2.75 mmol/L (>11 mg/dL) *Renal insufficiency*: creatinine clearance <40 ml/minute or serum creatinine >177 μmol/L (>2 mg/dL) Anemia: a hemoglobin value of >20 g/L below the lower limit of normal or a hemoglobin value <100 g/L *Bone lesions*: ~1 osteolytic lesion on skeletal radiography, CT, or PET/CT	Or ≥1 of the following biomarkers of malignancy: *Clonal bone marrow plasma cell percentage ≥ 60% An involved-to-uninvolved serum free light chain ratio ≥100 >1 focal lesion on MRI*

© Springer Nature Switzerland AG 2020
L. Zhang et al. (eds.), *Diagnostic Pathology of Hematopoietic Disorders of Spleen and Liver*,
https://doi.org/10.1007/978-3-030-37708-3_8

Etiology

There is no specific known etiology. However, extraosseous plasmacytoma may arise in recipients of solid organ transplantation as EBV-driven posttransplant lymphoproliferative disease (PTLD), monomorphic type [12].

The etiology of extramedullary myeloma is similar to that of PCM/PCL. Chronic antigen stimulation or exposure to toxins or radiation and genetic predisposition are postulated to be the causes.

Epidemiology

Primary plasmacytoma most commonly occurs in the head and neck regions. Primary plasmacytoma of the liver is rare and has been typically described as case reports in the literature [13, 14].

Myeloma or PCL occur more commonly in men than women, and African Americans are twice more susceptible than Caucasians or Asian Americans. Extramedullary myeloma is observed in 6–8% of myeloma cases at presentation and 30% of cases during the course of the disease overall [7]. The liver, skin, central nervous system (CNS), pleural cavity, kidneys, lymph nodes, and pancreas are organs susceptible to extramedullary spread, with the liver and pleura at the top of the list. Rarely, liver involvement is the only presenting sign of myeloma [15, 16]. Primary PCL comprises 1–2% of newly diagnosed cases of myeloma but 60% of all leukemic cases. Secondary PCL results from excessive tumor growth and represents 1% of all myeloma cases. Overall, even in cases without PCL, involvement of the liver, with or without elevated liver enzymes, is reported to be in 40% of patients [17, 18].

Since the introduction of novel therapies such as immunomodulatory drugs (IMiDs; thalidomide and lenalidomide), proteasome inhibitors (PI, bortezomib, carfilzomib), and more recently targeted therapy and immunotherapy that are aimed at destructing tumor cells as well as modifying tumor microenvironment, remarkable success has been achieved in eliminating myeloma cells in the bone marrow, but the incidence of extramedullary disease has not decreased [4, 6, 19, 20]. This is in part due to the factor that extramedullary myeloma tend to occur in high-risk myeloma highly resistant to current therapeutic strategies and in part due to better imaging studies with magnetic resonance imaging (MRI) and positron emission tomography (PET) scan that can detect small extramedullary diseases [21]. Features of high-risk myeloma will be discussed in more details in the sections of cytogenetics and molecular genetics of the chapter [9].

Clinical Presentations

Patients may have elevated serum transaminase or bilirubin. Most cases of primary plasmacytoma produce no detectable serum protein (<20%) and rarely evolve to myeloma.

To diagnose primary plasmacytoma of the liver, the case needs to meet the general criteria of plasmacytoma as proposed by the International Myeloma Working Group (IMWG). These include biopsy-proven solitary lesion with evidence of clonal plasma cells; absence of bone marrow or other involvement by biopsy and MRI, computed tomography (CT), or whole-body fluorodeoxyglucose/positron emission tomography-computed tomography (FDG/PET-CT) imaging; and absence of end-organ damage such as CRAB that can be attributed to myeloma. If accompanied by <10% of bone marrow monoclonal plasma cells, a diagnosis of plasmacytoma with minimal bone marrow involvement can be rendered. The role of MRI in excluding occult systemic disease has been heavily emphasized in the recent years. This is largely due to the fact that IMWG has recently proposed three biomarkers that are "myeloma-defining events," which are defined as follows: (a) clonal plasma cells of $\geq$60%, (b) involved-to-uninvolved serum light chain ratio of $\geq$100, and (c) more than one focal lesion of $\geq$5 mm by MRI exam (Table 8.1). Patients meeting more than one of the above three criteria are considered to have an ultrahigh risk of progressing to symptomatic myeloma despite absence of CRAB features, requiring systemic therapy.

In contrast to extraosseous plasmacytoma, liver or spleen involvement by myeloma or PCL usually shows features of advanced or refractory disease [22, 23]. These tumors may occur even after the patients have achieved complete remission when bone marrow is still free of myeloma, i.e., extramedullary myeloma of the liver presenting as the first sign of relapsed disease [24, 25].

In addition to CRAB as described above, serum M protein and Bence Jones protein are usually detected. Lactate dehydrogenase (LDH) levels may be elevated. Patients with liver involvement may present with painless jaundice, mild pruritus, and elevated liver enzyme mimicking cholestatic hepatitis, biliary obstruction, or ascites [26, 27]. Patients with splenic involvement may suffer from spontaneous rupture of the spleen [28, 29].

Morphology

Gross or Radiological Findings

The tumors are usually described as single or multiple mass lesions in the liver or spleen grossly or by imaging studies (Fig. 8.1) [30]. Primary plasmacytoma in the liver may mimic carcinoma [13, 31–34]. Splenic involvement usually

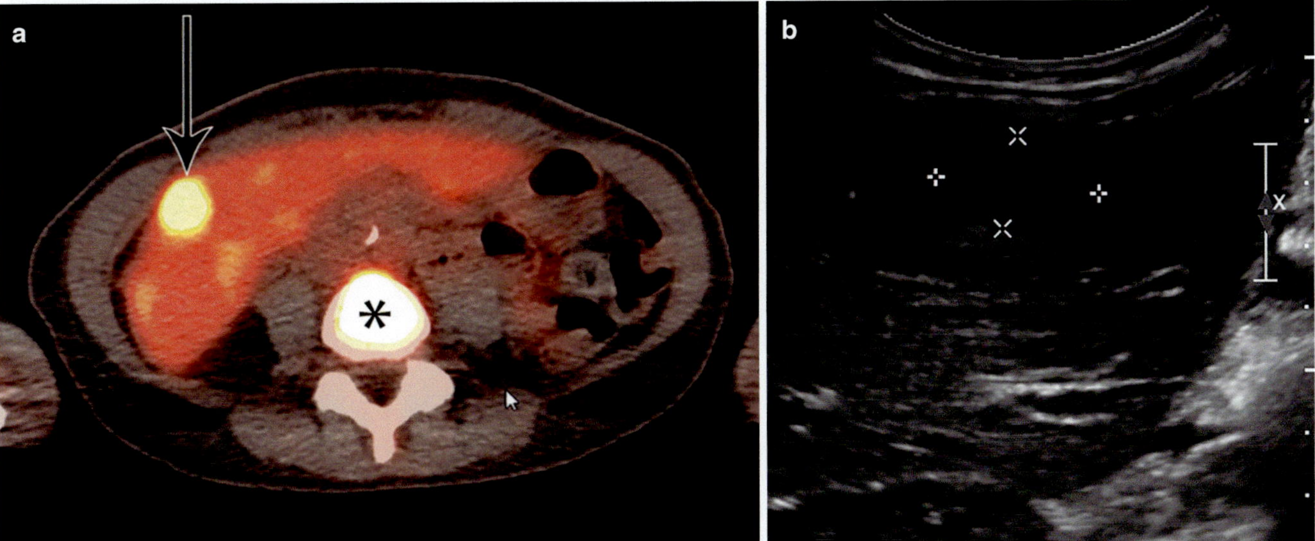

Fig. 8.1 (**a**) PET-CT image of extramedullary plasmacytoma involving the liver. Arrow points to plasmacytoma. (**b**) Ultrasound shows a single hypoechoic mass lesion in the liver

manifests as diffuse red pulp expansion resulting in splenomegaly [35, 36].

Microscopic Examination

In primary plasmacytoma, the neoplastic cells often form a mass and show mature cytological features, such as clock face nuclei and ample cytoplasm with perinuclear hof. Occasinally the neoplastic cells may show immature cytology or plasmablastic. In contrast, the neoplastic infiltrate in extramedullary spread of myeloma may form mass lesions (plasmacytomas) and/or dysplay a diffuse sinusoidal distribution, sparing the liver parenchyma. The tumor cells are usually highly aggressive with immature/plasmablastic or anaplastic morphology (Fig. 8.2).

Immunophenotyping

The neoplastic cells are typically positive for CD138, CD38, and MUM1. They also usually show cytoplasmic kappa or lambda immunoglobulin light chain restriction which can be demonstrated by immunohistochemical staining or in situ hybridization. PAX5, CD19, and CD45 are usually negative or weakly expressed. In cases where PAX5, CD19, or CD45 bright expressions are detected, an extranodal marginal zone lymphoma with marked plasmacytic differentiation should also be considered and ruled out. In posttransplant lymphoproliferative disorder (PTLD)-associated cases, EBV encoded RNA in situ hybridization is usually positive (EBER).

Secondary plasmacytoma also differs from primary cases in immunophenotype. Cyclin D1 is usually negative in primary plasmacytoma but positive in a subset of cases of secondary plasmacytoma. By flow cytometry immunophenotyping, the neoplastic plasma cells in extramedullary myeloma usually mirrow those in the bone marrow. They are usually negative or show decreased CD27 and CD81 expression. CD56, CD117, and CD20 are expressed in 60–75%, 25–30%, and 25–30% of myeloma cases, respectively. In contrast, CD56 is uncommonly or weakly expressed in primary plasmacytoma.

Cytogenetics

Primary plasmacytoma is rarely studied by conventional karyotyping. Most literature focuses on secondary involvement by myeloma. The most common immunoglobulin heavy chain gene (*IGH*) rearrangements seen in myeloma such as t(11;14)(q13;q32), t(4;14)(p16;q32), t(6;14)(p21;q32) have not been described primary plasmacytoma, and therefore, detection of these aberrations should raise the possibility of extramedullary involvement by a systemic disease.

Myeloma with high-risk features are more likely to spread beyond the bone marrow [5, 37]. Adverse features in myeloma include t(4;14)(p16;q32)/(*FGFR3-IGH*), t(14;16)(q32;q23)/(*IGH-MAF*), t(14;20)(q32;q12)(*IGH-MAFB*), del(17/17p)/*TP53*, *MYC* rearrangement and a non-hyperdiploid or complex karyotype. Each of these biomarkers is an independent prognostic factor, and coexistence of multiple factors confers an ultra-high risk. The del(17/17p)/*TP53* is enriched in extramedullary myeloma (secondary plasmacytoma) [9]. Interestingly,

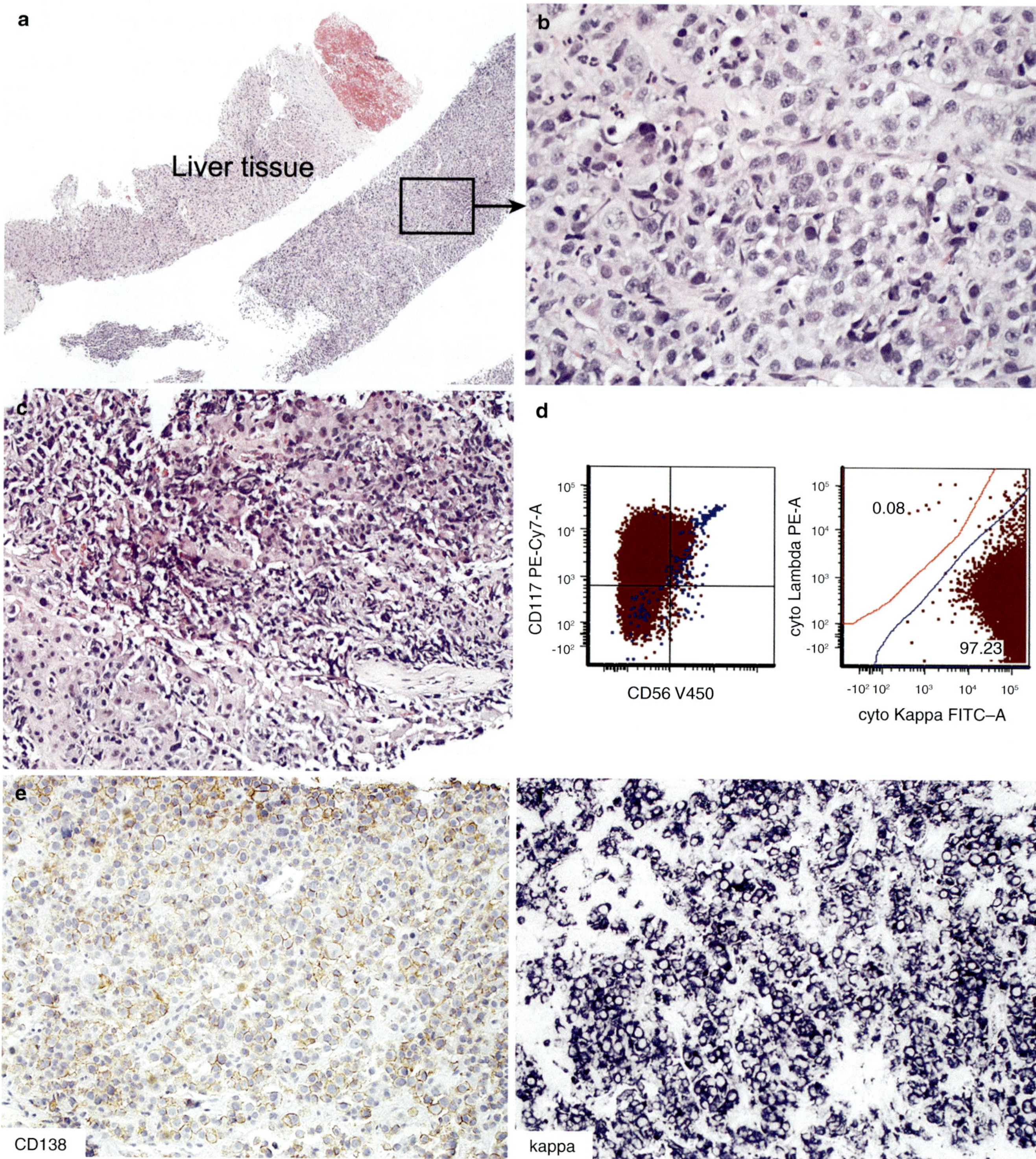

Fig. 8.2 Extramedullary myeloma (secondary plasmacytoma) involving the liver. (**a**) Needle core biopsy of the liver (H&E, 40×) showing neoplastic infiltrate; (**b**) the tumor cells have plasmablastic features with immature chromatin and prominent nucleoli (H&E, 400×); (**c**) portal tract areas are infiltrated by neoplastic cells with crush artifact, H&E, 200×; (**d**) flow cytometry showing the tumor cells are aberrantly positive for CD117 with cytoplasmic kappa light chain restriction. (**e**) CD138 immunostain highlights the plasmablastic cells. (**f**) In situ hybridization showing tumor cells are kappa light chain restricted

though t(11;14) by itself is a standard risk factor, it is the most common abnormality in primary PCL, which is a high risk factor for extramedullary spread [8].

Molecular Findings

Most literature focuses on extramedullary involvement by myeloma/PCL. Gene expression profiling has also identified high-risk gene expression profile (high proliferation) that may predict a propensity for a more widespread disease [38]. Recent studies also found a high frequency of *TP53* deletion and mutations as well as *RAS* mutation with upregulation of FAK (focal adhesion kinase) pathway in the extramedullary myeloma [4]. Furthermore, extramedullary myeloma may harbor deletions or mutations that differ from the primary clone originated in the bone marrow, as a result of natural selection upon therapeutic intervention. Of these, four genes (*ASPM, SLC19A1, TBRG4*, and *TMPO*) are particularly implicated [38]. These extramedullary lesions represent major challenges to treatment. The precise mechanisms of extramedullary spread, however, are unknown but are postulated to be related to an altered bone marrow microenvironment (hypoxia) and molecules such as high expression of CD44 and decreased expression of CD56 on the cell surface of myeloma cells. Lower expression of CXCR4 and its ligand CXCL12 which regulate plasma cells homing to the bone marrow may also promote dissemination.

Differential Diagnosis

Reactive plasmacytosis may contain a large number of plasma cells, but these cells are usually mature without cytological and nuclear atypia seen in extramedullary myeloma. These plasma cells also are polytypic. Primary plasmacytoma may morphologically consist of plasma cells devoid of nuclear and cytoplasmic atypia, but they are monotypic. As mentioned above, the most common *IGH* rearrangements seen in myeloma such as t(11;14), t(4;14), have not been described primary plasmacytoma, and therefore, detection of t(11;14)/cyclin D1 expression should raise the possibility of extramedullary involvement by a systemic disease.

When extramedullary myeloma shows a plasmablastic cytology, the differential diagnoses often include plasmablastic lymphoma (PL) or ALK+ large B cell lymphoma. In PL, EBER is often positive and can help confirm the diagnosis. Conversely, expression of cyclinD1 would favor extramedullary myeloma (though some high grade B cell lymphoma may express cyclinD1, usually variably rather than uniformly). In ALK+ large B cell lymphoma, CD138 is often positive and PAX5 can be dimly expressed, similar to myeloma; however, ALK expression may confirm the diagnosis. Examples of PL and ALK1+ large B cell lymphoma involving the liver are illustrated (Figs. 8.3 and 8.4).

Extranodal marginal zone lymphoma with marked plasmacytic differentiation usually shows some lymphoid components and is variably positive for CD19, CD45, and PAX5.

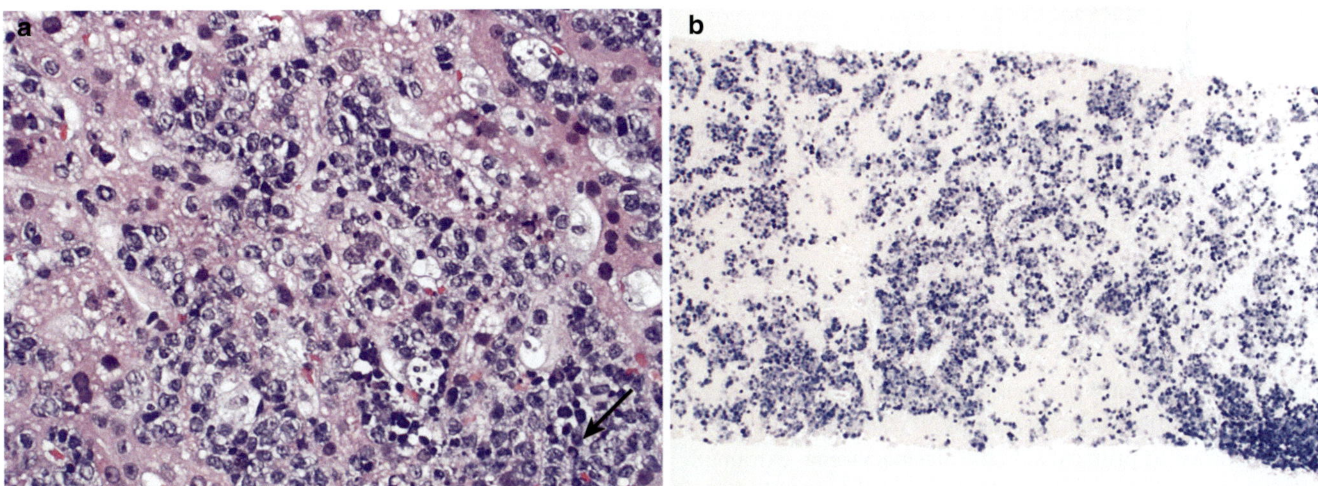

Fig. 8.3 (**a**) Plasmablastic lymphoma involving the liver (H&E, 400×), arrow points to apoptotic bodies. (**b**) The tumor cells are diffusely positive for EBER (Epstein-Barr virus-encoded RNA in situ hybridization, 100×)

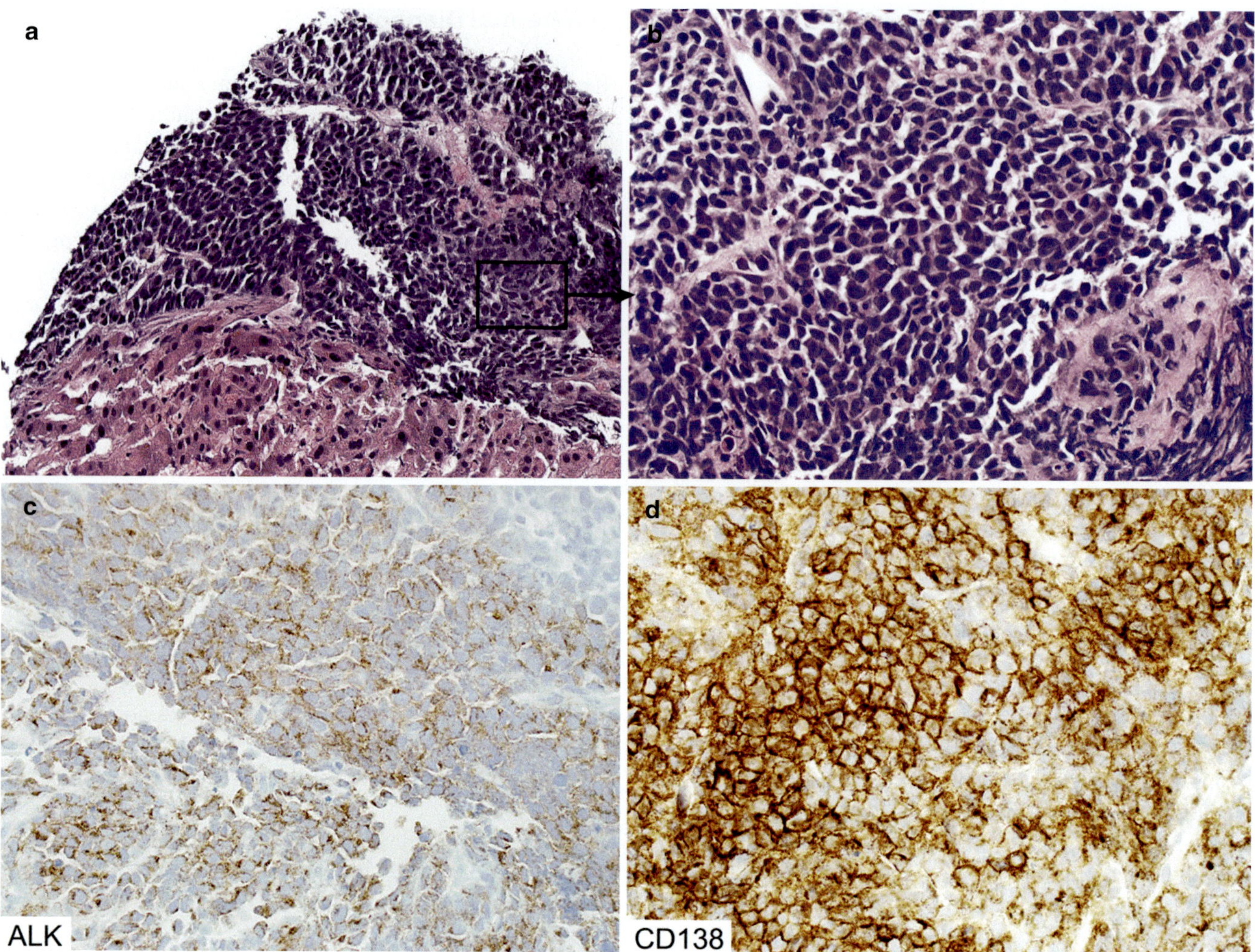

Fig. 8.4 ALK+ large B cell lymphoma. (**a**, **b**) Tumor cells infiltrating the liver (H&E, 200× and 400×, respectively); (**c**, **d**) immunostains show the tumor cells are ALK+ and CD138+ (400×)

Plasmacytoma can be distinguished from carcinoma by being negative for cytokeratin Cam 5.2. Plasma cells may show dot-like cytoplasmic positivity for AE1/AE3 but not diffuse and intense expression.

Prognosis

Patients with primary plasmacytoma usually have an excellent outcome after radiation therapy.

In contrast to primary solitary plasmacytoma, extramedullary myeloma is an independent adverse prognostic factor in myeloma patients receiving intensive therapy [23]. The median overall survival of patients who experience an extramedullary relapse is <6 months.

For patients with extramedullary myeloma, high-dose therapy followed by autologous stem cell transplantation (ASCT) and incorporation of novel agents including immunomodulatory drugs (IMiDs; thalidomide and lenalidomide) and a proteasome inhibitor (PI, bortezomib) have markedly improved the survival of patients. However high-risk patients still suffer high mortality and relapse is common. Newer generation of IMiD (pomalidomide) and PIs (carfilzomib, ixazomib, oprozomib, and marizomib); histone deacetylase inhibitor (panobinostat); monoclonal antibodies daratumumab, isatuximab, elotuzumab, BCL2 inhibitor (venetoclax), Bispecific T cell engagers (BiTEs) and CAR-T have been introduced to clinical trials, and improved survivals are expected in the future.

For transplant eligible patients are usually treated with three-drug combination followed by autologous stem cell transplant (ASCT), consolidation therapy, and maintenance with lenalidomide and/or bortezomib or other PI agents. Addition of monoclonal antibodies such as daratumumab or elotuzumab is being investigated as part of intensive up-front therapy in clinical trials. Transplant-ineligible patients are treated with bortezomib-melphalan-prednisone (VMP) with or without daratumumab or continuous lenalidomide plus dexamethasone (Len-Dex).

Diagnostic Caveats

- CD138 is expressed by epithelial tumor as well as plasmacytoma. Demonstration of immunoglobulin light chain restriction is essential in distinquishing plasmacytic/plasmablastic lesions from carcinoma.
- Cyclin D1 is usually absent in solitary plasmacytoma but can be seen in high-grade plasmablastic tumors such as plasmablastic lymphoma and diffuser large B cell lymphoma with immunoblastic/plasmablastic features, in the absence of t(11;14). Demonstration of cyclin D1 expression by immunohistochemistry is not equivalent to that of t(11;14) and therefore not a presumptive evidence of myeloma, except in the setting of differentiating primary vs. secondary plasmacytoma.
- Extranodal marginal zone lymphoma with marked plasmacytic differentiation usually shows variable lymphoid components and expression of CD19, PAX5, and CD45. In contrast, plasmacytoma shows uniform plasmacytic morphology and generally lacks CD19 or PAX5, with rare exceptions.

Amyloidosis Involving the Liver and Spleen

Definition

Accumulation of insoluble proteins with a β-pleated sheet configuration in the liver or spleen.

Etiology

Amyloidosis is caused by accumulation of insoluble proteins with a β-pleated sheet configuration. Primary amyloidosis (AL) is associated with PCNs, and the amyloid contains a part of the variable region of the light chain, most often λ (75%) and sometimes κ (25%). Rarely amyloid deposition may result from lymphoma with plasmacytic differentiation. Light chain (AL) amyloidosis is the most common form of systemic amyloidosis, accounting for 70% of patients with amyloidosis. Other causes of amyloidosis unrelated to PCNs are only discussed in the differential diagnosis in this chapter [39].

There is evidence to suggest AL has genetic predisposition. Single nucleotide polymorphisms (SNPs) study found splice variant rs9344 of *CCND1* gene and rs79419269 variant of *SMARCD3* (regulating chromatin remodeling) are enriched in AL patients [39].

Epidemiology

Amyloidosis can be seen in approximately 15% of patients with myeloma. The incidence of AL in the USA is 9–14 cases per million person years with a median age of 63 years at onset. There is a male predominance.

Clinical Presentations

The symptoms are vague and nonspecific in the early stage. The most common complaints are fatigue and malaise. Amyloid infiltrates cause organ damage and organ dysfunction. These include nephrotic syndrome or renal failure, restrictive cardiomyopathy or arrhythmia, gastrointestinal symptoms, peripheral neuropathy, and coagulopathy due to binding of the amyloid fibers with factor X.

Rarely, amyloidosis may cause rapidly progressive intrahepatic cholestasis leading to massive hepatomegaly, portal hypertension with splenomegaly, ascites, and varices [40].

Liver involvement may also cause elevation of alkaline phosphatase or liver enzyme, while splenic involvement causes splenomegaly and cytopenia and may rarely lead to spontaneous rupture [41].

In one third of patients with the AL, no distinct M spike is visible by serum protein electrophoresis (SPEP). *Immunofixation* electrophoresis (IFE) is more sensitive. Recently, mass spectrometry has been shown to be more sensitive than IFE for detection of M spike and is especially useful in follow up samples of patients treated with daratumumab. Serum free light chain (FLC) assays can determine the type of the M protein and confirm the diagnosis.

Morphology

Gross or Radiological Findings

Grossly, the involved organs appear to be waxy and stiff.

Microscopic Examination

On hematoxylin and eosin sections, the amyloid fibers have an amorphous, eosinophilic appearance often associated with cracking artifact and multinucleated giant cell reaction (Fig. 8.5a–d). The amyloid fibers appear apple-green birefringent when stained with Congo red and viewed under polarized light (Fig. 8.5e–f). Liver biopsy has a sensitivity level of 90% in confirming amyloid deposition.

By electronic microscopy (EM), amyloid fibers appear as a mass of nonbranching linear fibrils 7–10 nm in diameter and of variable length.

Immunophenotyping

The amyloid and monotypic plasma cells are best highlighted by immunohistochemistry or flow cytometry

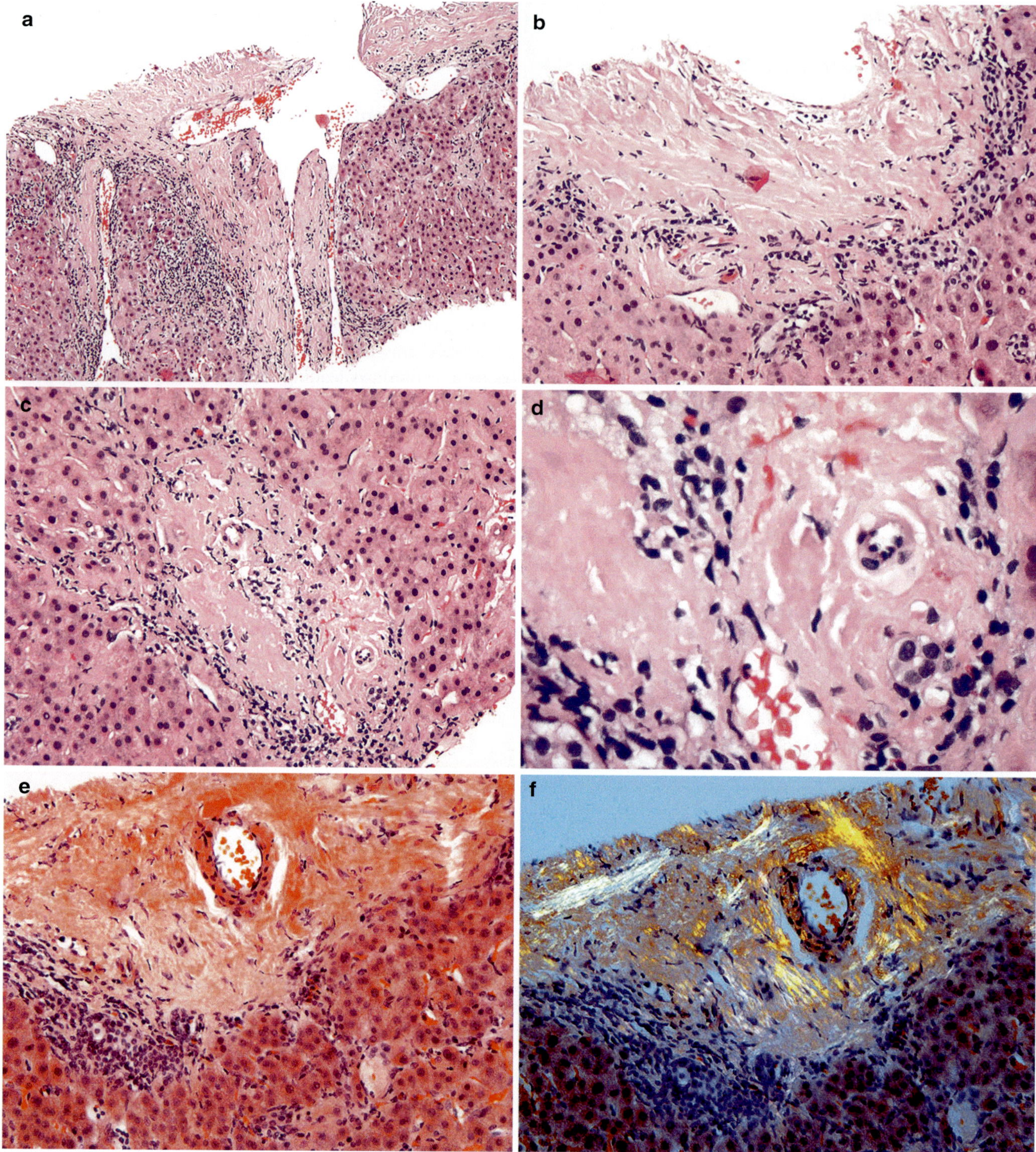

Fig. 8.5 (**a**, **d**) Massive amyloid deposition in the liver parenchyma and perivascular spaces (H&E, **a** 100×, **b**, **c**, 200×) associated with giant cell reaction to amyloid deposition (H&E, 600×); (**e**–**f**) Congo red stain highlights apple-green birefringent amyloid deposition

immunophenotyping using a panel of antibodies including CD138, in conjunction with immunoglobulin light chains. The AL amyloid can be detected using antibody specific for AL or amyloid P component.

Cytogenetics

Cytogenetic aberrations in AL are similar to those in myeloma; however, t(11;14) is particularly enriched in AL patients. The most frequent genetic abnormalities are t(11;14) (50%), monosomy 13/del(13q) (36%), and trisomies (26%). Other aberrations such as t(4;14) and t(14;16) and del(17p) are rare, accounting only for <5% of cases each [39].

Molecular Findings

Somatic mutations of the immunoglobulin light chain variable region (*IGLV*) result in reduced fold stability of native light chain. This leads to endoproteolysis and production of variable light chain domains that can cause amyloidosis. Light chain λ from *IGLV1-44* preferentially targets the heart, light chain λ from *IGLV6-57* targets the kidney, and light chain κ from *IGKV1-33* targets the liver [39].

Differential Diagnosis

AL should be distinguished from other types of amyloidosis, mainly AA, AF, and Aβ2M. Secondary amyloidosis (AA) is associated with chronic inflammation. AF is found in familial amyloidosis such as ATTRwt (senile systemic amyloidosis) and ATTR mutated (transthyretin V122I variant), whereas Aβ2m is related to hemodialysis. Molecular studies with polymerase chain reaction (PCR) amplification and DNA sequence analysis will detect patients with mutant transthyretin or mutated fibrinogen Aα-chain. High-performance liquid chromatography-mass spectrometry (HPLC-MS) allows specific typing of amyloid fibers and is considered the gold standard and a powerful ancillary tool.

Localized amyloid deposition can occur as part of lymphoma or plasmacytoma, sometimes with mass formation, the so-called amyloidoma. They are usually not associated systemic disease as AL.

The distinction between AL and light or heavy chain deposition diseases is discussed below.

Prognosis

The median survival of patients with AL is 1–2 years. The patients usually succumb to progressive organ failure. The prognosis largely depends on the dominant organ involvement. Cardiac involvement is the major prognostic factor for survival, and cardiac function can be assessed by monitoring NT-proBNP and troponin I. Congestive heart failure and fatal arrhythmia are the major cause of death. Although hepatic involvement is common, it does not usually affect prognosis.

Patients are treated with PI containing regimens, venetoclax, with or without autologous stem cell transplant (ASCT) for AL caused by PCNs. More recently years have seen three monoclonal antibodies targeting existing amyloid deposits: NEOD001, 11-1F4, and an anti-SAP antibody. Improved survivals are expected.

Diagnostic Caveats

- The diagnosis of AL requires direct evidence of amyloid-induced organ damage as a result of monoclonal plasma cell proliferation. Since patients with MGUS may also have secondary amyloidosis, the mere coexistence of monoclonal plasma cells and amyloid deposition are not sufficient for a diagnosis of AL.
- All of the following criteria need to be fulfilled to diagnose AL: (a) presence of amyloid-related systemic syndrome (such as renal, liver, heart, gastrointestinal tract, or peripheral nerve involvement) and (b) positive amyloid staining by Congo red or EM in any tissue, confirming that the amyloid is composed of Ig chain by immunostaining or mass spectrometry and detection of monoclonal plasma cell proliferation such as serum or urine M protein, abnormal FLC ratio, or monotypic plasma cells in bone marrow.
- The monoclonal immunoglobulin in AA can be IgM or non-IgM as well as light-chain-only type. As such, the organ dysfunction caused by amyloid deposition should not be taken as evidence of end-organ damage meeting the criteria for active PCM.
- Systemic amyloidosis should be distinguished from localized disease (amyloidoma) as the latter does not require systemic chemotherapy and has a very good prognosis.

Light Chain Deposition Disease or Light and Heavy Chain Deposition Diseases

Light chain deposition disease or light and heavy chain deposition diseases present with clinical features similar to those of AA, but ancillary studies such as Congo red or EM and mass spectrometry may confirm the nature of the deposited materials.

Summary

PCNs involving the liver and spleen may manifest as extramedullary plasmacytomas, amyloidosis, light chain deposition disease, or dissemination of advanced-stage myeloma or PCL. In the case of isolated primary plasmacytoma of the liver, the patient is usually treated with radiation therapy, and progression to a systemic disease is extremely rare. In cases of liver or splenic involvement due to advanced stage of myeloma or primary PCL, the tumor cells are usually of high grade with complex cytogenetic aberrations, *TP53* deletions, and other adverse genetic features. Extramedullary myeloma in the liver may exist as the initital presentation of relapsed myeloma. The prognosis of these patients is poor and response to current therapies is still suboptimal. Amyloidosis can be seen in approximately 15% of myeloma patients. Liver involvement in primary amyloidosis (AA) may lead to elevation of alkaline phosphatase or liver enzyme, while splenic involvement may lead to spontaneous rupture. Systemic therapy is usually needed to control the organ damages caused by amyloidosis and light chain deposition diseases.

References

1. Aguado B, Iñigo B, Sastre JL, Oriol A. Extramedullary plasmacytomas in the context of multiple myeloma. Adv Ther. 2011;28(Suppl 7):7–13.
2. Fotiou D, Dimopoulos MA, Kastritis E. How we manage patients with plasmacytomas. Curr Hematol Malig Rep. 2018;13(3):227–35.
3. Touzeau C, Moreau P. How I treat extramedullary myeloma. Blood. 2016;127(8):971–6.
4. Coo C, Chen X, Gao G. Progress in extramedullary disease in multiple myeloma. Cancer Res Clin. 2016;28(11):785–9.
5. Besse L, Sedlarikova L, Greslikova H, et al. Cytogenetics in multiple myeloma patients progressing into extramedullary disease. Eur J Haematol. 2016;97(1):93–100.
6. Weinstock M, Aljawai Y, Morgan EA, et al. Incidence and clinical features of extramedullary multiple myeloma in patients who underwent stem cell transplantation. Br J Haematol. 2015;169(6):851–8.
7. Weinstock M, Ghobrial IM. Extramedullary multiple myeloma. Leuk Lymphoma. 2013;54(6):1135–41.
8. Shin HJ, Kim K, Lee JJ, et al. The t(11;14)(q13;q32) translocation as a poor prognostic parameter for autologous stem cell transplantation in myeloma patients with extramedullary plasmacytoma. Clin Lymphoma Myeloma Leuk. 2015;15(4):227–35.
9. Deng S, Xu Y, An G, et al. Features of extramedullary disease of multiple myeloma: high frequency of P53 deletion and poor survival: a retrospective single-center study of 834 cases. Clin Lymphoma Myeloma Leuk. 2015;15(5):286–91.
10. Gonsalves WI, Kumar SK. Plasma cell leukemia. In: Zimmerman TM, editor. Biology and management of unusual plasma cell dyscrasias. New York: Springer; 2016. p. 1–16.
11. Malhotra P, Bhat P, Mahi S, Chauhan S, Rajwanshi A, Varma S. Evolution of hepatosplenic plasmacytoma in a patient with multiple myeloma receiving chemotherapy. Am J Hematol. 2005;78(1):82–3.
12. Trappe R, Zimmermann H, Fink S, et al. Plasmacytoma-like post-transplant lymphoproliferative disorder, a rare subtype of monomorphic B-cell post-transplant lymphoproliferation, is associated with a favorable outcome in localized as well as in advanced disease: a prospective analysis of 8 cases. Haematologica. 2011;96(7):1067–71.
13. Ghobrial PM, Goel A. Plasmacytoma of liver mimicking hepatocellular carcinoma at multiphasic computed tomography evaluation. J Comput Assist Tomogr. 2015;39(4):510–2.
14. Petrucci MT, Tirindelli MC, De Muro M, Martini V, Levi A, Mandelli F. Extramedullary liver plasmacytoma a rare presentation. Leuk Lymphoma. 2003;44(6):1075–6.
15. Coffey D, Fain B, Thompson C, Chan ED, Nawaz S. Liver failure as the only clinical manifestation of multiple myeloma. Ann Hematol. 2012;91(4):625–7.
16. Solves P, De La Rubia J, Jarque I, et al. Liver disease as primary manifestation of multiple myeloma in a young man. Leuk Res. 1999;23(4):403–5.
17. Perez-Soler R, Esteban R, Allende E, Tornos Salomo C, Julia A, Guardia J. Liver involvement in multiple myeloma. Am J Hematol. 1985;20(1):25–9.
18. Garfinkel D, Salamon F, Sidi Y, Ben-Bassat M, Lubin E, Pinkhas J. Multiple plasmacytomas of the liver and the spleen. Clin Nucl Med. 1985;10(11):819.
19. Varga C, Xie W, Laubach J, et al. Development of extramedullary myeloma in the era of novel agents: no evidence of increased risk with lenalidomide-bortezomib combinations. Br J Haematol. 2015;169(6):843–50.
20. Bladé J, Fernández de Larrea C, Rosiñol L. Extramedullary disease in multiple myeloma in the era of novel agents. Br J Haematol. 2015;169(6):763–5.
21. Kim DW, Kim WH, Kim MH, Choi KH, Kim CG. Detection of Extramedullary multiple myeloma in liver by FDG-PET/CT. Nucl Med Mol Imaging. 2014;48(2):166–8.
22. Muchtar E, Magen H, Gertz MA. High-risk multiple myeloma: a multifaceted entity, multiple therapeutic challenges. Leuk Lymphoma. 2017;58(6):1283–96.
23. Lee SE, Kim JH, Jeon YW, et al. Impact of extramedullary plasmacytomas on outcomes according to treatment approach in newly diagnosed symptomatic multiple myeloma. Ann Hematol. 2014;94(3):445–52.
24. da Silva RL, Monteiro A, Veiga J. Non-secretory multiple myeloma relapsing as extramedullary liver plasmacytomas. J Gastrointestin Liver Dis. 2011;20(1):81–3.
25. Rasche L, Bernard C, Topp MS, et al. Features of extramedullary myeloma relapse: high proliferation, minimal marrow involvement, adverse cytogenetics: a retrospective single-center study of 24 cases. Ann Hematol. 2012;91(7):1031–7.
26. Cohen R, Boulagnon C, Ehrhard F, et al. Portal hypertension with extensive fibrosis and plasma cell infiltration in multiple myeloma. Clin Res Hepatol Gastroenterol. 2016;40(6):e71–3.

27. Khan Y, Mansour I, Ong E, Shrestha M. Obstructive jaundice as initial presentation of multiple myeloma: case presentation and literature review. Case Rep Med. 2015;2015:1.
28. Magnoli F, Freguia S, Bernasconi B, et al. Fatal splenic rupture in a previously undiagnosed multiple myeloma: morphological, immunophenotypical and molecular cytogenetic analyses. Clin Lymphoma Myeloma Leuk. 2013;13(6):e22–5.
29. Veerappan R, Morrison M, Williams S, Variakojis D. Splenic rupture in a patient with plasma cell myeloma following G-CSF/GM-CSF administration for stem cell transplantation and review of the literature. Bone Marrow Transplant. 2007;40(4):361–4.
30. Saboo SS, Fennessy F, Benajiba L, Laubach J, Anderson KC, Richardson PG. Imaging features of extramedullary, relapsed, and refractory multiple myeloma involving the liver across treatment with cyclophosphamide, lenalidomide, bortezomib, and dexamethasone. J Clin Oncol. 2012;30(20):e175–9.
31. Okamoto Y, Ueda Y. Multiple myeloma mimicking liver metastases. Intern Med. 2015;54(16):2085–6.
32. Boumans D, Hoekstra R, Krukkert-Alberink AAM, Schot BW. Plasmablastic myeloma presenting with nodular liver lesions: rare but important to recognize. Eur J Gen Med. 2014;11(Suppl 1):48–50.
33. Simmons MZ, Miller JA, Levine CD, Glucksman WJ, Wachsberg RH. Myelomatous involvement of the liver: unusual ultrasound appearance. J Clin Ultrasound. 1997;25(3):145–8.
34. Thiruvengadam R, Penetrante RB, Goolsby HJ, Silk YN, Bernstein ZP. Multiple myeloma presenting as space-occupying lesions of the liver. Cancer. 1990;65(12):2784–6.
35. Kapoor P, Singh E, Radhakrishnan P, Mehta P. Splenectomy in plasma cell dyscrasias: a review of the clinical practice. Am J Hematol. 2006;81(12):946–54.
36. Perry-Thornton E, Verly GP, Karkala J, Walker M. An unusual presentation of multiple myeloma: primary plasmacytoma of the spleen. J Natl Med Assoc. 1989;81(10):1095.
37. Billecke L, Murga Penas EM, May AM, et al. Cytogenetics of extramedullary manifestations in multiple myeloma. Br J Haematol. 2013;161(1):87–94.
38. Sevcikova S, Paszekova H, Besse L, et al. Extramedullary relapse of multiple myeloma defined as the highest risk group based on deregulated gene expression data. Biomed Pap Med Fac Univ Palacky Olomouc Czech Repub. 2015;159(2):288–93.
39. Merlini G, Dispenzieri A, Sanchorawala V, et al. Systemic immunoglobulin light chain amyloidosis. Nat Rev Dis Primers. 2018;4(1):38.
40. Joseph M, TJS C. Review: amyloidosis and subacute liver failure. Gastroenterol Hepatol. 2012;8(3):208–11.
41. Renzulli P, Schoepfer A, Mueller E, Candinas D. Atraumatic splenic rupture in amyloidosis. Amyloid. 2009;16(1):47–53.

Michelle Don and Serhan Alkan

Definition

Hepatosplenic T-cell lymphoma (HSTL) is described as a subtype of aggressive peripheral T-cell lymphoma in the 2016 WHO classification. It is an extranodal lymphoma with poor response to chemotherapy and a poor prognosis. Typical cases present with hepatic or splenic enlargement and bone marrow infiltrate. There is sinusoidal infiltration of the liver and spleen and infiltration of the bone marrow by cytotoxic T-cells that most commonly express γ/δ T-cell receptor (TCR). Although less common, some of the patients may have a variant of HSTL that is associated with α/β receptor expressing cytotoxic T-cells. Unfortunately there is currently no standardized treatment or cure for HSTL.

Etiology

A great majority of HSTL arise *de novo*; however, a subset of cases, approximately 20–30%, occurs in the setting of iatrogenic immunosuppression and chronic antigenic stimulation [1, 2]. Long-term immunosuppression resulting in HSTL can occur in the posttransplant setting and in the setting of long-term immunomodulation [3]. HSTL occurring in the setting of immunomodulation has been most commonly associated with inflammatory bowel disease, primarily in patients with Crohn's disease. It has also been linked to patients who have been treated with thiopurines and/or tumor necrosis factor (TNF-α) inhibitors [1, 3]. It is less commonly associated with patients having psoriasis or rheumatoid arthritis [3]. Other examples of HSTL arising in association with immunosuppression, however rare, have been seen with pregnancy and in patients treated for acute leukemia and Hodgkin lymphoma [2].

The pathogenesis of HSTL is poorly understood. The normal cell counterpart is most commonly a γ/δ receptor cytotoxic T-cell of the innate immune system. γ/δ HSTL occurs at least 80% of the time; on rare occasions it is an α/β receptor cytotoxic T-cell that is the cell of origin [1–4]. Although both types result in a similar clinical presentation, morphologic and immunophenotypic profile, it is still likely that their true etiology is different.

Epidemiology

HSTL is a rare extranodal lymphoma that accounts for 1–2% of T/Natural killer cell lymphomas [3]. Classic γ/δ HSTL is associated with a male predominance (M:F = 5:1) and usually occurs in adolescents and young adults, with a median age of 35 years [2, 3]. In rare cases of α/β HSTL, women are more likely affected with a median age of 36 years [2]. HSTL most commonly occurs de novo but can also occur in the setting of chronic immunosuppression (see etiology).

Clinical Presentation

HSTL is often diagnosed late in the course of the disease, partly due to the usual lack of lymphadenopathy. Commonly presentation begins with B-symptoms which include fever, weight loss, night sweats, and fatigue [2]. Splenomegaly has been reported in 60–100% of cases [1, 2] and is the most commonly reported clinical finding, over hepatomegaly which is reported in 30–80% of cases [1, 2]. Lymphadenopathy has only been reported in 13–23% of cases [1, 2].

HSTL-associated laboratory findings include cytopenias, with thrombocytopenia being the most common. Anemia

M. Don · S. Alkan (✉)
Department of Pathology and Laboratory Medicine, Cedars-Sinai Medical Center, Los Angeles, CA, USA

© Springer Nature Switzerland AG 2020
L. Zhang et al. (eds.), *Diagnostic Pathology of Hematopoietic Disorders of Spleen and Liver*,
https://doi.org/10.1007/978-3-030-37708-3_9

and leukopenia are less commonly seen but also can occur [1, 2]. Increased severity of cytopenias has been correlated with disease progression [1]; however, the mechanism is unknown. Peripheral blood involvement can sometimes be identified with atypical lymphocytes present on the peripheral smear, but lymphocytosis is not commonly seen [1, 5]. Other reported laboratory findings include an increase in lactate dehydrogenase (LDH) which has been reported in 60–70% of patients [2]. Elevated bilirubin, beta-2 microglobulin, and elevation of liver function tests have also been associated [1, 6].

Rarely, leukemic transformation of HSTL has been identified. Laboratory changes associated with hemophagocytic syndrome [2] have also been seen, which is a well-known but rare related phenomenon that can be the presenting symptom of the patient or occur during the clinical course of the disease. Rare patients with an associated cold agglutinin disease have also been reported. Hemolytic anemia is extremely rare but has been reported as well [7].

Morphology and Immunophenotyping

HSTL most commonly involves the spleen, liver, and bone marrow. Grossly the spleen is usually enlarged ranging from 570 to 6500 grams [8]. Usually the cut surface of the spleen is grossly normal and homogeneously red-purple in appearance. The liver is often diffusely enlarged without any focal lesions and lymph nodes are often grossly normal [8]. Necrosis is only sometimes seen after therapy [2].

HSTL cells are known to initially involve sinuses and cords of the red pulp of the spleen [1, 2, 8]. There is infiltration of the lymphoma cells into the cords and sinusoids of the red pulp with eventual diffuse replacement of the spleen leaving the white pulp atrophic [1, 2, 8] (Fig. 9.1a, b). In the liver the lymphoma cells are seen invading the cords and sinusoids [3, 9] (Fig. 9.1c, d). Portal and periportal involvement may be present; however, it is usually mild and not predominant [9]. The lymphoma cells do not typically show any significant atypia, often causing one not to consider lymphoma in the initial differential diagnosis. Therefore, the differential diagnosis of HSTL should be included when there is significant sinusoidal lymphoid infiltrate.

Lymph node involvement is predominantly a sinusoidal pattern; however, diffuse replacement of the node by tumor cells can also be seen. Other extranodal sites that may be involved include the skin, mucosal surfaces, and kidney; however, HSTL in these sites is usually associated with advanced or recurrent disease. A more rare site includes the brain in one reported case [10].

Bone marrow involvement is identified at the time of diagnosis and typically shows hypercellularity with trilineage hematopoiesis. The lymphoma cells are located interstitially and within the sinusoids; however, due to the variability in the cytology, the lymphoma cells are not always easily identifiable. The aspirate smears can have a background of mild dyspoiesis [2]; however, this mild dysplasia is not known to contribute to any cytopenias identified in peripheral blood [2]. Thus, investigation of a possible coexistent myelodysplastic syndrome in this setting may be considered.

The lymphoma cells are usually intermediate in size; however, the cytology can vary in size and morphology. The lymphoma cells can range from small lymphocytes that appear mature with clumped chromatin and scant cytoplasm to larger lymphocytes with a blastic fine chromatin [11]. They can also be large and pleomorphic in appearance [1]. Typically the cytoplasm of lymphoma cells is pale and agranular and lacks azurophilic granules that are usually seen in large granular lymphocytic leukemia (T-LGL). In some cases cells may have features of acute leukemia due to the presence of fine chromatin and high nuclear-to-cytoplasmic ratio.

A well-known phenomenon that uncommonly occurs in the setting of the HSTL is hemophagocytosis. Only a very rare minority of patients actually present with hemophagocytic syndrome, and hemophagocytosis has been reported in 5% of patients.

The immunophenotype of HSTL can be determined by both immunohistochemistry and flow cytometry (Fig. 9.2). HSTL cells are positive for pan T-cell markers including surface CD2, CD3, CD7, and CD43. Most cases are negative for CD4 and CD8 but occasionally in a subset of cases, there is at least partial positivity for CD8. In fact, when someone encounters a double-negative (CD4$^-$/CD8$^-$) population, HSTL should be the first entity considered in the differential diagnosis; however, the phenotype could be seen in T-cell prolymphocytic leukemia (T-PLL), T- LGL, and T-cell acute lymphoblastic leukemia/lymphoma (T-ALL). HSTL cells usually lack CD5, CD1a, CD10, TDT, myeloid antigens, and B-cell antigens. CD56 is expressed in approximately 60% of cases. Surface γ/δ TCR is expressed in approximately 75% of cases and the remaining cases are either α/β TCR or negative for both. The HSTL cells usually express a mature, non-activated cytotoxic T-cell immunophenotype with expression of TIA-1 and granzyme M and negative for perforin. Positivity for granzyme B is seen in approximately 40% of cases. The proliferation rate is variable and results in a variable Ki-67. In situ hybridization using Epstein-Bar Virus encoded RNA (EBER) is negative.

In cases where TDT is positive, a diagnosis of T-ALL is likely. However, TDT-negative T-ALL cases may be difficult to differentiate since there is no specific marker known to differentiate T-ALL from γ/δ-LGL [12]. Further cytogenetic molecular studies may be quite helpful for immuno-

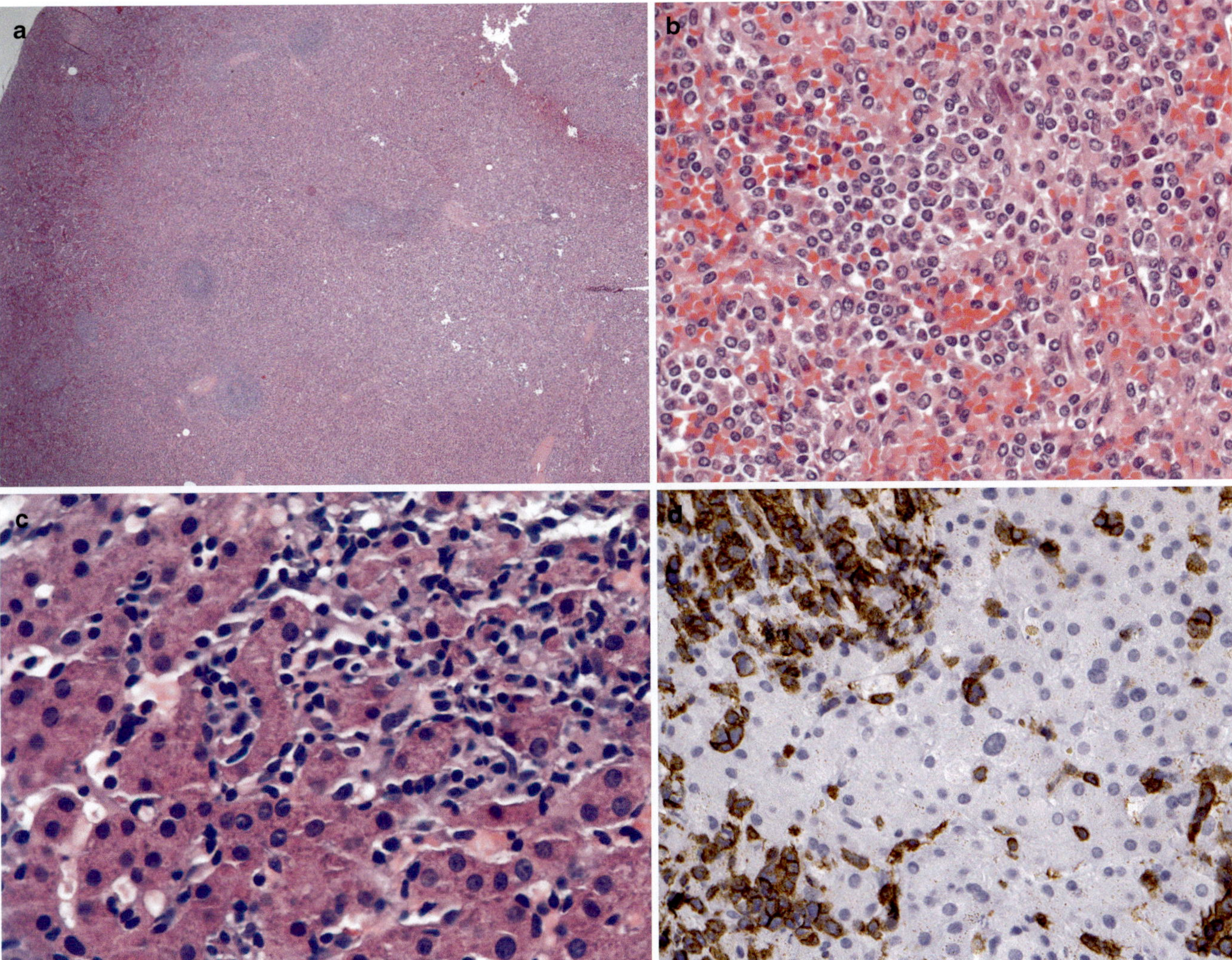

Fig. 9.1 Typical histologic features of spleen and liver involvement by hepatosplenic T-cell lymphoma are shown. (**a**, **b**) The spleen showing expansion of the red pulp by intermediate-sized lymphocytes. (**c**, **d**) Another case of HSTL involving the liver that shows small-size lymphocytes in the sinusoids. As observed here, insidious infiltrate may bring an inflammatory diagnosis in the differential. Therefore, careful review and further immunohistochemical analysis would be essential for characterization of a sinusoidal lymphocytic infiltrate. CD3 (**d**) staining highlights a sinusoidal lymphocytic infiltrate that could be further assessed by multiple T-cell markers including CD4, CD8, and cytotoxic markers

phenotypically challenging cases. T-PLL is usually CD4 positive with overexpression of TCL1, with approximately 25% of cases expressing both CD4 and CD8 [3].

Cytogenetics and Molecular Findings

The most common recurrent cytogenetic findings include isochromosome (7q), trisomy 8, and loss of the y chromosome [13, 14]. The recurrent finding of isochromosome (7q) is thought to be the primary chromosomal event which results in the deletion of the short arm of the chromosome causing loss of tumor suppressor genes located on 7p and loss of the TCRβ gene located at 7p15 [13, 14]. These specific cytogenetic findings are not known to be associated with other T-cell lymphomas [1] and are specific but not sensitive for HSTL. The frequency as to which these findings are detected in HSTL is variable, and that is attributed to varying methods of detection which include conventional karyotype vs. fluorescence in situ hybridization. The majority of prior studies have shown isochromosome 7 in greater than 50% of cases. Since this feature is highly characteristic of HSTL, ancillary studies, i.e., FISH or chromosomal microarray, could be performed when this disorder is in the differential diagnosis. Subsequently, there is duplication of the long arm which then leads to excess oncogenes that are located on 7q and the TCRγ gene located at 7q35 [13–15].

Trisomy 8 and the loss of chromosome y are not as frequent as isochromosome (7q) and thus considered secondary

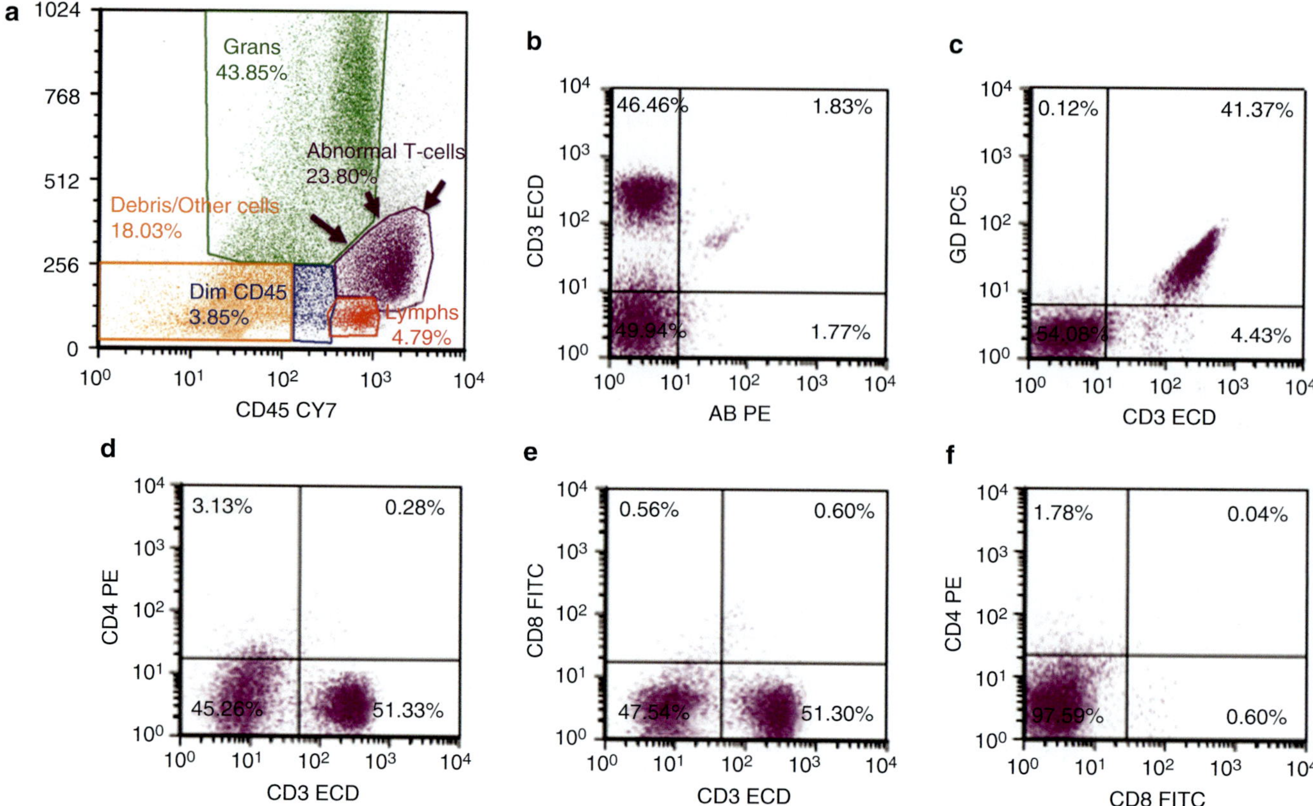

Fig. 9.2 Flow cytometry histograms in a case of hepatosplenic T-cell lymphoma (HSTL) show lymphoma cells with lower side scatter and bright CD45 (**a**) that are positive for CD3 (**b–e**) and negative for both CD4 and CD8 (**d–f**). A great majority of cases are observed in the location where monocytes are seen in CD45/SSC analysis. Therefore, careful analysis of this gate for a T-cell population would be useful for consideration of HSTL diagnosis. Typically, peripheral T-cell lymphomas reside in the lower SSC gate where the normal lymphocytes reside. As observed here, double-negative for CD4/CD8 and CD3 positive T-cell population is the most typical phenotype in HSTL cases

events [13]. The presence of these aberrations may be associated with progression of the disorder.

The γ/δ T-cells are thought to be a functionally immature clonal proliferation induced through the upregulation of the JAK/STAT pathway. Mutations of *STAT3* have been identified in 10% of cases and *STAT5b* in 30% of cases [1]. The presence of either *STAT3* or *STAT5B* mutation is thought to be mutually exclusive; however, a rare case report with both *STAT3* and *STAT5B* mutations has been reported in the literature [16, 17]. Both the *STAT3* and *STAT5B* mutations have been shown to be oncogenic driving mutations. This molecular profile is seen regardless of γ/δ vs. α/β origin [2]. The presence of *STAT3* and *STAT5b* mutations is important as there are targeted therapies available. Additionally, whole exome sequencing of 68 cases of HSTL again showed the presence of *STAT3* and *STAT5B* mutations as well as revealed mutations in chromatin modifiers including *SETD2*, *INO80*, *TET3*, *SMARCA2*, and *ARID1B1* [16]. Chromatin-modifying genes make up the majority (62%) of genes that are mutated in HSTL [16]. The most common of these, *SETD2*, a tumor suppressor gene, was seen in 25% of cases [16]. It has been suggested that *SETD2* has a tumor-suppressive function in

HSTL since 44% of patients had more than one mutation in *SETD2* with frequent biallelic loss of function mutations [1]. Other associated genes include *PIK3CD*, *TP53*, *UBR5*, and *IDH2* [16]. *PIK3CD* also has associated targeted therapies. It is notable that mutations which frequent other T-cell lymphomas in genes such as *RHOA*, *CD28*, and *CCR4* were absent or occurred at much lower frequency in HSTLs [16].

T-cell receptor gene rearrangements are identified showing monoclonal TCRδ rearrangements in most HSTL cases, particularly those with the γ/δ phenotype. In cases with the α/β TCR phenotype, T-cell receptor β gene rearrangements are identified [2].

Differential Diagnosis

The differential diagnosis of HSTL includes other hematopoietic neoplasms as well as some reactive/benign entities such as hepatitis. Morphologically, when identifying sinusoidal infiltration of the spleen by lymphocytes, splenic marginal zone lymphoma (SMZL) should be considered; however SMZL tends to prefer the white pulp, while HSTL involves the splenic red pulp. Diffuse involvement of the splenic red pulp by small lymphocytes brings in the differential of hairy cell leukemia; however, immunohistochemistry will distinguish these B-cell neoplasms from HSTL.

Other T-cell neoplasms (Table 9.1) also enter the differential diagnosis, as many can have overlapping features. Many extranodal T-cell lymphomas can express γ/δ TCR that include cutaneous γ/δ T-cell lymphoma and T-cell LGL expressing γ/δ TCR that are among other rare T-cell leukemias/lymphomas. In these cases, the sites of involvement and other clinical findings should be assessed, where HSTL involves the spleen, liver, and bone marrow and rarely cutaneous sites. The clinical course, histopathologic, phenotypic and cytogenetic findings favor HSTL when there is aggressive disease with hepatosplenomegaly characterized with sinusoidal lymphoid infiltrates lacking cytoplasmic azurophilic granules, CD4/CD8 negativity, expression of TIA-1, isochromosome 7q and/or trisomy of chromosome 8.

The presence of azurophilic granules and subsequent staining with cytotoxic markers brings into the differential T-LGL and additionally aggressive natural killer cell (NK-cell) leukemia. However in the case of NK-cell leukemia, IHC should reveal NK cell immunophenotype and EBV positivity.

T-PLL usually presents with hepatosplenomegaly and generalized lymphadenopathy, which can be seen in HSTL; however peripheral blood will have a lymphocyte count that is usually greater than 100×10^9/L, while HSTL usually does not present with a lymphocytosis [3]. Additionally, TCL1 positivity favors T-PLL. Hepatosplenomegaly and lymphadenopathy can also be seen in T-ALL; however, the presence of a mediastinal mass, high leukocyte count, and TDT positivity favors a diagnosis of T-ALL [3].

Prognosis

Overall the prognosis for HSTL is poor [3]. An elevated serum bilirubin (>1.5 mg/dL) and an elevated LDH are laboratory findings that are associated with a poor prognosis [1]. α/β HSTL is considered a variant of HSTL, with similar clinical, morphologic, immunophenotypic, and cytogenetic findings [1]; however, it appears to carry an even worst prognosis. Few studies with a small cohort size have stated that the presence of cytogenetic abnormalities including aberrancies in chromosome 7 and trisomy 8 are associated with a poorer prognosis; however, the true significance of this finding is still to be determined [16].

Diagnostic Caveats

HSTL has a well-defined presentation of sinusoidal infiltration of the lymphoma cells within the sinusoids of the spleen, liver, and bone marrow and is known to occur in younger individuals, usually male, and have a more aggressive course. However, there are still a number of various situations in which distinguishing HSTL from other entities can be a diagnostic challenge. As mentioned before, any significant sinusoidal infiltrate in the liver should bring about HSTL as a differential diagnosis, and further clinical as well as immunohistochemical assessment is warranted. Since the sinusoidal T-cell infiltrate in the bone marrow is very insidious, it could be easily missed. Unfortunately, bone marrow biopsy may be the first tissue biopsy pathologist may have to establish diagnosis. In this instance, a conversation with the clinician about the possibility of HSTL and obtaining tissue from the liver and/or spleen is essential for arriving correct diagnosis.

Table 9.1 Most common and pertinent findings in the differential diagnosis of hepatosplenic T-cell lymphoma

	HSTL	T-PLL	T-LGL	T-ALL	ATLL
Histologic findings	Small- to medium-sized lymphoid cells with agranular cytoplasm	Lymphoid cells with moderate cytoplasm and prominent nucleoli	Lymphoid cells with azurophilic granules and abundant cytoplasm	Blasts	Lymphoid cells with clover leaf nuclei
Splenomegaly	Yes	Yes	May present	Usually not	No
Lymphadenopathy	Usually not	No	No	Yes, mediastinal	No
Cytogenetics	Iso7q, trisomy 8, loss of y	t(14;14), inversion 14, Iso(8q)	No known abnormality	Abnormal karyotype, 14q11.2 (TCR α/β), 7q35 (TCR β), 7p14–15 (TCR γ)	No distinct abnormality, may have complex karyotype
Typical immunophenotypic findings	CD4$^-$, CD8$^-$	TCL1$^+$	CD8$^+$, CD16$^{+/-}$, CD57$^+$	TDT$^+$, CD34$^{+/-}$, CD1a$^+$, CD99$^+$, cytoplasmic CD3$^+$	CD4$^+$, CD25$^+$
Associated virus	–	–	–	–	HTLV1
Molecular findings	*STAT3*, *STAT5b*, *SETD2*, clonal *TCR* gene rearrangement	*ATM*, *TP53*	*STAT3*, *STAT5b*	*Myc*, *TAL1*, *RBTN2*, *HOX11*	*HBZ*, *CCR4*

HSTL hepatosplenic T-cell lymphoma, *T-PLL* T-cell prolymphocytic leukemia [18], *T-LGL* T-cell large granular lymphocyte leukemia [12], *T-ALL* T-cell acute lymphocytic leukemia, *ATLL* adult T-cell leukemia/lymphoma [19], *TCR* T-cell receptor

HSTL is most commonly of the γ/δ TCR type; however, in cases of α/β TCR subtype, T-LGL leukemia may be considered. Both can have sinusoidal infiltration of the spleen, occur in the presence of autoimmunity, are rarely associated with lymphadenopathy, have rarely azurophilic granules noted in HSTL, both are positive for cytotoxic markers (perforin expression favoring T-LGL), and can have *STAT3* and *STAT5B* mutations [3]. T-LGL is usually indolent and in older patients, while HSTL is more aggressive and usually in younger populations. However, T-LGL leukemia can present in younger patients with a subset having aggressive features that are commonly *STAT5b* positive, which can be particularly troubling when trying to tease these two entities apart. Cytogenetic studies may be of some utility in this situation as isochromosome (7q) is thought to be only present in HSTL, and identification of this chromosomal abnormality would favor HSTL.

The cytology of HSTL cells can be deceiving. In some cases the lymphoma cells have a high nuclear-to-cytoplasmic ratio and can mimic leukemic myeloid blasts [2]. In this setting acute myeloid leukemia may be considered; however, true myeloid blasts will not be increased. Flow cytometry and immunohistochemistry can be used to differentiate the HSTL cells from myeloid blasts [11].

1. Hepatosplenic T-cell lymphoma (HSTL) is described as a subtype of aggressive peripheral T-cell lymphoma. Typical cases present with hepatic or splenic enlargement and bone marrow infiltrate.
2. The majority of HSTL is γ/δ T-cell origin and the remaining is α/β type.
3. HSTL cells lack azurophilic granules, primarily involve sinuses and cords of the red pulp of the spleen and eventually diffuse replacement of the spleen. Similarly, in the liver the lymphoma cells are seen invading the cords and sinusoids. Portal and periportal involvement may be present; however, it is not predominant.
4. Isochromosome 7q is found in 50% of HSTL.
5. It is critical to distinguish between HSTL and T-LGL leukemia given their different clinical courses and outcomes. Phenotypically, the HSTL cells usually show double negative (CD4/CD8) population that express a mature non-activated cytotoxic T-cell immunophenotype with expression of TIA-1 and granzyme M and negative for perforin. T-LGL leukemia is typically CD8 positive and express perforin as well as TIA.

References

1. Yabe M, Miranda RN, Medeiros LJ. Hepatosplenic T-cell lymphoma: a review of clinicopathologic features, pathogenesis, and prognostic factors. Hum Pathol. 2018;74:5–16.
2. Medeiros L, O'Malley D, Caraway N, Vega F, Elenitoba-Johnson K, Lim M. AFIP atlas of tumor pathology. Washington, DC: American Registry of Pathology; 2017.
3. Swerdlow SHCE, Harris NL, Jaffe ES, Pileri SA, Stein H, Thiele J, Arber DA, Hasserjian RP, Le Beau MM, Orazi A, Siebert R. WHO classification of tumours of haematopoietic and lymphoid tissues. Lyon: International Agency for Research on Cancer; 2017.
4. McThenia SS, Rawwas J, Oliveira JL, Khan SP, Rodriguez V. Hepatosplenic gammadelta T-cell lymphoma of two adolescents: case report and retrospective literature review in children, adolescents, and young adults. Pediatr Transplant. 2018;22:e13213.
5. Belhadj K, Reyes F, Farcet JP, Tilly H, Bastard C, Angonin R, Deconinck E, Charlotte F, Leblond V, Labouyrie E, others. Hepatosplenic gammadelta T-cell lymphoma is a rare clinicopathologic entity with poor outcome: report on a series of 21 patients. Blood. 2003;102:4261–9.
6. Yabe M, Medeiros LJ, Tang G, Wang SA, K PP, Routbort M, Bhagat G, Bueso-Ramos CE, Jorgensen JL, Luthra R, others. Dyspoietic changes associated with hepatosplenic T-cell lymphoma are not a manifestation of a myelodysplastic syndrome: analysis of 25 patients. Hum Pathol. 2016;50:109–17.
7. Mavilia M, McAuliffe A, Hafeez S, Vaziri H. Hepatosplenic T cell lymphoma: a unifying entity in a patient with hemolytic anemia, massive splenomegaly, and liver dysfunction. Clin J Gastroenterol. 2018;11:364–70.
8. Shi Y, Wang E. Hepatosplenic T-cell lymphoma: a clinicopathologic review with an emphasis on diagnostic differentiation from other T-cell/natural killer-cell neoplasms. Arch Pathol Lab Med. 2015;139:1173–80.
9. Vega F, Medeiros LJ, Gaulard P. Hepatosplenic and other gammadelta T-cell lymphomas. Am J Clin Pathol. 2007;127:869–80.
10. Iijima S, Chiba T, Maruyama K, Saito K, Kobayashi K, Yamagishi Y, Shibahara J, Takayama N, Shiokawa Y, Nagane M. Hepatosplenic gammadelta T cell lymphoma involving the brain. World Neurosurg. 2018;118:139–42.
11. Pizzi M, Covey S, Mathew S, Liu YC, Ruan J, Leonard JP, Chadburn A. Hepatosplenic T-cell lymphoma mimicking acute myeloid leukemia. Clin Lymphoma Myeloma Leuk. 2016;16:e47–50.
12. Lamy T, Moignet A, Loughran TP Jr. LGL leukemia: from pathogenesis to treatment. Blood. 2017;129:1082–94.
13. Wlodarska I, Martin-Garcia N, Achten R, De Wolf-Peeters C, Pauwels P, Tulliez M, de Mascarel A, Briere J, Patey M, Hagemeijer A, Gaulard P. Fluorescence in situ hybridization study of chromosome 7 aberrations in hepatosplenic T-cell lymphoma: isochromosome 7q as a common abnormality accumulating in forms with features of cytologic progression. Genes Chromosomes Cancer. 2002;33:243–51.
14. Alonsozana EL, Stamberg J, Kumar D, Jaffe ES, Medeiros LJ, Frantz C, Schiffer CA, O'Connell BA, Kerman S, Stass SA, others. Isochromosome 7q: the primary cytogenetic abnormality in hepatosplenic gammadelta T cell lymphoma. Leukemia. 1997;11:1367–72.
15. Mandava S, Sonar R, Ahmad F, Yadav AK, Chheda P, Ramani M, Gupta AD, Das BR. Cytogenetic and molecular characterization of a hepatosplenic T-cell lymphoma: report of a novel chromosomal aberration. Cancer Genet. 2011;204:103–7.
16. McKinney M, Moffitt AB, Gaulard P, Travert M, De Leval L, Nicolae A, Raffeld M, Jaffe ES, Pittaluga S, Xi L, others. The genetic basis of hepatosplenic T-cell lymphoma. Cancer Discov. 2017;7:369–79.
17. Nicolae A, Xi L, Pittaluga S, Abdullaev Z, Pack SD, Chen J, Waldmann TA, Jaffe ES, Raffeld M. Frequent STAT5B mutations in gammadelta hepatosplenic T-cell lymphomas. Leukemia. 2014;28:2244–8.
18. Stengel A, Kern W, Zenger M, Perglerova K, Schnittger S, Haferlach T, Haferlach C. Genetic characterization of T-PLL reveals two major biologic subgroups and JAK3 mutations as prognostic marker. Genes Chromosomes Cancer. 2016;55:82–94.
19. Matutes E. Adult T-cell leukaemia/lymphoma. J Clin Pathol. 2007;60:1373–7.

Ling Zhang, Lugen Chen, and Serhan Alkan

Introduction

T-cell large granular lymphocytic leukemia (T-cell LGLL) is a clonal proliferation of circulating effector memory cytotoxic T-cells. It is often associated with autoimmune disorders. Neutropenia, secondary infection, and splenomegaly are the common clinical features. Anemia and thrombocytopenia can occur. Hepatomegaly and lymph node involvement are seen with an aggressive variant. The majority of T-LGLL appears more common in the elderly, with median age of 65, and has an indolent clinical course. Only 10% of patients died of disease's complication, e.g., severe infection. The median survival of T-LGLL is more than 10 years. It was previously proposed that a sustained antigen stimulation leads to an altered apoptotic pathway of LGLs. Recently people recognized that increased cytokine release (e.g., interleukin IL15) and acquired somatic mutations in *signal transducer and activator of transcription 3 (STAT3) and 5B (STAT5B)* or tumor necrosis factor alpha-induced protein 3 (*TNFA-IP3*) are the potent drivers of disease process. Immunophenotypically T-cell LGLLs are surface CD3 (+), dim CD5 (+), dim CD7 (+), CD8 (+), CD57 (+), and TCR $\alpha\beta$ (+) or $\gamma\delta$ (+) with partially coexpressing CD16. T-cell receptor (TCR) genes that are frequently rearranged. There are no recurrent cytogenetic abnormalities identified. However, notably approximately 50% of T-LGLL patients harbor *STAT3, STAT5B, TNF-AIP3* mutations, which may be helpful to distinguish between T-LGLL and reactive LGL expansions. The chapter will focus on the disease course of hepatosplenic involvement by T-LGLL.

Definition

According to 2016 World Health Organization classification of tumors of hematopoietic and lymphoid tissues, T-cell LGLL is defined by chronic lymphoproliferative disorder derived from terminally differentiated effector memory cytotoxic T-cells (CTLs) and clinically characterized by sustained cytopenia (> 6 months), splenomegaly, and persistent increase of circulating large granular lymphocytes (LGLs) (2×10^9/L) without any explainable etiology. It is often associated with autoimmune disorders [1–3]. A lower number of clonal T-LGLs (less than 1×10^9/L, usually >0.5×10^9/L) (normal count of T-LGLs in peripheral blood <0.3×10^9/L) in patients with symptomatic cytopenia or autoimmune disorder such as rheumatoid arthritis is also considered diagnostic for T-LGLL [3–7].

Epidemiology

Based on the 2010–2011 US Surveillance, Epidemiology and End Results (SEER) registration data, the incidence rate of T-cell LGLL is extremely low, accounting for 0.2 cases per 1,000,000 individuals [8]. Among all chronic lymphoproliferative disorders, LGLL represents approximately 2–5% of patients diagnosed in the United States and 5–6% in Asia [3, 9]. Although T-LGLL can affect subjects of any age, it is commonly diagnosed in adults, age between 45 and 75 years (median 65 years) [1], and has an indolent clinical course with median overall survival of >10 years [10]. In rare occasions (approximately 3%), T-cell LGLL is diagnosed in younger individuals (age <25 years). In general, there is no gender predilection [1]. Splenic involvement is found in approximately 35% of patients (ranging from 20% to 50%),

L. Zhang
Department of Pathology, H. Lee Moffitt Cancer Center and Research Institute, Tampa, FL, USA
e-mail: ling.zhang@moffitt.org

L. Chen
Department of Pathology, Tampa General Hospital, Tampa, FL, USA

S. Alkan (✉)
Department of Pathology and Laboratory Medicine, Cedars-Sinai Medical Center, Los Angeles, CA, USA
e-mail: serhan.alkan@cshs.org

© Springer Nature Switzerland AG 2020
L. Zhang et al. (eds.), *Diagnostic Pathology of Hematopoietic Disorders of Spleen and Liver*,
https://doi.org/10.1007/978-3-030-37708-3_10

while hepatic involvement has been reported but incidence rate is not well documented. T-LGLL is rarely presented with lymphadenopathy [4, 7].

Etiology and Pathogenesis

The exact etiopathogenesis of T-LGLL is unknown. However, it has been observed that abnormal or clonal proliferation of antigen-primed nature CTLs are able to escape activation-induced cell death (AICD) pathway and become long-term competent. Leukemic T-LGLs, similar to their normal counterpart, also show activation of multiple survival signalings [11–13]. Clinically T-cell LGLL is frequently associated with autoimmune disorders such as rheumatoid arthritis, Sjogren's syndrome, Felty's syndrome, systemic lupus erythematosus (SLE), pulmonary artery hypertension, and status post treatment response to antineoplastic or monoclonal antibody therapy and hematopoietic stem cell transplantation. It is hypothesized that T-LGLL occurs as a result of long-standing antigen stimulation with putative autoantigen or viral antigen and dysimmunoregulation leading to resistance to FAS-/FASL-mediated apoptosis and ultimately causing oligoclonal expansion of T-LGLs [3, 4, 6, 14–18]. Accompanying monoclonal gammopathy (MGUS) and B-cell lymphoproliferative disorders (e.g., chronic lymphocytic leukemia, follicular lymphoma, and hairy cell leukemia) are not uncommon, accounting for 3–9% and 2–5% of all T-LGLL, respectively, which could also support the above hypothesis of antigen stimulation [3, 6, 19–22]. Soluble Fas-L was found to be elevated in patients with T-LGLL [18]. As a consequence of chronic exposure to exogenous antigens and release of inflammatory cytokines such as IL15 and platelet-derived growth factor (PDGF), the survival pathways including JAK/STAT, MAPK, MEK1, RAS-RAF-1, PI3K (phosphatidylinositol 3-kinase)-Akt, NFkB (nuclear factor-kB), sphingolipid kinase 1 and NF kappa B are constitutively activated, eventually leading to malignant phenotype of T-LGLL [4, 13, 23–27]. Among the aforementioned pathways, it is recently consented that clonal expansion of T-LGLs with JAK/STAT (Janus kinase/signal transducer and activator of transcription) activation is the key mechanism for development of T-LGLL [4]. *STAT3* gene mutations have been reported in approximately 1/3 of T-LGLLs, and the key element in the pathway, STAT3 protein, is constitutively activated in T-LGLL when compared to normal circulating T-LGLs in healthy donors [12, 13, 28]. A blockage of STAT3 makes apoptosis restored in T-LGLs regardless of the mutation status [12]. The altered STAT3 signaling results in (1) sustained survival in T-LGLs via updated Mcl-1, IFN, MIP, and macrophage protein and resistances to apoptosis mediated by FAS/FAS-L and (2) release of proinflammatory cytokines (IL1β, IL1Rα, IL8, IL10,

IL12, IL18, INF-γ, RANTES, MIP1-alpha, and MIP1-beta) that attach to hematopoietic precursors, leading to alteration of immune response and related cytopenia [4, 23, 29, 30].

The spleen appears to be reservoir for T-LGLs, and the number of LGLs is significantly expanded during T-LGLLs leading to splenomegaly. However, the exact mechanism of splenic T-LGLL is unclear.

Clinical Features

There is a subpopulation of patients with T-LGLL that is asymptomatic at time of diagnosis [31], while the majority of them show symptoms related to cytopenias such as recurrent infections involving the skin, subcutaneous tissue, and urinary tract secondary to neutropenia and petechiae due to decreased platelets. Rarely bacteremia or perirectal abscesses can happen. Neutropenia is in variable degree with 16–28% of cases less than <0.5 × 10⁹/L, while anemia may or may not be present [32, 33]. When associated with hemolytic anemia or pure red blood cell aplasia, the subset of patients (approximately 20%) can often be accompanied with moderate to severe anemia [2]. Constitutional symptoms such as fevers, chills, and night sweats are noted in 20–30% of cases [31]. Approximately 20–30% of T-LGLL patients have palpable splenomegaly [34] and 10% of the patients have hepatomegaly [31, 35]. Lymphadenopathy is occasionally reported.

Increased number of circulating T-LGLs often is an incidental laboratory finding during work-up of asymptomatic lymphocytosis or investigation of cytopenias. Although according to WHO T-LGLL is defined as a clonal proliferation of T-LGLs greater than 2 × 10⁹/L lasting more than 6 months after exclusion of reactive T-LGL proliferation, clinically T-LGL count <1 × 10⁹/L can be seen in up to one third of patients with T-LGLL. A new cut-off LGL count of 0.5 × 10⁹/L is arbitrarily selected as the upper normal range of LGLs observed in normal subjects [5, 10, 31]. The LGL count beyond 0.5 × 10⁹/L has been adopted for diagnosis of T-LGLL for those who present with laboratory abnormalities or systemic symptoms characteristic for T-LGLL [32], in particular those with autoimmune disorder. Of note, in these patients with T-LGLL, the circulating LGL cells often constitute >50% of the circulating lymphocytes. Thus, to diagnose T-LGLL with lower LGL count, it is needed to correlate with clinical presentations and comprehensive immunophenotyping and molecular studies.

Initial evaluation of complete blood count with differential (CBC/Diff) and a review of peripheral blood smear are the most two important diagnostic methods. Neutropenia is the most common cytopenia that accompanies expanded clonal T-LGL cells in peripheral blood. It is not uncommon to see severe neutropenia with an absolute neutrophil count (ANC) less than 0.5 × 10⁹/L [3]. Since patients with T-LGLL can also have other autoimmune disorders, laboratory studies should include rheumatoid factor, autoantibodies (antinuclear antibody, antineutrophil antibody, antiplatelet antibody), circulating immune complexes, beta 2 macroglobulin, direct Coombs test, soluble Fas-ligand and protein electrophoresis for hyper- or hypogammaglobulinemia, and monoclonal gammopathy, which are often elevated in patients with T-LGLL [21, 36–38].

Laboratory virology tests commonly include the DNA copies of Epstein-Barr virus, cytomegalovirus, serology evaluation of anti-hepatitis A/B/C antibodies, enzyme-linked immunosorbent assay (ELISA) or Western blotting for human immunodeficiency virus (HIV), etc. to exclude secondary T-LGL proliferation. Parvovirus B-19 needs to be tested when bone marrow shows an erythroid aplasia. As far as human T-cell leukemia virus 1 (HTLV-1) is concerned, there is no definitive confirmation that this virus plays an important role in etiopathogenesis of T-LGLL. However, in selected patients from regions with high prevalence of HTLV-1 infection, this test can be useful [33].

Morphology

Gross and Radiological Findings

The spleen is moderately enlarged with median weight of 1300 grams [39]. The surface of the spleen is smooth, and cut surface is uniformly pink-pan with expanded red pulps with or without decreased white pulps.

Microscopic Findings

Peripheral Blood Smear Normal circulating LGLs are 15–18 μm in size, round to orally indented nuclei and contain reddish cytoplasmic cytotoxic granules and pale cytoplasm. T-LGL cells in patients with T-LGLL could resemble their normal counterparts without significant morphologic differences between each other. Peripheral blood smear of patients with T-LGLL reveals T-LGL cells are of medium size with round to oval nuclei, condense chromatin, smooth nuclear contour, inconspicuous nucleoli, and a moderate amount of clear cytoplasm containing rare to abundant reddish cytotoxic granules (Fig. 10.1). However, morphologic variants are also identified [31, 38, 40]. In some occasions cytotoxic granules in T-LGLs are decreased or even absent. In addition aggressive variant of T-LGLL it demonstrates more overt cytologic atypia, including nuclear irregularity, visible to prominent nucleoli, reduced cytoplasmic-to-nuclear ratio, and less condense chromatin (Fig. 10.2).

Bone Marrow The bone marrow aspirate smears from patients with T-LGLL contain a population of LGLs, morphologically similar to those noted in peripheral blood smear. These LGLs are admixed with other hematopoietic elements including normal-appearing reactive lymphocytes, which make it difficult to tell them apart, particularly when there is only a low-level involvement by T-LGLL. In view of core biopsy, the bone marrow involvement of T-LGLL is insidious, predominantly in interstitial or perisinusoidal distribution (Fig. 10.3). Without additional immunohistochemical staining, these T-LGL cells cannot be well recognized. T-LGLL with associated reactive lymphoid aggregates, monoclonal B-cell lymphocytosis, or polyclonal or monoclonal plasmacytosis has often been reported [19, 20]. Increased reticulin fibrosis is observed in a subset of T-LGLL patients [41]. The degree of bone marrow involvement by T-LGLL is variable, but most commonly 10–15% of total cellularity that could be discordant with the percentage involvement (the count of T-LGLL) and the degree of cytopenia in peripheral blood. Decreased myeloid precursors or myeloid maturation arrest, along with hypercellularity, is not uncommon, identified in 55% of patients with T-LGLL [21]. Moreover, T-LGLL can also be associated with reduction of single or multiple lineage hematopoietic precursors, resulting in lineage-specific hypoplasia [42, 43]. Sometimes confluent lymphoid infiltrate is also seen in indolent T-LGLL (Fig. 10.3). Aplastic anemia, pure red blood cell aplasia, paroxysmal nocturnal hemoglobinuria (PNH), and hypoplastic myelodysplastic syndromes (MDS) are the common hematopoietic disorders that coexist with T-LGLL that can be diagnosed by careful examination of bone marrow along with ancillary tests. These diseases can manifest with small LGL clones or develop overt disease of LGLL.

Lymph Node Nodal involvement by T-LGLL is very rare usually indicating more aggressive clinical behavior or transformation [44]. Without immunophenotyping morphologically the transformed could sometimes look like peripheral T cell lymphoma (PTCL) [44–46]. Occasionally the aggressive variant of LGLL also manifests with normal LGL morphology in lymph node. Then it would be misinterpreted with reactive counterparts. However, overtly increased number of peripheral LGLs associated with splenomegaly and cytopenia is helpful to decide whether there is lymph node involvement by T-LGLL.

Spleen and Liver Splenic involvement of T-LGLL is very common. The T-LGLL cells are mainly found in red pulps resulting in expansion of red pulps, while white pulps are identifiable or focally decreased depending on the level of involvement (Fig. 10.4). Focally white pulps could be dis-

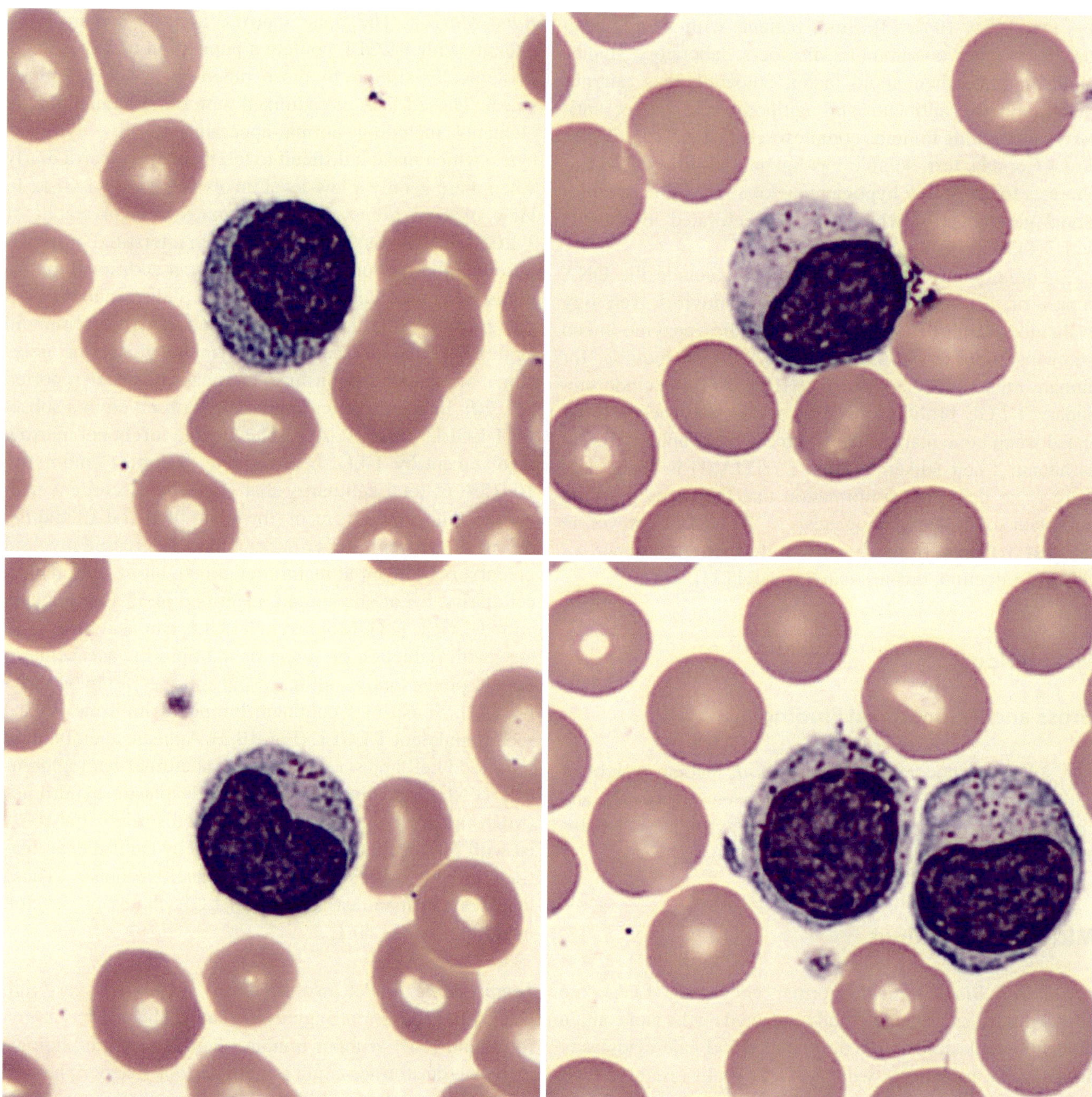

Fig. 10.1 Peripheral blood CellaVision from a patient with T-LGLL shows many small- to medium-sized mature-appearing lymphoid cells with round to oval nuclei, dense chromatin, invisible nucleoli, and cytoplasmic reddish granules

appearing when the degree of involvement is significant. T-LGLL cells in the spleen are also found in perisinusoidal arrangement. By touch imprint the morphology of T-LGLs is similar to those in the peripheral blood, medium in size and mature in appearance. There is a variable degree of cytologic atypia identified in either conventional or aggressive variant of T-LGLL. It is imperative to distinguish between splenic involvement of T-LGLL and hepatosplenic T-cell lymphoma (HSTCL). A preexisting T-LGLL history is usually a key diagnostic clue, while HSTCL shows more aggressive clinical nature. Furthermore, attention should also be paid to examine additional malignancies aside from T-LGLL. A concurrent diagnosis of T-LGLL with low-grade B-cell lymphoma and gamma heavy chain diseases has been reported [47]. Liver biopsy is rarely performed for diagnostic purpose of T-LGLL. Microscopic examination of the liver biopsies shows sinusoidal and portal infiltrates of T-LGLL.

Immunophenotyping

Flow Cytometry Analysis

T-LGLL cells usually express the following immunophenotype: CD2+, surface CD3+, CD8+, CD57+, dim CD5+, dim CD7+, CD45RA+, and HLA-DR+ [38, 40, 48] and CD4- and CD56- (Fig. 10.5). Of note, T-LGLL cases with expression of CD16 and CD57 account for more than ¾ of the cases, while CD56 is infrequently detected (reportedly 20%) [10, 31, 32]. Some study shows that approximately 90% of T-LGLL cells express surface CD57 marker. Other NK-associated markers CD16 and CD94/NKG2A are also identified in 80% and 50% of T-LGLL cells, respectively [32]; decreased or lost expression of other pan-T-cell markers such as CD2 (20% of patients) or CD3 (a minor subset) has also been observed in addition to decreased CD5 and CD7 expression [49, 50]. Loss of surface CD3 should be carefully separated from NK cells. Gamma-delta variant of T-LGLL is present in a minority of patients (<5%) [51, 52]. Phenotypically the variant of T-LGLL expresses surface CD3, dim CD5, dim CD7, and TCR γδ (Fig. 10.6). Additionally, dual CD4/CD8 negativity is the unique feature for the variant though dim CD8 expression has also been observed. Because lacking CD4 or dual CD4 and CD8 expression can also be HSTCL, a comprehensive phenotyping is necessary to distinguish between the two entities (see differential diagnosis) [53–55]. CD4+, dual CD4+/CD8+, and dual CD4-/CD8- (non-gamma-delta variant) T-LGLLs have been reported [1, 56, 57]. Keeping in mind there are overlapping immunophenotype features between reactive LGLs and T-LGLL. For example, weak expression of CD5 and CD7 can also be seen with reactive LGLs [58]. Correlation with clinical findings is needed to have an accurate diagnosis when a diagnosis of T-LGLL was previously established.

Of note, approximately 70% of LGLL cases display V beta restriction [59, 60, 61]. Although flow cytometric detection of variable β-chain repertoire is optional for assessment of clonality in addition to T-cell αβ and γδ gene rearrangement, the test is not widely used as a routine test.

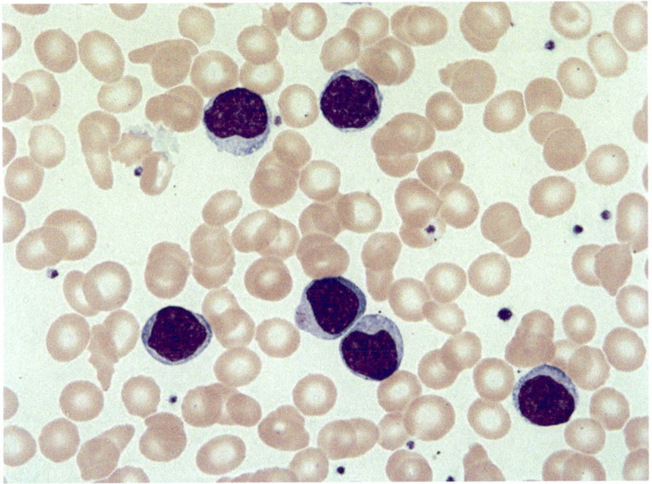

Fig. 10.2 T-LGLL with atypical cytology. Examination of the peripheral blood smear shows increased atypical lymphoid cells with decreased to absent cytotoxic granules; some shows irregular nuclear contour, visible to prominent nucleoli, and relatively reduced cytoplasmic-to-nuclear ratio (Wright stain, 1000×)

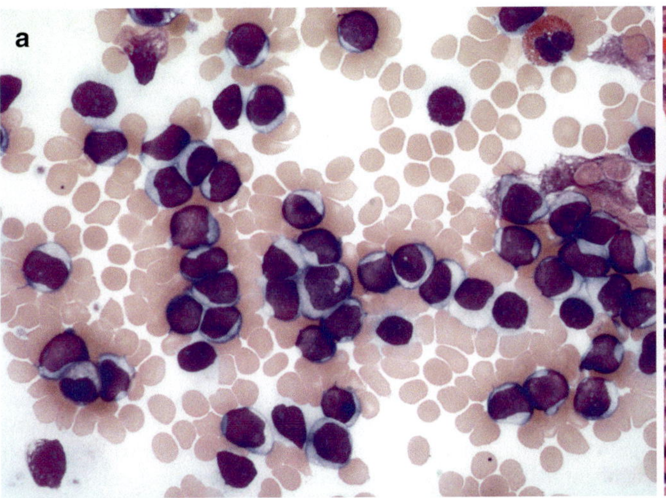
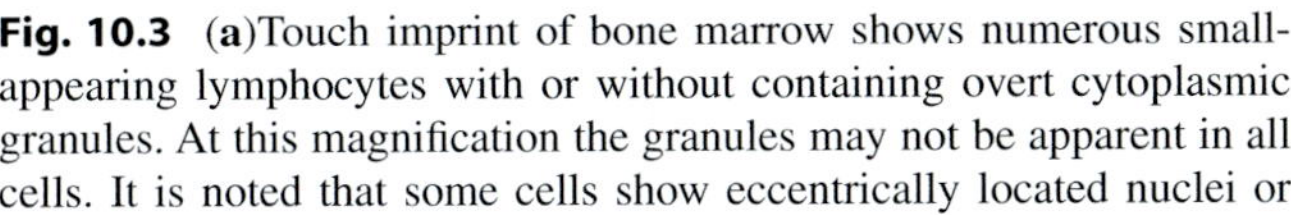
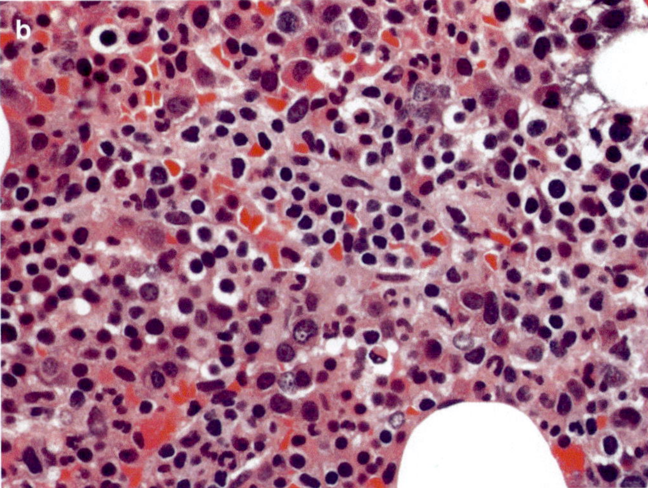

Fig. 10.3 (**a**)Touch imprint of bone marrow shows numerous small-appearing lymphocytes with or without containing overt cytoplasmic granules. At this magnification the granules may not be apparent in all cells. It is noted that some cells show eccentrically located nuclei or indented nuclear lobes (Wright Giemsa, 600×). (**b**)The submitted bone marrow core biopsy shows hypercellularity with interstitial or sinusoidal infiltration of atypical small lymphoid cells intermingling with background of trilineage hematopoietic precursors (H&E, 600×)

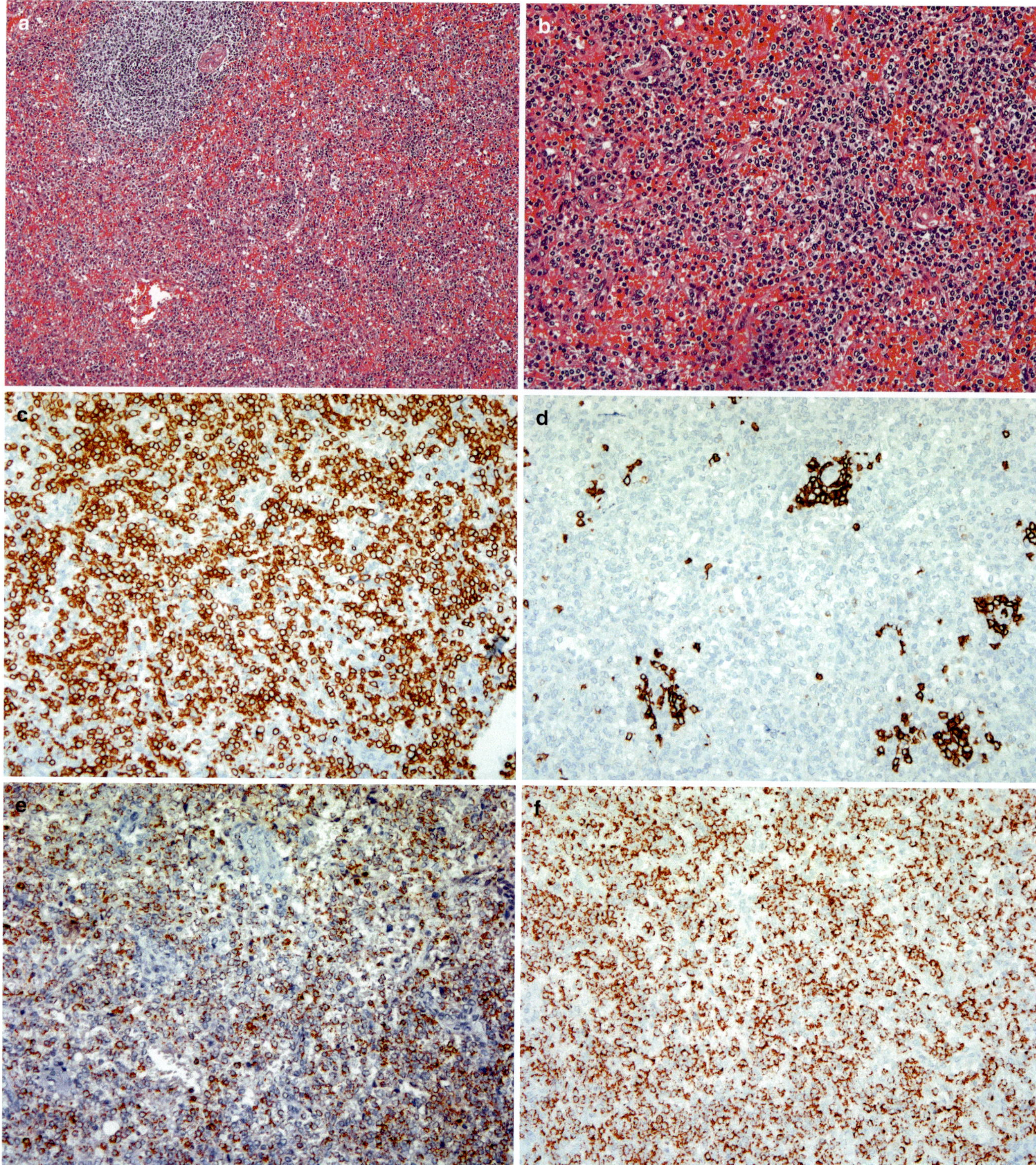

Fig. 10.4 A low-power view of splenic parenchyma (**a** and **b**; Wright Giemsa 100× and 200×) shows significant expansion of red pulp that are filled with small mature-appearing lymphoid cells, in a perisinusoidal distribution, associated with residual white pulp. These small-sized lymphoid cells show round to oval nuclei and scant eosinophilic to clear cytoplasm intermingled with sinus histiocytes and scattered mature plasma cells, endothelial cells, and red blood cells in intrasinusoidal space. (**c–f**) Immunohistochemical stains (immunoperoxidase, 200×) highlight the atypical lymphoid cells to be cytotoxic T-cell origin (**c**, CD3+; **e**, TIA+; and **f**, granzyme B+) and negative for CD20 (**d**)

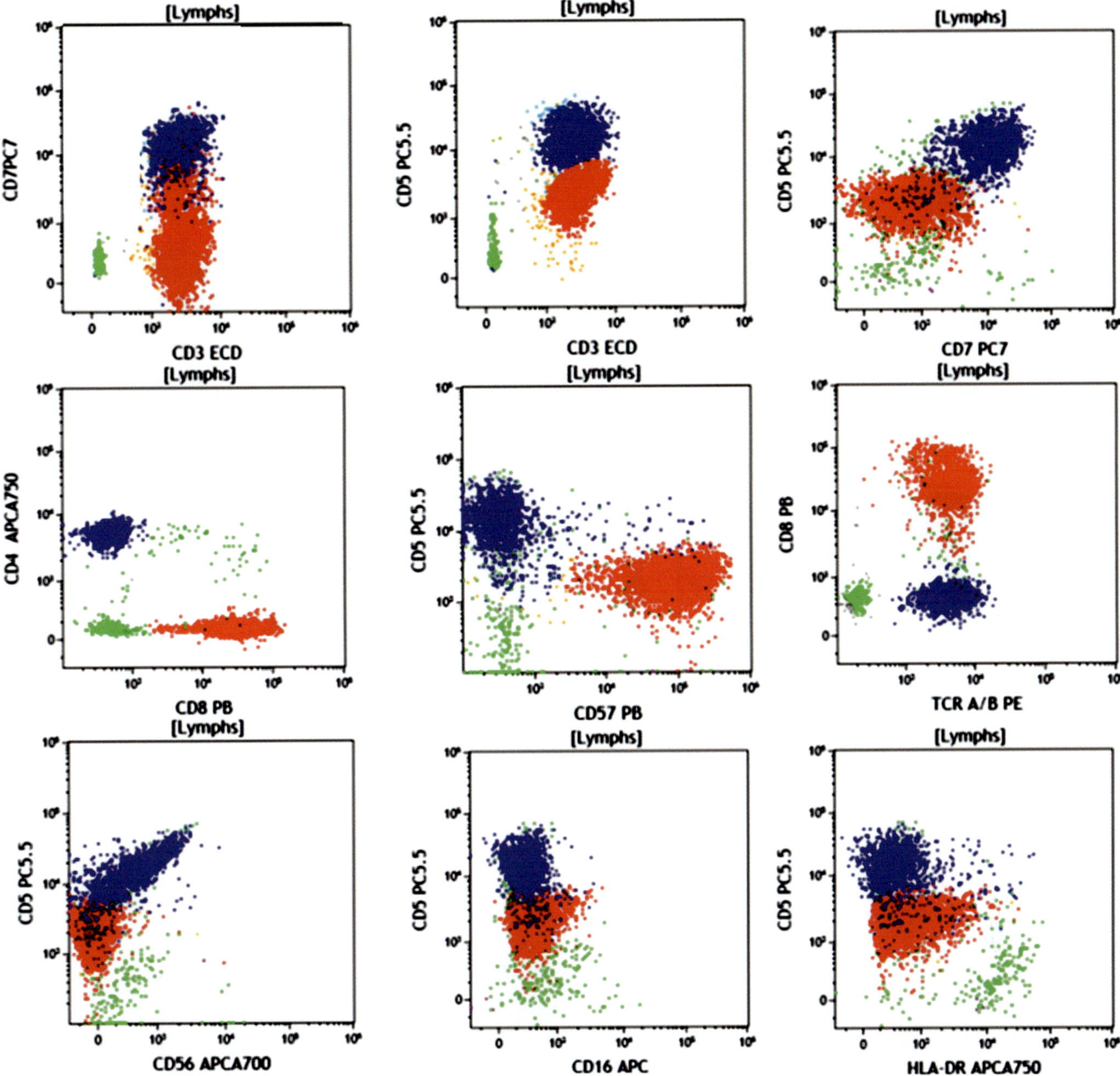

Fig. 10.5 Flow cytometric analysis reveals a distinct abnormal population of CD3+/CD8+ cytotoxic T-cells coexpressing CD2, CD57, TCRαβ, and dim HLA-DR with significantly decreased expression of CD5 and CD7

Immunohistochemical Staining

Using immunohistochemical (IHC) staining is more often ultilized in splenic sample than in bone marrow. In addition to aforementioned T-cell markers, IHC is particularly useful to detect cytotoxic granules including perforin, granzyme B, granzyme M, and TIA1 expressed in T-LGLL cells. Perforin, a member of serine protease family, functions as a pore-forming to induce cell lysis and release enzymes to the targeted cells [62]. Granzyme M or granzyme B is also a protease that leads to cell death via activating apoptotic pathway [63, 64]. TIA1 belongs to a member of a RNA-binding protein family that causes nucleolysis against cytotoxic lymphocyte target cells and eliminates LGL targeted cells [65, 66]. T-LGLL cells are immunophenotypically positive for CD2, CD3, CD8, CD57, TIA1, perforin, and granzyme B by IHC (Fig. 10.4) [38, 67, 68]. The IHC staining pattern is also useful to discriminate between active cytotoxic granules from splenic T-LGLL and inactive (immature) cytotoxic granules from HSTCL, which are usually TIA1(+), perforin(−), and granzyme B(−/+) [69–71].

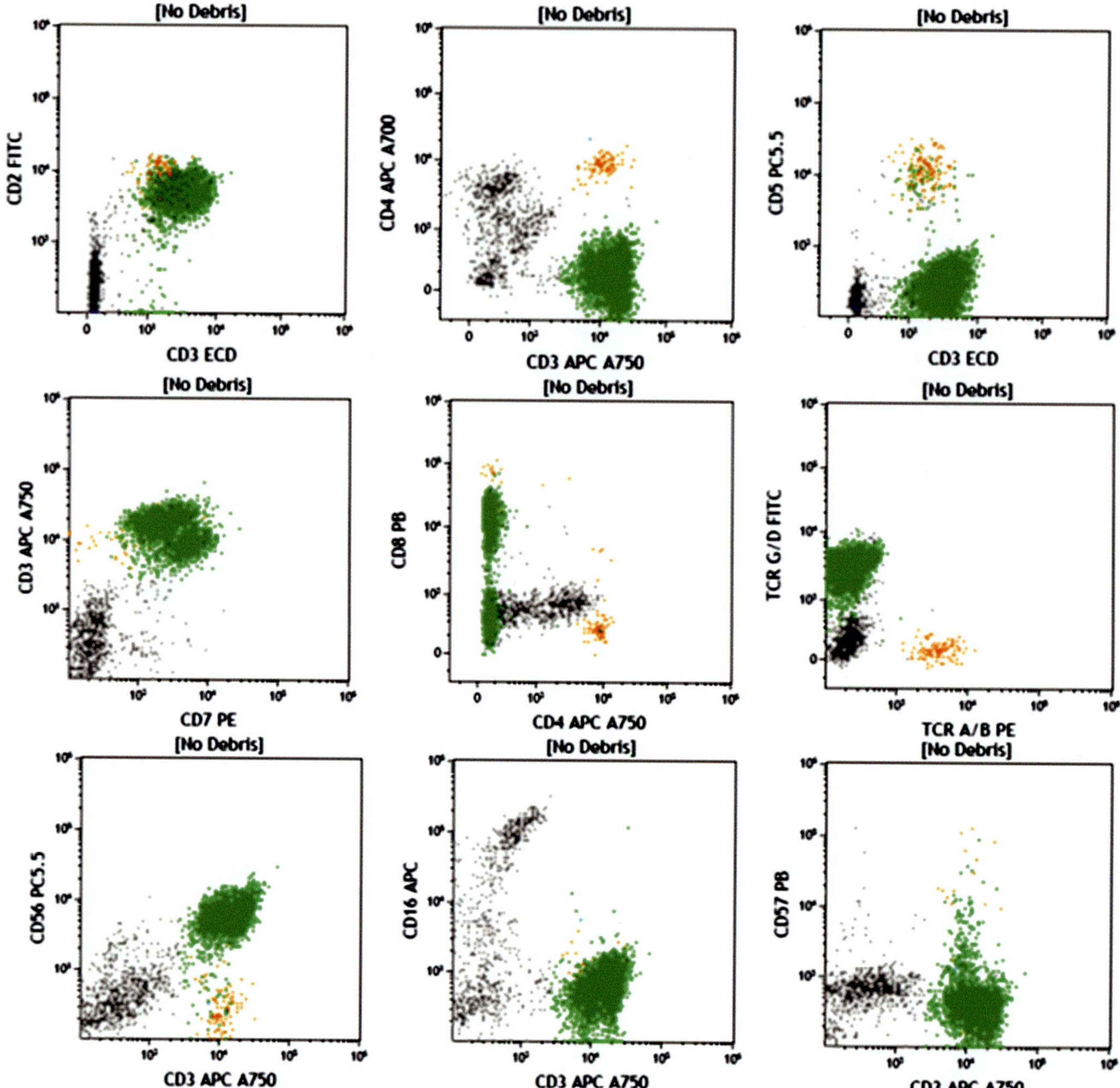

Fig. 10.6 Flow cytometry performed on peripheral blood from a patient with hepatosplenic gamma-delta T-cell lymphoma shows characteristic immunophenotypic findings: CD2+/surface CD3+/CD4-/CD5-/CD8-/TCRαβ/TCRγδ+/CD16-/CD56+/CD57-. In the present case, a subset of neoplastic T-cells shows no CD8 expression, while another subset of T-cells retains CD8 expression, which is not uncommon for the disease entity

Molecular Study

T-Cell Gene Rearrangements and Clonality of T-LGLL

The presence of clonal TCR gene rearrangement is also a feature of T-LGLL and may be useful to separate this disease from reactive LGL proliferations with increased circulating T-LGLs. However, interpretation of this test should be done with caution since a subset of T-LGLL patients does not exhibit TCR gene rearrangements [31, 32], while some reactive T-LGL proliferation could be monoclonal manifested by TCR gene rearrangements. Flow cytometry is an alternative way to identify T-cell clonality via measuring TCR beta V region restriction pattern although the method is not widely implicated [72, 73]. Traditionally, Southern Blot or PCR amplification of *TCR* genes are employed [31, 74]. How to correctly interpret the clonality remains challenging. A novel method of high-throughput sequencing by Next Generation of Sequening (NGS) of TCRβ gene might improve sensitivity of clonality testing in patients with T-LGLL [75].

Mutation Study

With expanded use of NGS, more variants have been detected in T-/NK cell lymphomas/leukemias. A number of gene mutations or alterations have been identified in NK/T-cell diseases such as *DDX3X, JAK3, STAT3, STAT5B, BCOR, MLL2, ASXL3, ARID1A,* and *EP300* [76]. It is noted that activation of the JAK/STAT pathway and overexpression of NK-κB and aurora kinase A play pistol roles in development of NK/T-cell lymphomas [77, 78] which could be attributed to mutations such as *JAK3, STAT3,* or *STAT5B* mutations [79–81]. *STAT3* mutations have been found frequently present in T-LGLL (25–78%, on average 50%) [12, 28, 82–84]. Mutated *STAT5B* gene is found in a minor subset (approximately 5%), which is mutual exclusively with *STAT3* mutations [83, 84]. Certain *STAT3* mutations may be predictable for a poorer therapeutic response, e.g., Y640E mutation to methotrexate as a frontline therapy, while N642 mutation is associated with an unfavorable clinical nature in CD3+/CD56+ aggressive T-LGLL [82, 85]. *STAT5B* mutation was also associated with aggressive CD3+/CD56+ T-LGLL [83, 86]. Tumor necrosis factor alpha-induced protein 3 (*TNFAIP*) mutation is detected in a small subset of T-LGLL (approximately 8%), which is an NF-kB signaling inhibitor [4]. Nonetheless, these mutations are not specific to T-LGLL, but may support a diagnosis of neoplastic LGL proliferation/leukemia over reactive LGL expansion if integrated with clinical and laboratory features.

Cytogenetic Study

Specific cytogenetic aberrations associated with T-LGLL have not been identified. A minority of cases (<10%) might harbor sporadic cytogenetic abnormalities involving 7p14-p15 (TCR-γ gene loci) and 14q11 (TCR-α/TCR-δ gene loci) [87]. The other abnormalities including +3, inv(4)(p14q12), del(5q), del(6)(q21), +8, inv(12p), inv(14q), +14, −X, or complex aberrations are present, however, of unclear clinical significance [2, 48, 88, 89].

Differential Diagnoses

Hepatosplenic T-Cell Lymphoma

Similar to T-LGLL, hepatosplenic T-cell lymphoma (HSTCL) may occur in immunocompromised subjects and manifest as cytopenias and hepatosplenomegaly [90]. The tissue-infiltrating pattern of HSTCL shows almost no differences from T-LGLL. Both neoplasms usually show interstitial and sinusoidal arrangement of T-cells and infrequent lymphoid aggregates in the bone marrow and liver and both cord and sinus involvement in the spleen [90]. Immunophenotyping is useful to distinguish between the two entities. HSTL frequently express T-cell receptor γδ phenotype, while a majority of T-LGLLs have αβ receptor expression [90]. Importantly, different from T-LGLL, HSTCL cells contain inactive cytotoxic granules in their cytoplasm that can be demonstrated by immunohistochemical study [70, 71]. HSTCL, frequently positive for surface CD2, CD3, and TCRγδ and negative for CD4, CD5, and CD8, could mimic T-LGLL, γδ variant. However, in contrast to T-LGLL, HSTL cells coexpress CD56, but lack CD57 expression that can be easily identified by flow cytometry study (Fig. 10.6). In addition, clinically HSTL shows a more aggressive clinical course and is often associated with HLH [90]. A multicenter study demonstrated that patients diagnosed with HSTCL often demonstrated massive hepatosplenomegaly, significantly increased atypical T-cells that are devoid of azurophilic cytoplasmic inclusion [53]. Moreover, cytogenetic abnormalities, in particular the presence of isochromosome 7q or other chromosome 7 anomalies, support a diagnosis of HSTL rather than T-LGLL [55, 91, 92].

Benign LGL Proliferation

There are many situations, e.g., post-viral infections (e.g., CMV, EBV, and hepatitis), post-solid organ or hematopoietic stem cell transplantation, post-immunotherapy, or concurrent with skin lesions, lymphomas, and solid tumors, that could link to proliferation of circulating LGLs, considering reactive processes [38, 93–97]. The count of LGLs in peripheral blood is usually less than $3–4 \times 10^9$/L, and the proliferation is usually polyclonal and lasts less than 6 months [31]. Increased T-LGL cells, monoclonal or polyclonal, can be seen in patients infected with a virus. In the viral situation, the increase of T-LGL is usually transient [98]. Importantly, benign LGL proliferation is not associated with cytopenia or splenomegaly.

Chronic Lymphoproliferation of NK Cells

Chronic lymphoproliferative disorder of NK cells (CLPD-NK) presents with sustainably increased circulating NK cells for more than 6 months after exclusion of viral infection and any other etiology. It is listed as a provisional entity in WHO classification. It is even rarer than T-LGLL [1, 99]. Clinically CLPD-NK has indolent clinical course with the median overall survival of 94% at 5 years, and it is usually diagnosed by flow cytometric analysis of peripheral blood and bone marrow specimens [100]. Hepatosplenic involvement is extremely rare. Similar to T-LGLL, CLPD-NK is also strongly associated with autoimmunity and hematopoietic neoplasms [100]. Immunophenotypically CLPD-NK is partially similar to T-LGLL by expressing CD16, CD8 (75%), and CD94 and being negative for CD56. These cells are unique by negative for surface CD3 expression and absence of expression of the KIR CD158a, CD158b, and CD158e and TCR $\alpha\beta$ or $\gamma\delta$ [32]. Also unlike aggressive NK cell leukemia, the majority of which display a clonal episomal form. EBV genome is never identified in CLPD-NK [99].

Aggressive NK Cell Leukemia

Aggressive NK cell leukemia (ANKL) is an extremely rare hematopoietic malignancy with a strong link to EBV infection or reactivation [101, 102]. ANKL is usually identified with rapidly increased circulating atypical lymphoid cells, hepatosplenomegaly, and bone marrow involvement and often associated with hemophagocytic lymphohistiocytosis (HLH) [103]. Different from T-LGLL (median age of 65), ANKL often occurs in younger adults (median age of 39 years) with equal male-to-female ratio. The clinical outcome is very poor with a median survival of about 2 months [1, 101, 102, 104, 105]. When compared with T-LGLL, ANKL cells usually show more atypical or bizarre cytology such as enlarged cell size, markedly irregular or lobated nuclei, frequent mitosis, karyolysis, karyorrhexis, pyknosis, and increased apoptosis although sometimes ANKL could look more plain resembling reactive LGLs. In addition, the presence of fever of unknown origin, progressive cytopenia (e.g., anemia, thrombocytopenia) and accompanying liver dysfunction, rapid hepatosplenomegaly, disseminated intravascular coagulation (DIC), HLH, and multiorgan failure is more associated with ANKL rather than T-LGLL.

ANKL also shows unique immunophenotype to distinguish from T-LGLL by lacking expression of surface CD3, CD4, CD5, CD8, CD57, TCR$\alpha\beta$, and TCR$\gamma\delta$ but strongly expressing CD45, CD2, CD7, cytoplasmic CD3, and CD56. CD8 can be variably positive in a subset of ANKL cells. ANKL cells show intact CD94 but have an entire loss of NK cell receptors (CD158a/h, CD158b, and CD158e) and a partial loss of CD161 in a subset of cases [106]. TCR gene germline configurations help to confirm the neoplastic cells to be of NK cell origin (CLPD-NK and ANKL) but not always the cases as the TCR β or γ gene rearrangement could be from the by-standing T-cells as a consequence of reactive process in tumor microenvironment [1, 107] (Table 10.1).

Peripheral T-Cell Lymphoma, NOS

Peripheral T-cell lymphoma, not otherwise specified (PTCL-NOS) is a nodal base lymphoma and rarely shows with splenic involvement [108]. The majority of PTCL, NOS is CD4 positive and CD8 negative. CD8 positive PTCL, NOS have also been reported in 15–30% of cases [109, 110]. In contrast to T-LGLL with peripheral blood, bone marrow, and splenic manifestation, PTCL, NOS is usually characteristic by generalized lymphadenopathy [1]. In addition, PTCL, NOS usually exhibits more aggressive clinical course than T-LGLL. Concurrent T-LGLL or clonal T-LGL proliferation with any subtype of PTCL, NOS or hematological malignancy is not uncommon [16, 111].

Table 10.1 Key clinical features identified in T-LGLL, CLPD-NK, ANKL, and HSTCL

	T-LGLL	CLPD-NK	ANKL	HSTCL
Cytopenia	Present	Present	Present, usually pancytopenia	Present
Circulating LGL	Granulated or partially loss of cytoplasmic granules	Granulated or partially loss of cytoplasmic granules	Plain or markedly atypical forms	Atypical lymphoid cells, some with fine cytoplasmic granules
Bone marrow infiltration	Interstitial and focally aggregate	Interstitial and focally aggregate	Interstitial and focally aggregate, often associated with hemophagocytosis	Sinusoidal infiltration of atypical lymphoid cells
Splenomegaly	Frequently	Infrequently	Frequent	All the time
Hepatomegaly	Can present	Can present	Frequent	Frequent
Immunophenotyping	CD2$^+$/sCD3$^+$/CD8$^+$/ CD5^{dim+}/CD7^{dim+}/ CD16^{-sub+}/CD56$^-$/CD57$^+$/ HLA-DR$^+$/TCR$\alpha\beta^+$	CD2$^+$/sCD3$^-$/cCD3$^+$/ CD4$^-$/CD8$^{-/+}$/CD5$^-$/CD7$^+$/ CD16$^+$/CD56$^{-/dim+}$/CD57$^-$/ HLA-DR$^{+/-}$/TCR$\alpha\beta^-$/TCR$\gamma\delta^-$	CD2$^+$/sCD3$^-$/cCD3$^+$/CD4$^-$/ CD8$^{-/+}$/CD7$^{+/-}$/CD16$^{-/dim+}$/ CD56^{b+}/CD57$^-$/HLD-DR$^+$/ TCR$\alpha\beta^-$/TCR$\gamma\delta^-$	CD2$^+$/sCD3$^+$/CD4$^-$/CD8$^{-/dim+}$/ CD5$^+$/CD7$^+$/CD16$^-$/CD56$^-$/ CD57$^-$/HAL-DR$^{+/-}$/TCR$\alpha\beta^-$/ TCR$\gamma\delta^+$
PCR for TCR gene rearrangement	TCR$\alpha\beta$ and/or TCR $\gamma\delta$ gene rearranged	TCR gene germline configuration	TCR gene germline configuration	TCR $\gamma\delta$ and/or TCR$\alpha\beta$ genes rearranged
Clinical outcomes	OS 7 years	OS >7 years	OS 2.2 months	OS 28.3 months

Prognosis and Treatment

Many patients with T-LGLL are put on observation when they are asymptomatic or have a mild degree of cytopenias. Severe neutropenia with absolute neutrophil count (ANC) level of 500/uL, moderate neutropenia (ANC >500 but <1500/uL) with clinical symptoms such as recurrent infection, anemia (symptomatic or required transfusion), and accompanying autoimmune disorders are indicated for treatment. The mainstream therapy includes methotrexate, cyclophosphamide, and cyclosporine [112]. Splenectomy is indicated when patients have severe refractory cytopenias, resistant to conventional therapy, or present with a symptomatic splenomegaly [39]. Splenectomy will improve the counts and symptoms (e.g., fullness, early satiety, and pain-related to enlarged spleen) in the majority of patients [39].

Diagnostic Caveats

1. T-LGLL has an indolent clinical course that is often manifested by asymptomatic or symptomatic cytopenia (predominantly neutropenia) and recurrent bacterial infection.
2. Splenomegaly, with or without hepatomegaly, is one of common clinical features of T-LGLL. Splenectomy is indicated for the patients who are refractory to conventional therapy or symptomatic splenomegaly. Peripheral blood specimen is usually harvested for flow cytometric analysis of circulating T-LGLs. Bone marrow, but not liver biopsy, is frequently performed for diagnosis of T-LGLL.
3. T-LGLL is commonly associated with autoimmune disorders such as rheumatoid arthritis, Felty's syndrome, pure red cell aplasia, and immune thrombocytopenia purpura (ITP).
4. T-LGLL or T-LGL proliferation can be present with concomitant B-cell lymphoma or other malignancies.
5. It is critical to distinguish T-LGLL from HSTCL in that they have totally different clinical courses and outcomes. The presence of cytotoxic markers, e.g., TIA1, perforin, and granzyme B, favors T-LGLL over HSTCL. T-LGLL is more frequently TCRαβ type and rarely expresses TCRγδ in which HSTCL shows opposite pattern: more TCR γδ variant than TCR αβ subtype.

References

1. Chan WC, Foucar K, Morice WG, Catovsky D. T-cell large granular lymphocytic leukemia. In: Swerdlow SH, Elias C, Harris NL, et al., editors. WHO classification of tumours of haematopoietic and lymphoid tissues. 4th ed. Lyon: IARC Press, WHO Publications Center; 2008. p. 272–3.
2. Loughran TP Jr, Kadin ME, Starkebaum G, et al. Leukemia of large granular lymphocytes: association with clonal chromosomal abnormalities and autoimmune neutropenia, thrombocytopenia, and hemolytic anemia. Ann Intern Med. 1985;102(2):169–75.
3. Lamy T, Loughran TP Jr. How I treat LGL leukemia. Blood. 2011;117(10):2764–74.
4. Lamy T, Moignet A, Loughran TP Jr. LGL leukemia: from pathogenesis to treatment. Blood. 2017;129(9):1082–94.
5. Semenzato G, Zambello R, Starkebaum G, Oshimi K, Loughran TP Jr. The lymphoproliferative disease of granular lymphocytes: updated criteria for diagnosis. Blood. 1997;89(1):256–60.
6. Bareau B, Rey J, Hamidou M, et al. Analysis of a French cohort of patients with large granular lymphocyte leukemia: a report on 229 cases. Haematologica. 2010;95(9):1534–41.
7. Mohan SR, Maciejewski JP. Diagnosis and therapy of neutropenia in large granular lymphocyte leukemia. Curr Opin Hematol. 2009;16(1):27–34.
8. Shah MV, Hook CC, Call TG, Go RS. A population-based study of large granular lymphocyte leukemia. Blood Cancer J. 2016;6(8):e455.
9. Zhang R, Shah MV, Loughran TP Jr. The root of many evils: indolent large granular lymphocyte leukaemia and associated disorders. Hematol Oncol. 2010;28(3):105–17.
10. Matutes E. Large granular lymphocytic leukemia. Current diagnostic and therapeutic approaches and novel treatment options. Expert Rev Hematol. 2017;10(3):251–8.
11. Sokol L, Loughran TP Jr. Large granular lymphocyte leukemia. Oncologist. 2006;11(3):263–73.
12. Epling-Burnette PK, Liu JH, Catlett-Falcone R, et al. Inhibition of STAT3 signaling leads to apoptosis of leukemic large granular lymphocytes and decreased Mcl-1 expression. J Clin Invest. 2001;107(3):351–62.
13. Schade AE, Wlodarski MW, Maciejewski JP. Pathophysiology defined by altered signal transduction pathways: the role of JAK-STAT and PI3K signaling in leukemic large granular lymphocytes. Cell Cycle. 2006;5(22):2571–4.
14. Epling-Burnette PK, Sokol L, Chen X, et al. Clinical improvement by farnesyltransferase inhibition in NK large granular lymphocyte leukemia associated with imbalanced NK receptor signaling. Blood. 2008;112(12):4694–8.
15. Rossoff LJ, Genovese J, Coleman M, Dantzker DR. Primary pulmonary hypertension in a patient with CD8/T-cell large granulocyte leukemia: amelioration by cladribine therapy. Chest. 1997;112(2):551–3.
16. Viny AD, Maciejewski JP. High rate of both hematopoietic and solid tumors associated with large granular lymphocyte leukemia. Leuk Lymphoma. 2015;56(2):503–4.
17. Wlodarski MW, O'Keefe C, Howe EC, et al. Pathologic clonal cytotoxic T-cell responses: nonrandom nature of the T-cell-receptor restriction in large granular lymphocyte leukemia. Blood. 2005;106(8):2769–80.
18. Liu JH, Wei S, Lamy T, et al. Blockade of Fas-dependent apoptosis by soluble Fas in LGL leukemia. Blood. 2002;100(4):1449–53.
19. Matos DM, de Oliveira AC, Tome Mde N, Scrideli CA. Monoclonal B-cell lymphocytosis MBL, CD4+/CD8 weak T-cell large granular lymphocytic leukemia (T-LGL leukemia) and monoclonal gammopathy of unknown significance (MGUS): molecular and flow cytometry characterization of three concomitant hematological disorders. Med Oncol. 2012;29(5):3557–60.
20. Viny AD, Lichtin A, Pohlman B, Loughran T, Maciejewski J. Chronic B-cell dyscrasias are an important clinical feature of T-LGL leukemia. Leuk Lymphoma. 2008;49(5):932–8.
21. Dhodapkar MV, Li CY, Lust JA, Tefferi A, Phyliky RL. Clinical spectrum of clonal proliferations of T-large granular lymphocytes: a T-cell clonopathy of undetermined significance? Blood. 1994;84(5):1620–7.

22. Papadaki T, Stamatopoulos K, Kosmas C, et al. Clonal T-large granular lymphocyte proliferations associated with clonal B cell lymphoproliferative disorders: report of eight cases. Leukemia. 2002;16(10):2167–9.

23. Zhang R, Shah MV, Yang J, et al. Network model of survival signaling in large granular lymphocyte leukemia. Proc Natl Acad Sci U S A. 2008;105(42):16308–13.

24. Mishra A, Liu S, Sams GH, et al. Aberrant overexpression of IL-15 initiates large granular lymphocyte leukemia through chromosomal instability and DNA hypermethylation. Cancer Cell. 2012;22(5):645–55.

25. Yang J, Liu X, Nyland SB, et al. Platelet-derived growth factor mediates survival of leukemic large granular lymphocytes via an autocrine regulatory pathway. Blood. 2010;115(1):51–60.

26. Epling-Burnette PK, Bai F, Wei S, et al. ERK couples chronic survival of NK cells to constitutively activated Ras in lymphoproliferative disease of granular lymphocytes (LDGL). Oncogene. 2004;23(57):9220–9.

27. Shah MV, Zhang R, Irby R, et al. Molecular profiling of LGL leukemia reveals role of sphingolipid signaling in survival of cytotoxic lymphocytes. Blood. 2008;112(3):770–81.

28. Koskela HL, Eldfors S, Ellonen P, et al. Somatic STAT3 mutations in large granular lymphocytic leukemia. N Engl J Med. 2012;366(20):1905–13.

29. Teramo A, Gattazzo C, Passeri F, et al. Intrinsic and extrinsic mechanisms contribute to maintain the JAK/STAT pathway aberrantly activated in T-type large granular lymphocyte leukemia. Blood. 2013;121(19):3843–3854, S3841.

30. Kothapalli R, Nyland SB, Kusmartseva I, Bailey RD, McKeown TM, Loughran TP Jr. Constitutive production of proinflammatory cytokines RANTES, MIP-1beta and IL-18 characterizes LGL leukemia. Int J Oncol. 2005;26(2):529–35.

31. Lamy T, Loughran TP Jr. Clinical features of large granular lymphocyte leukemia. Semin Hematol. 2003;40(3):185–95.

32. Morice WG. T-cell and NK-cell large granular lymphocyte proliferations. In: Jaffe ES, Arber DA, Campo DA, Harris NL, Quintanilla-Martinez L, editors. Hematopathology. Philadelphia: Elsevier; 2017. p. 599–608.

33. Loughran TP Jr, Hadlock KG, Perzova R, et al. Epitope mapping of HTLV envelope seroreactivity in LGL leukaemia. Br J Haematol. 1998;101(2):318–24.

34. Neben MA, Morice WG, Tefferi A. Clinical features in T-cell vs. natural killer-cell variants of large granular lymphocyte leukemia. Eur J Haematol. 2003;71(4):263–5.

35. Agnarsson BA, Loughran TP Jr, Starkebaum G, Kadin ME. The pathology of large granular lymphocyte leukemia. Hum Pathol. 1989;20(7):643–51.

36. O'Malley DP. T-cell large granular leukemia and related proliferations. Am J Clin Pathol. 2007;127(6):850–9.

37. Bassan R, Pronesti M, Buzzetti M, et al. Autoimmunity and B-cell dysfunction in chronic proliferative disorders of large granular lymphocytes/natural killer cells. Cancer. 1989;63(1):90–5.

38. Loughran TP Jr. Clonal diseases of large granular lymphocytes. Blood. 1993;82(1):1–14.

39. Subbiah V, Viny AD, Rosenblatt S, Pohlman B, Lichtin A, Maciejewski JP. Outcomes of splenectomy in T-cell large granular lymphocyte leukemia with splenomegaly and cytopenia. Exp Hematol. 2008;36(9):1078–83.

40. Lamy T, Loughran TP Jr. Current concepts: large granular lymphocyte leukemia. Blood Rev. 1999;13(4):230–40.

41. Mailloux AW, Zhang L, Moscinski L, et al. Fibrosis and subsequent cytopenias are associated with basic fibroblast growth factor-deficient pluripotent mesenchymal stromal cells in large granular lymphocyte leukemia. J Immunol. 2013;191(7):3578–93.

42. Zhang X, Sokol L, Bennett JM, Moscinski LC, List A, Zhang L. T-cell large granular lymphocyte proliferation in myelodysplastic syndromes: Clinicopathological features and prognostic significance. Leuk Res. 2016;43:18–23.

43. Hansen RM, Lerner N, Abrams RA, Patrick CW, Malik MI, Keller R. T-cell chronic lymphocytic leukemia with pure red cell aplasia: laboratory demonstration of persistent leukemia in spite of apparent complete clinical remission. Am J Hematol. 1986;22(1):79–86.

44. Matutes E, Wotherspoon AC, Parker NE, Osuji N, Isaacson PG, Catovsky D. Transformation of T-cell large granular lymphocyte leukaemia into a high-grade large T-cell lymphoma. Br J Haematol. 2001;115(4):801–6.

45. Tagawa S, Mizuki M, Onoi U, et al. Transformation of large granular lymphocytic leukemia during the course of a reactivated human herpesvirus-6 infection. Leukemia. 1992;6(5):465–9.

46. Brito-Babapulle V, Matutes E, Foroni L, Pomfret M, Catovsky D. A t(8;14)(q24;q32) in a T-lymphoma/leukemia of CD8+ large granular lymphocytes. Leukemia. 1987;1(12):789–94.

47. Zhang L, Sotomayor EM, Papenhausen PR, et al. Unusual concurrence of T-cell large granular lymphocytic leukemia with Franklin disease (gamma heavy chain disease) manifested with massive splenomegaly. Leuk Lymphoma. 2013;54(1):205–8.

48. Dallapiccola B, Alimena G, Chessa L, et al. Chromosome studies in patients with T-CLL chronic lymphocytic leukemia and expansions of granular lymphocytes. Int J Cancer. 1984;34(2):171–6.

49. Morice WG, Kurtin PJ, Leibson PJ, Tefferi A, Hanson CA. Demonstration of aberrant T-cell and natural killer-cell antigen expression in all cases of granular lymphocytic leukaemia. Br J Haematol. 2003;120(6):1026–36.

50. Lundell R, Hartung L, Hill S, Perkins SL, Bahler DW. T-cell large granular lymphocyte leukemias have multiple phenotypic abnormalities involving pan-T-cell antigens and receptors for MHC molecules. Am J Clin Pathol. 2005;124(6):937–46.

51. Yabe M, Medeiros LJ, Wang SA, et al. Clinicopathologic, immunophenotypic, cytogenetic, and molecular features of gammadelta T-cell large granular lymphocytic leukemia: an analysis of 14 patients suggests biologic differences with alphabeta T-cell large granular lymphocytic leukemia. [corrected]. Am J Clin Pathol. 2015;144(4):607–19.

52. Sandberg Y, Almeida J, Gonzalez M, et al. TCRgammadelta+ large granular lymphocyte leukemias reflect the spectrum of normal antigen-selected TCRgammadelta+ T-cells. Leukemia. 2006;20(3):505–13.

53. Yabe M, Medeiros LJ, Wang SA, et al. Distinguishing between hepatosplenic T-cell lymphoma and gammadelta T-cell large granular lymphocytic leukemia: a clinicopathologic, immunophenotypic, and molecular analysis. Am J Surg Pathol. 2017;41(1):82–93.

54. Morice WG, Macon WR, Dogan A, Hanson CA, Kurtin PJ. NK-cell-associated receptor expression in hepatosplenic T-cell lymphoma, insights into pathogenesis. Leukemia. 2006;20(5):883–6.

55. Benjamini O, Jain P, Konoplev SN, et al. CD4(−)/CD8(−) variant of T-cell large granular lymphocytic leukemia or hepatosplenic T-cell lymphoma: a clinicopathologic dilemma. Clin Lymphoma Myeloma Leuk. 2013;13(5):610–3.

56. Karasawa M, Mitsui T, Isoda A, et al. TCR Vbeta repertoire analysis in CD56+ CD16(dim/−) T-cell large granular lymphocyte leukaemia: association with CD4 single and CD4/CD8 double positive phenotypes. Br J Haematol. 2003;123(4):613–20.

57. Olteanu H, Karandikar NJ, Eshoa C, Kroft SH. Laboratory findings in CD4(+) large granular lymphocytoses. Int J Lab Hematol. 2010;32(1 Pt 1):e9–16.

58. Gorczyca W, Weisberger J, Liu Z, et al. An approach to diagnosis of T-cell lymphoproliferative disorders by flow cytometry. Cytometry. 2002;50(3):177–90.

59. Qiu ZY, Shen WY, Fan L, et al. Assessment of clonality in T-cell large granular lymphocytic leukemia: flow cytometric T cell receptor Vbeta repertoire and T cell receptor gene rearrangement. Leuk Lymphoma. 2015;56(2):324–31.

60. Morice WG, Kimlinger T, Katzmann JA, et al. Flow cytometric assessment of TCR-Vbeta expression in the evaluation of peripheral blood involvement by T-cell lymphoproliferative

disorders: a comparison with conventional T-cell immunophenotyping and molecular genetic techniques. Am J Clin Pathol. 2004;121(3):373–83.

61. Feng B, Jorgensen JL, Hu Y, Medeiros LJ, Wang SA. TCR-Vbeta flow cytometric analysis of peripheral blood for assessing clonality and disease burden in patients with T cell large granular lymphocyte leukaemia. J Clin Pathol. 2010;63(2):141–6.

62. Voskoboinik I, Smyth MJ, Trapani JA. Perforin-mediated target-cell death and immune homeostasis. Nat Rev Immunol. 2006;6(12):940–52.

63. Liu CC, Young LH, Young JD. Lymphocyte-mediated cytolysis and disease. N Engl J Med. 1996;335(22):1651–9.

64. Bolitho P, Voskoboinik I, Trapani JA, Smyth MJ. Apoptosis induced by the lymphocyte effector molecule perforin. Curr Opin Immunol. 2007;19(3):339–47.

65. McAlinden A, Liang L, Mukudai Y, Imamura T, Sandell LJ. Nuclear protein TIA-1 regulates COL2A1 alternative splicing and interacts with precursor mRNA and genomic DNA. J Biol Chem. 2007;282(33):24444–54.

66. Anderson P, Nagler-Anderson C, O'Brien C, et al. A monoclonal antibody reactive with a 15-kDa cytoplasmic granule-associated protein defines a subpopulation of CD8+ T lymphocytes. J Immunol. 1990;144(2):574–82.

67. Lauria F, Foa R, Migone N, et al. Heterogeneity of large granular lymphocyte proliferations: morphological, immunological and molecular analysis in seven patients. Br J Haematol. 1987;66(2):187–91.

68. Oshimi K, Shinkai Y, Okumura K, Oshimi Y, Mizoguchi H. Perforin gene expression in granular lymphocyte proliferative disorders. Blood. 1990;75(3):704–8.

69. Shi Y, Wang E. Hepatosplenic T-cell lymphoma: a clinicopathologic review with an emphasis on diagnostic differentiation from other T-cell/natural killer-cell neoplasms. Arch Pathol Lab Med. 2015;139(9):1173–80.

70. Gaulard P, Jaffe ES, Krenacs L, Macon WR. Hepatosplenic T-cell lymphoma. In: Swerdlow SH, Campo E, Jaffe ES, Pileri SA, Thiele J, Vardiman JW, editors. WHO classification of tumours of haematopoietic and lymphoid tissue. Lyon: WHO Press; 2008. p. 292–3.

71. Vega F, Medeiros LJ, Gaulard P. Hepatosplenic and other gammadelta T-cell lymphomas. Am J Clin Pathol. 2007;127(6):869–80.

72. Langerak AW, van Den Beemd R, Wolvers-Tettero IL, et al. Molecular and flow cytometric analysis of the Vbeta repertoire for clonality assessment in mature TCRalphabeta T-cell proliferations. Blood. 2001;98(1):165–73.

73. van den Beemd R, Boor PP, van Lochem EG, et al. Flow cytometric analysis of the Vbeta repertoire in healthy controls. Cytometry. 2000;40(4):336–45.

74. Behlke MA, Spinella DG, Chou HS, Sha W, Hartl DL, Loh DY. T-cell receptor beta-chain expression: dependence on relatively few variable region genes. Science. 1985;229(4713):566–70.

75. Qu Y, Huang Y, Liu D, et al. High-throughput analysis of the T cell receptor beta chain repertoire in PBMCs from chronic hepatitis B patients with HBeAg seroconversion. Can J Infect Dis Med Microbiol. 2016;2016:8594107.

76. Tse E, Kwong YL. Diagnosis and management of extranodal NK/T cell lymphoma nasal type. Expert Rev Hematol. 2016;9(9):861–71.

77. Wang SS, Vose JM. Epidemiology and prognosis of T-cell lymphoma. In: Foss F, editor. T-cells lymphomas, contemporary hematology. New York: Springer Science + Business Media; 2013. p. 25–39.

78. Iqbal J, Weisenburger DD, Chowdhury A, et al. Natural killer cell lymphoma shares strikingly similar molecular features with a group of non-hepatosplenic gammadelta T-cell lymphoma and is highly sensitive to a novel aurora kinase A inhibitor in vitro. Leukemia. 2011;25(2):348–58.

79. Koo GC, Tan SY, Tang T, et al. Janus kinase 3-activating mutations identified in natural killer/T-cell lymphoma. Cancer Discov. 2012;2(7):591–7.

80. Kucuk C, Jiang B, Hu X, et al. Activating mutations of STAT5B and STAT3 in lymphomas derived from gammadelta-T or NK cells. Nat Commun. 2015;6:6025.

81. Lee S, Park HY, Kang SY, et al. Genetic alterations of JAK/STAT cascade and histone modification in extranodal NK/T-cell lymphoma nasal type. Oncotarget. 2015;6(19):17764–76.

82. Rajala HL, Porkka K, Maciejewski JP, Loughran TP Jr, Mustjoki S. Uncovering the pathogenesis of large granular lymphocytic leukemia-novel STAT3 and STAT5b mutations. Ann Med. 2014;46(3):114–22.

83. Rajala HL, Eldfors S, Kuusanmaki H, et al. Discovery of somatic STAT5b mutations in large granular lymphocytic leukemia. Blood. 2013;121(22):4541–50.

84. Andersson EI, Rajala HL, Eldfors S, et al. Novel somatic mutations in large granular lymphocytic leukemia affecting the STAT-pathway and T-cell activation. Blood Cancer J. 2013;3:e168.

85. Loughran TP Jr, Zickl L, Olson TL, et al. Immunosuppressive therapy of LGL leukemia: prospective multicenter phase II study by the Eastern Cooperative Oncology Group (E5998). Leukemia. 2015;29(4):886–94.

86. Gentile TC, Uner AH, Hutchison RE, et al. CD3+, CD56+ aggressive variant of large granular lymphocyte leukemia. Blood. 1994;84(7):2315–21.

87. Wong KF, Chan JC, Liu HS, Man C, Kwong YL. Chromosomal abnormalities in T-cell large granular lymphocyte leukaemia: report of two cases and review of the literature. Br J Haematol. 2002;116(3):598–600.

88. Pittman S, Morilla R, Catovsky D. Chronic T-cell leukemias. II. Cytogenetic studies. Leuk Res. 1982;6(1):33–42.

89. Brito-Babapulle V, Matutes E, Parreira L, Catovsky D. Abnormalities of chromosome 7q and Tac expression in T cell leukemias. Blood. 1986;67(2):516–21.

90. Chen YH, Peterson L. Differential diagnosis of CD4-/CD8- gammadelta T-cell large granular lymphocytic leukemia and hepatosplenic T-cell lymphoma. Am J Clin Pathol. 2012;137(3):496–7.

91. Jaffe ES, Arber DA, Campo E, Harris NL, Quintanilla-Martinez L. Hematopathology. Philadelphia: Elsevier; 2017.

92. Feldman AL, Law M, Grogg KL, et al. Incidence of TCR and TCL1 gene translocations and isochromosome 7q in peripheral T-cell lymphomas using fluorescence in situ hybridization. Am J Clin Pathol. 2008;130(2):178–85.

93. Mohty M, Faucher C, Vey N, et al. Features of large granular lymphocytes (LGL) expansion following allogeneic stem cell transplantation: a long-term analysis. Leukemia. 2002;16(10):2129–33.

94. Gentile TC, Hadlock KG, Uner AH, et al. Large granular lymphocyte leukaemia occurring after renal transplantation. Br J Haematol. 1998;101(3):507–12.

95. Mohty M, Faucher C, Vey N, et al. High rate of secondary viral and bacterial infections in patients undergoing allogeneic bone marrow mini-transplantation. Bone Marrow Transplant. 2000;26(3):251–5.

96. Semenzato G, Pandolfi F, Chisesi T, et al. The lymphoproliferative disease of granular lymphocytes. A heterogeneous disorder ranging from indolent to aggressive conditions. Cancer. 1987;60(12):2971–8.

97. Oshimi K, Yamada O, Kaneko T, et al. Laboratory findings and clinical courses of 33 patients with granular lymphocyte-proliferative disorders. Leukemia. 1993;7(6):782–8.

98. Rossi D, Franceschetti S, Capello D, et al. Transient monoclonal expansion of CD8+/CD57+ T-cell large granular lymphocytes after primary cytomegalovirus infection. Am J Hematol. 2007;82(12):1103–5.

99. Villamor N, Morice WG, Chan WC, Foucar K. Chronic lymphoproliferative disorders of NK cells. Lyon: IARD; 2008.

100. Poullot E, Zambello R, Leblanc F, et al. Chronic natural killer lymphoproliferative disorders: characteristics of an international cohort of 70 patients. Ann Oncol. 2014;25(10):2030–5.

101. Suzuki R. Treatment of advanced extranodal NK/T cell lymphoma, nasal-type and aggressive NK-cell leukemia. Int J Hematol. 2010;92(5):697–701.

102. Kwong YL. Natural killer-cell malignancies: diagnosis and treatment. Leukemia. 2005;19(12):2186–94.

103. Cheuk W, Chan JKC. NK-cell neoplasm. In: Jaffe ES, editor. Hematopathology. Lyon: Saunders/Elsevier; 2011. p. 473–91.

104. Kwong YL. The diagnosis and management of extranodal NK/T-cell lymphoma, nasal-type and aggressive NK-cell leukemia. J Clin Exp Hematop. 2011;51(1):21–8.

105. Kwong YL, Anderson BO, Advani R, et al. Management of T-cell and natural-killer-cell neoplasms in Asia: consensus statement from the Asian Oncology Summit 2009. Lancet Oncol. 2009;10(11):1093–101.

106. Li Y, Wei J, Mao X, et al. Flow cytometric immunophenotyping is sensitive for the early diagnosis of de novo Aggressive Natural Killer Cell Leukemia (ANKL): a multicenter retrospective analysis. PLoS One. 2016;11(8):e0158827.

107. Yabe M, Medeiros LJ, Tang G, et al. Prognostic factors of Hepatosplenic T-cell lymphoma: clinicopathologic study of 28 cases. Am J Surg Pathol. 2016;40(5):676–88.

108. Vose J, Armitage J, Weisenburger D, International TCLP. International peripheral T-cell and natural killer/T-cell lymphoma study: pathology findings and clinical outcomes. J Clin Oncol. 2008;26(25):4124–30.

109. Hastrup N, Ralfkiaer E, Pallesen G. Aberrant phenotypes in peripheral T cell lymphomas. J Clin Pathol. 1989;42(4):398–402.

110. Went P, Agostinelli C, Gallamini A, et al. Marker expression in peripheral T-cell lymphoma: a proposed clinical-pathologic prognostic score. J Clin Oncol. 2006;24(16):2472–9.

111. Zhang L, Van den Bergh M, Sokol L. CD4-positive T-cell large granular lymphocytosis mimicking Sezary syndrome in a patient with mycosis Fungoides. Cancer Control. 2017;24(2):207–12.

112. Steinway SN, LeBlanc F, Loughran TP Jr. The pathogenesis and treatment of large granular lymphocyte leukemia. Blood Rev. 2014;28(3):87–94.

Mariko Yabe and Ahmet Dogan

Introduction

Common T-cell leukemias/lymphomas frequently involving the spleen and liver include entities such as T-cell prolymphocytic leukemia, aggressive NK-cell leukemia, and hepatosplenic T-cell lymphoma. The involvement of the spleen and liver by other nodal or extranodal T-cell or NK-/T-cell lymphomas is less common and mostly as part of disseminated disease. The clinicopathologic features of these uncommon mature T-cell lymphomas in the spleen and liver, including peripheral T-cell lymphoma, NOS, adult T-cell leukemia/lymphoma, angioimmunoblastic T-cell lymphoma, ALK-positive and ALK-negative anaplastic large cell lymphoma, and extranodal NK-/T-cell lymphoma, nasal type, are discussed in this chapter. Spleen and liver biopsies are typically not obtained in these lymphomas, as diagnosis is typically made on lymph node or other primary sites of involvement. In the few reported cases, the morphological and immunophenotypic features of these lymphomas are the same as that of nodal or extranodal disease.

Peripheral T-Cell Lymphoma, Not Otherwise Specified

Definition

The term peripheral T-cell lymphoma (PTCL) is used to describe lymphoid neoplasm of mature T-cell lineage, as opposed to neoplasms of thymic origin. In the current version of the WHO classification, peripheral T-cell lymphoma not otherwise specified (PTCL-NOS) is in part a diagnosis of exclusion: a lymphoma of mature T-cell lineage that does not

fit into other specific categories of T-cell lymphoma [1]. Excluded from this category are tumors with a T-follicular helper (TFH) cell phenotype (discussed later in the section of angioimmunoblastic T-cell lymphoma), as defined by the expression of at least two (ideally three) of the following markers: CD10, BCL6, PD1, CXCL13, CXCR5, ICOS, and SAP [1].

Epidemiology

Most patients with PTCL-NOS are adults, with a median age ranging from 51 to 68 years in various studies, with a male predominance [1–3].

Clinical Presentation

Patients usually present with lymphadenopathy, but extranodal sites of disease are common including the skin, liver, spleen, Waldeyer's ring, and lung. Most patients (70%) have advanced-stage disease, 67% presented with an intermediate to high International Prognostic Index (IPI), and approximately 50% patients have B symptoms [4]. A subset of patients can present with eosinophilia, pruritus, or hemophagocytic syndrome [5]. Primary hepatic PTCL is rare but has been reported. Ramai D et al. reported a similar case with EBV infection [6].

Morphology

Most patients present with peripheral lymph node involvement, but any site can be affected including the liver and spleen. Vascular proliferation is common, and many inflammatory cells are often admixed with the lymphoma cells. Cytologically, the neoplastic cells of PTCL-NOS show a spectrum of sizes from small cells to large cells and can have

M. Yabe (✉) · A. Dogan
Department of Pathology, Memorial Sloan Kettering Cancer Center, Hematopathology Service, New York, NY, USA
e-mail: yabem@mskcc.org; dogana@mskcc.org

© Springer Nature Switzerland AG 2020
L. Zhang et al. (eds.), *Diagnostic Pathology of Hematopoietic Disorders of Spleen and Liver*,
https://doi.org/10.1007/978-3-030-37708-3_11

abundant clear cytoplasm. Reed-Sternberg-like cells may be also found. Mitotic figures are usually easily identified and are often numerous. Although the spleen and liver are involved by PTCL-NOS cases, the morphological and immunophenotypic features at these locations have not been systematically studied. When these sites are involved, the histological and immunophenotypic features mimic other sites of involvement. In the liver, the involvement is most commonly portal with rare cases showing intrasinusoidal involvement mimicking hepatosplenic T-cell lymphoma. In the spleen, the involvement is typically nodular but sinusoidal infiltration can be seen (Fig. 11.1) [7]. Ramai's case showed clusters of atypical lymphoid cells with nuclear irregularity [6].

Immunophenotyping

Immunophenotypic studies have shown that PTCL-NOS are of mature T-cell lineage. Thus, the neoplastic cells express pan-T-cell antigens, usually TCR-$\alpha\beta$, and approximately 75% of cases exhibit an aberrant T-cell immunophenotype with frequent loss of CD5 and CD7, which is useful for diagnosis. Rare cases of PTCL-NOS have been reported to express B-cell antigens (e.g., CD20, CD79a) (Fig. 11.1) [1, 7]. Proliferation is usually high, and Ki-67 proliferation index exceeding 80% is associated with a worse prognosis [3].

Cytogenetics

The genetic findings of PTCL-NOS are heterogeneous. Conventional cytogenetic analysis commonly shows an abnormal karyotype, with a high frequency of complex karyotypes [8]. There are no consistent cytogenetic abnormalities in PTCL-NOS, and the most common abnormalities, in general, are copy number changes. Comparative genomic hybridization analysis of PTCL-NOS had shown a number of gains and losses [9, 10].

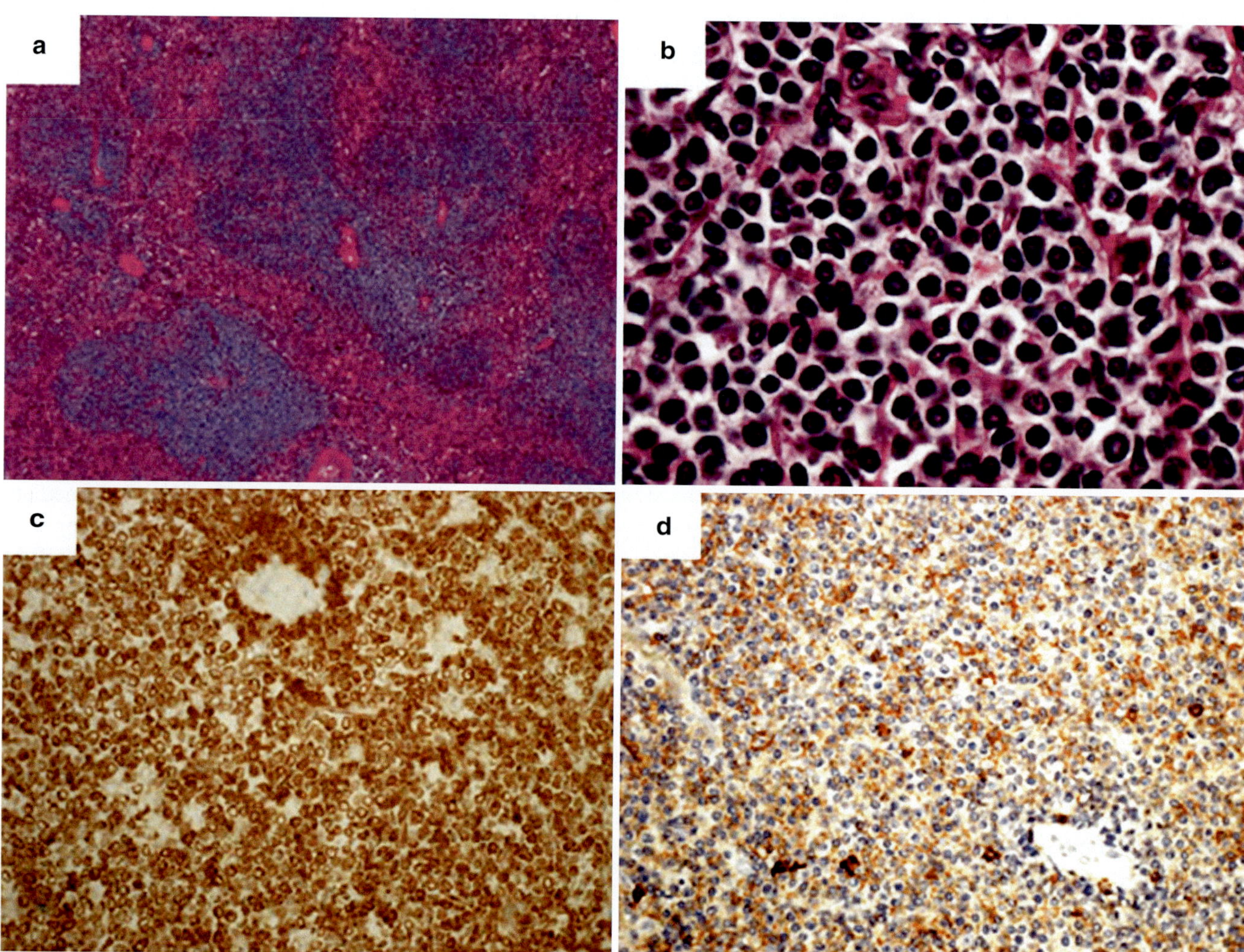

Fig. 11.1 Histological findings of the spleen of a patient with PTCL-NOS. Hematoxylin-eosin staining (**a**, ×40; **b** ×1000) demonstrated the enlarged white pulp of the spleen occupied by small lymphoid cells in a diffuse or pseudonodular pattern. Immunological staining showed strong CD3 positivity (**c**) and weak CD20 positivity (**d**). (Adopted from Ichikawa et al. [7])

Molecular Findings

Recent gene expression profiling studies have identified two major subgroups of PTCL-NOS, based on overexpression of *GATA3* or *TBX21/Tbet*, with poorer or better prognosis, respectively [11]. Poor clinical outcomes were also observed when *TBX21*-associated cases express a cytotoxic T-cell gene signature [12]. A study of targeted sequencing was reported in PTCL-NOS, which included 237 genes chosen for their relevance in other hematologic malignancies. This study demonstrated mutations were most commonly observed in epigenetic mediators (e.g., *KMT2D*, *TET2*, *DNMT3A*), but also in genes involved in T-cell receptor signaling pathways (e.g., *TNFAIP3*, *APC*, *CHD8*) and tumor suppressor genes (e.g., *TP53*, *ATM*) [13].

Prognosis

Patients with PTCL-NOS have a poor overall prognosis; the 5-year survival in different studies has ranged from 25% to 50% [1, 3].

Adult T-Cell Lymphoma/Leukemia

Definition

Adult T-cell lymphoma/leukemia (ATLL) is a type of mature T-cell lymphoma that is caused by infection by the human T-cell leukemia/lymphoma retrovirus (HTLV-1).

Etiology

HTLV-1 is a single-stranded RNA retrovirus that is lymphotropic for T-lymphocytes [14]. The virus is transmitted by breast milk, sexual intercourse, shared needles among intravenous drug users, and transfusion of blood products. The incubation period for development of ATLL in HTLV-1 individuals ranges from 20 to 40 years [14]. The hallmark for the diagnosis of ATLL is the demonstration of HTLV-1 infection. Molecular identification of HTLV-1 is ideal for this purpose as the virus clonally integrates into the host cell genome in a random fashion [14]. The site of HTLV-1 integration into the genome appears to be similar in most cases; unusual sites of viral integration may correlate with a poorer prognosis [15]. The mechanisms to explain how HTLV-1 is involved in lymphomagenesis are not well worked out. The TAX viral protein and HTLV-1 basic leucine zipper factor (HBZ) are thought to be involved [16].

Epidemiology

Endemic regions for HTLV-1 infection include south-western Japan, Brazil, and Caribbean countries, and cases are also reported, although infrequent, in Europe and the United States. Patients with ATLL are usually adults, with a median age between 58 and 62 years and a male-to-female ratio ranging from 1.2–1.5 to 1 [17, 18].

Clinical Presentation

Patients usually present with one of four variants: acute, lymphomatous, chronic, and smoldering [19]. Patients with acute ATLL, the most common form of the disease, have generalized lymphadenopathy, hepatosplenomegaly, skin lesions, peripheral blood involvement with high leukocyte counts, lytic bone lesions, and hypercalcemia [17]. The lungs and central nervous system are also commonly involved. Patients with the lymphomatous form of ATLL present with prominent lymphadenopathy and tumors in other organs without hepatosplenomegaly or hypercalcemia. Skin lesions are common. Many patients with the acute form of ATLL, and a lesser number with lymphomatous ATLL, have evidence of immunodeficiency and opportunistic infections. The IPI predicts prognosis in patients with acute/lymphomatous ATLL [18]. These patients respond to chemotherapy, but remissions are short and overall survival is usually poor [20]. Patients who present with chronic variant ATLL have an absolute lymphocytosis and cytologically abnormal cells in the blood. Skin lesions, lymphadenopathy, and involvement of other viscera may occur [17, 19]. Patients who have the smoldering form of ATLL have chronic disease for years, usually skin lesions with minimal peripheral blood involvement; the viscera are usually spared. Patients with the chronic and smoldering variants of ATLL do not usually require therapy but should be carefully followed as approximately 25% of patients transform to acute or lymphomatous variant ATLL [17, 20].

Morphology

Histologically, ATLL diffusely replaces lymph nodes or extranodal sites. Lymph node shows expanded paracortical areas containing a diffuse infiltrate of small- to medium-sized lymphoid cells with nuclear irregularities and may exhibit classic Hodgkin lymphoma or angioimmunoblastic T-cell lymphoma-like morphology [17]. Pleomorphic small cell type, pleomorphic medium and large cell type, and anaplastic large cell type are also seen [21]. Involvement of the liver is mainly seen in the portal area, which shows infiltration of atypical medium- to large-sized lymphoid cells with irregular nuclei, occasional destruction of limiting plates, and in some cases sinus infiltration, but rarely fibrosis [21] (Fig. 11.2) [22]. Skin lesions are seen in more than 50% of patients with ATLL. Epidermal infiltration with Pautrier-like microabscess is common, which can mimic mycosis fungoides. Some cases are indistinguishable from other T-cell lymphoma subtypes without knowledge of HTLV-1 infection. The neoplastic cells in the peripheral blood smear in patients with acute or lymphomatous ATLL are characteristic [17]. The circulating neoplastic cells are medium-sized with basophilic cytoplasm and markedly irregular, multilobulated nuclei, including cloverleaf shapes, also known as *flower cells*.

Immunophenotyping

Immunophenotypic studies have shown that ATLLs have a mature T-cell immunophenotype [17]. The neoplastic cells express the pan-T-cell antigens CD2, CD3, CD5, and the TCR αβ receptor but are usually negative for CD7. Most cases of ATLL are CD4$^+$ CD8$^-$. The lymphoma cells intensely express the CD25, and approximately 40% of ATLLs are positive for CCR4 and FOXP3, markers of regulatory T-cells [23].

Cytogenetics

Conventional cytogenetic studies have shown a wide range of abnormalities in cases of ATLL. Usually multiple abnormalities are identified per individual neoplasm, at least six in one study [24]. These results suggest a multistep pathogenesis for ATLL and are consistent with the known long incubation period from time of infection to onset of tumor. Several studies with array-based comparative genomic hybridization show frequent losses at chromosomes 6q and 13q; frequent gains at chromosomes 14q, 7q, and 3p, as well as aneuploidy (+3, +7, +21, −X, −Y); and translocations involving 14q11 and 14q32 (*TCR* α and δ, respectively). Increased number of chromosomal imbalances was associated with a significantly shorter survival [25].

Molecular Findings

Genomic profiling of ATLL has been studied to date. One study reported that in a comparison of acute and chronic variants of ATLL, there were differences in the gene expression profile and in chromosome copy numbers. Expression of MET was high in acute variant ATLL suggest-

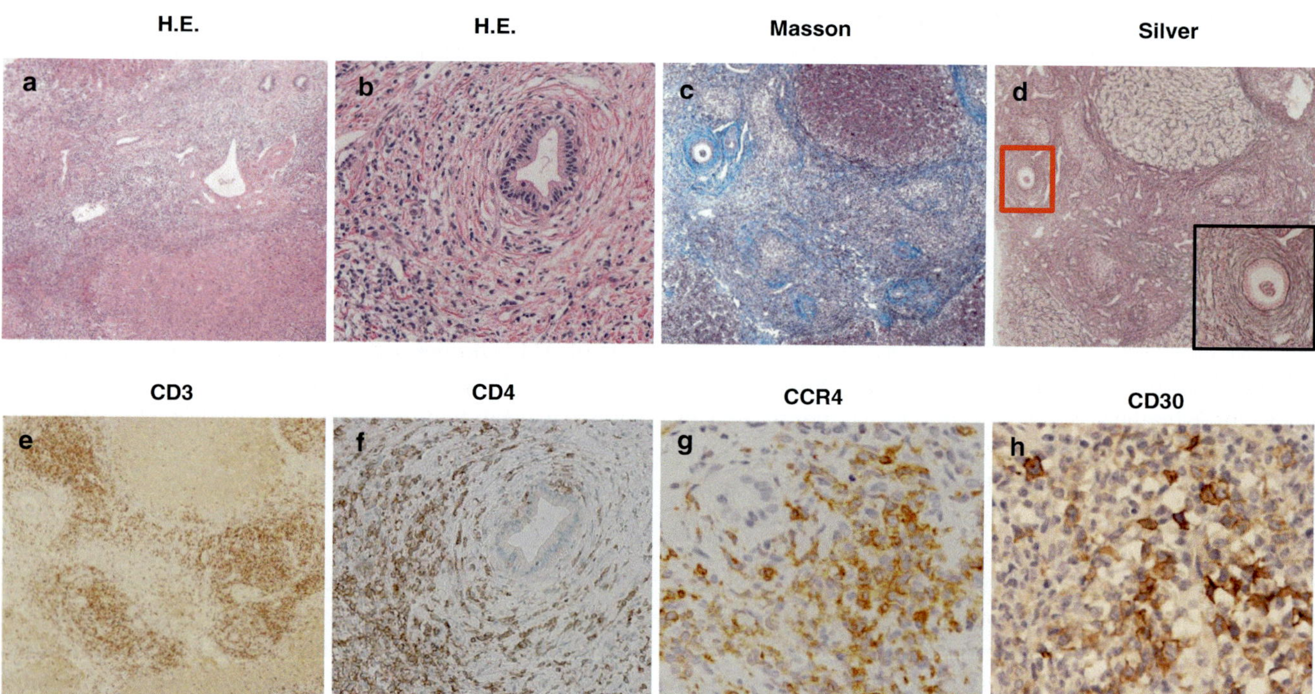

Fig. 11.2 Histopathologic features of the liver of a patient with ATLL with H&E stain (**a**, ×40; **b**, ×200), Masson Trichrome stain (**c**, ×40), silver staining (**d**, ×40, and *inset*, ×200), and immunohistochemical stain including CD3 (**e**, ×40), CD4 (**f**, ×200), CC chemokine receptor 4 (CCR4) (**g**, ×400), and CD30 (**h**, ×400). ATLL cells infiltrated mainly in the portal area (**a**, **b**, and **e**) and presented with prominent portal fibrosis (**c** and **d**). Magnified image showed fibrosis surrounding interlobular bile duct (**d**). ATLL cells expressed CD3, CD4, CCR4, and CD30 (**e–h**). (Reprinted with permission from Kawano et al. [22])

ing a potential therapeutic target [26]. Recent study of an integrated molecular analysis of a total of 426 ATLL cases identified alterations of NF-κB signaling [27]. Other notable features include a predominance of activating mutations (*PLCG1*, *PRKCB*, *CARD11*, *VAV1*, *IRF4*, *FYN*, *CCR4*, *CCR7*) and gene fusions (*CTLA4-CD28* and *ICOS-CD28*) [27]. Frequent intragenic deletions involving *IKZF2*, *CARD11*, and *TP73* and mutations in *GATA3*, *HNRNPA2B1*, *GPR183*, *CSNK2A1*, *CSNK2B*, and *CSNK1A1* were also observed [27].

Prognosis

The survival time for the acute and lymphomatous variants ranges from 2 weeks to >1 year. The chronic and smoldering forms have a more protracted clinical course and better survival but can progress to an acute phase with an aggressive course in approximately 25% of patients [17].

Angioimmunoblastic T-Cell Lymphoma

Definition

Angioimmunoblastic T-cell lymphoma (AITL) is one of the most common specific types of T-cell lymphoma in Western nations, representing 15–20% of all cases of PTCL [28]. It is a neoplasm of mature T-follicular helper (TFH) cells.

Epidemiology

Patients with AITL are elderly, with a median age in the seventh decade [28, 29].

Clinical Presentation

AITL is commonly a systemic disease at its onset characterized by advanced-stage disease, immunodysregulation, and immunodeficiency. Many patients have constitutional symptoms such as fever, chills, night sweats, malaise, and arthralgias. Patients usually have peripheral lymphadenopathy, often generalized, and extranodal sites of disease are common including involvement of the liver, spleen, skin, lungs, and bone marrow. Various laboratory abnormalities are common including polyclonal hypergammaglobulinemia, anemia, cold agglutinins, circulating immune complexes, cryoglobulins, antinuclear antibodies, eosinophilia, and elevated serum LDH levels.

Patients with AITL are at risk for developing B-cell lymphomas, particularly diffuse large B-cell lymphoma (DLBCL), and less frequently classic Hodgkin lymphoma or plasmacytoma [30]. A subset of cases of DLBCL and most classic Hodgkin lymphoma arising in this setting are EBV⁺. One possible explanation for this phenomenon is that EBV infection prolongs B-cell lifespan, increasing the likelihood of secondary molecular aberrations that result in lymphoma. In some patients, the diagnosis of DLBCL can precede the diagnosis of AITL. These B-cell lymphoproliferative disorders may present at extranodal sites which may include the spleen and the liver. Therefore, the histopathology work-up should not only address the T-cell lymphoma but also investigate the possibility of a B-cell process.

Morphology

Histology of AITL can show three general, often overlapping patterns designated as types I, II, and III [28, 31]. In the type I pattern, the overall architecture is partially preserved and many hyperplastic lymphoid follicles are present. In types II and III, there is progressive or complete replacement, respectively, of the lymph node architecture, and small and atrophic germinal centers can be present. A mixture of patterns can occur at presentation, or patients may relapse with a different pattern [31]. The cytological features of AITL are broad, as there is usually an abundant and variable inflammatory infiltrate associated with the neoplastic cells [28, 31]. In fact, in many cases of AITL, the neoplastic cells are a minority component in the biopsy specimen. As a result, the histologic appearance of AITL is polymorphous composed of neoplastic small- and medium-sized lymphoid cells, often with clear cytoplasm, associated with reactive plasma cells, eosinophils, histiocytes, and B-immunoblasts. Arborizing small blood vessels are present and usually numerous in AITL. In the spleen the pattern of involvement is nodular and histological features closely mimic the morphology seen in the lymph nodes. In the liver portal tracts are typically involved with similar features. At these locations, it may be impossible to identify the neoplastic by morphology, and immunophenotyping is essential.

Immunophenotyping

Immunophenotypic studies of AITL have shown that these tumors are of mature T-cell lineage, expressing a variety of pan-T-cell antigens and negative for Ig and B-cell antigens [28]. In addition, most cases of AITL lesions have an immunophenotype closely akin to that of normal follicular T-helper cells [32]. Therefore, the neoplastic cells are CD4⁺ and CD8⁻ and are often positive for CXCL13, CD10, Bcl-6, PD-1, or

CXCR5 [28, 33]. The immunodysregulation and immunodeficiency associated with AITL also may explain the common presence of EBV in nonneoplastic B-immunoblasts in many AITL biopsy specimens.

Cytogenetics

Conventional cytogenetic studies have shown a wide variety of numerical and structural abnormalities in approximately 75% of cases of AITL. Trisomies of chromosomes 3, 5, 21, and X and loss of 6q are most common [34]. The presence of a complex karyotype correlates with a poorer prognosis. Comparative genomic hybridization studies have further increased the frequency of detection of chromosomal alterations, identified in up to 90% of AITL cases.

Molecular Findings

Gene rearrangement studies have demonstrated that most AITL cases have *TCR* gene rearrangements. The *IGH* gene is rearranged in 10–20% of cases [28]. Gene expression profiling studies of AITL have further confirmed the concept that AITL is a neoplasm of follicular T-helper cells [35]. In addition, approximately 90% of the gene signatures in AITL are contributed by reactive cells in these lesions, particularly B-cells.

Recently, additional discoveries of the genetic basis for AITL were made. Mutations in the epigenetic regulators *TET2*, *DNMT3A*, and *IDH2* frequently occur in AITL, but are not specific [36, 37]. Most specific to AITL is a point mutation in the Ras homolog gene family member A (*RHOA* G17V) in almost 70% of AITL samples, resulting in a disruption of RHOA signaling [38]. These studies proposed that these mutations may be acquired in a multistep manner, because all the *RHOA*-mutated samples are *TET2* mutated, and the smaller percentage of *IDH2*-mutated tumors harbored both *TET2* and *RHOA* mutations [38].

Prognosis

The median survival for all patients with AITL is <3 years, but a subset of patients, approximately 25%, have a more indolent course with better long-term survival [28].

Anaplastic Large Cell Lymphoma, ALK-Positive

Definition

In the current WHO classification, there are four categories of disease that include the term anaplastic large cell lymphoma (ALCL): ALCL, ALK-positive (ALK$^+$ ALCL) and ALCL, ALK-negative (ALK$^-$ ALCL), which are their own entities; cutaneous ALCL, being a well-established, separate category of disease; and breast implant-associated ALCL which is currently considered a provisional entity [39–42]. ALK$^+$ ALCL is defined as a T-cell lymphoma, usually composed of anaplastic cells, associated with molecular alterations of the *ALK* gene, ALK overexpression, and uniform expression of CD30 [39].

Epidemiology

ALK$^+$ ALCL affects children and adults, with a wide age range, but is most common in the first three decades of life [39, 43].

Clinical Presentations

B symptoms are common in ALK$^+$ ALCL patients, particularly high fever, and approximately 75% of patients have advanced-stage disease. Lymph nodes are the most common site of involvement, but extranodal sites are commonly involved, most often the skin, soft tissue, bones, lungs, and liver [39]. Bone marrow is involved in approximately 20% of patients with ALK$^+$ ALCL if searched for diligently using immunohistochemical analysis. Leukemic involvement is uncommon in patients with ALK$^+$ ALCL. ALK$^+$ ALCL is clinically aggressive and patients require combination chemotherapy; however, prognosis is favorable. In disseminated disease, it is likely that the liver and spleen are also involved, but the pathological features have not been documented as these sites are rarely biopsied.

Morphology

Histologically, ALK$^+$ ALCL can partially or completely replace lymph node architecture [39, 43]. In partially involved lymph nodes, the tumor tends to infiltrate sinuses or preferentially replaces the nodal paracortex. Necrosis is common and there are high numbers of apoptotic cells and mitotic figures. Cytologically, ALK$^+$ ALCL can exhibit a remarkably wide spectrum, and the current WHO classification recognizes five variants: common (60%), lymphohistiocytic (10%), small cell (5–10%), Hodgkin-like (3%), and composite (15%) [39]. The lymphohistiocytic variant is composed of relatively few neoplastic cells associated with numerous lymphocytes and histiocytes. In the small cell variant, large anaplastic neoplastic cells are infrequent, and many small cells are present. Small cell and lymphohistiocytic components are reported to be associated with poorer response to therapy in pediatric population [44]. In most cases of ALK+ ALCL, irrespective of the variant, at least some hallmark cells are present, cells with a horseshoe- or kidney-shaped nucleus with vesicular chromatin and prominent nucleoli, abundant and basophilic cytoplasm, and a paranuclear clear area or hof [39].

Immunophenotyping

Immunophenotypic studies have shown that all cases of ALK+ ALCL express CD30, with a membranous and paranuclear pattern, as well as ALK [39]. Virtually all cases of ALK+ ALCL strongly express CD25, and most cases express EMA, T-cell antigens (most often CD2, CD4, CD5, CD43), and cytotoxic antigens (granzyme B and TIA-1). Ki-67 immunostaining shows a variable but usually high proliferation rate. Bcl-2 is virtually always absent, as is EBV (either EBER or LMP1) and CD117/KIT, and CD15 is very rarely expressed [39, 45]. ALK+ ALCLs are negative for Ig and B-cell antigens. Approximately 10–20% of cases of ALK+ ALCL are immunophenotypically "null cell" without any T-cell antigens being expressed. This occurs more often when only immunohistochemical analysis is used, as a lesser number of antibodies are available, and this method is less sensitive than flow cytometry.

Cytogenetics and Molecular Findings

Conventional cytogenetic studies initially showed the t(2;5) (p23;q35) translocation in a subset of cases of ALCL [46]. The breakpoints of this translocation were then cloned, showing the *ALK* gene locus at chromosome 2p23 and the nucleophosmin (*NPM*) gene at chromosome 5q35 [47]. These genes are disrupted to create a novel *NPM-ALK* fusion gene [47]. There are many additional molecular alterations of *ALK* including reciprocal translocations and one inversion [43]. These *ALK* gene abnormalities are now known to be characteristic of ALK+ ALCL and are included in the definition of this neoplasm. The t(2;5)(p23;q35) is most common, identified in approximately 80% of cases of ALK+ ALCL. The t(1;2)(q25;p23) involving *TPM3* occurs in approximately 10% of ALK+ ALCLs, and all other known translocations are uncommon, in the range of <1 to approximately 2% [39]. One study identified a novel *TRAF1-ALK* fusion using deep RNA sequencing [48]. The discovery of this *TRAF1-ALK* fusion expands the diversity of known ALK fusion partners and highlights the power of deep sequencing for fusion transcript discovery.

The pattern of ALK expression, as shown by immunohistochemical analysis, correlates with the molecular abnormalities present [39]. Tumors carrying the t(2;5) have a nuclear and cytoplasmic pattern of ALK expression. This is because NPM can migrate from the cytoplasm into the nucleus. The rare t(2;X)(p23;q11-12) involves *moesin (MSN)*. Tumors with this translocation have a membranous pattern of ALK expression, because *MSN* is located in the membrane. All other translocations result in a cytoplasmic pattern of ALK expression. The t(2;17)(p23;q23) involving *clathrin (CLTC)* is distinctive because the ALK expression pattern appears flocculent. This is true because CLTC is normally located in the membranes of cytoplasmic vesicles.

ALK+ ALCLs usually carry *TCR* gene rearrangements, including most of the "null cell' cases. The *perforin* gene was reported to be mutated in a subset of cases [49]. The *SHP1* and *RB* genes are commonly inactivated or deleted [50]. Gene expression profiling has shown that ALK+ ALCL has a different signature than ALK− ALCL, with overexpression of over 100 genes [51]. The top four genes were *BCL-6*, *PTPN12*, *CEBPbeta*, and *serpin A1*. A number of studies have elucidated pathways that are active in ALK+ ALCL including pathways involved globally in proliferation, ribosome synthesis, survival, apoptosis evasion, angiogenesis, and cytoarchitectural organization.

The NPM-ALK fusion protein activates various signaling pathways in ALK+ ALCL cells, including the JAK/STAT3, PI3K/AKT/mTOR, RAS/ERK, and PLCγ pathways. Rearrangements of *MYC* have been reported in ALK+ ALCL. All these patients with dual *ALK* and *MYC* rearrangements demonstrated an aggressive clinical course, with systemic and extranodal presentation, early tumor relapse, and bone marrow involvement during the course of the disease [52, 53].

Prognosis

The long-term survival rate associated with ALK+ ALCL approaches 80% and is better overall than that of ALK− ALCL [39].

Anaplastic Large Cell Lymphoma, ALK-Negative

Definition

This disease is defined in the WHO classification as a CD30+ T-cell lymphoma "not reproducibly distinguishable on morphological grounds from ALK-positive ALCL, but lacks ALK protein" [40]. Recent clinical, pathologic, and genetic data have revealed significant heterogeneity in ALK− ALCL [54].

Epidemiology

Patients with ALK− ALCL can be any age, but most patients are adults 40–65 years of age. The male-to-female ratio is 1.5 to 1 [40].

Clinical Presentation

Lymph nodes are most commonly involved, but extranodal sites (40–60% of patients) can be involved, although extranodal sites are less commonly involved than in ALK+ ALCL. In disseminated disease, it is likely that the liver and spleen are also involved, but the pathological features have not been documented as these sites are rarely biopsied. Patients often have B symptoms, advanced-stage disease, and an aggressive clinical course requiring combination chemotherapy [40, 55]. Primary hepatic ALCL is rare. A case with solitary liver lesion without lymphadenopathy, splenomegaly, or bone marrow involvement is reported [56]. The other two primary hepatic ALCLs presenting with acute liver failure and one identified by fine needle aspirate/needle core biopsy (Fig. 11.3) have also been found in the literature [57, 58].

Morphology

Histologically, most cases of ALK− ALCL resemble the common variant of ALK+ ALCL [40, 54]. The neoplasm tends to infiltrate lymph node sinuses. The lymphoma cells are large and often more pleomorphic, and Hallmark cells are present.

Immunophenotyping

Immunophenotypic studies show uniform expression of CD30 in a membranous and paranuclear pattern and absence of ALK expression [40]. ALK− ALCLs express T-cell antigens, and most cases are positive for cytotoxic molecules and clusterin. Many cases of ALK− ALCL express Bcl-2 and approximately 50% of cases express survivin. A subset of cases can express EMA or CD15, and all cases are negative for Ig and B-cell antigens [40].

Cytogenetics and Molecular Findings

Until recently, the genetics of ALK− ALCL has been unknown. A recent study by Parrilla and colleagues identified *DUSP22* and *TP63* rearrangements in 30% and 8% of systemic ALK− ALCLs, respectively [54]. The former involves the *DUSP22-IRF4* locus on 6p25.3 and is most commonly present as t(6;7)(p25.3;q32.3) [59]. *DUSP22* is a dual-specificity phosphatase that inhibits T-cell receptor signaling by inactivating MAP/ERK [60]. Most frequent partner gene of *TP63* is *TBL1XR1* [61]. *TP63* encodes the p53 family member, p63, and the gene rearrangements encode p63 fusion proteins which have putative oncogenic function [61]. These rearrangements were mutually exclusive and are uniformly absent in ALK+ ALCL.

Prognosis

In ALK-negative ALCL, *DUSP22*-rearranged cases have favorable outcomes similar to ALK+ ALCL. *TP63*-rearranged ALCLs have a poor prognosis.

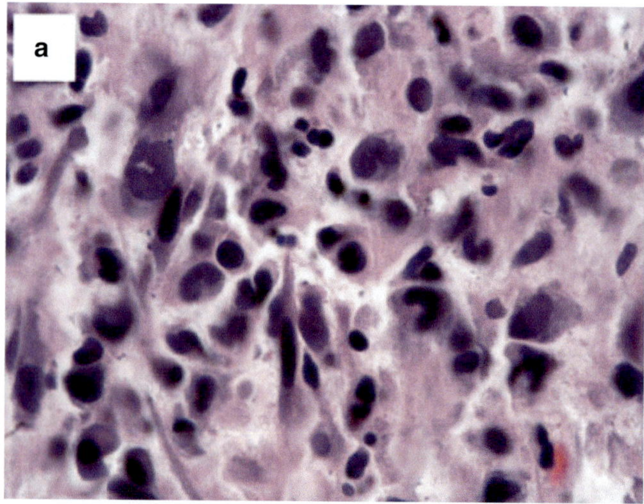
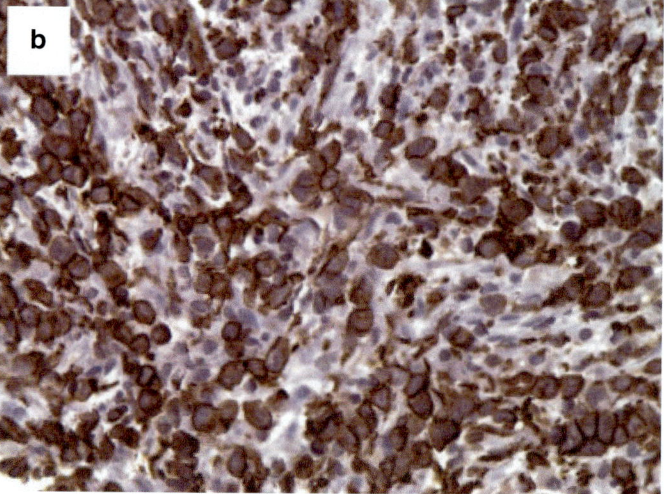

Fig. 11.3 Histological findings of the liver of a patient with ALCL, ALK−. The core biopsy shows lymphoid infiltrate composed of predominantly large cells with characteristic hallmark cell morphology, admixed with small lymphocytes (**a**, H&E stain, ×1000). These lymphoma cells are immunoreactive with CD30 in a membranous and Golgi pattern (**b** CD30 immunohistochemistry, ×400). Microscopic photos courtesy of Dr. Filiz Sen, Memorial Sloan Kettering Cancer Center, New York, NY

Extranodal NK-/T-Cell Lymphoma, Nasal Type

Definition

Extranodal NK-/T-cell lymphoma, nasal type (NK-/T-cell lymphoma) is a predominantly extranodal lymphoma of NK-cell or T-cell lineage, characterized by vascular damage and destruction, prominent necrosis, cytotoxic phenotype, and association with EBV [62].

Etiology

The very strong association with EBV, irrespective of the ethnic origin of the patients, suggests a pathogenic role of the virus [62].

Epidemiology

NK-/T-cell lymphoma exhibits marked geographic variation, with a high frequency in Asia and the indigenous population of Mexico and Central and South America [62].

Clinical Presentation

Clinically, NK-/T-cell lymphomas have a marked propensity for involving extranodal sites, most commonly the nasal cavity, nasopharynx, and palate [62, 63]. In a subset of patients, the disease involves non-aerodigestive tract sites (so-called non-nasal type), commonly in the skin, soft tissue, gastrointestinal tract, and testis [63]. Extranodal NK-/T-cell lymphomas involving the upper aerodigestive tract are predominantly localized processes at onset and may be present for years prior to diagnosis, but widespread dissemination can occur including lymph nodes and bone marrow [62, 64]. In disseminated disease the spleen and liver are often involved but rarely biopsied. A subset of patients developed hemophagocytic lymphohistiocytosis (HLH) [62, 65]. Primary splenic extranodal NK-/T-cell lymphoma is rarely reported [66].

Morphology

Grossly the spleen is usually enlarged with homogeneous surface (Fig. 11.4) [66]. Histologically, NK-/T-cell lymphomas are diffuse, destructive tumors that almost invariably are

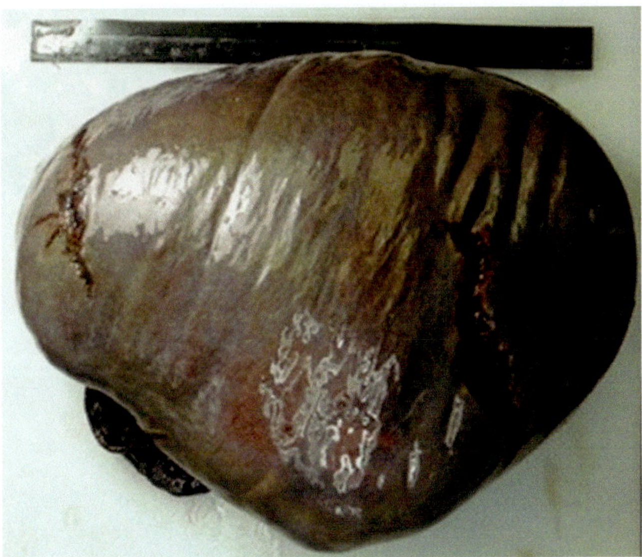

Fig. 11.4 Macroscopic appearance of the significantly enlarged 18.0 cm × 15.0 cm × 10.0 cm spleen of a patient with primary spleen extranodal NK-/T-cell lymphoma, nasal type. Surface and cut-surface of the spleen showed diffuse grayish crimson without nodules. (Adopted form Cao et al. [66])

associated with necrosis and commonly exhibit angioinvasion and angiodestruction [62, 67]. The cytologic spectrum of NK-/T-cell lymphomas is very wide and neoplasms can be composed of small or very large cells. A prominent inflammatory cell background is also usually present, but eosinophils and neutrophils are rare or absent. Splenic extranodal NK-/T-cell lymphoma shows more diffuse infiltrating pattern and contains a heterogeneous population of lymphoma cells (Fig. 11.5) [66].

Immunophenotyping

Immunophenotypic studies of NK-/T-cell lymphomas have shown that most cases are of NK-cell origin, although a subset of cases are of T-cell lineage [62, 67]. Virtually all cases of NK-/T-cell lymphoma are positive for EBER [62]. Most cases also express the NK-cell-associated antigen CD56 and NK-/T-cell-associated antigens such as CD2 and CD7. All cases of NK-/T-cell lymphomas express cytoplasmic CD3 epsilon; NK-cell tumors are negative for T-cell-specific antigens such as surface CD3, CD5, and TCRs, whereas T-cell tumors express these T-cell markers. Most NK-/T-cell lymphomas express cytotoxic markers (e.g., perforin, TIA-1, and granzyme B) [62]. CD16 and CD57 are usually negative, and Ig and B-cell antigens are negative.

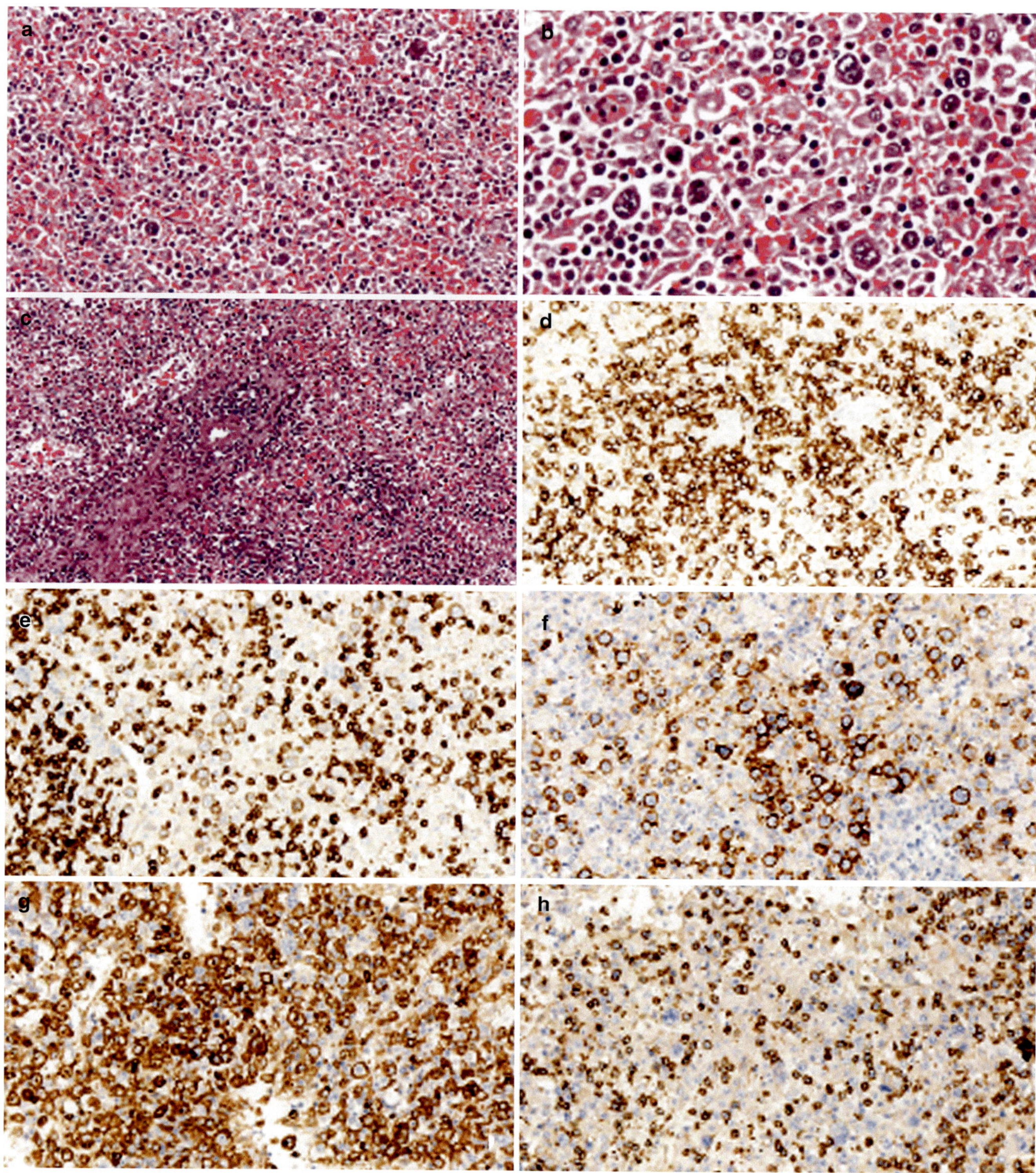

Fig. 11.5 Microscopic features of the spleen and the bone marrow of a patient with primary spleen extranodal NK-/T-cell lymphoma, nasal type (same case with Fig. 11.4). (**a**) The structure of spleen white and red pulp was destroyed by the diffusely infiltrating neoplastic cells (HE×100). (**b**) The size of the neoplastic cells was from medium to large with irregular pleomorphic hyperchromatin nuclei and conspicuous nucleoli. Giant tumor cells and apoptotic bodies were easily observed (HE×200). (**c**) A splenic artery was infiltrated and destroyed by the lymphomatous cells (HE×40); tumor cells were positive for CD2 (**d**), CD3ε (**e**), CD56 (**f**), CD4 (**g**), CD8 (**h**), and CD30 (**i**) (Envision×100). (**j**) Tumor cells were positive for EBERs by in situ hybridization. (**k**) Bone marrow biopsy showed scattered medium-sized tumor cells (arrow) (HE×100). (**l**) Tumor cells of bone marrow were positive for CD56 (Envision×100). (Adopted form Cao et al. [66])

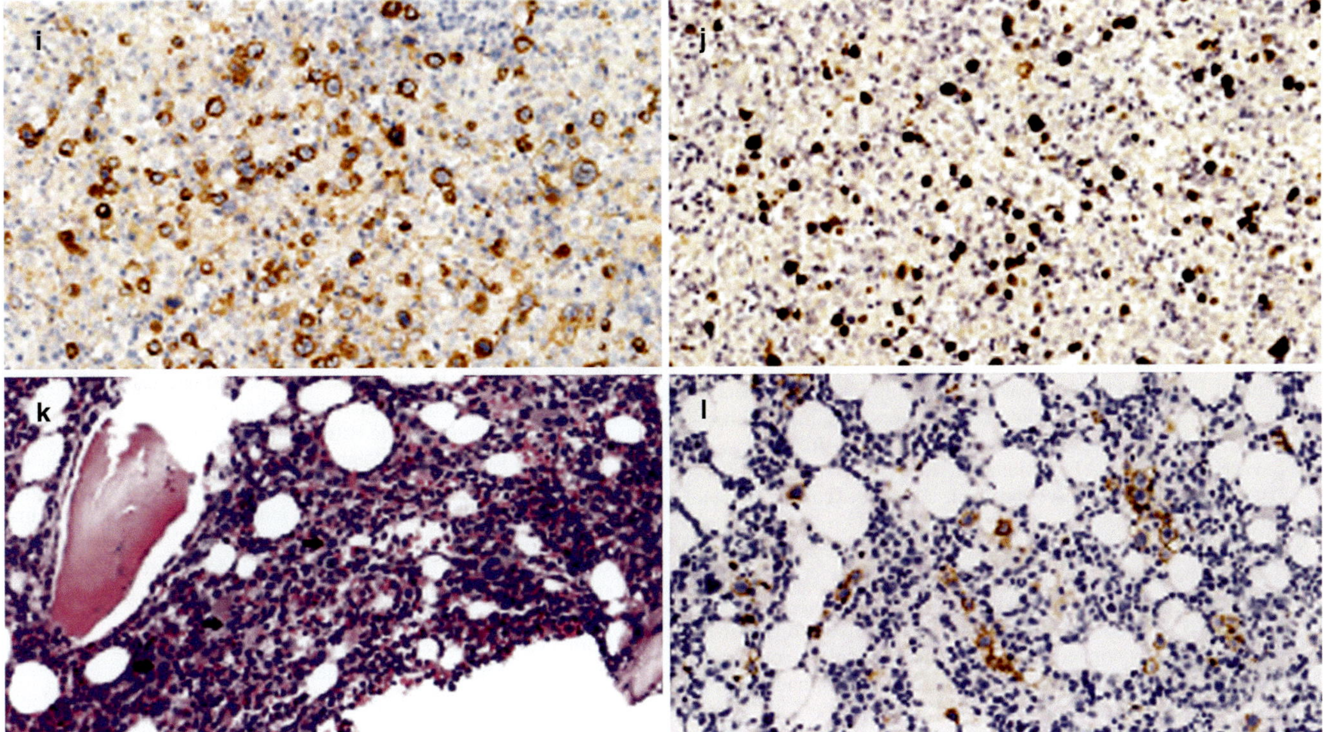

Fig. 11.5 (continued)

Cytogenetics and Molecular Findings

Molecular studies of NK-/T-cell lymphomas have shown an absence of *TCR* and *IG* rearrangements in NK cases and *TCR* gene rearrangements in T-cell cases [62]. EBV genomes have been identified in the neoplastic cells using Southern blot, PCR, and in situ hybridization techniques. The virus also has been shown to be present in monoclonal form indicating that EBV is present prior to clonal expansion. Comparative genomic hybridization studies of these neoplasms have shown gains of chromosome 2q and many losses involving chromosomal 1p, 4q, 5q, 6q, 7q, 12q, and 15q [68]. Deletion of chromosome 6q (6q21–6q25) is found in 40–50% of NK-/T-cell lymphoma cases, several putative tumor suppressor genes (*HACE1*, *PRDM1*, *ATG5*, *AIM1*, *FOXO3*) were identified in the 6q21–q25 region, and their roles as a potential tumor suppressors were suggested [69–71]. Many other gene alterations are reported, involving angiogenic genes, platelet-derived growth factor alpha (*PDGFRA*), tumor suppressor genes including *TP53*, and deregulation of the AKT, JAK-STAT, and NF-κB pathways. Among these, *TP53* mutations appear to correlate with large cell morphology and more advanced-stage disease [72].

Prognosis

The prognosis of patients with NK-/T-cell lymphomas involving the aerodigestive tract has improved with chemotherapy and radiotherapy [73, 74]. The prognosis of patients with non-nasal NK-/T-cell lymphomas is much poorer [63].

Diagnostic Caveats

1. Primary hepatic or splenic T-/NK-cell lymphomas are extremely rare.
2. Secondary involvement to the liver and/or spleen by T-cell prolymphocytic leukemia, aggressive NK-cell leukemia, and hepatosplenic T-cell lymphoma is more common.
3. The involvement of the spleen and liver by nodal or extranodal T-cell or NK-/T-cell lymphomas is less common and mostly as part of disseminated disease.
4. Liver or splenic biopsy is seldom performed. A diagnosis of these T-/NK-cell lymphoma/leukemias is usually made by a biopsy performed on the enlarged lymph nodes or evaluation of a peripheral blood sample in conjunction with morphology, immunophenotype, cytogenetics, and molecular study.

References

1. Pileri SA, Sng I, Muller-Hermelink HK, Chan WC, Jaffe ES. Peripheral T-cell lymphoma, NOS. In: Swerdlow SH, Campo E, Harris NL, Jaffe ES, Pileri SA, Stein H, Thiele J, editors. WHO classification of tumours of haematopoietic and lymphoid tissues. Lyon: IARC; 2017. p. 403–7.
2. Gallamini A, Stelitano C, Calvi R, et al. Peripheral T-cell lymphoma unspecified (PTCL-U): a new prognostic model from a retrospective multicentric clinical study. Blood. 2004;103(7):2474–9.
3. Vose J, Armitage J, Weisenburger D, International TCLP. International peripheral T-cell and natural killer/T-cell lymphoma study: pathology findings and clinical outcomes. J Clin Oncol. 2008;26(25):4124–30.
4. Zinzani PL, Broccoli A. T-cell lymphoproliferative disorders. In: Hoffbrand V, Higgs D, Keeling DEA, editors. Postgraduate hematology. Hoboken: Wiley BLackwell; 2016. p. 524–36.
5. Savage KJ, Ferreri AJ, Zinzani PL, Pileri SA. Peripheral T-cell lymphoma–not otherwise specified. Crit Rev Oncol Hematol. 2011;79(3):321–9.
6. Ramai D, Ofori E, Nigar S, Reddy M. Primary hepatic peripheral T-cell lymphoma associated with Epstein-Barr viral infection. World J Hepatol. 2018;10(2):347–51.
7. Ichikawa S, Hatta S, Saito Y, et al. CD20-positive and CD4/CD8-double-negative peripheral T-cell lymphoma of spleen complicated with severe disseminated intravascular coagulation and enteropathy. J Clin Exp Hematop. 2012;52(2):133–6.
8. Lepretre S, Buchonnet G, Stamatoullas A, et al. Chromosome abnormalities in peripheral T-cell lymphoma. Cancer Genet Cytogenet. 2000;117(1):71–9.
9. Thorns C, Bastian B, Pinkel D, et al. Chromosomal aberrations in angioimmunoblastic T-cell lymphoma and peripheral T-cell lymphoma unspecified: a matrix-based CGH approach. Genes Chromosomes Cancer. 2007;46(1):37–44.
10. Nelson M, Horsman DE, Weisenburger DD, et al. Cytogenetic abnormalities and clinical correlations in peripheral T-cell lymphoma. Br J Haematol. 2008;141(4):461–9.
11. Iqbal J, Wright G, Wang C, et al. Gene expression signatures delineate biological and prognostic subgroups in peripheral T-cell lymphoma. Blood. 2014;123(19):2915–23.
12. Sandell RF, Boddicker RL, Feldman AL. Genetic landscape and classification of peripheral T cell lymphomas. Curr Oncol Rep. 2017;19(4):28.
13. Schatz JH, Horwitz SM, Teruya-Feldstein J, et al. Targeted mutational profiling of peripheral T-cell lymphoma not otherwise specified highlights new mechanisms in a heterogeneous pathogenesis. Leukemia. 2015;29(1):237–41.
14. Franchini G. Molecular mechanisms of human T-cell leukemia/lymphotropic virus type I infection. Blood. 1995;86(10):3619–39.
15. Shimamoto Y, Suga K, Shibata K, Matsuzaki M, Yano H, Yamaguchi M. Clinical importance of extraordinary integration patterns of human T-cell lymphotropic virus type I proviral DNA in adult T-cell leukemia/lymphoma. Blood. 1994;84(3):853–8.
16. Tsukasaki K, Tobinai K. Human T-cell lymphotropic virus type I-associated adult T-cell leukemia-lymphoma: new directions in clinical research. Clin Cancer Res. 2014;20(20):5217–25.
17. Ohshima K, Yoshino T, Siebert R. Adult T-cell leukemia/lymphoma. In: Swerdlow SH, Campo E, Harris NL, Jaffe ES, Pileri SA, Stein H, Thiele J, editors. WHO classification of tumours of haematopoietic and lymphoid tissues. Lyon: IARC; 2017. p. 363–7.
18. Suzumiya J, Ohshima K, Tamura K, et al. The International Prognostic Index predicts outcome in aggressive adult T-cell leukemia/lymphoma: analysis of 126 patients from the International Peripheral T-Cell Lymphoma Project. Ann Oncol. 2009;20(4):715–21.
19. Shimoyama M. Diagnostic criteria and classification of clinical subtypes of adult T-cell leukaemia-lymphoma. A report from the Lymphoma Study Group (1984–87). Br J Haematol. 1991;79(3):428–37.
20. Tobinai K. Current management of adult T-cell leukemia/lymphoma. Oncology (Williston Park). 2009;23(14):1250–6.
21. Ohshima K. Pathological features of diseases associated with human T-cell leukemia virus type I. Cancer Sci. 2007;98(6):772–8.
22. Kawano H, Wakahashi K, Ebara S, et al. Unusual hepatic involvement with significant fibrosis in adult T cell leukemia. Ann Hematol. 2014;93(5):897–8.
23. Karube K, Aoki R, Sugita Y, et al. The relationship of FOXP3 expression and clinicopathological characteristics in adult T-cell leukemia/lymphoma. Mod Pathol. 2008;21(5):617–25.
24. Itoyama T, Chaganti RS, Yamada Y, et al. Cytogenetic analysis and clinical significance in adult T-cell leukemia/lymphoma: a study of 50 cases from the human T-cell leukemia virus type-1 endemic area, Nagasaki. Blood. 2001;97(11):3612–20.
25. Oshiro A, Tagawa H, Ohshima K, et al. Identification of subtype-specific genomic alterations in aggressive adult T-cell leukemia/lymphoma. Blood. 2006;107(11):4500–7.
26. Choi YL, Tsukasaki K, O'Neill MC, et al. A genomic analysis of adult T-cell leukemia. Oncogene. 2007;26(8):1245–55.
27. Kataoka K, Nagata Y, Kitanaka A, et al. Integrated molecular analysis of adult T cell leukemia/lymphoma. Nat Genet. 2015;47(11):1304–15.
28. Dogan A, Jaffe ES, Muller-Hermelink HK, de Leval L. Angioimmunoblastic T-cell lymphoma and other nodal lymphomas of T follicular helper cell origin. In: Swerdlow SH, Campo E, Harris NL, Jaffe ES, Pileri SA, Stein H, Thiele J, editors. WHO classification of tumours of haematopoietic and lymphoid tissues. Lyon: IARC; 2017. p. 407–12.
29. Mourad N, Mounier N, Briere J, et al. Clinical, biologic, and pathologic features in 157 patients with angioimmunoblastic T-cell lymphoma treated within the Groupe d'Etude des Lymphomes de l'Adulte (GELA) trials. Blood. 2008;111(9):4463–70.
30. Willenbrock K, Brauninger A, Hansmann ML. Frequent occurrence of B-cell lymphomas in angioimmunoblastic T-cell lymphoma and proliferation of Epstein-Barr virus-infected cells in early cases. Br J Haematol. 2007;138(6):733–9.
31. Attygalle AD, Kyriakou C, Dupuis J, et al. Histologic evolution of angioimmunoblastic T-cell lymphoma in consecutive biopsies: clinical correlation and insights into natural history and disease progression. Am J Surg Pathol. 2007;31(7):1077–88.
32. de Leval L, Gisselbrecht C, Gaulard P. Advances in the understanding and management of angioimmunoblastic T-cell lymphoma. Br J Haematol. 2010;148(5):673–89.
33. Grogg KL, Attygalle AD, Macon WR, Remstein ED, Kurtin PJ, Dogan A. Expression of CXCL13, a chemokine highly upregulated in germinal center T-helper cells, distinguishes angioimmunoblastic T-cell lymphoma from peripheral T-cell lymphoma, unspecified. Mod Pathol. 2006;19(8):1101–7.
34. Schlegelberger B, Zhang Y, Weber-Matthiesen K, Grote W. Detection of aberrant clones in nearly all cases of angioimmunoblastic lymphadenopathy with dysproteinemia-type T-cell lymphoma by combined interphase and metaphase cytogenetics. Blood. 1994;84(8):2640–8.
35. de Leval L, Rickman DS, Thielen C, et al. The gene expression profile of nodal peripheral T-cell lymphoma demonstrates a molecular link between angioimmunoblastic T-cell

lymphoma (AITL) and follicular helper T (TFH) cells. Blood. 2007;109(11):4952–63.

36. Couronne L, Bastard C, Bernard OA. TET2 and DNMT3A mutations in human T-cell lymphoma. N Engl J Med. 2012;366(1):95–6.

37. Odejide O, Weigert O, Lane AA, et al. A targeted mutational landscape of angioimmunoblastic T-cell lymphoma. Blood. 2014;123(9):1293–6.

38. Sakata-Yanagimoto M, Enami T, Yoshida K, et al. Somatic RHOA mutation in angioimmunoblastic T cell lymphoma. Nat Genet. 2014;46(2):171–5.

39. Falini B, Campo E, Jaffe ES, Gascoyne RD, Stein H, Muller-Hermelink HK, Kinney MC. Anaplastic large cell lymphoma, ALK-positive. In: Swerdlow SH, Campo E, Harris NL, Jaffe ES, Pileri SA, Stein H, Thiele J, editors. WHO classification of tumours of haematopoietic and lymphoid tissues. Lyon: IARC; 2017. p. 413–8.

40. Feldman AL, Stein H, Campo E, Kinney MC, Jaffe ES, Falini B, Inghirami GG, Pileri SA. Anaplastic large cell lymphoma, ALK-negative. In: Swerdlow SH, Campo E, Harris NL, Jaffe ES, Pileri SA, Stein H, Thiele J, editors. WHO classification of tumours of haematopoietic and lymphoid tissues. Lyon: IARC; 2017. p. 418–21.

41. Feldman AL, Stein H, Campo E, Kinney MC, Jaffe ES, Falini B, Inghirami GG, Pileri SA. Breast implant-associated anaplastic large cell lymphoma. In: Swerdlow SH, Campo E, Harris NL, Jaffe ES, Pileri SA, Stein H, Thiele J, editors. WHO classification of tumours of haematopoietic and lymphoid tissues. Lyon: IARC; 2017. p. 421–2.

42. Willemze R, Kadin ME. Primary cutaneous CD30-positive T-cell lymphoproliferative disorders. In: Swerdlow SH, Campo E, Harris NL, Jaffe ES, Pileri SA, Stein H, Thiele J, editors. WHO classification of tumours of haematopoietic and lymphoid tissues. Lyon: IARC; 2017. p. 392–6.

43. Medeiros LJ, Elenitoba-Johnson KS. Anaplastic large cell lymphoma. Am J Clin Pathol. 2007;127(5):707–22.

44. Lamant L, McCarthy K, d'Amore E, et al. Prognostic impact of morphologic and phenotypic features of childhood ALK-positive anaplastic large-cell lymphoma: results of the ALCL99 study. J Clin Oncol. 2011;29(35):4669–76.

45. Rassidakis GZ, Sarris AH, Herling M, et al. Differential expression of BCL-2 family proteins in ALK-positive and ALK-negative anaplastic large cell lymphoma of T/null-cell lineage. Am J Pathol. 2001;159(2):527–35.

46. Kaneko Y, Frizzera G, Edamura S, et al. A novel translocation, t(2;5)(p23;q35), in childhood phagocytic large T-cell lymphoma mimicking malignant histiocytosis. Blood. 1989;73(3):806–13.

47. Morris SW, Kirstein MN, Valentine MB, et al. Fusion of a kinase gene, ALK, to a nucleolar protein gene, NPM, in non-Hodgkin's lymphoma. Science. 1994;263(5151):1281–4.

48. Feldman AL, Vasmatzis G, Asmann YW, et al. Novel TRAF1-ALK fusion identified by deep RNA sequencing of anaplastic large cell lymphoma. Genes Chromosomes Cancer. 2013;52(11):1097–102.

49. Cannella S, Santoro A, Bruno G, et al. Germline mutations of the perforin gene are a frequent occurrence in childhood anaplastic large cell lymphoma. Cancer. 2007;109(12):2566–71.

50. Rassidakis GZ, Lai R, Herling M, Cromwell C, Schmitt-Graeff A, Medeiros LJ. Retinoblastoma protein is frequently absent or phosphorylated in anaplastic large-cell lymphoma. Am J Pathol. 2004;164(6):2259–67.

51. Lamant L, de Reynies A, Duplantier MM, et al. Gene-expression profiling of systemic anaplastic large-cell lymphoma reveals differences based on ALK status and two distinct morphologic ALK+ subtypes. Blood. 2007;109(5):2156–64.

52. Liang X, Branchford B, Greffe B, et al. Dual ALK and MYC rearrangements leading to an aggressive variant of anaplastic large cell lymphoma. J Pediatr Hematol Oncol. 2013;35(5):e209–13.

53. Moritake H, Shimonodan H, Marutsuka K, Kamimura S, Kojima H, Nunoi H. C-MYC rearrangement may induce an aggressive phenotype in anaplastic lymphoma kinase positive anaplastic large cell lymphoma: identification of a novel fusion gene ALO17/C-MYC. Am J Hematol. 2011;86(1):75–8.

54. Parrilla Castellar ER, Jaffe ES, Said JW, et al. ALK-negative anaplastic large cell lymphoma is a genetically heterogeneous disease with widely disparate clinical outcomes. Blood. 2014;124(9):1473–80.

55. Falini B. Anaplastic large cell lymphoma: pathological, molecular and clinical features. Br J Haematol. 2001;114(4):741–60.

56. Cerban R, Gheorghe L, Becheanu G, Serban V, Gheorghe C. Primary focal T-cell lymphoma of the liver: a case report and review of the literature. J Gastrointestin Liver Dis. 2012;21(2):213–6.

57. Saikia UN, Sharma N, Duseja A, Bhalla A, Joshi K. Anaplastic large cell lymphoma presenting as acute liver failure: a report of two cases with review of literature. Ann Hepatol. 2010;9(4):457–61.

58. Cai G, Inghirami G, Moreira A, Sen F. Primary hepatic anaplastic large-cell lymphoma diagnosed by fine-needle aspiration biopsy. Diagn Cytopathol. 2005;33(2):106–9.

59. Feldman AL, Dogan A, Smith DI, et al. Discovery of recurrent t(6;7)(p25.3;q32.3) translocations in ALK-negative anaplastic large cell lymphomas by massively parallel genomic sequencing. Blood. 2011;117(3):915–9.

60. Alonso A, Merlo JJ, Na S, et al. Inhibition of T cell antigen receptor signaling by VHR-related MKPX (VHX), a new dual specificity phosphatase related to VH1 related (VHR). J Biol Chem. 2002;277(7):5524–8.

61. Vasmatzis G, Johnson SH, Knudson RA, et al. Genome-wide analysis reveals recurrent structural abnormalities of TP63 and other p53-related genes in peripheral T-cell lymphomas. Blood. 2012;120(11):2280–9.

62. Chan JK, Ferry JA. Extranodal NK/T-cell lymphoma, nasal type. In: Swerdlow SH, Campo E, Harris NL, Jaffe ES, Pileri SA, Stein H, Thiele J, editors. WHO classification of tumours of haematopoietic and lymphoid tissues. Lyon: IARC; 2017. p. 368–71.

63. Au WY, Weisenburger DD, Intragumtornchai T, et al. Clinical differences between nasal and extranasal natural killer/T-cell lymphoma: a study of 136 cases from the International Peripheral T-Cell Lymphoma Project. Blood. 2009;113(17):3931–7.

64. Shet T, Suryawanshi P, Epari S, et al. Extranodal natural killer/T cell lymphomas with extranasal disease in non-endemic regions are disseminated or have nasal primary: a study of 84 cases from India. Leuk Lymphoma. 2014;55(12):2748–53.

65. Takahashi N, Miura I, Chubachi A, Miura AB, Nakamura S. A clinicopathological study of 20 patients with T/natural killer (NK)-cell lymphoma-associated hemophagocytic syndrome with special reference to nasal and nasal-type NK/T-cell lymphoma. Int J Hematol. 2001;74(3):303–8.

66. Cao Q, Huang Y, Ye Z, Liu N, Li S, Peng T. Primary spleen extranodal NK/T cell lymphoma, nasal type, with bone marrow involvement and CD30 positive expression: a case report and literature review. Diagn Pathol. 2014;9:169.

67. Li S, Feng X, Li T, et al. Extranodal NK/T-cell lymphoma, nasal type: a report of 73 cases at MD Anderson Cancer Center. Am J Surg Pathol. 2013;37(1):14–23.

68. Ko YH, Choi KE, Han JH, Kim JM, Ree HJ. Comparative genomic hybridization study of nasal-type NK/T-cell lymphoma. Cytometry. 2001;46(2):85–91.

69. Huang Y, de Reynies A, de Leval L, et al. Gene expression profiling identifies emerging oncogenic pathways operating in extranodal NK/T-cell lymphoma, nasal type. Blood. 2010;115(6):1226–37.

70. Iqbal J, Kucuk C, Deleeuw RJ, et al. Genomic analyses reveal global functional alterations that promote tumor growth and novel tumor suppressor genes in natural killer-cell malignancies. Leukemia. 2009;23(6):1139–51.

71. Huang Y, de Leval L, Gaulard P. Molecular underpinning of extranodal NK/T-cell lymphoma. Best Pract Res Clin Haematol. 2013;26(1):57–74.

72. Quintanilla-Martinez L, Kremer M, Keller G, et al. p53 Mutations in nasal natural killer/T-cell lymphoma from Mexico: association with large cell morphology and advanced disease. Am J Pathol. 2001;159(6):2095–105.

73. Liang R. Advances in the management and monitoring of extranodal NK/T-cell lymphoma, nasal type. Br J Haematol. 2009;147(1):13–21.

74. Wang ZY, Li YX, Wang WH, et al. Primary radiotherapy showed favorable outcome in treating extranodal nasal-type NK/T-cell lymphoma in children and adolescents. Blood. 2009;114(23):4771–6.

Joo Young Song and Saba Fatima Ali

Introduction

According to the World Health Organization (WHO), Hodgkin lymphomas are divided into two subtypes: classic Hodgkin lymphoma (CHL) (approximately 95% of cases) and nodular lymphocyte-predominant Hodgkin lymphoma (NLPHL). CHL rarely arises as an isolated lymphoma confined to a single organ or tissue, but nodular lymphocyte-predominant Hodgkin lymphoma (NLPHL) may present as localized disease. Clinically patients with CHL present with generalized lymphadenopathy, particularly in cervical and axillary lymph nodes and mediastinum. The liver and spleen are frequently involved in the advanced stage, and modern-day practice uses imaging to guide detection and assessment of stage as staging laparotomy has long since been obsolete. Only very rare cases of primary splenic lymphoma of Hodgkin's disease have been reported, and none of the liver. CHL is characterized by identifiable Reed-Sternberg cells or Hodgkin cells (CD45$^-$/CD30$^+$/CD15$^+$/CD20$^{-/+}$ and PAX-5^{dim+}) in a matrix of inflammatory cells with or without extensive fibrosis, while NLPHL is manifested by expansive vague nodule of small lymphocytes intermingling with sparse large LP cells (lymphocyte-predominant cells, or popcorn cells) (CD45$^+$/CD20$^+$/PAX-5$^{strong+}$/CD15$^-$/CD30$^-$). Here we outline the generalized features of the Hodgkin lymphomas and highlight characteristics specific to liver and spleen (primary and secondary) involvement.

Definition

Hodgkin lymphoma is a group of mature B-cell neoplasms composed of a small component of large neoplastic cells with varying degrees of reactive background polymorphous inflammatory cells. Hodgkin lymphoma was first described by Thomas Hodgkin in 1832 in a series of autopsy reports of patients with massive enlargement of the lymph nodes and spleen [1]. Originally subclassified into distinct histologic subtypes according to Lukes and Butler and later modified by Rye [2, 3], the current classification is defined by the World Health Organization (WHO) Classification of Tumors of Hematopoietic and Lymphoid Tissues (2017) and includes two main types: nodular lymphocyte-predominant Hodgkin lymphoma (NLPHL) and classic Hodgkin lymphoma (CHL) [4]. Classic Hodgkin lymphoma is further subdivided based on the background inflammatory infiltrate, epidemiologic and etiologic factors, and architectural features: nodular sclerosis, lymphocyte-rich, mixed-cellularity, and lymphocyte-depleted subtypes. Immunohistochemistry expressions in all histologic subtypes of CHL are similar and representative of the underlying decrease of the B-cell program (decrease or loss of PAX5 and CD20 expression). In contrast, NLPHL maintains expression of B-cell lineage-specific markers such as CD20, CD79a, and transcription factors such as PAX5 and Oct2. Although there are striking phenotypic differences between the tumor cells of NLPHL and CHL, they are both believed to be derived from germinal center B-cells [4–7].

Epidemiology

General

Classic Hodgkin lymphomas comprise 0.5% of all newly diagnosed cancer cases in the United States of America (USA). The annual incidence of CHL is approximately 2.5 per 100,000 new cases/year on average with 0.3 per 100,000 deaths/year on average. The 5-year survival rate from 2008 to 2014 is a reported 86.6%. Although the annual incidence has remained constant, newer screening tools and advances in therapy have shown a change in death rate statistics, decreasing 2.8% per year from 2005 to 2015 [8]. NLPHL accounts for 3–8% of Hodgkin lymphomas [9, 10].

J. Y. Song (✉) · S. F. Ali
Department of Pathology and Laboratory Medicine, City of Hope National Medical Center, Duarte, CA, USA
e-mail: josong@coh.org

© Springer Nature Switzerland AG 2020
L. Zhang et al. (eds.), *Diagnostic Pathology of Hematopoietic Disorders of Spleen and Liver*,
https://doi.org/10.1007/978-3-030-37708-3_12

Classic Hodgkin lymphoma presents with a bimodal age distribution, occurring in younger patients between the ages of 20 and 34 and in older patients between the ages of 75 and 84 [4, 6]. CHL is rare in children, and approximately 12% of cases occur in patients less than 20 years of age [8]. The median age at death is 67 years, with approximately 22% of deaths occurring in the older age group. In contrast, deaths attributed to the younger age group comprise 10.7% of all cases [8]. The peak incidence for NLPHL is the fourth decade [10].

Hodgkin lymphoma has a slightly greater predilection for men (2.9/100,000 per year) than women (2.2/100,000 per year) [8] in age-adjusted statistics regardless of race for all histological subtypes except nodular sclerosis, which is more common in younger females [4, 7]. The number of new cases per year is slightly higher in black males (3.1/100,000/ per year) than white males (3.0/100,000/ per year), and the incidence decreases in the Hispanic and Asian races [8]. In contrast, NLPHL has a male predominance of 2.4:1 [10].

The majority of CHL cases present in stage II (40%), with the lymphoma localized to the regional lymph nodes. The 5-year survival rate for stage II cancer is 93.4%. Approximately 20% of patients present in stage III with splenic involvement, and the relative 5-year survival for all races and both genders with stage III disease is 83%. Distant metastasis with potential hepatic involvement accounting for stage IV lymphoma is the presenting stage in approximately 20% of patients, with a 5-year relative survival of 72.9% [8]. NLPHL usually presents with isolated lymphadenopathy, and there is frequent involvement of the cervical and axillary nodes with mediastinal being a rare site [9, 11]. Classic Hodgkin lymphoma accounts for almost 90% of cases [4]. The most common subtype of CHL is the nodular sclerosis subtype, which frequently presents in younger patients with a predilection for females [4, 7]. Mixed cellularity occurs in older patients and has a greater association with Epstein-Barr virus (EBV) [4, 7, 8]. Lymphocyte-rich CHL accounts for up to 5% of all CHL, occurs in older individuals (median age 38 years), and often presents in the early stages of disease (80% stage I and stage II) [9, 12]. Lymphocyte-depleted CHL is rare and occurs in less than 1% of cases. NLPHL accounts for 3–8% [9] of all cases of Hodgkin lymphoma, occurs in the older age group (median age 40) [4, 8, 9], and often presents in the early stages of disease, similar to lymphocyte-rich CHL [9, 12].

Familial Hodgkin Lymphoma

Familial Hodgkin lymphoma only contributes to a minority of cases and is infrequent; however studies have proved first-degree relatives have an increased risk for developing lymphoma [7]. In a study by Mack et al., 10/179 monozygotic twins both developed Hodgkin lymphoma. However cytoge-netic evidence is lacking and further studies are needed to define specific genetic links [13].

Viral-Related Hodgkin Lymphoma

In westernized developed countries, the incidence of Hodgkin lymphoma is higher [4, 8, 14]. Studies have shown this is in part due to the association of viral risk factors, primarily Epstein-Barr virus, and the timing of childhood exposure, with an increased risk for Hodgkin lymphoma for those exposed at a later age. Hence, the incidence is increased in smaller families with fewer children as compared to larger families who have a higher probability of previous viral exposure. Additionally, the incidence of Hodgkin lymphoma is increased in families with parents who have a higher level of education and thus a more affluent family background [14–16]. These epidemiologic findings are similar to other Epstein-Barr virus-related diseases, including poliomyelitis and infectious mononucleosis, thus supporting the relationship of EBV and HL [15, 16].

Incidence of HL Confined to the Spleen and Liver

Hodgkin lymphoma involving the spleen is frequently a secondary phenomenon and rarely a primary site of involvement. The incidence of Hodgkin lymphoma confined to the spleen is extremely rare and is estimated to be <1% [13, 17, 18]. Between 1968 and 1997, only five cases of PSL-HD were reported [19]. In a study by Kraemer on primary splenic lymphoma, only 1 case out of 49 was Hodgkin lymphoma [20]. The frequency of involvement of the spleen correlates with histologic subtype: nodular sclerosis 39%, mixed cellularity 62%, lymphocyte depletion 66%, and lymphocyte predominant 23% [21]. There have been no reports on Hodgkin lymphoma confined to the liver only. When the liver is involved, it occurs in the advanced stages of the disease and always with previously documented or concurrent splenic involvement [22]. A small subset of NLPHL has been reported to be involved in the spleen (8%), liver (3%), and rarely other body sites such as the bone (2%) and lung (1%) during the natural course of disease.

Etiology and Pathogenesis

Although the driving factor behind all cases of Hodgkin lymphoma remains to be defined, viral infection is considered the main etiology. In 1966 MacMahon proposed an infectious agent as a contributing factor in young adults [14]. Since then, studies have hinted the possible oncogenetic role of Epstein-Barr virus (EBV), which is detected in at least 30–50% of Hodgkin lymphoma cases [23]. EBV has a greater association in young adults with infectious mononucleosis (IM); some studies have reported as much as sevenfold increased risk. This is controversial, as other studies show a risk of developing HL after IM infection in only 1 in 1000 persons and other confounding factors are likely responsible for the development of lymphoma [24]. Additionally EBV is not demonstrated in all of the cases associated with IM, although this may be due to loss of EBV in the RS cells [24]. EBV-associated CHL has a geographic predilection for developing countries, where it is present in >90% of cases. Histologic subtypes frequently associated with EBV include mixed cellularity, particularly in the older age group, and lymphocyte depleted [3, 4, 23–26]. NLPHL is rarely affected with EBV [4].

EBV in HL is present in memory B-cells and can be present in the serum and plasma as naked viral DNA and within Hodgkin/Reed-Sternberg (HRS) cells [26]. EBV remains latent in HRS cells in the type II form, with expression of EBV early RNA (EBER)-1, EBER-2, and BamHI, as well as protein expression of latent membrane protein (LMP)-1, latent membrane protein-2, and EBNA1 [23, 26]. It is postulated LMP-1 and LMP-2 assist in B-cell transformation by activating the NFkB pathway, a pro-inflammatory and anti-apoptotic transcription factor. BCL-2 protein expression is augmented by NFkB. RANK and IL-13 also reportedly increase NFkB transcription. In addition to NFkB providing the HRS with antiapoptotic benefits, another reported mechanism HRS escape death is through Fas resistance. HRS cells are believed to be crippled germinal center B-cells, and the normal physiologic response to abnormal affinity maturation, lack of surface immunoglobulin expression, and clonal Ig rearrangement of the HRS cells lead to Fas-mediated destruction. Thus a poorly defined mechanism to escape death in the germinal center by Fas-mediated apoptosis contributes to the immortality of the neoplastic HRS cells [23].

Genetic analysis has shown the risk of EBV-associated HL may be linked to HLA1 alleles. The risk of EBV-positive Hodgkin lymphoma after IM was increased with HLA-A∗01 alleles and decreased with HLA-A∗02 alleles [27].

Immunosuppression leads to uncontrolled EBV infection and increases the risk of EBV-related CHL; these cases have a much higher mortality rate than non-immunosuppressed patients [28]. The incidence of death due to Hodgkin lymphoma can largely be attributed to individuals infected with both HIV and EBV, accounting for 8% of deaths in males and 1% of deaths in females [4, 27, 28].

Clinical Presentation

Spleen

As discussed above, isolated involvement of the spleen by Hodgkin lymphoma is an extremely rare occurrence, accounting for less than 1% of cases. Historically, primary splenic involvement is controversial since microscopic involvement of lymph nodes or an extranodal site cannot

confidently be excluded [17]. Modern-day imaging using positron emission tomography-computed tomography (PET-CT) may be helpful in ruling out extrasplenic lymphoma involvement and supporting the diagnosis. Because splenomegaly is a nonspecific finding, in the absence of disseminated disease, an accurate diagnosis of Hodgkin lymphoma can easily be missed. Depending on the histologic subtype, the incidence of splenic involvement varies and the majority of the time involvement is not isolated. NLPHL tends to have a more indolent clinical course, and the incidence of splenic spread is low (<10%; constitutional symptoms are infrequent) [9, 12]. Splenic involvement is a frequent presenting feature of lymphocyte-depleted Hodgkin lymphoma as a secondary site in the advanced stage [4, 13].

Primary Splenic Hodgkin Lymphoma

Primary splenic Hodgkin lymphoma (PS-HL) was first described in 1931 by Symmers et al. [17, 29]. Since many reports regarding the criteria for an accurate diagnosis of PS-HL have been reported. Das Gupta described criteria required for the diagnosis of PS-HL, which include splenomegaly as a presenting symptom, absence of lymphoma at other sites, negative laparotomy liver and lymph node biopsies, and a disease-free interval of 6 months after splenectomy [18]. Generally, the clinical presentation of primary splenic lymphoma is nonspecific and includes upper quadrant abdominal pain, bi- or pancytopenia, malaise, generalized weakness, and fever [17, 20]. In1965 specific qualifications for the diagnosis of PS-HL were defined by Gebauer and include (1) enlarged spleen, (2) Pel-Ebstein fever, (3) weight loss, and (4) anemia, leukopenia, thrombocytopenia, and lymphocytosis. In cases of extreme anemia, the clinical picture is related and can include dyspnea and non-pitting edema. This anemia does not respond to blood transfusions and marked thrombocytopenia is frequently apparent. In 1984, Kraemer reported three main criteria including splenomegaly, bicytopenia, and no lymphadenopathy [20]. Despite such criteria, the clinical presentation of splenomegaly in some reports is inconsistent. In a study by Rosenberg, half of the patients with splenomegaly had histological involvement by Hodgkin lymphoma. The remainder of cases did not have lymphoma involvement, weighed up to 400 g, and microscopic examination demonstrated vascular congestion and granulomata formation as the cause for enlargement. The probability of lymphoma in the spleen is increased above 400 g. Additionally, Rosenberg reported about a quarter of patients will have splenic involvement of CHL without splenomegaly [22].

Splenic rupture in HD-PSL is an extremely rare occurrence with a high mortality; symptoms include fever, acute weight loss, cytopenias, and cardiogenic shock [30]. Rarely primary splenic Hodgkin lymphoma can occur in association with chronic and hereditary granulomatous disease [31], hemorrhagic ascites, or chronic pruritus [32]. The bone marrow is typically normal.

Secondary Splenic Hodgkin Lymphoma

Systemic symptoms and splenic involvement are typically seen in advanced stages of Hodgkin lymphoma. Histological evaluation of traditional staging laparotomy specimens showed splenic disease by contiguous spread in up to at least 40% of cases at initial diagnosis. In a study of 13 patients, Aisenberg et al. reported the spleen is the first abdominal organ involved and spread to the surrounding lymph nodes occurs subsequently, likely through the bloodstream because the spleen lacks a lymphatic supply [33]. The possibility of initial involvement of the lymph nodes and retrograde spread to the spleen, however, is also a plausible mechanism for splenic lymphoma. Patients in advanced-stage disease have symptoms resulting from splenomegaly, painless enlargement of supradiaphragmatic lymph nodes, bulky mediastinal disease, and generalized nonspecific symptoms such as malaise and fatigue [32, 33]. Per the Ann Arbor staging, the spleen is a "nodal" site, and involvement confers stage III disease and may manifest B symptoms (fever, night sweats, weight loss). The presence of B-symptoms in Hodgkin lymphoma confers a poor prognosis [34].

Liver

Liver involvement in Hodgkin disease rarely occurs without concurrent splenic lymphoma, and a positive correlation between increasing splenic weight and greater likelihood of hepatic involvement exists [22]. Clinical signs and symptoms including palpable hepatomegaly, abnormal laboratory tests (such as elevated aspartate aminotransferase, AST, and alanine aminotransferase, ALT), and imaging studies including magnetic resonance imaging (MRI), CT, and ultrasound showing diffuse hepatic enlargement are nonspecific and have low accuracy, with a sensitivity of about 40% for the liver and spleen [22, 35, 36]. Histological confirmation is required for diagnosis; however false negatives may occur due to limited biopsy specimens and small focal lesions. Lymphocyte-rich Hodgkin lymphoma involves the liver more often than the spleen (2% of cases) [12] in contrast to other CHL.

Morphology

Gross Features

Spleen: Gross examination of the spleen when involved by Hodgkin lymphoma shows a variable appearance. Autopsy reports and examination of laparotomy specimens report features of subtle congestion, firm parenchymal consistency, and the presence of infarcts and increased fibrosis [17]. More obvious lesions show large single or multifocal tumor masses [20] or single small parenchymal nodules [32]. During gross examination, serial sections of 1–1.5 cm [37] are crucial to avoid missing smaller lymphoma deposits. These may present as small gross enlargements of Malpighian corpuscles [2, 38]. Extensive fibrosis results in an adherence to the surrounding visceral organs, particularly the stomach, pancreas, and liver [19]. The average weight of the spleen is 258 grams with a range of 55–3290 grams. An interesting correlation between splenic weight and erythrocyte sedimentation rate shows a higher probability of lymphoma involvement with a splenic weight of at least 300 grams and an ESR of >50 mmHg [38].

Liver: The liver may be enlarged, either due to vascular congestion or a benign reactive lymphocytic infiltrate rather than true involvement by lymphoma. Similarly to the spleen, obvious lesions may present as large tumor masses or small miliary nodules [39, 40].

Microscopic Features

Spleen

Splenic histology is largely dependent upon the degree of involvement and subclassification can often be difficult. In cases with minimal involvement, at low power, the splenic architecture is generally preserved in both red and white pulp [37]. The initial foci of HL can be identified next to the white pulp and blood vessels, within the marginal zones and peri-arteriolar lymphoid sheaths [37, 40]. A variable cellular reaction is present in the background, with eosinophils, plasma cells, histiocytes, and fibrosis. Hodgkin and Reed-Sternberg cells may be difficult to find, but they show the classic morphology of large atypical cells with vesicular chromatin, irregular nuclear contours, and prominent nucleoli with occasional Reed-Sternberg cells (Figs. 12.1 and 12.2) [31]. Necrosis may be seen in association with nodular sclerosis and mixed-cellularity types in a third of cases, and many atypical histiocytes and HRS cells are present around these areas [38]. Reactive germinal centers and hemorrhage are present, and rare vascular invasion may be seen, particularly in cases of nodular sclerosis [38].

Nodular lymphocyte-predominant Hodgkin lymphoma is rare in the spleen. Even positive for imaging finding, a biopsy of enlarged lymph node is diagnostic. Splenectomy is not an indication.

Immunohistochemistry studies are required to distinguish NLPHL and CHL as they are morphologically similar in the spleen [37].

Histological subclassification in the spleen is not a therapeutic implication and thus is not necessary. Histologic discordance may be seen in the spleen and other sites of lymphoma. Non-caseating granulomata when present consist of large clusters of epithelioid histiocytes that replace the

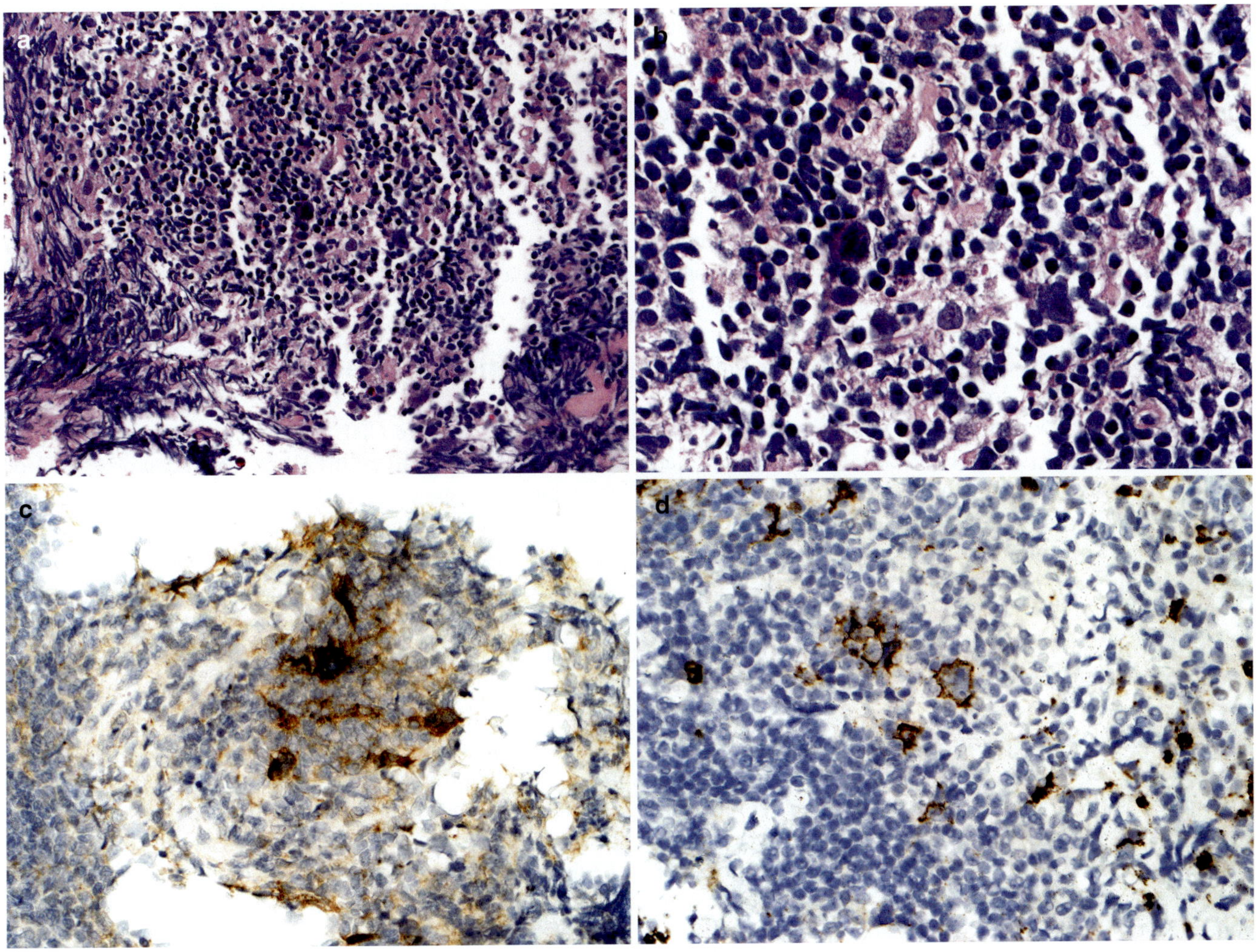

Fig. 12.1 Classic Hodgkin lymphoma. H&E section of the spleen showing a dense lymphocytic infiltrate and scattered large Hodgkin/Reed-Sternberg (HRS) cells (**a**, 400× magnification). Higher power showing the HRS cells with round nuclear contours, fine chroma- tin, variably prominent nucleoli, and scant to moderate cytoplasm (**b**, 600×). The HRS show membranous staining for CD30 (**c**, 400× magnification) and CD15 (**d**, 400× magnification)

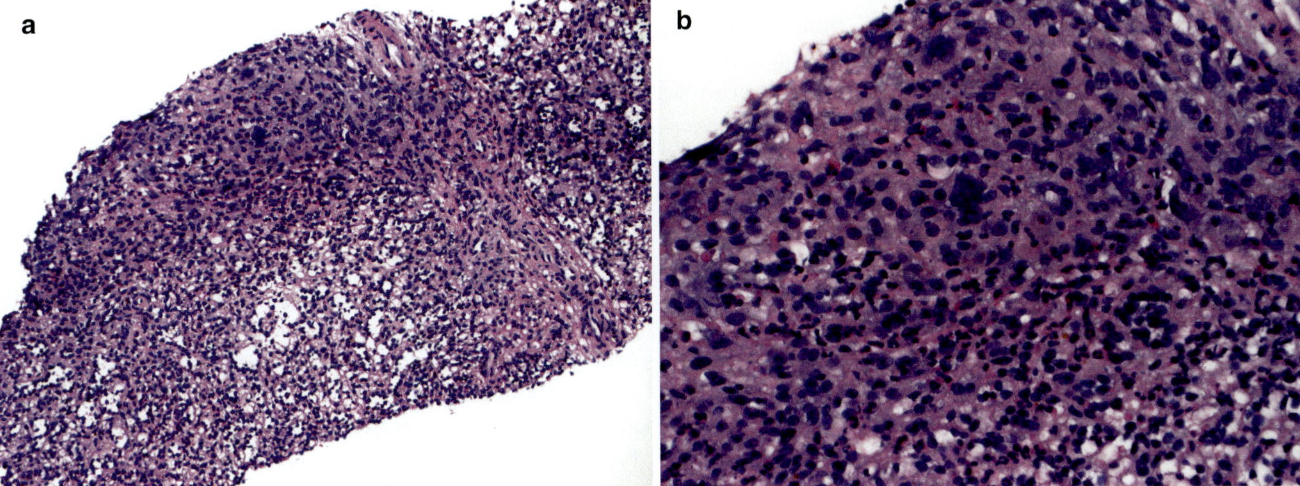

Fig. 12.2 Classic Hodgkin lymphoma. H&E section of the spleen showing Hodgkin/Reed-Sternberg (HRS) cells of variable sizes in a background of lymphocytes, eosinophils, neutrophils, and histiocytes. The surrounding splenic architecture is preserved and fibrosis is limited (200× magnification). The same HRS cells (**b**) at higher magnification (400× magnification). Immunostains (not shown) demonstrate expres- sion with CD15 and CD30

white pulp around periarteriolar lymphoid sheaths [38]. These findings imply a positive prognosis [40]. The granulomata lack Schaumann/asteroid bodies and when extensive can be identified in the red pulp in a subendothelial location [37].

Liver

Hodgkin lymphoma in the liver in the early stage is confined to the portal tracts; lobular involvement occurs with progressive disease. Although definitive Reed-Sternberg cells are difficult to identify, a frequent observation in many aggregates of atypical histiocytes and Hodgkin cells in a rich inflammatory background, some consider this enough for a diagnosis of liver involvement with the proper immunostains highlighting the Hodgkin cells [4, 40] (Fig. 12.3). These histiocytes are not to be confused with epithelioid histiocytes, a frequent finding in CHL and NLPHL. Reactive hepatitis composed of a small lymphocytic infiltrate can be identified within the lobules as well as small bile ductule proliferation [2].

Immunophenotyping

Classic Hodgkin Lymphoma

Hodgkin/Reed-Sternberg (HRS) cells in CHL lack expression of CD20; however weak expression in a subset of the HRS cells and variants may be seen in 20–40% of cases [40]. B-cell program is shown by expression of PAX-5 in greater than 90% of cases [4], which shows weak expression when compared to background small lymphocytes. CD79a, OCT-2, and BOB1 are infrequently expressed. Membranous and Golgi staining for CD15 (75–85%) and CD30 is present in nearly all cases [4, 40], and CD45 is typically absent (Fig. 12.1). Other more recently identified markers such as HGAL and LMO2 have also been described in some cases. A small number of cases demonstrate expression of CD21 and CD35, although weak and variable [41]. Immunoglobulin light chains may be expressed in the HRS cytoplasm. Aberrant expressions of T-cell-associated antigens are present in a few cases, usually with nodular sclerosis subtype, and indicate a poorer prognosis. CD4 (80%) and CD2 (77%), followed by CD5 and CD8, are most commonly expressed [42]. T-cell receptor gene rearrangements are negative in these cases.

Nodular lymphocyte-predominant Hodgkin lymphoma LP cells express all markers specific to the mature B-cell lineage, including CD20, CD79a, PAX-5, OCT-2, and BOB-1. IgD is present in a subset of cases in mainly young males with neck adenopathy [4]. In contrast to CHL, CD15 is rarely expressed but CD30 can be present in a subset [40].

Detection of EBV

In formalin-fixed, paraffin-embedded tissue, the "gold standard" for detection of EBV is demonstration by nuclear in situ hybridization for EBER, which is highly sensitive [27]. Immunohistochemistry for LMP-1 expression in a membranous and cytoplasmic pattern may also be utilized; however poor fixation may hinder accurate results. Additionally, background staining of eosinophils and plasma cells with LMP-1 may lead to difficulty in interpretation [23].

Cytogenetic and Molecular Findings

Molecular analysis of CHL was initially difficult to investigate due to the scarcity of the HRS, which comprise <3% of the total cells. Single-cell PCR analysis shows Hodgkin cells in CHL have clonal immunoglobulin gene rearrangements [23] in almost all cases [4]. The HRS cells show hypermutation in the variable region and lack immunoglobulin transcription and surface immunoglobulin [4]. In contrast, in NLPHL the neoplastic cells show ongoing mutation and immunoglobulin transcription.

Recent studies using comparative genomic hybridization show HRS have recurrent gains or losses resulting in activation of transcription factors or loss of tumor suppression that ultimately inhibit apoptosis and promote cell growth. The loci that play a major role are present on the chromosomes 12 and 22 regions. Losses include tumor suppressor genes *SPRY1*, *NELL1*, and *ID4*, and gains of *FOXC2*, *NOTCH 1*, *TRAF2*, and *SHH*, among others [43].

HRS cells lack transcription factors specific to the B-cell lineage (*POU2F2*, *POU2AF1*, and *PU.1*).

Cytogenetic studies of NLPHL often show a complex karyotype, with gains of 1, 2q, 3, 4q, 5q, 6, 8q, 11q, 12q, and X. Rearrangements of the *BCL6* gene have been detected by FISH studies, along with *BCL2* translocations [40].

Differential Diagnoses

The differential diagnosis of HL in the spleen and liver is largely with a reactive process, e.g., granulomatous changes, EBV-related lymphoproliferative disorders, and some B-cell lymphomas expressing CD30, particularly when HRS cells are scarce and fibrosis with a paucicellular nonneoplastic inflammatory background is present. Additionally, the presence of many granulomata may obscure HRS and suggest chronic granulomatous inflammation rather than lymphoma. Application of immunohistochemistry study helps in identifying HRS cells in the spleen and liver.

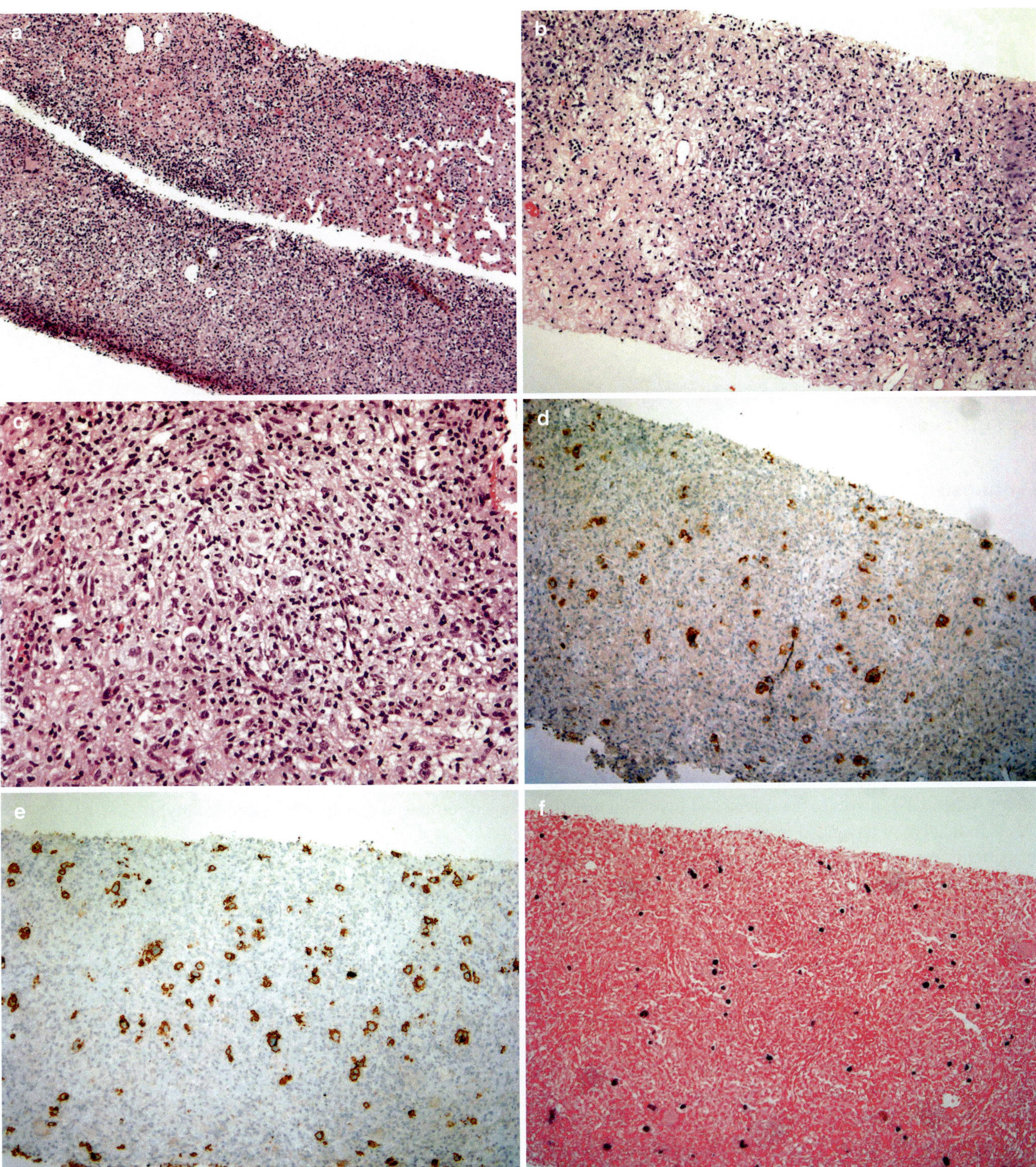

Fig. 12.3 Classic Hodgkin lymphoma involving the liver. (**a**, **b**) The H&E sections patchy atypical cellular infiltrate composed of lymphocytes, histiocytes, and large forms (40× magnification, 100× magnification, respectively). (**c**) A higher-power view of the infiltrating cells containing large hyperchromatic forms showing single large nuclei, one to two prominent nuclei, and clear to foamy cytoplasm. The background histiocytes display vesicular nuclei and abundant eosinophilic cytoplasm. Small reactive lymphocytes are present (H&E, 200× magnification). (**d**, **e**) Immunohistochemical stains with CD30 and CD15 highlight increased Hodgkin cells (200× magnification). (**f**) EBER (Epstein-Bar virus-encoded viral RNA) in situ hybridization (ISH) confirmed the presence of EBV-positive neoplastic cells (ISH, 200× magnification). (**g**, **h**) CD20 and CD45 immunohistochemical stains show negative staining in the Hodgkin cells (H&E, 100× and 200× magnification, respectively)

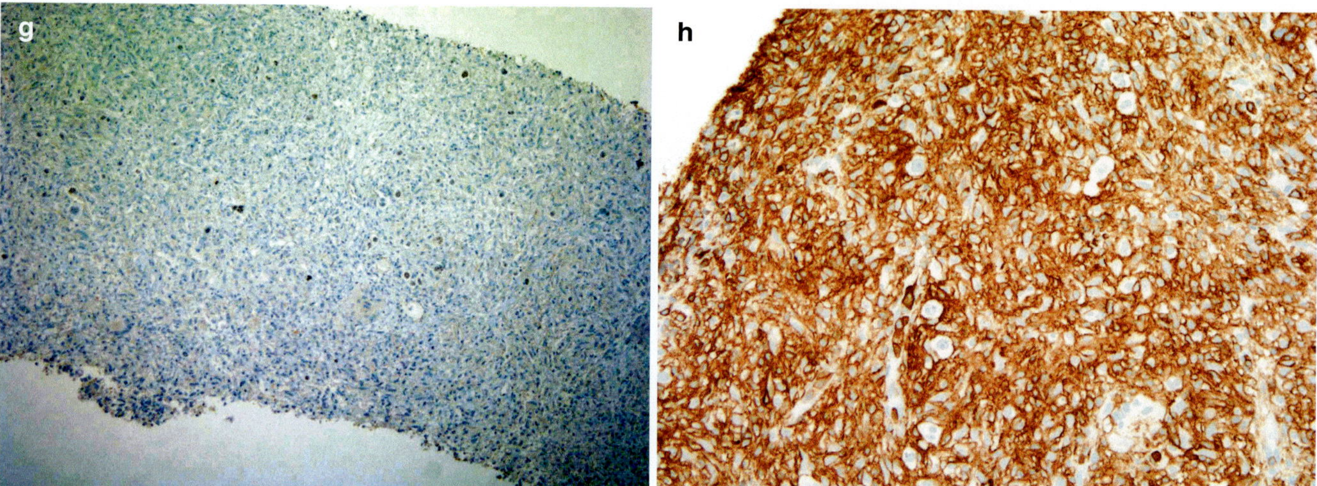

Fig. 12.3 (continued)

Prognosis

The prognoses of CHL and NLPHL in general are dependent on epidemiologic factors including the age of the patient, the stage at presentation, and the immune status of the patient. As discussed above, splenic or liver involvement by Hodgkin lymphoma is seen in advance stages. In general, the majority of cases have a good prognosis, with a 5-year survival of ~86%, particularly in young adults, with standard chemotherapy. Lymphocyte-rich CHL has the best prognosis as it presents in the earlier stage. It is postulated the rich lymphocytic background plays a role in immunologic control of the tumor. When CHL involves the spleen and liver concurrently, this is indicative of advanced-stage disease and less than half of patients survive. However, isolated splenic involvement has a reportedly excellent prognosis and can be treated with chemoradiation or rarely splenectomy. Partial splenectomy is not recommended because microfoci of tumor may be overlooked [44]. In cases with aberrant expression of T-cell markers, the overall survival is decreased [42]. Conflicting studies of the impact of EBV status on overall survival have been investigated, and in one study by Levine et al., it was found EBV titers are higher in untreated patients with advanced-stage disease and indicates a poorer overall prognosis and shorter survival; however a causative role for EBV was not detected [45]. Other studies have shown an increased overall survival in early-stage patients with EBV-positive CHL and LMP-1 expression [45, 46].

Conclusion/Summary

In summary, primary involvement of the spleen and liver by either CHL or NLPHL is extremely rare, with virtually no identifiable primary cases of the liver and only <1% of primary splenic lymphomas reported to be Hodgkin lymphoma in the last century. Extranodal involvement is present in the advanced stage of HL, and the incidence of spread to the liver and spleen is dependent on the histologic subtype. Of the CHL, lymphocyte-rich is least likely to involve the spleen and liver, whereas mixed-cellularity and lymphocyte-depleted CHL present in the spleen. Similar to LRCHL, NLPHL infrequently involves the spleen. Morphologically, CHL and NLPHL usually have a similar appearance in the spleen, and immunohistochemistry studies are needed to accurately distinguish the two. Overall, the prognosis of CHL and NLPHL is dependent on the summation of patient age, immune status, and histologic subtype.

Diagnostic Caveats

- Primary splenic Hodgkin lymphoma (PSL-HD) is a rare diagnosis and definitively ruling out other sites of involvement is difficult. More commonly, the liver and spleen are involved in the advanced stages of lymphoma.
- On gross examination, the presentation of PSL-HD varies from large tumor macronodules to small microscopic foci that may be difficult to visualize, and serial sections (1–1.5 cm) are necessary for thorough examination.
- The gross weight of the spleen correlates with the likelihood of lymphoma involvement, with reports showing greater than 400 grams is indicative of PSL-HL. However splenomegaly may also occur due to congestion, granulomata, and reactive changes, and lymphoma cannot be assumed.
- In PSL-HD, histological subclassification may be difficult, and HRS cells are not easily found and when present are near the marginal zones and PALS. The splenic architecture is generally preserved. Immunohistochemistry helps in the diagnosis and highlighting HRS cells.

- Primary hepatic Hodgkin lymphoma has never been reported.
- The liver can show nonspecific reactive change in HD including lobular lymphocytic infiltrates and small bile ductule proliferation; lymphoma involvement presents similar to the spleen.
- EBV has a greater association with the mixed-cellularity and lymphocyte-depleted subtypes of CHL, which are found in patients from less well-developed countries and more commonly present with splenic involvement.
- The incidence of death from HL is greater in patients who are immunosuppressed.
- EBV is present in the B-cells in the type II latent form and can be demonstrated using in situ hybridization for EBER RNA and immunostains for LMP-1.
- The prognosis of PSL-HD is excellent and can be treated with chemoradiation or splenectomy; partial splenectomy is not advised. In advanced-stage splenic/liver lymphoma, the prognosis depends on the histological subtype and epidemiologic factors including age and immune status.

References

1. Hodgkin. On some morbid appearances of the absorbent glands and spleen. Med Chir Trans. 1832;17:68–114.
2. Lukes RJ. Criteria for involvement of lymph node, bone marrow, spleen, and liver in Hodgkin's disease. Cancer Res. 1971;31(11):1755–67.
3. Rappaport H, Berard CW, Butler JJ, Dorfman RF, Lukes RJ, Thomas LB. Report of the committee on histopathological criteria contributing to staging of Hodgkin's disease. Cancer Res. 1971;31(11):1864–5.
4. The 2016 revision of the World Health Organization classification of lymphoid neoplasms.
5. Pinkus GS, Said JW. Hodgkin's disease, lymphocyte predominance type, nodular–a distinct entity? Unique staining profile for L&H variants of Reed-Sternberg cells defined by monoclonal antibodies to leukocyte common antigen, granulocyte-specific antigen, and B-cell-specific antigen. Am J Pathol. 1985;118(1):1–6.
6. Pinkus GS, Said JW. Hodgkin's disease, lymphocyte predominance type, nodular–further evidence for a B cell derivation. L & H variants of Reed-Sternberg cells express L26, a pan B cell marker. Am J Pathol. 1988;133(2):211–7.
7. Thomas RK, Re D, Zander T, Wolf J, Diehl V. Epidemiology and etiology of Hodgkin's lymphoma. Ann Oncol. 2002;13(Suppl 4):147–52.
8. Noone AM, Howlader, N, Krapcho M, Miller D, Brest A, Yu M, Ruhl J, Tatalovich Z, Mariotto A, Lewis DR, Chen HS, Feuer EJ, Cronin KA (eds). SEER cancer statistics review 1975–2015. Bethesda: National Cancer Institute (2018).
9. Diehl V, Sextro M, Franklin J, Hansmann ML, Harris N, Jaffe E, et al. Clinical presentation, course, and prognostic factors in lymphocyte-predominant Hodgkin's disease and lymphocyte-rich classical Hodgkin's disease: report from the European Task Force on Lymphoma Project on Lymphocyte-Predominant Hodgkin's Disease. J Clin Oncol. 1999;17(3):776–83.
10. Poppema S, Kaiserling E, Lennert K. Epidemiology of nodular paragranuloma (Hodgkin's disease with lymphocytic predominance, nodular). J Cancer Res Clin Oncol. 1979;95(1):57–63.
11. Miettinen M, Franssila KO, Saxen E. Hodgkins-disease, lymphocytic predominance nodular – increased risk for subsequent non-Hodgkins lymphomas. Cancer. 1983;51(12):2293–300.
12. Shimabukuro-Vornhagen A, Haverkamp H, Engert A, Balleisen L, Majunke P, Heil G, et al. Lymphocyte-rich classical Hodgkin's lymphoma: clinical presentation and treatment outcome in 100 patients treated within German Hodgkin's Study Group trials. J Clin Oncol. 2005;23(24):5739–45.
13. Zellers RA, Thibodeau SN, Banks PM. Primary splenic lymphocyte-depletion Hodgkin's disease. Am J Clin Pathol. 1990;94(4):453–7.
14. MacMahon B. Epidemiology of Hodgkin's disease. Cancer Res. 1966;26(6):1189–201.
15. Gutensohn N, Cole P. Childhood social environment and Hodgkin's disease. N Engl J Med. 1981;304(3):135–40.
16. Chang ET, Zheng T, Weir EG, Borowitz M, Mann RB, Spiegelman D, et al. Childhood social environment and Hodgkin's lymphoma: new findings from a population-based case-control study. Cancer Epidemiol Biomark Prev. 2004;13(8):1361–70.
17. Isaacson NH, Spatt SD, Grayzel DM. Primary splenic Hodgkin's disease without lymph node involvement. Ann Intern Med. 1947;27(2):294–301.
18. Kattepur AK, Rohith S, Shivaswamy BS, Babu R, Santhosh CS. Primary splenic lymphoma: a case report. Indian J Surg Oncol. 2013;4(3):287–90.
19. Midorikawa Y, Kubota K, Mori M, Watanabe S, Koyama H, Kajiura N. Advanced primary Hodgkin's disease of the spleen cured by surgical resection: report of a case. Surg Today. 1999;29(4):367–70.
20. Kraemer BB, Osborne BM, Butler JJ. Primary splenic presentation of malignant lymphoma and related disorders. A study of 49 cases. Cancer. 1984;54(8):1606–19.
21. Dorfman RF. Relationship of histology to site in Hodgkin's disease. Cancer Res. 1971;31(11):1786–93.
22. Rosenberg SA. A critique of the value of laparotomy and splenectomy in the evaluation of patients with Hodgkin's disease. Cancer Res. 1971;31(11):1737–40.
23. Gandhi MK, Tellam JT, Khanna R. Epstein-Barr virus-associated Hodgkin's lymphoma. Br J Haematol. 2004;125(3):267–81.
24. Hjalgrim H, Askling J, Rostgaard K, Hamilton-Dutoit S, Frisch M, Zhang J-S, et al. Characteristics of Hodgkin's lymphoma after infectious mononucleosis. N Engl J Med. 2003;349(14):1324–32.
25. Glavina-Durdov M, Jakic-Razumovic J, Capkun V, Murray P. Assessment of the prognostic impact of the Epstein–Barr virus-encoded latent membrane protein-1 expression in Hodgkin's disease. Br J Cancer. 2001;84(9):1227–34.
26. Jarrett RF. Risk factors for Hodgkin's lymphoma by EBV status and significance of detection of EBV genomes in serum of patients with EBV-associated Hodgkin's lymphoma. Leuk Lymphoma. 2003;44(Suppl 3):S27–32.
27. Hjalgrim H. On the aetiology of Hodgkin lymphoma. Dan Med J. 2012;59(7):B4485.
28. Shiels MS, Koritzinsky EH, Clarke CA, Suneja G, Morton LM, Engels EA. Prevalence of HIV Infection among U.S. Hodgkin lymphoma cases. Cancer Epidemiol Biomark Prev. 2014;23(2):274–81.
29. Symmers D. Certain unusual lesions of the lymphatic apparatus: Including a description of primary Hodgkin's disease of the spleen and a case of gastrointestinal pseudoleukemia. Arch Intern Med. 1909;IV(3):218–37.
30. Dobrow RB. Spontaneous (pathologic) rupture of the spleen in previously undiagnosed Hodgkin's disease: report of a case with survival. Cancer. 1977;39(1):354–8.
31. Geramizadeh B, Alborzi A, Hosseini M, Ramzi M, Foroutan H. Primary splenic Hodgkin's disease in a patient with chronic granulomatous disease, a case report. Iran Red Crescent Med J. 2010;12(3):319–21.
32. Kosari F, Ghaffari F. Primary splenic Hodgkin lymphoma presenting with chronic pruritus. Arch Iran Med. 2016;19(6):446–8.

33. Aisenberg AC, Goldman JM, Raker JW, Wang CC. Spleen involvement at the onset of Hodgkin's disease. Ann Intern Med. 1971;74(4):544–7.

34. Younes A, Johnson P, Dabaja B, Ansell S, Kuruvilla J. Chapter 102: Hodgkin's lymphoma. In: DeVita VT, Lawrence TS, Rosenberg SA, editors. DeVita, Hellman, and Rosenberg's Cancer: principles and practice of oncology. 10th ed. Philadelphia: Lippincott Williams & Wilkins; 2015.

35. Biemer JJ. Hepatic manifestations of lymphomas. Ann Clin Lab Sci. 1984;14(4):252–60.

36. Toma P, Granata C, Rossi A, Garaventa A. Multimodality imaging of Hodgkin disease and non-Hodgkin lymphomas in children. Radiographics. 2007;27(5):1335–54.

37. O'Malley DP. Atlas of spleen pathology. New York: Springer; 2013.

38. Kadin ME, Glatstein E, Dorfman RF. Clinicopathologic studies of 117 untreated patients subjected to laparotomy for the staging of Hodgkin's disease. Cancer. 1971;27(6):1277–94.

39. Rueffer U, Sieber M, Stemberg M, Gossmann A, Josting A, Koch T, et al. Spleen involvement in Hodgkin's lymphoma: assessment and risk profile. Ann Hematol. 2003;82(7):390–6.

40. Arber DA, Elias C, Harris NL, Jaffe ES, Quintanilla-Martinez L. Hematopathology. Philadelphia, PA: Elsevier, 2017.

41. Nakamura S, Nagahama M, Kagami Y, Yatabe Y, Takeuchi T, Kojima M, et al. Hodgkin's disease expressing follicular dendritic cell marker CD21 without any other B-cell marker: a clinicopathologic study of nine cases. Am J Surg Pathol. 1999;23(4):363–76.

42. Venkataraman G, Song JY, Tzankov A, Dirnhofer S, Heinze G, Kohl M, et al. Aberrant T-cell antigen expression in classical Hodgkin lymphoma is associated with decreased event-free survival and overall survival. Blood. 2013;121(10):1795–804.

43. Slovak ML, Bedell V, Hsu YH, Estrine DB, Nowak NJ, Delioukina ML, et al. Molecular karyotypes of Hodgkin and Reed-Sternberg cells at disease onset reveal distinct copy number alterations in chemosensitive versus refractory Hodgkin lymphoma. Clin Cancer Res. 2011;17(10):3443–54.

44. Brox A, Bishinsky JI, Berry G. Primary non-Hodgkin lymphoma of the spleen. Am J Hematol. 1991;38(2):95–100.

45. Levine PH, Ablashi DV, Berard CW, Carbone PP, Waggoner DE, Malan L. Elevated antibody titers to Epstein-Barr virus in Hodgkin's disease. Cancer. 1971;27(2):416–21.

46. Flavell KJ, Murray PG. Hodgkin's disease and the Epstein-Barr virus. Mol Pathol. 2000;53(5):262–9.

David C. Gajzer, Lugen Chen, and Ling Zhang

Introduction

B-cell acute lymphoblastic leukemia (B-ALL)/lymphoblastic lymphoma (LBL) is an abnormal proliferation of hematopoietic progenitors (blasts) committed to the B-cell lineage. B-ALL accounts for >75% of ALL, while solitary B-LBL involving the nodal or non-nodal tissues is less common. Both liver and spleen are common sites to be involved by B-ALL/LBL, though biopsies of these organs are not commonly collected for primary diagnosis. Splenectomy is usually not performed for diagnosis of B-ALL. Morphologically, B-ALL and T-cell acute lymphoblastic leukemia (T-ALL) are almost indistinguishable from one another. Phenotypically, B-ALL/LBL expresses immature B-cell markers including TdT, CD34, CD10, CD19, surface or cytoplasmic CD22, cytoplasmic CD79a, and partial CD20. B-ALL/LBL also harbors a wide spectrum of cytogenetic and molecular alterations. Correct diagnosis and subclassification of B-ALL relies on assessment of morphology, immunophenotype, cytogenetics, and molecular signatures [1]. Emerging next-generation genome-wide profiles have brought novel molecular insights into B-ALL and further help to refine the subclassifications of B-ALL, e.g., BCR-ABL1-like subtype [2]. The acquired molecular signatures will also be used to perform risk stratification, design therapeutic targets, and monitor treatment response [2–4]. The chapter will review the updated epidemiology, etiology, pathogenesis, and clinical and pathologic findings of B-ALL/-LBL, focusing on hepatosplenic involvements.

Definition

B-lymphoblastic leukemia/lymphoma is an abnormal proliferation of B-cell progenitors, which can be further subclassified according to the predominantly involved site. B-ALL manifests as extensive peripheral blood and bone marrow involvement (at least 20% lymphoblasts), while B-LBL shows rapidly enlarged lymph nodes or extranodal masses with limited spread to peripheral blood and/or bone marrow, with the peripheral blood being more commonly involved than bone marrow [1].

Epidemiology

B-ALL or LBL is the number one hematological malignancy in children. It also shows a bi-model age distribution, with the first peak at age 3.5 years (ranging from 2–5 years) and the second peak at age 50 [3, 5]. The early-onset B-ALL in children and young adults (<20 years) comprises approximately 70% of all B-ALL, of which the majority of patients are younger than 15 years [6–8]. In accordance with the 2012 American Cancer Society cancer statistics, there are 6050 new cases of ALL diagnosed in the United States per year [9]. Approximately 80% of these ALL cases are B-ALL [9]. Primary liver or splenic presentation of B-ALL without extrahepatic or extrasplenic involvement is extremely rare. Two large cohorts (Berlin/Cologne 1994–2003) composed of 205 liver biopsies with lymphoma manifestations showed that only 2 cases (1%) had B-ALL/-LBL and their median age was 22, ranging from 18–28 years with a male-to-female ratio of 1:1 [10]. The incidence of primary splenic involvement is unclear due to the paucity of cases reported.

D. C. Gajzer (✉) · L. Zhang
Department of Pathology, H. Lee Moffitt Cancer Center and Research Institute, Tampa, FL, USA
e-mail: david.gajzer@moffitt.org; ling.zhang@moffitt.org

L. Chen
Department of Pathology, Tampa General Hospital, Tampa, FL, USA

© Springer Nature Switzerland AG 2020
L. Zhang et al. (eds.), *Diagnostic Pathology of Hematopoietic Disorders of Spleen and Liver*,
https://doi.org/10.1007/978-3-030-37708-3_13

Etiology

The etiology is thought to be multifactorial and associated with environmental toxins and infection exposure, endogenous gene mutations, as well as immune dysregulation [3]. It takes two steps to develop pediatric ALL. The first hit usually occurs during fetal development that potentially forms abnormal gene fusion or changes in diploidy, while the second hit leads to a preleukemic clone that can progress to leukemia. Only 1% of children who harbor a preleukemic clone eventually transform to overt leukemia [11]. It is recognized that the second hit can be triggered by infection. The etiology in adult ALL is not well known.

Clinical Presentation

In general, patients with B-ALL usually present with pallor, fatigue, weakness, fever, arthralgia, weight loss, and bone pain [12]. Some patients can be asymptomatic. A series of nausea, pressure vomiting, headache, and altered mental status are indicative of central nervous system (CNS) involvement by B-ALL [12]. Extramedullary involvement is not uncommon. When it does occur, skin, soft tissue, bone, and lymph nodes are the most commonly involved sites [12]. The liver and spleen are also considered two common extramedullary organs invaded by B-ALL or B-LBL in addition to several sanctuary sites including the male testis and CNS [12]. Non-tender hepatomegaly can be found by physical examination and imaging study [13]. Jaundice (skin and/or icteric sclera) and its accompanying signs and symptoms (itching, loss of appetite, nausea, vomiting, or passing clay-colored stools) could hint to hepatic and biliary infiltration by B-ALL/-LBL [13–17]. A distinguishing factor from T-cell LBL is the fact that B-cell LBL seldom involves the mediastinum [1].

Patients with B-ALL often develop pancytopenia secondary to impaired hematopoiesis from a marrow-occupying lesion – diffuse proliferation of leukemic blasts. Thus, early laboratory findings include mild normocytic, normochromic anemia and thrombocytopenia. B-ALL patients can present with either leukopenia or leukocytosis, mainly blastosis [12]. Pancytopenia is not uncommon. Accompanying eosinophilia can occur in some B-ALL, in particular with *BCR-ABL1* translocation or t(5;14)/*IgH-IL5* gene rearrangement [1].

Morphology

Gross and Radiologic Findings

There is limited information on gross pictures of the spleen and liver removed from patients with B-ALL/-LBL. One autopsy report of a 5-year-old patient with B-LBL/-ALL showed the spleen was twice the size (130 grams) of normal. The liver showed an abnormal lobulated cut surface. The central zones appeared dark red, while the peripheral zones were yellow and associated with diffuse necrosis [18].

A right upper quadrant sonogram and CT scan revealed diffuse enlargement of both organs. Ultrasonography showed a liver-occupying lesion with diffuse increased echogenicity. Biliary obstruction manifested by intra- or extrahepatic biliary duct dilatation could be observed [13].

Microscopic Examination

Examination of peripheral blood shows many circulating lymphoblasts, which are small to medium in size and show delicate chromatin, inconspicuous to small nucleoli, and invisible to scant cytoplasm (Fig. 13.1). Occasional large forms with or without cytoplasmic vacuoles are seen. Some lymphoblasts display "hand-mirror" changes characterized by a cytoplasmic tail extending out from one pole of the nucleus. The blasts in bone marrow aspirate smears are similar to those in peripheral blood. The bone marrow core biopsy is usually packed with lymphoblasts with fairly high nuclear-to-cytoplasmic ratio, and normal trilineage hematopoiesis is diminished (Fig. 13.2a–d). Sometimes small lymphoblasts are difficult to tell apart from small mature lymphocytes, blastoid mantle cell lymphoma, or acute myeloid leukemia with minimal differentiation, in particular when the blast count is low. Lymphoblasts with cytoplasmic vacuoles could also represent Burkitt lymphoma.

Microscopically, B-LBL/-ALL involving the liver and/or spleen exhibits a typical sinusoidal infiltrating pattern [17]. In the liver, similar to other leukemias, the immature precursors percolate intrasinusoidal space and often also fill portal tracts (Fig 13.3a, b). Adjacent hepatic cell necrosis has been

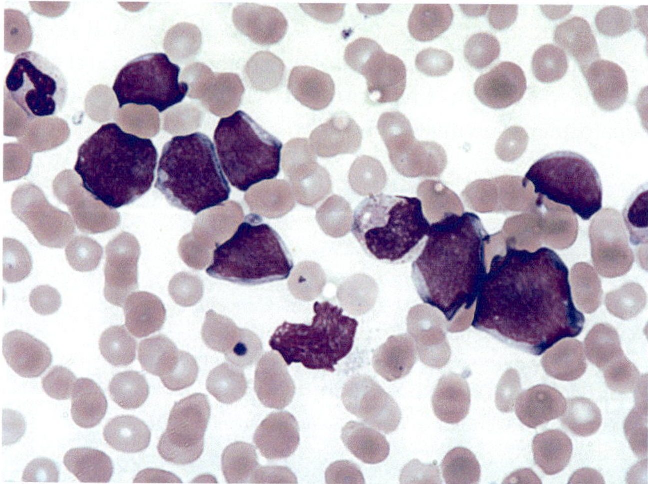

Fig. 13.1 Peripheral blood smear of B-ALL (Giemsa stain, 1000×)

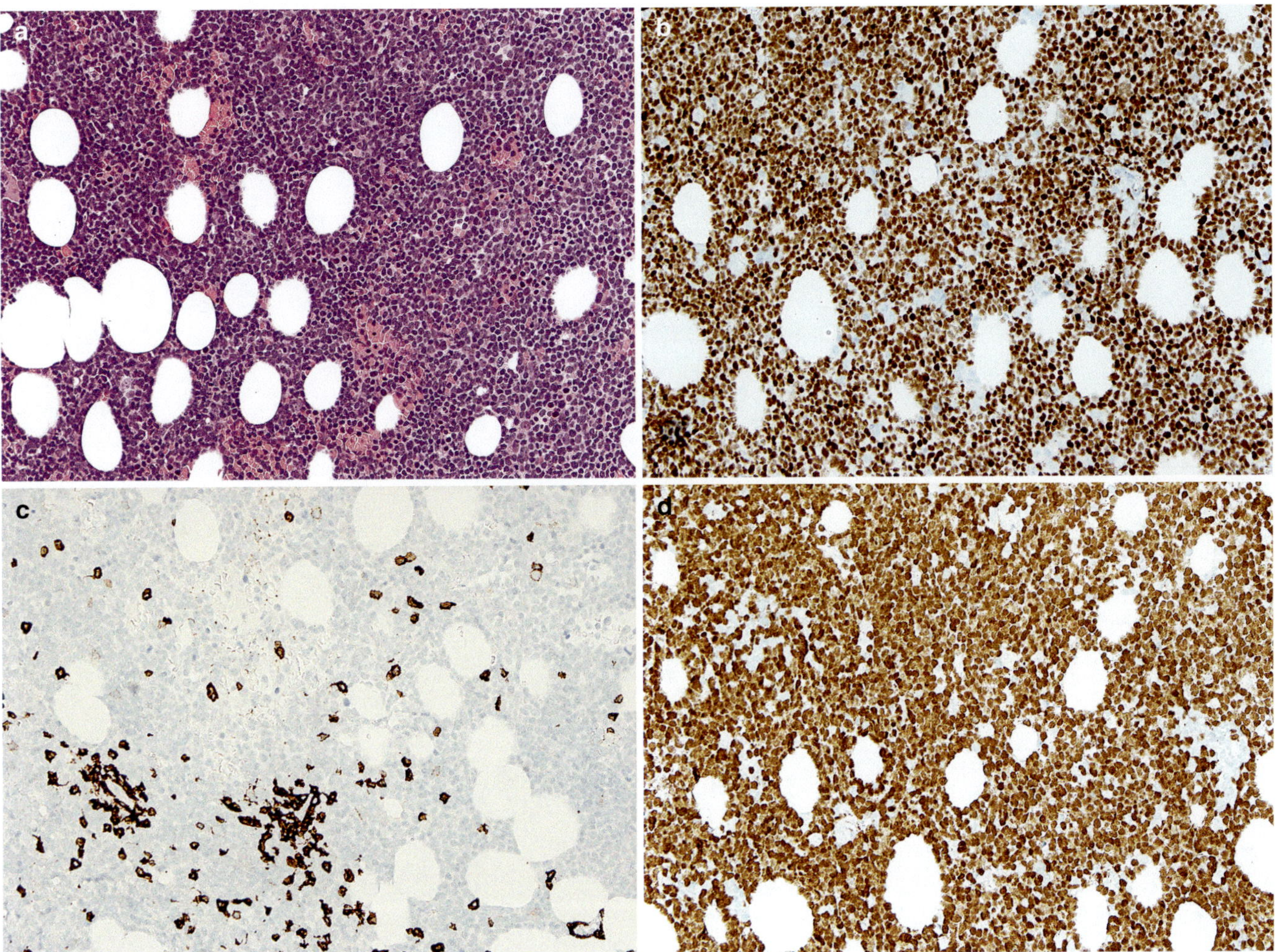

Fig. 13.2 Bone marrow core biopsy findings of B-ALL/-LBL. (**a**) Bone marrow core biopsy with diffuse infiltrate by lymphoblasts (H&E, 200×). (**b–d**) Immunostains show the lymphoblasts to be positive for PAX-5 (**b**) and TdT (**d**) and negative for CD20 (**c**) (immunoperoxidase, 200×)

documented [13, 18]. Cholestasis can occur secondary to dense portal infiltration [18]. In the spleen, sinuses are loaded with leukemic cells (pictures not shown).

Touch imprint (Wright-Giemsa stain) shows typical lymphoblasts that could be small or mixed small to medium in size, with or without cytoplasmic vacuoles. Principally, all forms exhibit fine chromatin and a very high N:C ratio. Nucleoli are inconspicuous to conspicuous (similar to those identified in the nodal or extranodal sites).

Immunophenotyping

Immunohistochemical (IHC) staining is preferred to flow cytometry for detection of B-ALL/-LBL involving the liver due to limited tissue harvested from a liver biopsy. Similar to the leukemia/lymphoma present in peripheral blood or bone marrow, these immature B-cell precursors/blasts are positive for B-cell-specific markers [CD19, PAX-5, CD22 (surface and

cytoplasmic), CD24, CD79a, and fully or partially CD20] along with CD10 and other markers indicating immaturity or stem cell origin such as CD99, CD34, and TdT (Fig. 13.3c–g). Flow cytometry identifies a similar pattern if it is applicable, usually performed on a peripheral blood specimen (Fig. 13.4) [1, 19, 20]. Expression of CD20 is seen in 30–50% of patients with B-ALL. A positive result was considered to be associated with an adverse clinical outcome before standard anti-CD20 monoclonal antibody (rituximab) therapy [21, 22]. As CD34 or TdT is identified in an early stage of B-cell development, it is usually identified in a subset of B-ALL/-LBL, e.g., pro-B phase, and lost in the late phase of B-ALL [4]. Another important marker is CD10, strongly positive in B-ALL/-LBL [4]. However, CD10 is also frequently found in other B-cell lymphomas with germinal center origin. Therefore, it could be difficult to diagnose B-ALL in a liver biopsy when the B-LBL blasts lack both CD34 and TdT expression. Also keeping in mind is that in normal liver, a CD10 stain shows bile canalicular pattern [23]. In addition, a subset of B-ALL also express myeloid markers such as CD13

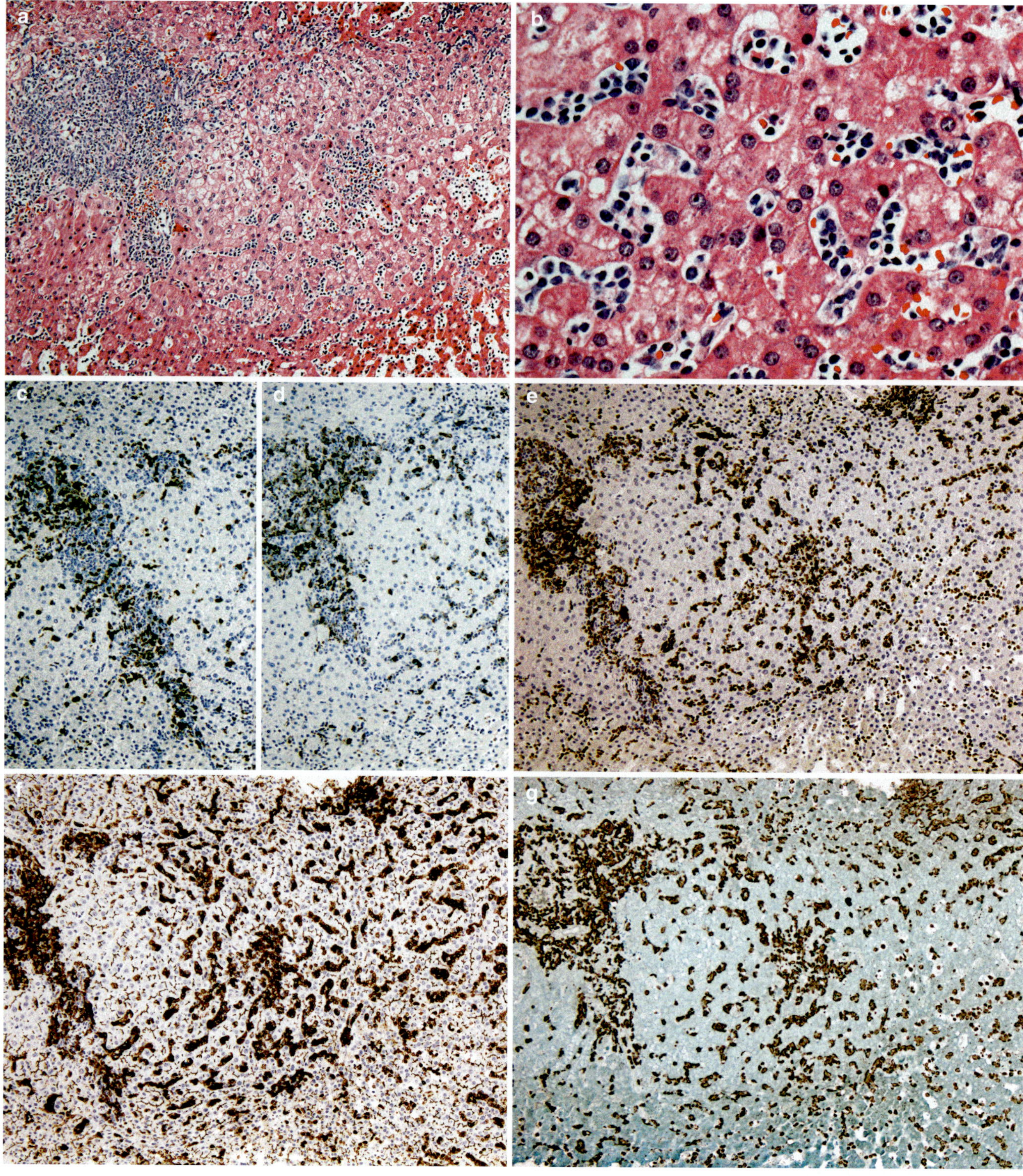

Fig. 13.3 Hepatic involvement by B-ALL/-LBL. (**a**, **b**) Microscopic examination reveals normal hepatocytes associated with sinusoidal infiltration by small immature precursors and peripheral portal dense lymphoid aggregates composed of mostly similar cells (H&E, 100× and 400×, respectively). (**c–g**) A panel of immunohistochemical stains performed on the liver biopsy proved the neoplastic infiltrate to be negative for CD3 (**c**, 100×) and positive for CD20 (a small subset) (**d**, 100×), CD79a (**e**, 100×), CD10 (**f**, 100×), and TdT (**g**, 100×)

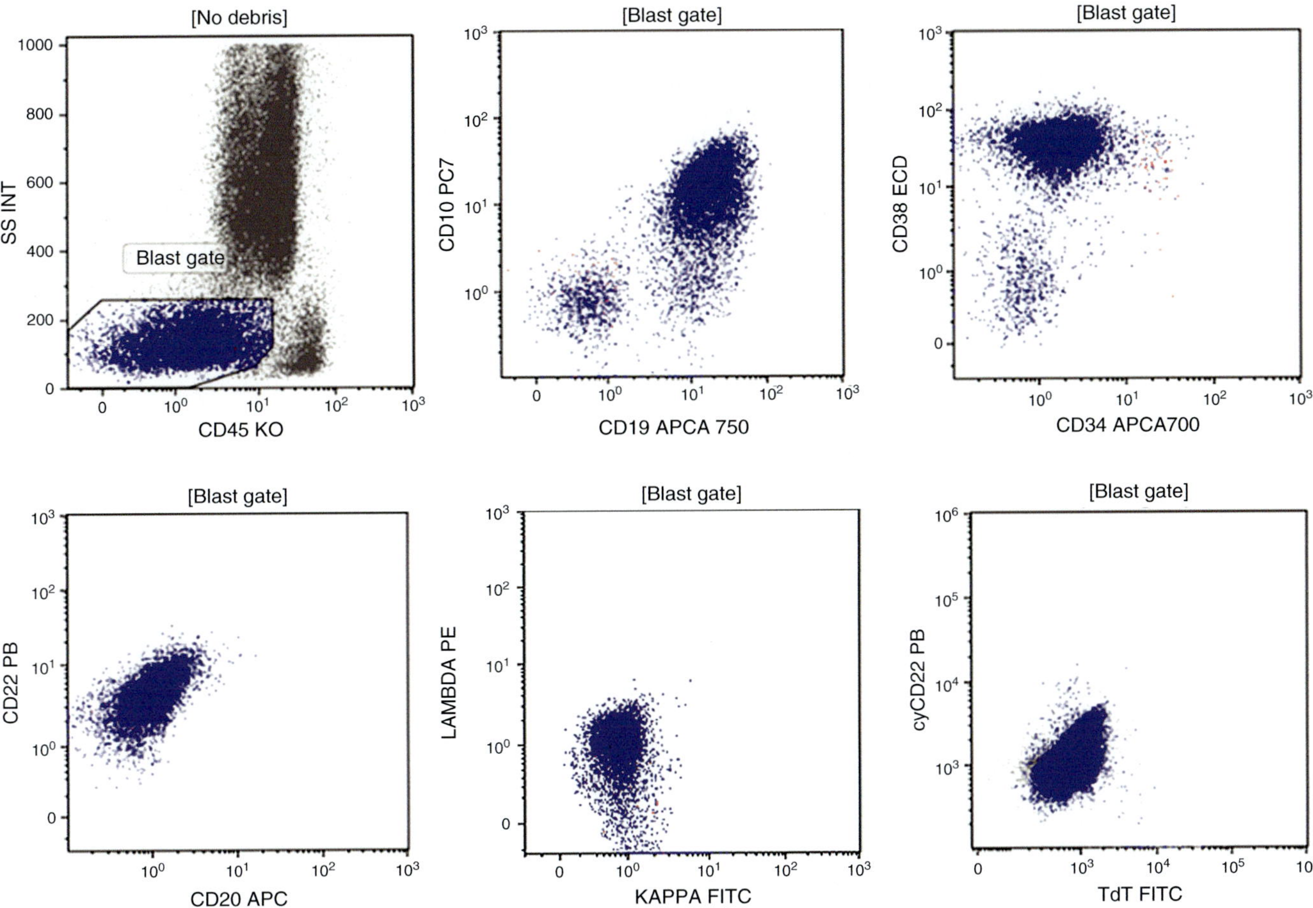

Fig. 13.4 Flow cytometric analysis of B-lymphoblastic leukemia (peripheral blood)

and CD33 but not CD117. The latter can be used to differentiate between ALL and AML without MPO expression [4]. Coexpression of dim CD38 and HLA-DR on B-ALL cells can also be identified. These markers (CD13, CD33, HLA-DR, and CD38) are usually tested by flow cytometry rather than by IHC because only few laboratories perform IHC for these markers. If clinically highly suspicious for B-ALL/-LBL, a fresh tissue biopsy of the liver is feasible for flow cytometric analysis. An 8- or 10-parameter flow cytometry panel consisting of necessary markers should be adopted given the pauci-cellularity of liver fine needle aspirate specimens.

During practice, caution must also be given for CD19-negative B-ALL/-LBL [24], particularly in the setting of post-chimeric antigen receptor T-cell (CAR-T) therapy targeting CD19. Changing the gating strategy to the surface CD22-positive cell population will repopulate the neoplastic cells. An early-phase CD45-negative B-ALL could be missed if only paying attention to the dim CD45 positive blast region [25, 26].

Cytogenetic and Molecular Diagnosis

Cytogenetics and molecular studies are recommended to be carried out on peripheral blood or bone marrow specimens. The recurrent cytogenetic abnormalities listed in the 2017 WHO classification (hyperdiploidy, hypodiploidy, *BCR-ABL1*, *KMT 2A/MLL*, t(11;22)/*ETV6-RUNX1*, t(5;14)/*IL3-IgH*, t(1;19)/*TCR3-PBX1*, and intrachromosomal amplification of AMP21) should be tested for B-ALL by using conventional karyotyping or specific FISH probes (Table 13.1). BCR-ABL1-like genetic signature testing such as *IGH-CRLF2, NUP214 -ABL1, EBF1-PDGFRB, BCR-JAK2, STRN3-JAK2, IGH-EPOR, CRLF2,* and *IKZF1* deletion) is possibly performed by using next generation sequencing (NGS) [27–30]. BCR-ABL1-like ALL accounts for approximately 15% of B-ALL, either adult or pediatric group, and associated with a poor prognosis [4, 30].

Table 13.1 Updated WHO classification of B-ALL/-LBL [1]

Main category	Subcategory	Unique features
B-lymphoblastic leukemia/lymphoma, not otherwise specified (NOS)	B-lymphoblastic leukemia/lymphoma, not otherwise specified (NOS)	May include genetic signature of BCR-ABL1-like B-ALL. The specific variant has a poorer clinical outcome when compared with B-ALL, NOS patients without such genetic aberrancy in the sample group
B-lymphoblastic leukemia/lymphoma with recurrent abnormalities	B-lymphoblastic leukemia/lymphoma with t(9;22) (q34.1;q11.2); *BCR-ABL1*	Occurs more frequently in adults than children Blasts contain cytoplasmic granules Blasts coexpress myeloid markers, e.g., CD13, CD33 Suitable for tyrosine kinase inhibitor treatment, e.g., imatinib, dasatinib
	B-lymphoblastic leukemia/lymphoma with t(v;11q23.3); *KMT2A/MLL*-rearranged	Less frequent (<5%) *De novo* or therapy related CD10−, CD15+/CD19+ blasts Adverse clinical outcome
	B-lymphoblastic leukemia/lymphoma with t(12;21) (p13.2;q22.1); *ETV6-RUNX1*	Mostly found in pediatric group Make up ¼ of pediatric B-ALL/-LBL Good prognosis
	B-lymphoblastic leukemia/lymphoma with hyperdiploidy	>50 chromosomes (usually <66), more common in childhood than adulthood Good prognosis
	B-lymphoblastic leukemia/lymphoma with hypodiploidy	Uncommonly encountered The following three subgroups are associated with a poor prognosis: 23–29 chromosomes: near-haploid ALL 33–39 chromosomes: low hypodiploid ALL 40–43 chromosomes: high hypodiploid ALL
	B-lymphoblastic leukemia/lymphoma with t(5;14) (q31.1;q32.1); *IgH/IL3*	Rare (<1%) Circulating blasts may not be identified Associated with eosinophilia
	B-lymphoblastic leukemia/lymphoma with t(1;19)(q23;p13.3); *TCF3-PBX1*	CD9+/CD34−/cytoplasmic µ+ blasts
	B-lymphoblastic leukemia/lymphoma, BCR-ABL1-like	Approximately ¼ of cases Poor prognosis Benefit from tyrosine kinase inhibitor therapy
	B-lymphoblastic leukemia/lymphoma with iAMP21	Positive *RUNX1* amplification (typically ≥5, or ≥3 copies), can be detected by FISH study

Differential Diagnosis

It is critical to differentiate B-LBL of the liver from other diseases that could lead to hepatic dysfunction, benign or malignant. Cytologically, B-LBL shows blastoid chromatin and is frequently associated with brisk mitosis and increased apoptosis. By comprehensive immunophenotyping, B-LBL/-ALL should be able to be told apart from other mature B-cell lymphomas/leukemias that commonly involve the liver or spleen. These B-cell lymphomas can be distinguished from B-LBL/-ALL by certain cytologic features, different infiltrating patterns, immunophenotyping, and unique cytogenetic/molecular aberrations (Table 13.2).

Immature B-Cell Precursors/Hematogones

A recent study observed a very interesting phenomenon: Dual TdT/PAX-5 expression, indicating the presence of immature B-cell precursors, can be present in the liver when biopsied from healthy adults or children. In adults, 6% of liver biopsies (2 of 31 cases) show immature B-cell precursors, while in the pediatric group, up to 40% (4 of 10 cases, all neonates) of liver biopsies contain the same cell population [31], which warrants a careful interpretation in these settings. Certainly, confluent involvement by such an immature B-cell population, dual positivity of PAX-5/TdT, or multifocal involvement require further exclusion of B-ALL/-LBL. In bone marrow specimens, it is important to distinguish between B-ALL and hematogones that are small in size and express CD19/CD10. However, hematogones usually show an identifiable maturation pattern from phases 1–3 by gradual gain of CD20 and loss of CD34 that can be detected by flow cytometry [32].

T-Lymphoblastic Leukemia/Lymphoma

Liver or spleen involvement by T-ALL is also very rare, yet given the similarity to B-ALL in cytology and infiltrating pattern, this entity is included in the differential diagnosis. T-ALL/-LBL is derived from T-cell progenitors and expresses the T-cell lineage-specific marker, CD3 (cytoplasmic or surface), along with certain other surface T-cell markers (CD1a, CD2, CD5, CD7, CD4, CD8) and immature precursor

Table 13.2 Cytomorphologic and immunophenotypic patterns of B-cell lymphomas/leukemias involving the liver and spleen [10]

	Cytology	Histologic infiltrating pattern	Immunophenotyping	Other diagnostic features
B-LBL/B-ALL	Small, high N:C ratio, immature chromatin	Sinusoidal pattern (liver and spleen)	CD19+, PAX-5+, CD79a+, CD10+/−, TdT+, CD34−/+	*BCR-ABL1* or other B-ALL-related translocations
SMZL	Small, high N:C ratio, condensed chromatin, plasmacytoid differentiation, cytoplasmic projections	White pulp expansion with red pulp spotting (spleen) Dense periportal lymphoid aggregates and scattered interstitial infiltrate (liver)	CD20+, PAX-5+, CD5−, CD10−, CD23−, CD43+, CD21+(residual follicular dendritic meshworks)	
Follicular lymphoma	Medium size, cleaved nuclei, relative low N:C ratio	White pulp expansion, back to back (spleen) Dense periportal lymphoid aggregates and scattered interstitial infiltrates (liver)	CD20+, PAX-5+, CD10+, BCL-2+/−, BCL-6+	t(14;18)/*BCL2-IgH*
DLBCL	Large size, vesicular chromatin, irregular nuclear contours, peripherally or centrally located prominent nucleoli, abundant cytoplasm	Micro- or macronodular to diffuse infiltrating pattern	CD20+, PAX-5+, CD10+/−, BCL-2+/−, BCL-6+/−, MUM1−/+, TdT−, CD34−	t(14;18), trisomy 3, gains of 3q
Burkitt lymphoma	Uniformly medium size, dispersed chromatin, multiple small nucleoli, and a small amount of cytoplasm	Big nodular to diffuse infiltrating pattern	CD20+, PAX-5+, CD10+, BCL-2−, BCL-6+, MUM1−, TdT−, CD34−	t(8;22); t(814) or t(2;8)-*MYC* gene-related rearrangements
High-grade B-cell lymphomas (double or triple-hit, or NOS)	Small to large size, dispersed to blastoid chromatin, high N:C ratio, and scant cytoplasm	Usually diffuse infiltrating pattern	CD20+, PAX-5+, TdT−, CD34−, GCB (75–90%, CD10+ and/or BCL-6+) or non-GCB type	*MYC* and *BCL-2* and/or *BCL6* gene rearrangements for subclassification of double or triple - hit lymphoma
HCL	Medium size, kidney-bean shaped nuclei, inconspicuous nucleoli, abundant cytoplasm, and radiated cytoplasmic hairy projections	Sinusoidal pattern	CD20+, PAX-5+, DBA.44+, CD5−, CD10−, CD23−, CD25+, TRAP+, CD11c+, CD103+, cyclin D1+/−, and annexin 1+	*BRAF V600E* mutation
B-CLL	Small size, clumped chromatin, round nuclei, and scant cytoplasm	White pulp expansion (spleen) Dense periportal lymphoid aggregates and scattered interstitial infiltrates (liver)	CD20 dim+, PAX-5+, CD5+, CD10−, CD23+, cyclinD1−, CD43+, LEF1+	11q/ATM, -13q, trisomy 13, del(17p)/TP53
MCL	Small size, condensed chromatin, prominent nucleoli, and scant cytoplasm	White pulp expansion (spleen) Dense periportal lymphoid aggregates and scattered interstitial infiltrate (liver)	CD20+, PAX-5+, CD5+, CD23−, CD10−, cyclin D1+, SOX-11+	t(11;14)/*IgH-BCL1*

markers (CD99, TdT, and/or CD34) [33]. Upon its maturation, T-ALL can be further subclassified into pro-T, pre-T, cortical T- and mature T-cells. Certain pro-T or pre-T types can now be reclassified as early T-cell precursor lymphoblastic leukemia (ETP-ALL), if phenotypically compatible (CD1a-, CD5 dim+/−, CD8-, plus at least one myeloid marker and/or one stem cell marker, e.g., CD34, TdT) [4, 34].

Mixed Phenotype Acute Leukemia (B-/Myeloid)

Mixed phenotype acute leukemia (B-/myeloid) is a rare subtype of leukemia. At first, it is critical for pathologists to identify B-lymphoblasts from blasts with myeloid or monocytic differentiation and then determine whether the blasts are biphenotypic. Useful markers indicative of myeloid phenotype include MPO, and for monocytic phenotype CD11c, CD14, CD64, lysozyme, and non-specific esterase (NSE) [4].

High-Grade B-Cell Lymphomas

Certain high-grade B-cell lymphomas (e.g., blastoid variant of mantle cell lymphoma, Burkitt lymphoma, high-grade B-cell lymphomas, double or triple hit, or high-grade lymphoma, NOS) often exhibit a blastoid chromatin pattern and lack surface light chain expression, thus mimicking B-ALL. In this case, identification of CD34 or TdT expression is helpful in differentiating B-ALL from lymphoma. As CD34 is not always positive in B-ALL, TdT becomes a more critical marker, as TdT-negative B-ALLs are rare [35], while mature B-cell lymphomas are always negative for these two markers.

CD45-Negative Neoplasms

CD45-negative B-ALL/-LBL should be carefully separated from other CD45-negative neoplasms, e.g., metastatic carcinoma, melanoma, and leukemic plasmacytoma. These neoplasms are similar to B-ALL and also show a sinusoidal pattern [10]. The differential diagnosis should also include so-called small blue cell neoplasms involving the liver or spleen, such as Ewing sarcoma, metastatic small cell carcinoma of the lung, and Merkel cell carcinoma. Cytokeratin and TTF-1 are usually positive for small cell carcinoma of the lung. However, both B-ALL/-LBL and Ewing sarcoma could be positive for CD99 and negative for CD45. Therefore, a comprehensive panel including all B- and stem cell markers should be performed. Ewing sarcoma is essentially negative for CD19, CD20, PAX-5, TdT, and CD34 but shows immunoreactivity to FLI-1 and partially neuron-specific markers such as NSE, synaptophysin, and S100 [36]. Merkel cell carcinoma is a great mimic to B-ALL, as it also expresses TdT and PAX-5. Additional IHC staining with CK20 and CAM5.2 helps to differentiate between Merkel cells (positive, dot-like staining pattern) and B-ALL (negative) [37].

Others

Of note, B-LBL could concur with chronic liver disease such as hepatitis B or C and autoimmune hepatitis that should be additionally excluded. A laboratory investigation using hepatitis B or C surface and core antigens, antinuclear antibodies, anti-smooth muscle antibodies, anti-mitochondrial antibodies, etc. may provide diagnostic clues.

Prognosis

Accurate assessment of prognosis is central to the management of ALL. Risk stratification allows the physician to determine the most appropriate initial treatment regimen as well as when to consider allogeneic hematopoietic stem cell transplantation (allo-HSCT).

A variety of factors impact the clinical outcome of B-ALL, including demographics, immunophenotype, cytogenetic features, individual drug metabolism, and early treatment response [12, 38]. Historically, age and white blood cell count at the time of diagnosis have been used to risk stratify patients. Increasing age portends a worsening prognosis. Patients over the age of 60 have particularly poor outcomes, with only 10–15% long-term survival [21]. Age is at least in part a surrogate for other prognosticators as the elderly tend to have disease with intrinsic unfavorable biology (e.g., Philadelphia chromosome positive (Ph+), hypodiploidy and complex karyotype), more medical comorbidities, and inability to tol-

erate standard chemotherapy regimens, but it helps guide therapy nonetheless. The largest prospective trial to determine optimal treatment, MRC UKALL XII/ECOG E2993, found a significant difference in both disease-free survival (DFS) and overall survival (OS) based on age using a cutoff of 35 in Philadelphia chromosome negative (Ph-) disease [22]. Similarly, their study found that an elevated white blood cell count at diagnosis, defined as $>30 \times 10^9$ for B-ALL or $>100 \times 10^9$ for T-ALL, is an independent prognostic factor for DFS and OS [22].

Although clinical factors play an important role in guiding therapy, cytogenetic changes, e.g., harboring t(9;22)/Ph chromosome, have implications both in terms of prognosis and for treatment. Historically, Ph+ ALL has a 1-year survival of around 10%. However, with the development of tyrosine kinase inhibitors (TKIs), overall survival has improved. Other poor prognostic indicators include t(4;11), *KMT2A/MLL*, t(8;14)/*IgH-MYC*, complex karyotype (≥ 5 chromosomal abnormalities), and low hypodiploidy (30–39 chromosomes)/near triploidy (60–78 chromosomes). In contrast, patients with hyperdiploidy and del(9p) have a significantly better outcome [24]. In a later study, the Southwest Oncology Group (SWOG) showed that among the 200 study patients, cytogenetic profile was a more important prognostic factor than age or WBC count [25]. Ph-like ALL has been associated with poor response to induction chemotherapy, elevated minimal residual disease, and poor survival [13, 14, 26].

In addition to disease characteristics at the outset, it has long been recognized that response to initial therapy predicts outcome. Recently, molecular techniques such as flow cytometry and PCR to evaluate patients for minimal residual disease (MRD) have become standard practice [27]. Several studies have shown the importance of MRD in assigning risk [28–33]. Brüggemann et al. [38] re-stratified standard-risk patients to low risk, intermediate risk, and high risk with relapse rates of 0%, 47%, and 94%, respectively, based on the persistence of elevated MRD, defined as $>10^{-4}$. In a multivariate analysis of 326 adolescent and adult patients with high-risk Ph-negative ALL treated in the Programa Espanol de Tratamientos en Hematologia (PETHEMA ALL-AR-03), Ribera et al. [39] showed that poor MRD clearance, defined as levels $>1 \times 10^{-3}$ after induction and levels $>5 \times 10^{-4}$ after early consolidation chemotherapy measured by flow cytometry, was the only significant prognostic factor for DFS and OS.

On the basis of what is known about prognostic factors in adult ALL, the National Comprehensive Cancer Network (NCCN) has developed recommendations to approach risk stratification [16]. The National Cancer Institute (NIH) defines adolescent and young adults to be those aged 15–39 years. The NCCN recognizes that adolescent and young adults may benefit from treatment with pediatric-inspired regimens and thus are considered separately from adults >40 years [40].

Diagnostic Caveats

- It is more common for the liver and/or spleen to be secondarily involved by B-ALL/-LBL than to be a primary site.
- Diagnosis should usually rely on flow cytometric analysis of peripheral blood and/or bone marrow specimens because solitary liver or spleen manifestation is extremely rare and a biopsy of the liver or spleen is not usually performed.
- If a liver biopsy is performed, given the limited amount of tissue, IHC study is preferred over flow cytometry. Following effective cytoreduction therapy, splenectomy is usually not indicated for these patients.
- If available, FISH results (e.g., *BCR-ABL1*) and information on a specific molecular signature (e.g., BCR-ABL1-like) provide disease prognosis and benefit treatment decision-making.

References

1. Borowitz MJ, Chan J, Downing J, Arber DA. B-lymphoblastic leukemia/lymphoma. In: Swerdlow SH, Campo E, Harris NL, et al., editors. WHO classification of tumors of haematopoietic and lymphoid tissues (2017 revised edition). Geneva: WHO Press; 2017. p. 199–213.
2. Terwilliger T, Abdul-Hay M. Acute lymphoblastic leukemia: a comprehensive review and 2017 update. Blood Cancer J. 2017;7(6):e577.
3. Inaba H, Greaves M, Mulligan CG. Acute lymphoblastic leukaemia. Lancet. 2013;381(9881):1943–55.
4. Chiaretti S, Zini G, Bassan R. Diagnosis and subclassification of acute lymphoblastic leukemia. Mediterr J Hematol Infect Dis. 2014;6(1):e2014073.
5. Paul S, Kantarjian H, Jabbour EJ. Adult acute lymphoblastic leukemia. Mayo Clin Proc. 2016;91(11):1645–66.
6. Medeiros LJ, O'Malley DP, Caraway NP, Vega F, Felnitoba-Johnson KSJ, Lim M. B-lymphoblastic leukemia/lymphoma. In: Tumors of the lymph nodes and spleen. Washington, DC: ARP Press; 2017. p. 149–63.
7. Bassan R, Hoelzer D. Modern therapy of acute lymphoblastic leukemia. J Clin Oncol. 2011;29(5):532–43.
8. Hunger SP, Lu X, Devidas M, et al. Improved survival for children and adolescents with acute lymphoblastic leukemia between 1990 and 2005: a report from the children's oncology group. J Clin Oncol. 2012;30(14):1663–9.
9. Siegel R, Naishadham D, Jemal A. Cancer statistics, 2012. CA Cancer J Clin. 2012;62(1):10–29.
10. Loddenkemper C, Longerich T, Hummel M, et al. Frequency and diagnostic patterns of lymphomas in liver biopsies with respect to the WHO classification. Virchows Arch. 2007;450(5):493–502.
11. Greaves M. A causal mechanism for childhood acute lymphoblastic leukaemia. Nat Rev Cancer. 2018;18(8):471–84.
12. Pui CH, Robison LL, Look AT. Acute lymphoblastic leukaemia. Lancet. 2008;371(9617):1030–43.
13. Siddique MN, Popalzai M, Aoun N, Maroun R, Awasum M, Dai Q. Precursor B-cell acute lymphoblastic leukemia presenting as obstructive jaundice: a case report. J Med Case Rep. 2011;5:269.
14. Alvaro F, Jain M, Morris LL, Rice MS. Childhood acute lymphoblastic leukaemia presenting as jaundice. J Paediatr Child Health. 1996;32(5):466–8.
15. Daniel SV, Vani DH, Smith AM, Hill QA, Menon KV. Obstructive jaundice due to a pancreatic mass: a rare presentation of acute lymphoblastic leukaemia in an adult. JOP. 2010;11(1):72–4.
16. Chang LS, Yu HR, Chen YC, et al. Acute lymphoblastic leukemia presented as severe jaundice and hyperferritinemia: a case report. J Pediatr Hematol Oncol. 2011;33(3):e117–9.
17. Takamatsu T. Preferential infiltration of liver sinusoids in acute lymphoblastic leukemia. Rinsho Ketsueki. 2001;42(12):1181–6.
18. McCord RG, Gilbert EF, Joo PJ. Acute leukemia presenting as jaundice with acute liver failure. Clin Pediatr (Phila). 1973;12(12):17A passim.
19. Coustan-Smith E, Behm FG, Sanchez J, et al. Immunological detection of minimal residual disease in children with acute lymphoblastic leukaemia. Lancet. 1998;351(9102):550–4.
20. Janossy G, Coustan-Smith E, Campana D. The reliability of cytoplasmic CD3 and CD22 antigen expression in the immunodiagnosis of acute leukemia: a study of 500 cases. Leukemia. 1989;3(3):170–81.
21. Thomas DA, O'Brien S, Jorgensen JL, et al. Prognostic significance of CD20 expression in adults with de novo precursor B-lineage acute lymphoblastic leukemia. Blood. 2009;113(25):6330–7.
22. Maury S, Huguet F, Leguay T, et al. Adverse prognostic significance of CD20 expression in adults with Philadelphia chromosome-negative B-cell precursor acute lymphoblastic leukemia. Haematologica. 2010;95(2):324–8.
23. Shousha S, Gadir F, Peston D, Bansi D, Thillainaygam AV, Murray-Lyon IM. CD10 immunostaining of bile canaliculi in liver biopsies: change of staining pattern with the development of cirrhosis. Histopathology. 2004;45(4):335–42.
24. Bansal S, Sharma U, Jain A, Sharma R, Yagnik B. CD19-negative B-lineage acute lymphoblastic leukemia: a diagnostic and therapeutic challenge. Indian J Pathol Microbiol. 2017;60(4):596–8.
25. Seegmiller AC, Kroft SH, Karandikar NJ, McKenna RW. Characterization of immunophenotypic aberrancies in 200 cases of B acute lymphoblastic leukemia. Am J Clin Pathol. 2009;132(6):940–9.
26. Sedek L, Bulsa J, Sonsala A, et al. The immunophenotypes of blast cells in B-cell precursor acute lymphoblastic leukemia: how different are they from their normal counterparts? Cytometry B Clin Cytom. 2014;86(5):329–39.
27. Holmfeldt L, Wei L, Diaz-Flores E, et al. The genomic landscape of hypodiploid acute lymphoblastic leukemia. Nat Genet. 2013;45(3):242–52.
28. Haferlach T, Kohlmann A, Schnittger S, et al. Global approach to the diagnosis of leukemia using gene expression profiling. Blood. 2005;106(4):1189–98.
29. Chiaretti S, Li X, Gentleman R, et al. Gene expression profiles of B-lineage adult acute lymphocytic leukemia reveal genetic patterns that identify lineage derivation and distinct mechanisms of transformation. Clin Cancer Res. 2005;11(20):7209–19.
30. Harvey RC, Mulligan CG, Wang X, et al. Identification of novel cluster groups in pediatric high-risk B-precursor acute lymphoblastic leukemia with gene expression profiling: correlation with genome-wide DNA copy number alterations, clinical characteristics, and outcome. Blood. 2010;116(23):4874–84.
31. Wen KW, Gill RM. Immature terminal deoxynucleotidyl transferase positive B cells are detected in a subset of adult and pediatric liver biopsies. Appl Immunohistochem Mol Morphol. 2019;27(4):319–24.
32. Sevilla DW, Colovai AI, Emmons FN, Bhagat G, Alobeid B. Hematogones: a review and update. Leuk Lymphoma. 2010;51(1):10–9.

33. Borowitz MJ, Chan JKC, Bene MC, Arber DC. T-lymphoblastic leukemia. In: Swerdlow SH, Campo E, Harris NL, et al., editors. WHO classification of tumours of haematopoietic and lymphoid tissues. Geneva: WHO Press; 2017. p. 209–13.

34. Coustan-Smith E, Mullighan CG, Onciu M, et al. Early T-cell precursor leukaemia: a subtype of very high-risk acute lymphoblastic leukaemia. Lancet Oncol. 2009;10(2):147–56.

35. Faber J, Kantarjian H, Roberts MW, Keating M, Freireich E, Albitar M. Terminal deoxynucleotidyl transferase-negative acute lymphoblastic leukemia. Arch Pathol Lab Med. 2000;124(1):92–7.

36. Nilsson G, Wang M, Wejde J, Kreicbergs A, Larsson O. Detection of EWS/FLI-1 by immunostaining. An adjunctive tool in diagnosis of Ewing's sarcoma and primitive neuroectodermal tumour on cytological samples and paraffin-embedded archival material. Sarcoma. 1999;3(1):25–32.

37. Kolhe R, Reid MD, Lee JR, Cohen C, Ramalingam P. Immunohistochemical expression of PAX5 and TdT by Merkel cell carcinoma and pulmonary small cell carcinoma: a potential diagnostic pitfall but useful discriminatory marker. Int J Clin Exp Pathol. 2013;6(2):142–7.

38. Brüggemann M, Raff T, Flohr T, et al. Clinical significance of minimal residual disease quantification in adult patients with standardrisk acute lymphoblastic leukemia. Blood. 2006;107(3):1116–23.

39. Ribera JM, Oriol A, Morgades M, et al. Treatment of high-risk Philadelphia chromosome-negative acute lymphoblastic leukemia in adolescents and adults according to early cytologic response and minimal residual disease after consolidation assessed by flow cytometry: final results of the PETHEMA ALL-AR-03 trial. J Clin Oncol. 2014;32(15):1595–604.

40. Vrooman LM, Silverman LB. Childhood acute lymphoblastic leukemia: update on prognostic factors. Curr Opin Pediatr. 2009;21(1):1–8.

T-Lymphoblastic Leukemia/Lymphoma Involving the Spleen or Liver

David C. Gajzer and Ling Zhang

Definition

T-lymphoblastic leukemia/lymphoma is characterized by an abnormal proliferation of T-cell progenitors, phenotypically expressing stem cell markers (e.g., TdT) as well as T-cell antigens [1, 2]. It constitutes an aggressive subset of T-lymphoblasts that involves the bone marrow as well as additional organs. T-lymphoblastic lymphoma (T-LBL) is characterized by a bulky mediastinal or cervical mass leading to compression of adjacent organs or tissues in approximately 75% of cases. When T-LBL spreads to the peripheral blood and/or bone marrow, it enters the leukemic phase. Isolated T-cell acute lymphoblastic leukemia or T-lymphoblastic leukemia (T-ALL), defined as >25% T-lymphoblasts in peripheral blood and/or bone marrow without accompanying T-LBL is less common. Clinically, T-ALL usually shows marked leukocytosis composed of mainly circulating lymphoblasts [3]. The blast morphology in T-ALL and T-LBL are indistinguishable [1]. However, gene expression profiling has shown differential expression of genes involved in chemotactic responses, angiogenesis, and homotypic cell-cell adhesion (e.g., *BCL2*, *EPAS1*, *SIPR1*, and *ICAM1*), suggesting a role in tumor cell localization, which may explain the differences in clinical manifestation [4, 5]. Hepatosplenic involvement by T-LBL has been frequently documented, but has rarely been reported presenting as a sole lesion involving these organs at initial presentation [6].

Epidemiology

Approximately 6000 cases of ALL are diagnosed in the United States annually, and T-ALL accounts for 10–15% of pediatric and 20–25% of ALL in the Western hemisphere, although the incidence diminishes with older age [7]. T-LBL comprises approximately 85–90% of all lymphoblastic lymphomas, much higher than B-lymphoblastic lymphoma (B-LBL). However, T-ALL is less common than B-ALL. T-ALL often presents in patients that are male, black, older, and less likely to be Hispanic than patients with B-ALL. T-LBL tends to affect young patients in the second and third decades of life [8].

A recently described subgroup of T-ALL, early T-cell precursor lymphoblastic leukemia (ETP-ALL), accounts for approximately 10% of pediatric T-ALL, yet its incidence increases with age, accounting for approximately 40–50% of adult T-ALL [9]. Originally, patients with ETP-ALL were described as a high-risk group with a higher rate of extramedullary infiltration and increased incidences of failure to obtain complete hematological remission, a higher prevalence of hematological relapse, and significantly reduced overall survival in children and adults [9]. However, recent clinical series suggest that the grave prognosis associated with childhood ETP-ALL can be overcome with intensified treatment strategies.

Etiology and Pathogenesis

The etiology of T-ALL/-LBL is unclear, but suggestive of underlying genetic instability or mutations. A recent familial T-ALL study (monozygotic twins) disclosed an identified T-cell receptor (TCR) gene rearrangement [10]. It results from a transformation process during thymocyte development caused by genetic alterations that disrupt key oncogenic, tumor suppressor, and developmental pathways

D. C. Gajzer · L. Zhang (✉)
Department of Pathology, H. Lee Moffitt Cancer Center and Research Institute, Tampa, FL, USA
e-mail: ling.zhang@moffitt.org

© Springer Nature Switzerland AG 2020
L. Zhang et al. (eds.), *Diagnostic Pathology of Hematopoietic Disorders of Spleen and Liver*,
https://doi.org/10.1007/978-3-030-37708-3_14

responsible for cell growth, proliferation, survival, and differentiation.

The biology, risk factors, and pathogenesis of T-LBL are still elusive. Recent studies have brought new insights into molecular signatures of T-ALL/-LBL via identification of *NOTCH* gene dysregulation and other genes controlling T-cell proliferation and differentiation, e.g., *FBXW7*, which play critical roles in initiation and development of T-ALL/-LBL. These genes will be discussed in the genetic and molecular sections [8, 11].

Clinical Findings

When compared with B-LBL, T-LBL patients present more frequently with mediastinal tumors. Clinically, T-LBL can present with fatigue, dyspnea, and dysphagia secondary to fast-growing bulky mass(es) involving the anterior mediastinum resulting in compression of the respiratory tract and/or esophagus. Superior vena cava syndrome (SVCS) may occur when the superior vena cava is partially blocked or compressed by T-LBL located in the chest [8]. Cervical, supraclavicular, and axillary lymph nodes are often involved. It is not uncommon for T-LBL to be associated with pleural or cardiac effusions leading to functional compromise of the lung and heart. Besides the mediastinum, peripheral blood, and bone marrow, other body sites can also be involved such as the skin, tonsil, spleen, liver, and central nervous system (CNS) [8].

Reports on hepatosplenic involvement by T-LBL are variable in rate and one review considered it an unusual finding [8]. However, other reports stated that hepatosplenomegaly is found in 40–70% of T-ALL and often accompanies progressive disease [12, 13]. Clinically, >80% of patients are categorized as stage III or stage IV disease. Serum lactate dehydrogenase (LDH) is usually elevated and approximately 50% of patients have B-symptoms [14]. Involvement of the testis (male) or uterus (female) has also been reported. CNS involvement occurs especially if the neoplasm is left untreated [7].

Patients with T-ALL present with profound leukocytosis (often >50 × 10^9/L and thus much higher than in B-ALL) as well as peripheral lymphadenopathy and hepatosplenomegaly [1, 15]. Anemia and thrombocytopenia are noted. Leukopenia with a very low tumor burden in the peripheral blood or bone marrow (<20% T-lymphoblasts) warrants further verification before a diagnosis is rendered [2].

Initial presentation with liver or spleen disease by T-ALL/-LBL is even more rarely reported than that by B-ALL. Cholestatic jaundice, associated with nausea, pale stools, dark urine, weight loss, and anorexia, has been documented in one patient with liver involvement by T-ALL/-LBL. A CT scan in this case revealed massive hepatomegaly and a mediastinal bulky mass (16.0 × 10.0 cm) as well [6].

Similar to B-LBL, the St. Jude Children's Research Hospital staging system and the Ann Arbor system are utilized for staging [16, 17].

Morphology

Microscopic Examination

Microscopic examination reveals a lymphoblast population which tends to be homogeneous, with individual blast cells having a central, mostly round, sometimes indented nucleus and high nucleocytoplasmic ratio. The nuclear chromatin is fine, with dispersed condensation and inconspicuous nucleoli. The cytoplasm is scant and basophilic, sometimes with a single long projection which confers the name hand-mirror cell (Fig. 14.1). Cytoplasmic granules are rarely present and always negative for peroxidase, esterase, and toluidine blue by histochemistry. Cytoplasmic vacuoles can be present, while Auer rods are always absent [1, 2, 18]. T-LBL involving the mediastinum and/or lymph nodes usually shows a diffuse infiltrate by sheets of lymphoblasts with oval to irregular nuclei, less prominent nucleoli, fine or slightly coarse chromatin, and a scant to moderate amount of pale blue cytoplasm. Mitotic activity is brisk. The background cellularity consists of eosinophils and histiocytes/macrophages. Sometimes, associated geographic necrosis or a starry sky pattern are identified, not different from other high turnover lymphomas, e.g., Burkitt lymphoma [2, 18] (Fig. 14.2a).

Liver involvement by T-ALL/-LBL is mainly located in periportal and perivascular regions. Scattered sinusoidal manifestation, patchy necrosis, or secondary fibrosis are also

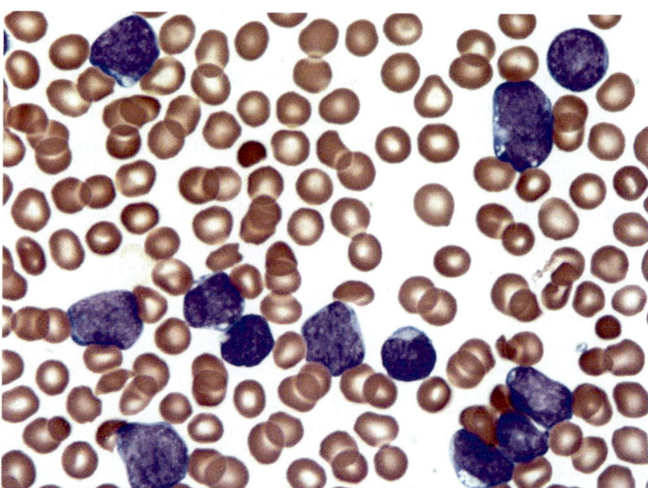

Fig. 14.1 Peripheral blood involvement by T-lymphoblastic leukemia. The circulating T-lymphoblasts are variable in size and display hyperchromatic nuclei, round to irregular nuclear contours, one to multiple nucleoli, and a small amount of cytoplasm with or without cytoplasmic vacuoles (Wright stain, 1000×)

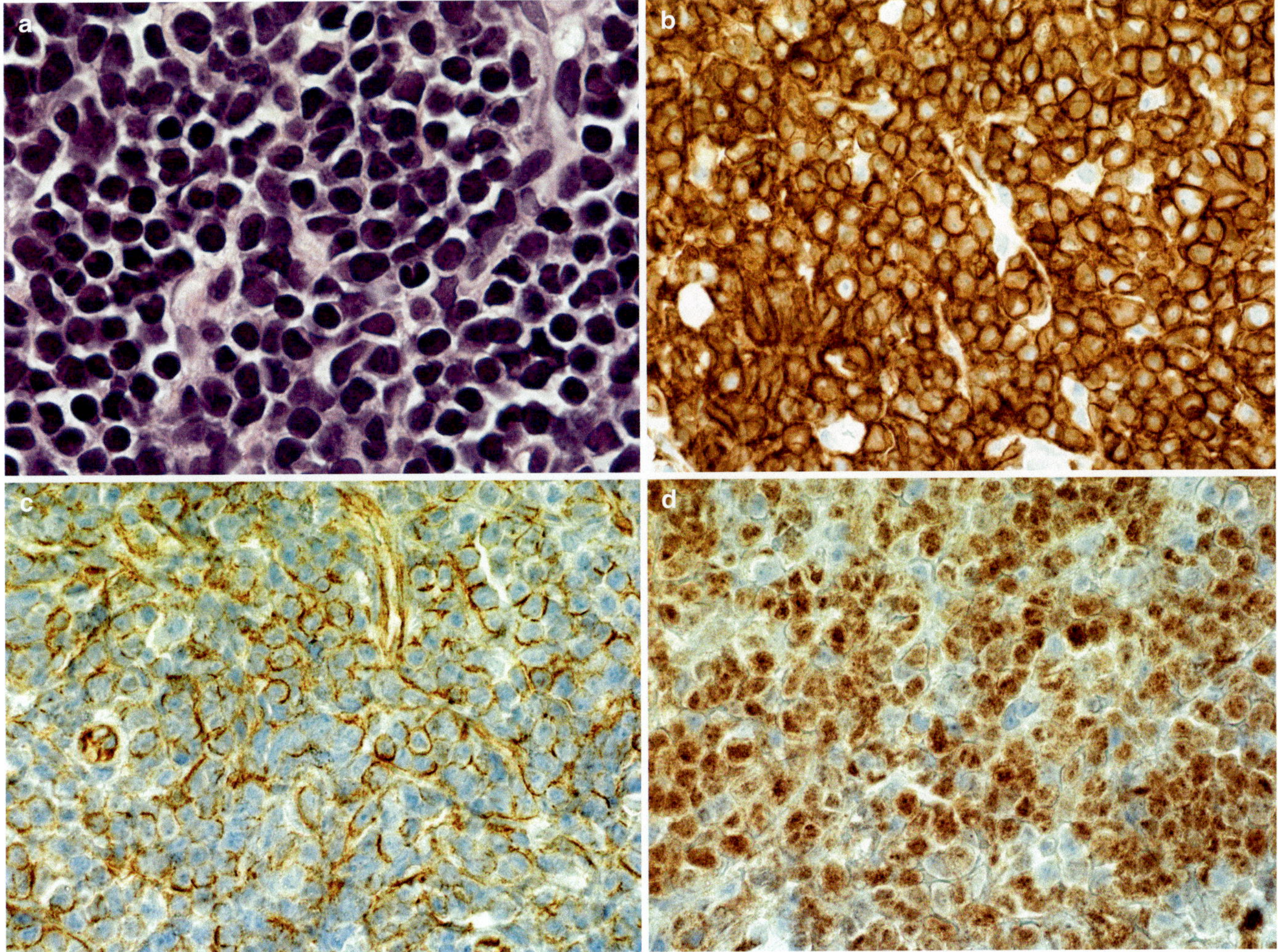

Fig. 14.2 Mediastinal manifestation of T-lymphoblastic lymphoma. The lymphoma cells are small to medium in size with nuclear irregularity and high N:C ratio (**a** - H&E stain, 600×). Immunohistochemical stains show diffuse cytoplasmic CD3 (**b**), CD99 (**c**), and TdT (**d**) expression (immunoperoxidase, 600×)

observed (Fig. 14.3a–c). Bile stasis can be present. The background hepatocytes show normal histomorphology or a variable degree of pathologic changes secondary to the patients' original liver disease. Splenic involvement with packed white blood cells may lead to infarction. Sections of splenic parenchyma reveal diffuse red-pulp expansion and are filled with T-ALL/-LBL (Fig. 14.4a–d). Cytologically, the immature precursors are not different from B-LBL on the touch imprint. Residual B-cell follicles can still be identified.

Immunophenotyping

The WHO defines lymphoblasts in T-ALL as TdT positive with variable expression of CD1a, CD2, CD3, CD4, CD5, CD7, and CD8, depending on individual stages of intrathymic differentiation [8]. Cytoplasmic CD3 and surface CD7 are often positive. CD2, CD5, and CD7 antigens are markers of the most immature T-cells, but none of them is absolutely lineage-specific, so that diagnosis of T-ALL rests on the demonstration of surface and cytoplasmic CD3; the latter is more common [8]. CD10 expression is quite common (25%) and not specific; CD34 can be expressed, mostly found in the pro-T and pre-T stage. Upon the maturation stage, T-ALL blasts show slightly variable expression of stem cell markers and T-cell antigens (Table 14.1). Tumor cells positive for cytoplasmic CD3, CD99, and TdT expression by immunostains are diagnostic of T-LBL (Fig. 14.2b–d) when a flow cytometry study is not available. Identification of cytoplasmic CD3 and TdT by immunostains is sufficient to support a diagnosis of liver or splenic involvement (Fig. 14.3d and f) when a diagnosis of T-ALL is rendered in other sites. Of note, aberrant expression of myeloid markers (e.g., CD13, CD33, CD117) or B-cell markers (CD9, CD21, and CD24) or partial loss of pan T-cell markers can be identified in T-ALL/-LBL [1], which are

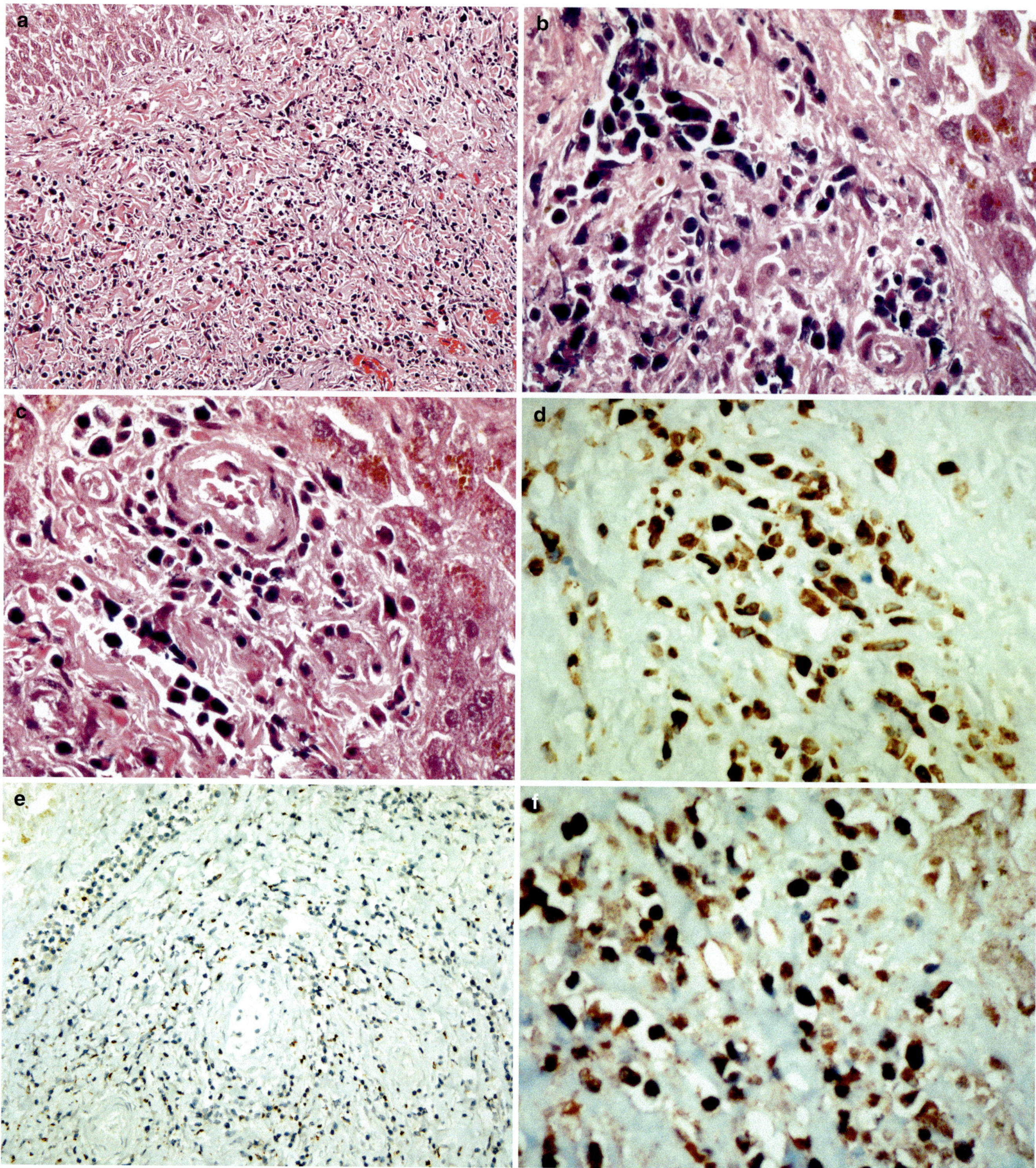

Fig. 14.3 **Autopsy case of T-ALL/-LBL involving the liver**. The H&E sections of liver parenchyma (**a**) show involvement of lymphoblasts with hyperchromatic nuclei, irregular nuclear contours, and scant cytoplasm associated with partially autolyzed hepatocytes (200×). Higher-power views (**b** and **c**, 600×) demonstrate these neoplastic cells with intravascular or peripheral infiltrating pattern. Immunohistochemical study reveals that T-LBL cells are positive for CD3 (cytoplasmic staining pattern) (**d**, immunoperoxidase, 600×) and TdT (nuclear stain) (**f**, immunoperoxidase, 600×), and negative for CD20 (**e**, immunoperoxidase, 600×)

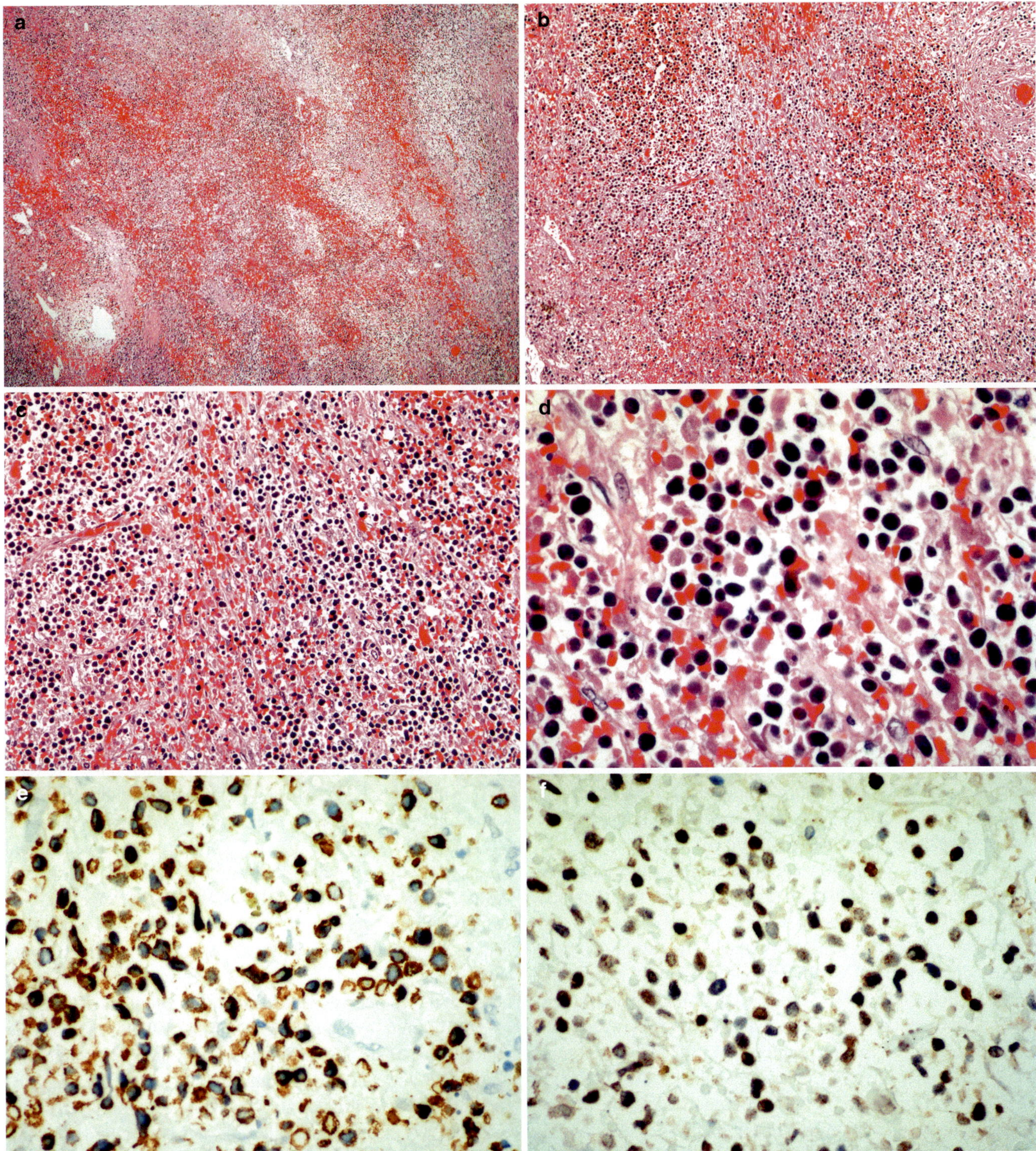

Fig. 14.4 Autopsy case of T-ALL/-LBL involving the spleen. (**a–c**) Low- to medium-power view of the splenic parenchyma shows complete effacement by loss of the normal white pulp and extensive expansion of the red pulp associated with congestion and infiltration by leukemic blasts (H&E stain, 40×, 100×, and 200×, respectively). (**d**) A high power view of the H&E section (600×) shows the sinusoidal spaces are loaded with lymphoblasts, slightly variable in size with round to oval nuclei and hyperchromasia. Immunohistochemical stains proved the neoplastic cells to be T-lymphoblasts expressing cytoplasmic CD3 (**e**, immunoperoxidase, 600×) and nuclear TdT (**f**, immunoperoxidase, 600×)

Table 14.1 Phenotypic findings of T-ALL/-LBL at various stages of intrathymic differentiation

	cCD3	CD1a	CD2	CD4	CD7	CD8	CD34	TdT	TCR (PCR)
Pro-T	+	−	−	−	+	−	+/−	+	Germline
Pre-T	+	−	+	−	+	−	+/−	+/−	Rearranged
Cortical T	+	+	+	+	+	+	−	+/−	Rearranged
Medullary T	+	−	+	Variable	+	+	−	−	Rearranged

Table 14.2 Differential diagnoses of common small blue cell neoplasms involving the mediastinum

	Common sites	Morphology	IHC/flow cytometry findings	Note
Thymoma	Mediastinum or ectopic sites include the neck, gastrointestinal tract, etc. Rarely involves the liver or spleen.	Admixed epithelial cells with oval nuclei, pale chromatin and abundant cytoplasm and maturing T-cells with high N:C ratio and oval to irregular nuclei.	Cytokeratin highlights epithelial cells.	Different patterns based on WHO classification of thymoma: lymphocyte predominant, mixed lymphocytes and epithelial cells, and spindle cell form.
SCLC	Mediastinal lymph node; it can metastasize to the peripheral lymph nodes, liver, spleen, and bone marrow.	Two-fold larger than small lymphocytes, fine, "salt-pepper" chromatin, high N:C ratio, and scant cytoplasm, often associated with nuclear molding or rosette formation.	Neural and neuroendocrine markers, e.g., chromogranin, synaptophysin, CD56, nonspecific esterase (NSE).	Large-cell variant is also identified. Extensive crush artifact or crushed nuclei are common.
T-ALL/-LBL	Primarily found in mediastinum, lymph node, peripheral blood, and bone marrow. The liver and spleen are secondarily involved.	Variable in size, small to large, with immature chromatin, finely granulated or less clumped chromatin, prominent nucleoli, and a small amount of basophilic cytoplasm.	Negative for above listed neuroendocrine markers except for synaptophysin. Selectively positive for TdT, CD34, CD1a, CD4, CD8, CD5 and frequently positive for cytoplasmic CD3, surface CD2, and CD7.	A variant of indolent T-LBL has been reported that could be found extra-mediastinally. [9]

useful to distinguish it from other cytologic mimickers, e.g., thymoma, in addition to cytokeratin. T-LBL cells involving the liver may aberrantly express a neuroendocrine marker, synaptophysin, leading to a diagnostic pitfall [6].

Early T-cell precursor acute lymphoblastic leukemia (ETP-ALL) shows a distinct phenotype that is frequently CD34+, CD1a-, cytoplasmic CD3+, dim or loss of CD5+, dual CD4- and CD8-, while cortical T-LBL exhibits a more mature phenotype by usually lacking CD34 and expressing CD1a, cytoplasmic CD3, CD4, or CD8 or both in addition to other T-cell markers [9, 19]. ETP-ALL often aberrantly expresses stem cell markers such as CD34, TdT (subset), and HLA-DR and/or myeloid markers such as CD11b, CD13, CD33, and CD117 [2, 7]. Recent studies have shown the majority of previously called pro-T or pre-T T-ALL/-LBL now fall into the ETP-ALL category.

Differential Diagnoses

T-ALL/-LBL is usually readily identifiable by morphologic assessment of the bone marrow and multiparameter flow cytometry evaluation, with no need for additional tests, since ancillary studies such as genetics/cytogenetics/genomics are available at a later stage but they cannot be employed for purely diagnostic

purposes. It may sometimes be difficult to differentiate between T-ALL including ETP-ALL, AML, and mixed phenotypic leukemia, T/myeloid, due to phenotypic overlapping. Of note, CD117, CD13, CD33, and TdT are not discriminative markers because all of them can be identified in both T-ALL and AML. No reactivity to Susan Black B (SBB) or myeloperoxidase (MPO) histochemical stains is characteristic of T-ALL cells (<3% positive) [19]. Diffuse strong MPO positivity favors AML over T-ALL. This rule also applies for the distinction between mixed phenotypic leukemia, T/myeloid, and T-ALL.

The differential diagnosis of T-ALL/-LBL also includes the majority of small blue cell tumors with fine chromatin and high nuclear-to-cytoplasmic ratio such as small cell lung cancer (SCLC) and thymoma. The neoplasms are frequently found in the mediastinum and adjacent lymph nodes. Small cell lung cancer (SCLC) metastasizing to the liver is also very common. A comprehensive immunohistochemical staining panel is necessary to differentiate between T-ALL/-LBL and other tumors. The common cytomorphologic and immunophenotypic features of T-ALL/-LBL in comparison to other neoplasms that frequently involve the mediastinum, liver, and spleen are summarized in Table 14.2. Figure 14.5a depicts a Merkel cell carcinoma with liver involvement, morphologically resembling T-ALL/-LBL. Additional immunostaining with CK20, pancytokeratin, and synaptophysin (Fig. 14.5b–d)

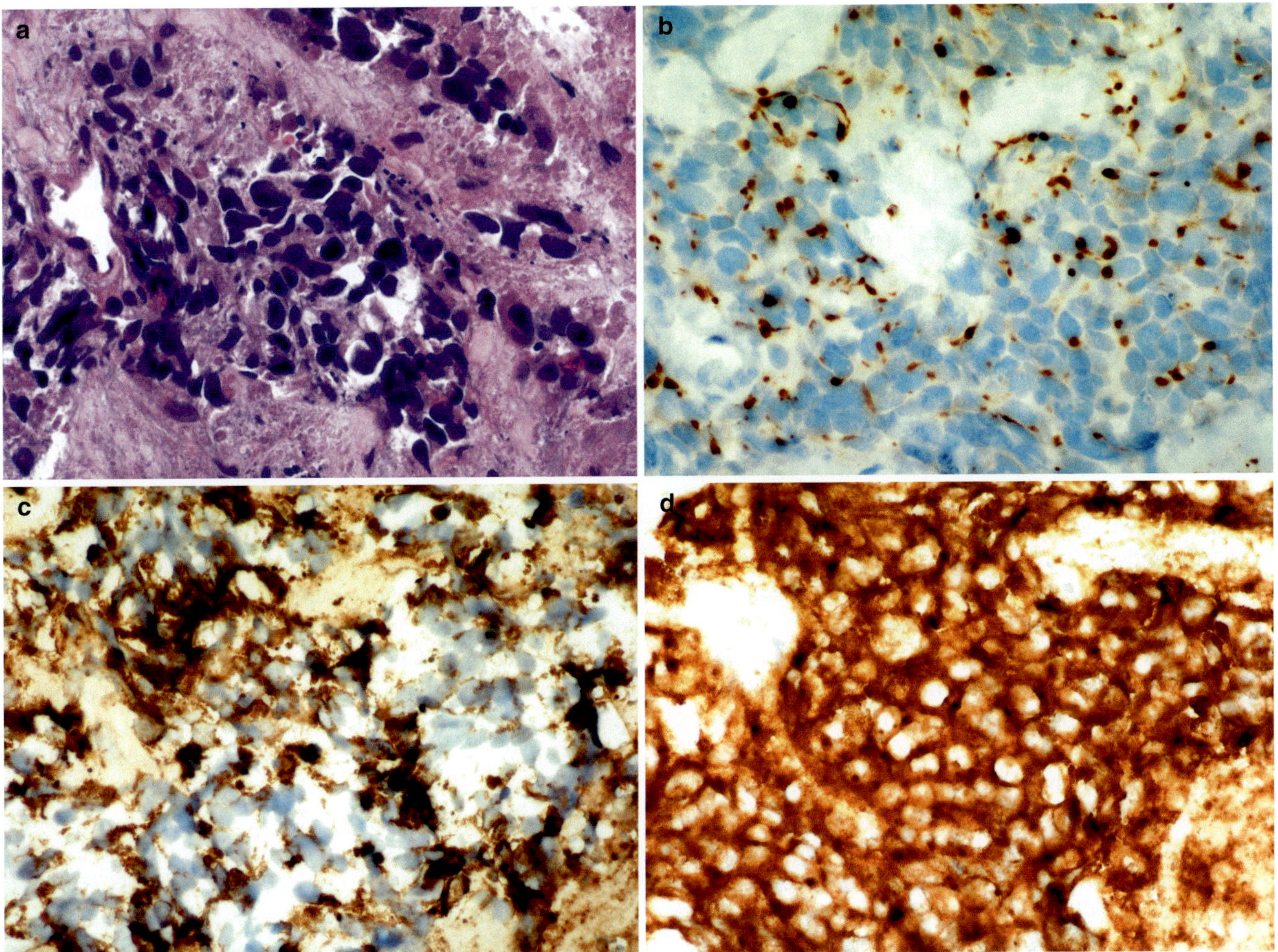

Fig. 14.5 Merkel cell carcinoma metastasizing to the liver. (**a**) The H&E section of liver biopsy shows clusters of neoplastic cells in the background of extensive necrosis. These cells show hyperchromatic nuclei, high N:C ratio, and markedly irregular nuclear contours that could resemble T-LBL (H&E stain, 600×). Immunohistochemical stains highlight the tumor cells as positive for CK20 (**b**), AE1/AE3/Cam5.2 (**c**), and synaptophysin (**d**) (**b-d**, immunoperoxidase, 600×)

or other neuroendocrine markers helps differentiate the tumor from T-ALL/-LBL.

Of note, the presence of T-cell receptor γ or β chain gene rearrangements present in the majority of T-ALL cases is not used for lineage assignment or as an additional tool for differentiation between T-ALL and a myeloid neoplasm [8].

Cytogenetics

T-ALL/-LBL is a highly heterogeneous neoplasm based on conventional cytogenetic analysis and undated molecular studies [9]. Approximately 60% of T-ALL/-LBL harbor cytogenetic abnormalities [2].

Translocations involving the T-cell receptor (TCR) regions 14q11 (TCRA/D) and 7q34 (TCRB) can be detected in approximately 35% of patients [20, 21]. These juxtapose enhancer elements of the TCR genes with transcription factors involved in T-cell differentiation, with deregulation of lymphopoiesis.

T-ALL oncogenes include activated transcription factors such as basic helix-loop-helix genes (*bHLH*), LIM-only domain (*LMO1 and LMP2*) genes, homeobox genes (*HOXA*, *TLX1/HOX11*, *TLX3/HOX11L2*, and *NKX2–5*), the *CALM-AF10*, and *MLL/KMT2A* fusions, and proto-oncogenes (e.g., *MYB*) [11, 20, 22].

The most common translocations involve T-cell leukemia homeobox genes *TLX1* (*HOX11*) and *TLX3* (*HOX11L2*). Translocations involving *TLX1* are present in up to 30% of adults and 7% of children and involve t(10;14)(q24;q11) and t(7;10)(q34;q24) [20]. These chromosomal translocations place *TLX1* under the control of strong enhancers in the

TCRA and *TCRD* loci, thus inducing high levels of TLX1 expression in T-ALL lymphoblasts. TLX1 expression is associated with an early cortical phenotype and has a more favorable outcome. The cryptic translocation t(5;14) (q35;q32) induces TLX3 expression and is detected in 20% of children and 13% of adults [20]. The rearrangement does not involve the *TCR* loci but instead places the *TLX3* oncogene under the control of strong T-cell regulatory elements in the *BCL11B* locus.

Translocations t(7;11)(q34;p15) and t(11;14)(p13;q11) involving the LIM domain-only proteins LMO1 and LMO2 induce aberrant expression of these proteins and are detected in 5–10% of T-ALL [9].

Cytogenetic aberrations involving other known oncogenes include the Homeobox A (*HOXA*) cluster subgroup, T-cell acute leukemia 1 (*TAL1*), and lymphoblastic leukemia associated hematopoiesis regulator 1 (*LYL1*) genes [23]. Aberrations in the *HOXA* subgroup are detected in approximately 5% of T-ALL and include several lesions, such as *MLL/KMT2A* rearrangements and inversion of chromosome 7, inv(7)(p15q34), and t(10;11)(p13;q23) resulting in *CALM-AF10* rearrangement as well as the cryptic deletion del(9)(q34.11q34.13) leading to *SET-NUP214* [24–26].

The bHLH gene group is composed of *TAL1, TAL2, LYL1,* and *BHLHB1* [9]. Aberrant TAL1 expression due to cytogenetic aberrations is detected in approximately 20–30% of T-ALL, and in a small subset of patients can be secondary to t(1;14)(p32;q11) (3%) or more often due to a submicroscopic interstitial deletion, resulting in the *SIL-TAL1* fusion gene [27, 28]. Aberrant TAL1 expression may interfere with differentiation and proliferation through the inhibition of the transcriptional activity of E47/HEB. Aberrant LYL1 expression is detected in approximately 1% of T-ALL. It is involved in t(7;19)(q34;p13) [9, 20].

T-ALL with t(6;7)(q23;q34) shows activation of *MYB*, an oncogenic leucine zipper transcription factor, with resultant increased expression of proliferation and mitosis related genes [29].

Cytogenetic aberrations in T-ALL involving tyrosine kinases include *ABL1* as well as Janus kinases *JAK1* and *JAK2*. A translocation also involving *ABL1* in T-ALL, t(9;14)(q34;q32), leads to the *EML1-ABL1* fusion gene [30].

Chromosomal deletions involving the *CDKN2A* locus in the short arm of chromosome 9 result in loss of p16INK4A and p14ARF in approximately 70% of T-ALL [2].

A normal karyotype is less commonly found in patients with ETP-ALL, which, instead, is usually associated with complex cytogenetic aberrations [9].

Molecular Findings

Microarray gene expression studies have established a close association between differentiation arrest gene expression signatures, immunophenotype, and activation of oncogenic pathways, enriching our understanding of T-ALL heterogeneity from that gained from immunophenotype-only-based classifications [31]. Though many genes have been identified by next generation sequencing, emerging data has demonstrated a strong association between *NOTCH* and *CDKN1/2* genes and conventional T-ALL, but not linking to the subtype, ETP-ALL [31–33]. Other gene pathways altered in T-ALL include cell cycle abnormalities, cell growth transcription factors, tumor suppressors, signal transduction and chromatin remodeling [9].

NOTCH1, a class I transmembrane glycoprotein functioning as a ligand-activated transcription factor, directly transduces extracellular signals at the cell membrane into transcriptional changes in specific target genes in the nucleus, and activation of the NOTCH1 receptor in the thymus is crucial for early T-cell fate specification and thymocyte development. As a transmembrane receptor, it is expressed on T-cell precursors and plays a critical role in development of T-ALL/-LBL [9]. While first described in T-ALL harboring t(7;9) (q34;q34.3), which leads to the expression of a truncated and constitutively active form of NOTCH1, it is mainly activating mutations that disrupt specific domains responsible for controlling the initiation and termination of NOTCH1 [35]. Activating mutations of *NOTCH1* or inactivating mutations of *FBXW7* gene, a negative regulator of NOTCH1, are identified in 60% of T-ALL [33, 36].

Analysis of direct NOTCH1 target genes and NOTCH1-regulated gene expression profiles demonstrated ability to directly transcriptionally upregulate anabolic pathways [37]. The MYC oncogene represents a direct target of NOTCH1, and its upregulation also induces activation of anabolic pathways [38]. Hairy and enhancer of split 1 homologue (HES1), an evolutionarily conserved transcriptional repressor functioning downstream of NOTCH1, is of particular importance for T-cell development and NOTCH1-induced leukemogenesis and leukemia cell survival [39]. The NOTCH1-HES1 regulatory axis activates PI3K and NFkB pathways [40].

Recent studies have proposed the splenic microenvironment may be different from the bone marrow and have a direct influence on T-ALL. In a NOTCH-induced T-ALL animal model, Ma S et al. had observed a higher level of MIP-3 beta cytokine expression in splenic microenvironments than in bone marrow microenvironments. The consequence of increased MIP-3 beta expression is to further recruit the T-ALL cells with high MIP-3 beta receptors (CCR7) into the spleen [41]. Further study demonstrated that the tumor-associated macrophages harvested from the liver infiltrate by NOTCH1 exhibited their unique proinflammatory (M1) pattern, which may play a critical role in the microenvironments [42].

Loss of cell cycle control plays a major role in T-ALL development. Aside from loss of CDKN2A (see above), 15% of T-ALL harbor chromosomal deletions involving the *RB1* locus on chromosome 13q14.2 [11]. Additional cytogenetic aberrations involve *CDKN1B* which encodes p27KIP1, an inhibitor of cyclin E–CDK2 and cyclin D–CDK4 complexes [43, 44].

ETP-ALL exhibits its unique genetic signatures that can be subgrouped according to their functions, more frequently involving the RAS signaling pathway and controlling cytokines (*NRAS, KRAS, BRAF, JAK1, JAK3, SH2B3, FLT3, IL7R*), inactivating mutations in transcription factors that regulate hematopoiesis (*GATA3, RUNX1, IKZF1*, and *ETV6*), and methylation/histone modification genes (*EZH2, EED, SUZ12, SETD2*, and *EP300*) [9, 32, 34]. Certain genes involving myeloid or stem cell profiles including *CD34, KIT, GATA2, CD44*, and *CEBPA* are overexpressed, and other genes that are frequently mutated in myeloid neoplasms such as *FLT3, IDH1/2*, and *DNMT3A* are also found in ETP-ALL [19, 32, 34, 45, 46], while gene mutations more associated with T-ALL (*NOTCH1* and *CDKN1/2*) are infrequent. Overexpression of LYL1 was reported to be associated with early precursors [23].

Prognosis

T-ALL/-LBL shows a more aggressive clinical course when compared with B-ALL/-LBL, in particular when the T-ALL/-LBL patients have high-risk clinical features, for example, elderly individual, high white blood cell count (predominantly lymphoblasts), or high tumor loads such as massive mediastinal lymphadenopathy [9]. In the series of T-ALL patients treated in the MRC/ECOG trial, the traditional prognostic factor of a leukocyte count >100×10^9/L resulted in a shorter overall survival (OS) at 5 years, compared with patients with a leukocyte count <100×10^9/L. Patients with a complex cytogenetic karyotype (more than five chromosomal abnormalities) had a significantly lower OS at 5 years, compared with patients with simple or normal karyotypes (19% vs 51%, $P = 0.006$), and this impact was not affected by a higher leukocyte count or age. Patients with T-ALL/T-LBL involving the CNS, although not as frequently seen as in B-ALL, usually have a poor prognosis by a reduced rate of long-term remission [7].

Recent molecular studies have shed some light on the prognostic value of T-ALL. Multiple studies in both pediatric and adult patients have shown that mutations in *NOTCH1* and *FBXW7* are associated with an improved early treatment response and increased sensitivity to corticosteroid therapy [31, 47]. According to the Group for Research on Adult Acute Lymphoblastic Leukemia (GRAALL), the adult T-ALL patients who harbored *NOTCH1* and/or *FBXW7* gene mutations had a better prognosis than those who did not [48]. Further studies of patients with *NOTCH1/FBXW7* mutations have shown that patients within these subgroups who have *K-RAS, N-RAS*, and *PTEN* mutations or deletions have a poorer prognosis than patients who are without mutations in these other genes [49].

The strongest prognostic factor emerging for patients with ALL is minimal residual disease (MRD) [50–52] which can be assessed by flow cytometry, ClonoSeq, or TCR gene rearrangements. *LYL1, TAL1*, or *TLX3* gene alteration predicts a poorer prognosis, whereas *TLX1* activation is associated with a favorable clinical outcome [31].

Diagnostic Caveats

- T-LBL constitutes 85–90% of all LBL and affects predominantly adolescent males.
- The mediastinum (thymus) is the most common site for T-LBL followed by lymph nodes, skin, tonsils, liver, spleen, CNS, and testes.
- Primary hepatosplenic T-ALL/-LBL without other site involvements is very rare.
- T-ALL is diagnosed by identifying T-lymphoblasts in peripheral blood and bone marrow.
- The phenotype of T-ALL varies according to the stage of intrathymic differentiation: Pro-T, pre-T, and cortical T- and medullary T-cells. Many pro-T and pre-T lymphoblastic leukemias are considered ETP-ALL based on their genetic profile.

References

1. Duffield AS, Racke FK, Borowitz MJ, Precursor B. T-cell neoplasms. In: Jaffe ES, Arber DA, Campa E, Harris NL, Quintanilla-Martinez L, editors. Hematopathology. Philadelphia: Elsevier; 2016. p. 761–74.
2. Borowitz MJ, Chan JKC, Bene MC, Arber DA. T-lymphoblastic leukemia/lymphoma. In: Swerdlow SH, Campa E, Harris NL, et al., editors. WHO classification of tumors of haematopoietic and lymphoid tissues. Lyon: WHO Press; 2017. p. 209–12.
3. Hoelzer D, Gokbuget N. T-cell lymphoblastic lymphoma and T-cell acute lymphoblastic leukemia: a separate entity? Clin Lymphoma Myeloma. 2009;9(Suppl 3):S214–21.
4. Feng H, Stachura DL, White RM, et al. T-lymphoblastic lymphoma cells express high levels of BCL2, S1P1, and ICAM1, leading to a blockade of tumor cell intravasation. Cancer Cell. 2010;18(4):353–66.

5. Basso K, Mussolin L, Lettieri A, et al. T-cell lymphoblastic lymphoma shows differences and similarities with T-cell acute lymphoblastic leukemia by genomic and gene expression analyses. Genes Chromosomes Cancer. 2011;50(12):1063–75.

6. Patel KJ, Latif SU, de Calaca WM. An unusual presentation of precursor T cell lymphoblastic leukemia/lymphoma with cholestatic jaundice: case report. J Hematol Oncol. 2009;2:12.

7. Vadillo E, Dorantes-Acosta E, Pelayo R, Schnoor M. T cell acute lymphoblastic leukemia (T-ALL): new insights into the cellular origins and infiltration mechanisms common and unique among hematologic malignancies. Blood Rev. 2018;32(1):36–51.

8. Cortelazzo S, Ponzoni M, Ferreri AJ, Hoelzer D. Lymphoblastic lymphoma. Crit Rev Oncol Hematol. 2011;79(3):330–43.

9. You MJ, Medeiros LJ, Hsi ED. T-lymphoblastic leukemia/lymphoma. Am J Clin Pathol. 2015;144(3):411–22.

10. Ford AM, Pombo-de-Oliveira MS, McCarthy KP, et al. Monoclonal origin of concordant T-cell malignancy in identical twins. Blood. 1997;89(1):281–5.

11. Van Vlierberghe P, Ferrando A. The molecular basis of T cell acute lymphoblastic leukemia. J Clin Invest. 2012;122(10):3398–406.

12. Kai T, Ishii E, Matsuzaki A, et al. Clinical and prognostic implications of bone lesions in childhood leukemia at diagnosis. Leuk Lymphoma. 1996;23(1–2):119–23.

13. Chiaretti S, Foa R. T-cell acute lymphoblastic leukemia. Haematologica. 2009;94(2):160–2.

14. Murakami J, Shimizu Y. Hepatic manifestations in hematological disorders. Int J Hepatol. 2013;2013:484903.

15. Racke FK, Borowitz MJ. Precursor B- and T-cell neoplasms. In: Jaffe ES, Harris NL, Vardiman JW, Campo E, Arber DA, editors. Hematopathology. Philadelphia: Elsevier; 2011. p. 629–39.

16. Murphy SB, Fairclough DL, Hutchison RE, Berard CW. Non-Hodgkin's lymphomas of childhood: an analysis of the histology, staging, and response to treatment of 338 cases at a single institution. J Clin Oncol. 1989;7(2):186–93.

17. Coleman CN, Picozzi VJ Jr, Cox RS, et al. Treatment of lymphoblastic lymphoma in adults. J Clin Oncol. 1986;4(11):1628–37.

18. Cortelazzo S, Ferreri A, Hoelzer D, Ponzoni M. Lymphoblastic lymphoma. Crit Rev Oncol Hematol. 2017;113:304–17.

19. Coustan-Smith E, Mullighan CG, Onciu M, et al. Early T-cell precursor leukaemia: a subtype of very high-risk acute lymphoblastic leukaemia. Lancet Oncol. 2009;10(2):147–56.

20. Graux C, Cools J, Michaux L, Vandenberghe P, Hagemeijer A. Cytogenetics and molecular genetics of T-cell acute lymphoblastic leukemia: from thymocyte to lymphoblast. Leukemia. 2006;20(9):1496–510.

21. Han X, Bueso-Ramos CE. Precursor T-cell acute lymphoblastic leukemia/lymphoblastic lymphoma and acute biphenotypic leukemias. Am J Clin Pathol. 2007;127(4):528–44.

22. Armstrong SA, Look AT. Molecular genetics of acute lymphoblastic leukemia. J Clin Oncol. 2005;23(26):6306–15.

23. Meijerink JP. Genetic rearrangements in relation to immunophenotype and outcome in T-cell acute lymphoblastic leukaemia. Best Pract Res Clin Haematol. 2010;23(3):307–18.

24. Dik WA, Brahim W, Braun C, et al. CALM-AF10+ T-ALL expression profiles are characterized by overexpression of HOXA and BMI1 oncogenes. Leukemia. 2005;19(11):1948–57.

25. Soulier J, Clappier E, Cayuela JM, et al. HOXA genes are included in genetic and biologic networks defining human acute T-cell leukemia (T-ALL). Blood. 2005;106(1):274–86.

26. Van Vlierberghe P, van Grotel M, Tchinda J, et al. The recurrent SET-NUP214 fusion as a new HOXA activation mechanism in pediatric T-cell acute lymphoblastic leukaemia. Blood. 2008;111(9):4668–80.

27. Brown L, Cheng JT, Chen Q, et al. Site-specific recombination of the tal-1 gene is a common occurrence in human T cell leukemia. EMBO J. 1990;9(10):3343–51.

28. Janssen JW, Ludwig WD, Sterry W, Bartram CR. SIL-TAL1 deletion in T-cell acute lymphoblastic leukemia. Leukemia. 1993;7(8):1204–10.

29. Clappier E, Cuccuini W, Kalota A, et al. The C-MYB locus is involved in chromosomal translocation and genomic duplications in human T-cell acute leukemia (T-ALL), the translocation defining a new T-ALL subtype in very young children. Blood. 2007;110(4):1251–61.

30. Hagemeijer A, Graux C. ABL1 rearrangements in T-cell acute lymphoblastic leukemia. Genes Chromosomes Cancer. 2010;49(4):299–308.

31. Ferrando AA, Neuberg DS, Staunton J, et al. Gene expression signatures define novel oncogenic pathways in T cell acute lymphoblastic leukemia. Cancer Cell. 2002;1(1):75–87.

32. Zhang J, Ding L, Holmfeldt L, et al. The genetic basis of early T-cell precursor acute lymphoblastic leukaemia. Nature. 2012;481(7380):157–63.

33. Weng AP, Ferrando AA, Lee W, et al. Activating mutations of NOTCH1 in human T cell acute lymphoblastic leukemia. Science. 2004;306(5694):269–71.

34. Van Vlierberghe P, Ambesi-Impiombato A, Perez-Garcia A, et al. ETV6 mutations in early immature human T cell leukemias. J Exp Med. 2011;208(13):2571–9.

35. Chiaramonte R, Basile A, Tassi E, et al. A wide role for NOTCH1 signaling in acute leukemia. Cancer Lett. 2005;219(1):113–20.

36. Fogelstrand L, Staffas A, Wasslavik C, et al. Prognostic implications of mutations in NOTCH1 and FBXW7 in childhood T-ALL treated according to the NOPHO ALL-1992 and ALL-2000 protocols. Pediatr Blood Cancer. 2014;61(3):424–30.

37. Borggrefe T, Oswald F. The Notch signaling pathway: transcriptional regulation at Notch target genes. Cell Mol Life Sci. 2009;66(10):1631–46.

38. Weng AP, Millholland JM, Yashiro-Ohtani Y, et al. c-Myc is an important direct target of Notch1 in T-cell acute lymphoblastic leukemia/lymphoma. Genes Dev. 2006;20(15):2096–109.

39. Wendorff AA, Koch U, Wunderlich FT, et al. Hes1 is a critical but context-dependent mediator of canonical Notch signaling in lymphocyte development and transformation. Immunity. 2010;33(5):671–84.

40. Espinosa L, Cathelin S, D'Altri T, et al. The Notch/Hes1 pathway sustains NF-kappaB activation through CYLD repression in T cell leukemia. Cancer Cell. 2010;18(3):268–81.

41. Ma S, Shi Y, Pang Y, et al. Notch1-induced T cell leukemia can be potentiated by microenvironmental cues in the spleen. J Hematol Oncol. 2014;7:71.

42. Yang X, Feng W, Wang R, et al. Hepatic leukemia-associated macrophages exhibit a pro-inflammatory phenotype in Notch1-induced acute T cell leukemia. Immunobiology. 2018;223(1):73–80.

43. Karrman K, Andersson A, Bjorgvinsdottir H, et al. Deregulation of cyclin D2 by juxtaposition with T-cell receptor alpha/delta locus in t(12;14)(p13;q11)-positive childhood T-cell acute lymphoblastic leukemia. Eur J Haematol. 2006;77(1):27–34.

44. Tosi S, Mostafa Kamel Y, Owoka T, Federico C, Truong TH, Saccone S. Paediatric acute myeloid leukaemia with the t(7;12)(q36;p13) rearrangement: a review of the biological and clinical management aspects. Biomark Res. 2015;3:21.

45. Neumann M, Coskun E, Fransecky L, et al. FLT3 mutations in early T-cell precursor ALL characterize a stem cell like leukemia and imply the clinical use of tyrosine kinase inhibitors. PLoS One. 2013;8(1):e53190.

46. Neumann M, Heesch S, Schlee C, et al. Whole-exome sequencing in adult ETP-ALL reveals a high rate of DNMT3A mutations. Blood. 2013;121(23):4749–52.

47. Aifantis I, Raetz E, Buonamici S. Molecular pathogenesis of T-cell leukaemia and lymphoma. Nat Rev Immunol. 2008;8(5):380–90.

48. Ben Abdelali R, Asnafi V, Leguay T, et al. Pediatric-inspired intensified therapy of adult T-ALL reveals the favorable outcome of

NOTCH1/FBXW7 mutations, but not of low ERG/BAALC expression: a GRAALL study. Blood. 2011;118(19):5099–107.

49. Trinquand A, Tanguy-Schmidt A, Ben Abdelali R, et al. Toward a NOTCH1/FBXW7/RAS/PTEN-based oncogenetic risk classification of adult T-cell acute lymphoblastic leukemia: a Group for Research in Adult Acute Lymphoblastic Leukemia study. J Clin Oncol. 2013;31(34):4333–42.

50. van Dongen JJ, van der Velden VH, Bruggemann M, Orfao A. Minimal residual disease diagnostics in acute lymphoblastic leukemia: need for sensitive, fast, and standardized technologies. Blood. 2015;125(26):3996–4009.

51. Bassan R, Spinelli O. Minimal residual disease monitoring in adult ALL to determine therapy. Curr Hematol Malig Rep. 2015;10(2):86–95.

52. Willemse MJ, Seriu T, Hettinger K, et al. Detection of minimal residual disease identifies differences in treatment response between T-ALL and precursor B-ALL. Blood. 2002;99(12):4386–93.

David C. Gajzer and Ling Zhang

Introduction

Aggressive natural killer-cell leukemia (ANKL) originates from a natural killer-cell and is a very rare neoplasm typically associated with the Epstein-Barr virus (EBV). It follows an aggressive clinical course and can involve the liver and spleen, however, a biopsy of the two organs is infrequently performed. Phenotypically, ANKL cells express cytoplasmic CD3, surface CD2, CD7, CD16, CD56, and cytotoxic markers, and lack CD4, CD8, and TCR-alpha/beta and TCR-gamma/delta expression. The presence of circulating atypical cells with phenotypic findings compatible with NK-cell origin, in conjunction with an aggressive clinical course, coexistence of hemophagocytic lymphohistiocytosis (HLH) or multiorgan failure and identified EBV infection or reactivation place ANKL on top of the list of differential diagnoses. T-cell prolymphocytic leukemia (T-PLL) is a rare and aggressive T-cell leukemia involving the peripheral blood, bone marrow, lymph nodes, liver, spleen, and skin. The leukemia shows its unique immunophenotype (mature T-cell markers, frequently intact surface CD2, CD3, CD4, CD5, CD7, and TCL1 expression, lacking TdT and CD1a) and often harbors cytogenetic abnormalities [e.g., inv(14)(q11q23) or t(14;14)(q11;q32)]. Diagnosis is primarily made according to cytologic and phenotypic findings of circulating atypical lymphocytes with or without cytogenetics study. This chapter will discuss aggressive natural killer-cell leukemia and T-cell prolymphocytic leukemia, two rare and highly aggressive lymphoproliferative disorders that typically involve the liver and spleen.

D. C. Gajzer · L. Zhang (✉)
Department of Pathology, H. Lee Moffitt Cancer Center
and Research Institute, Tampa, FL, USA
e-mail: ling.zhang@moffitt.org

Aggressive Natural Killer-Cell Leukemia

Definition

Aggressive natural killer-cell leukemia is a highly aggressive and extremely rare malignant neoplasm originating from natural killer-cells, typically associated with the Epstein-Barr virus (EBV), and follows an aggressive clinical course [1]. The revision of the fourth edition of the World Health Organization (WHO) Classification of Tumours of Hematopoietic and Lymphoid Tissues distinguishes ANKL [1] from the following EBV-positive NK-cell neoplasms: extranodal NK/T-cell lymphoma, nasal type (ENKTL) [2], hydroavacciniforme-like lymphoproliferative disorder, a rare cutaneous T-cell or sometimes NK-cell lymphoma of children and adolescents [3], as well as a provisional entity, the so-called chronic lymphoproliferative disorder of NK cells (CLPD-NK) [4]. Hepatosplenic involvement by ANKL is very common [1], however, a biopsy of liver or spleen for diagnosis is rarely performed.

Etiology

ANKL is a rare disease and not well understood, but its striking association with EBV suggests a pathogenetic role of the virus [5]. Chronic EBV infection has been suspected to cause the disease in younger patients [6–8]. Some cases are transformed from preexisting chronic lymphoproliferative disorder of NK cells [9, 10]. It is debatable whether ANKL represents a leukemic counterpart of ENKTL, an entity histomorphologically and immunophenotypically very similar to ANKL but usually involving the nose and upper aerodigestive tract and other body sites as an angiodestructive lesion [2]. Disseminated ENKTL involving skin, peripheral blood or bone marrow can occur. ANKL typically presents as systemic disease with multiorgan and bone marrow involvement, and

© Springer Nature Switzerland AG 2020
L. Zhang et al. (eds.), *Diagnostic Pathology of Hematopoietic Disorders of Spleen and Liver*,
https://doi.org/10.1007/978-3-030-37708-3_15

this overlap in clinical presentation adds to the difficulty in distinguishing ANKL from ENKTL [11].

Epidemiology

The term NK-cell leukemia was initially used by Fernandez et al. in 1986 in the first report of an aggressive NK-cell leukemia in an adult with the establishment of a leukemia cell line [12]. Imamura et al. then named this hematologic malignancy aggressive NK-cell leukemia/lymphoma in 1990 [13]. Its prevalence is significantly higher in Asia and Central and South America than in other geographic regions [5]. Patients are typically young to middle-aged adults, with a median age of 40 years ranging from 30 to 50 years [8, 14–17] with a male to female ratio of approximately 1:1 [5, 11, 13, 15–22]. An extremely rare disease, relevant information so far has been gained mostly from case reports, and its underlying molecular mechanisms have not been extensively studied.

Clinical Presentations

The clinical presentation typically includes fever, cytopenia, hepatosplenomegaly, and occasional lymphadenopathy. The neoplastic cell burden in the bone marrow and peripheral blood can range from low to high, from a few to greater than 80% of leukocytes. The terminal illness is characterized by fulminant liver failure and often renal failure following an aggressive clinical course and involvement mainly of the bone marrow, peripheral blood, liver, and spleen, whereas the skin is rarely involved. Coagulopathy, hemophagocytic lymphohistiocytosis (HLH) (60% of cases) and multiorgan failure are characteristic complications [13, 15–18, 20, 23, 24]. Patients have initially presented with flu-like signs or symptoms but rapidly progressed with blurred vision, dyspnea on exertion, lower extremity edema, or jaundice. B-symptoms are not uncommon and include fever and night sweats.

Morphology

Microscopic Examination

Morphologic diagnosis of ANKL usually relies on careful examination of atypical cells in the peripheral blood and bone marrow. In the peripheral blood, the neoplastic cells are large and feature irregular nuclei with open, transcriptionally active chromatin, distinct nucleoli and abundant blue cytoplasm with azurophilic granules. Sometimes, it can be difficult to distinguish the neoplastic cells from benign large granular lymphocytes. In the bone marrow, the neoplastic cells range from small and monotonous to large and pleomorphic and show

a perivascular and interstitial infiltrative pattern. The nuclei tend to be monotonous but can sometimes be pleomorphic, and apoptosis and necrosis are common (Fig. 15.1). Similar to ENKTL, the distinctive histopathologic feature in ANKL is a polymorphic neoplastic infiltrate with angiocentricity, angiodestruction, and necrosis of the tissues and organs (e.g., liver and spleen) involved [25]. (Figs. 15.2 and 15.3).

Immunophenotyping

By immunohistochemistry, the neoplastic cells are typically positive for CD2, cytoplasmic CD3-ε, and CD56, while being negative for surface CD3 [17]. CD11b may be expressed, and CD57 is typically negative [11, 26]. Aberrant loss of expression of CD2, CD7, or CD45 is possible [15]. Reactivity for cytotoxic granules (TIA1, granzyme B and perforin) varies, and tumor cells are typically negative for CD4, CD5, and CD8. The neoplastic cells express FAS ligand (also known as CD95L). High levels of this ligand have been detected in the serum of affected patients, and binding of FAS ligand with its receptor on individual cells of FAS-bearing tissues, such as hepatocytes in liver, induces apoptosis [27–29]. CD16 has been frequently reported (75%) in ANKL. Epstein-Barr virus-encoded RNA can be reliably highlighted by in situ hybridization [30]. Of note, CD56-negative cases of ANKL have been reported [31]. There have also been reports on EBV-negative ANKL which described the neoplastic cell phenotype as similar but not identical to that of the classic, EBV-positive ANKL, in that it uniformly lacks surface CD3 and is positive for CD2, CD56, and granzyme B, and in some cases positive for CD8 and CD30, but negative for CD4, CD5, TCR beta-F1, TCR-gamma, and EBV- LMP1 [32, 33].

Cytogenetics

No consistent cytogenetic abnormalities are known for ANKL; however, various clonal cytogenetic abnormalities have been identified, including deletions involving the long arm of chromosomes 6, e.g., del(6)(q21q25) [34], and del(11q) [22]. Yang et al. reported losses and gains of chromosome 7p as the most common aberration in their case series, whereas the deletion of chromosome 6q was not seen [30]. Overall, cytogenetic aberrations were more commonly found in ANKL (75%) than ENKTL (25%) [30], and the overall cytogenetic abnormality rate of 45% (9/20) was similar to that of another study (46%; 6/13) [35]. Suzuki et al. reported on cytogenetic abnormalities in 10 of 22 cases of their series of ANKL and these involved mostly chromosomes 7 and 6, but without deletion of chromosome 6q [17]. Nakashima and colleagues reported on array comparative genomic hybridization-based identification of significant differences in genomic alteration patterns between ANKL and ENKTL; in particular, recurrent genetic changes identified in ANKL include gains of 1q and loss of 7p15.1–p22.3 and 17p13 [36].

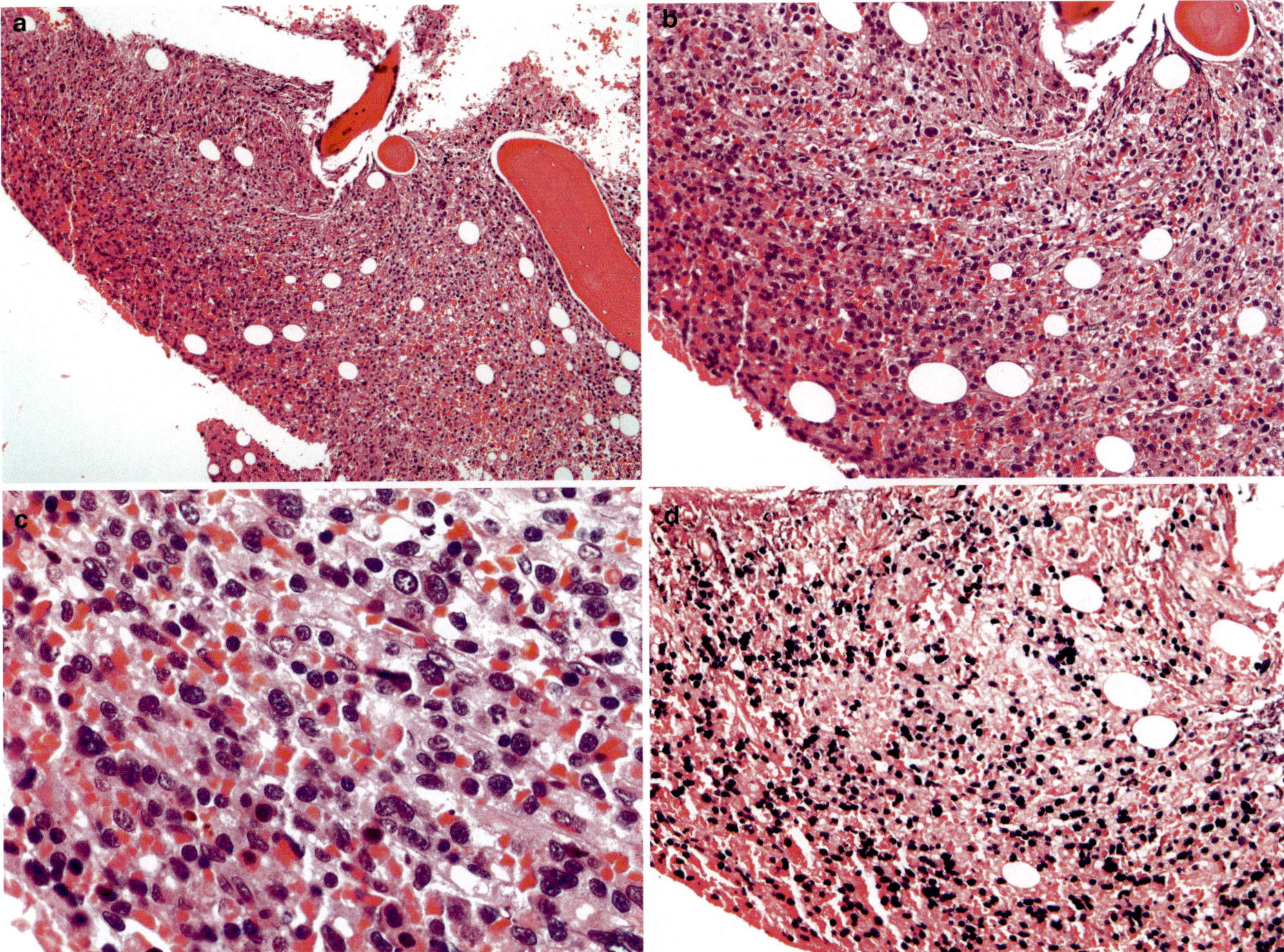

Fig. 15.1 **Bone marrow manifestation of ANKL**. (**a–c**) The sections from the bone marrow core demonstrates altered and diminished normal bone marrow hematopoietic cellular distribution with a significant increase in atypical lymphoid cells composed of medium- to large-sized cells with open chromatin and some with small visible nucleoli (H&E stain, 100×, 200×, and 600×, respectively). Hemophagocytosis is only occasionally identified (not shown in the figure). (**d**) Numerous EBV-positive cells are highlighted by in situ hybridization using EBV encoded RNA probe (in situ hybridization, 600×)

Molecular Findings

In ANKL, the T-cell receptor (*TCR*) genes are in germline configuration [37]. Unlike ENKTCL, molecular aberrations have not been as extensively studied, although few copy number aberration analyses and more recent targeted sequencing studies of small patient cohorts have been performed. Loss of tumor suppressor genes including *PRDM1, ATG5, AIM1*, and *HACE1* in 6q21 are commonly reported [38].

Karube et al. in 2011 reported on two tumor suppressor genes (*PRDM1*, PR domain zinc finger protein 1, and *FOXO3*, encoding the transcription factor forkhead box O-3) involved in the pathogenesis of NK-cell neoplasms including ANKL [39]. Nonsense mutations of *PRDM1* could result in functional inactivation of NK cells [39]. In vitro studies showed that the expression of FOXO3 inhibited cell growth in NK-cell lines via AKT activation [40]. Dufva and col-

leagues have recently increased our understanding of the mutational landscape of ANKL using a whole-exome sequencing (WES)-based approach on material from 14 patients diagnosed with ANKL (4 tumor-normal pairs and 10 tumor-only samples) [41]. Here, the authors identified alterations involving the JAK-STAT pathway, in particular STAT3 (21%), with the majority of mutations previously reported as activating, localizing to exons 20 and 21 which encode the SH2 domain responsible for its dimerization and activation. Gain-of-function mutations involving the RAS-MAPK pathway were present in roughly one fifth of patients (21%), including those leading to constitutive RAS activation as well as *BRAF* mutation. The same study also identified mutations in epigenetic regulators and histone-modifying enzymes in 50% of patients, including *BCOR, MLL2, SETD2*, and *TET2*. *BCOR* and *KMT2A2/MLL2* were previ-

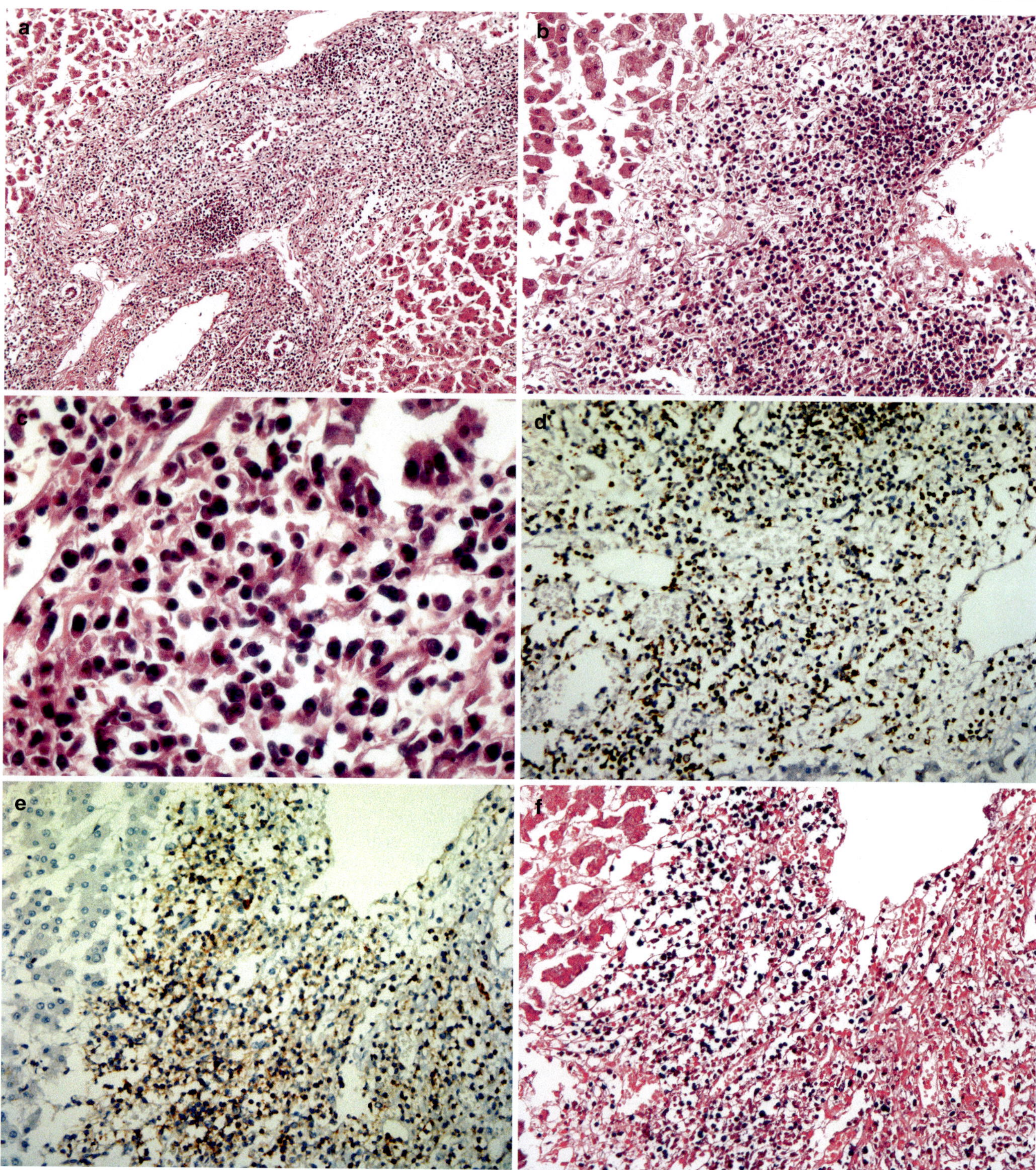

Fig. 15.2 Liver involvement by ANKL. (**a**, **b**) H&E section of liver shows peripheral vascular dense infiltrate by atypical lymphoid cells and partially persevered hepatocyte architecture (100× and 200×, respectively). (**c**) H&E section demonstrates the atypical lymphoid cells with hyperchromatic nuclei associated with increased vasculature in the background and infiltration to small bile duct (600x). (**d**, **e**) Immunohistochemical staining shows cytoplasmic CD3 staining pattern (**d**, 200×) and surface CD56 staining pattern (**e**, 200×). (**f**) In situ hybridization using EBV probe proves the presence of EBV virus genome in the neoplastic cells (200×)

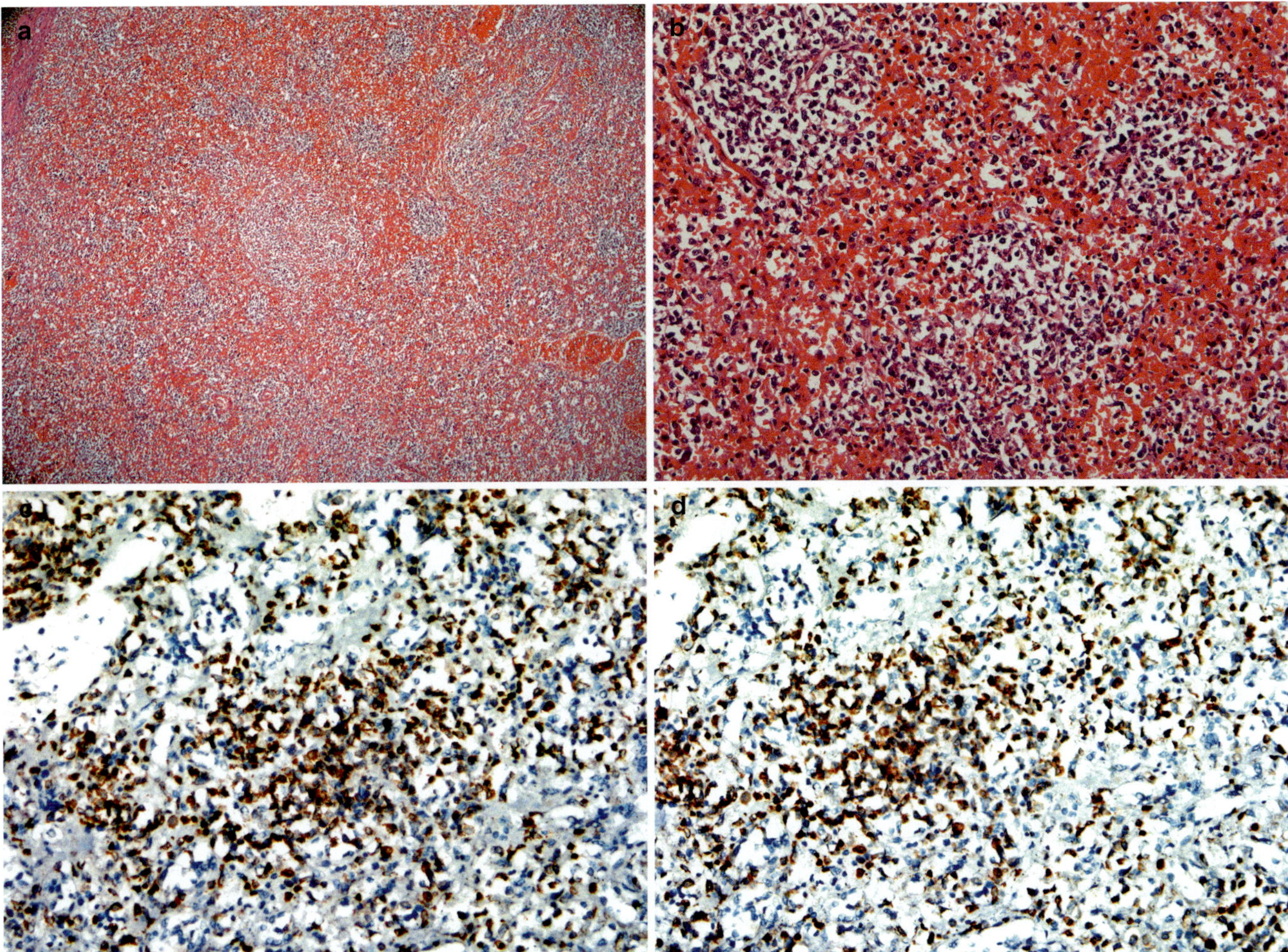

Fig. 15.3 **Splenic involvement by ANKL**. (**a**) Low power view of the submitted H&E section from an autopsy splenic specimen reveals diffuse red pulp expansion filled with atypical lymphoid cells (H&E stain, 100×). (**b**) Increased magnification shows these atypical lymphoid cells with condensed chromatin and irregular nuclei forming small clusters in association with small capillaries (H&E, 200×). (**c**, **d**) The neoplastic infiltrating cells are highlighted by cytoplasmic CD3 staining and CD56 surface staining (immunoperoxidase, 200×, respectively)

ously described as mutated in ENKTL. *DDX3X*, an RNA helicase commonly mutated in ENKTL, showed mutations in 29% of patients. While there was a markedly higher fraction of reads mapping to the EBV genome in tumor samples of ANKL and ENKTL compared to controls, no connections were evident between EBV status and mutational signatures [41]. Another study pointed out that even EBV infection/reactivation may play a role in disease progression of ANKL, but it may not be oncogenic [42].

Differential Diagnosis

The differential diagnosis of ANKL includes T-cell large granular lymphocytic leukemia (T-LGLL), an abnormal proliferation of T-cell large granular lymphocytes in an indolent clinical course and distint immimophenotype (surface CD3+, dim CD5, dim CD7, CD8+, CD57+ and TCR+), but with regard to EBV association as the common denominator, ENKTL, hydroa-vacciniforme-like lymphoma, and fulminant EBV-positive lymphoproliferative disease must be excluded [43].

ENKTL represents the most important differential diagnosis with respect to neoplastic cell immunophenotype, clinical course, and prognosis. Although CD16 is frequently positive in ANKL (75%) [17], the marker is not useful in distinguishing ANKL from ENKTL, since positivity varies between 14% and 100% in ENKTL. Yang and co-authors reported in their study on the rates of positivity between ANKL (50%) and ENKTL (40%) as not being significantly different [30]. Clinically, ANKL tends to affect teenagers and young adults with systemic involvement frequently involving liver and spleen but rarely skin and lymph nodes, and featuring hemophagocytic syndrome earlier in the course of disease, whereas ENKTL typically is seen in middle-aged patients and follows a locally angiodestructive course, and while it can involve multiple organs, it does not typically culminate in multiorgan failure [1, 2].

Novel molecular studies have revealed differences in mutational signatures identified between ANKL and ENKTL, indicating at least a partial difference in the evolution of the two entities [5, 11]. The results support the notion that these neoplasms are actually two separate entities rather than ANKL representing the leukemic phase of ENKTL.

Prognosis

ANKL is a highly aggressive neoplasm with a fulminant clinical course. The median survival is less than 2 months [11, 15–17, 22, 44]. Chemotherapy does not usually prove effective and, due to its rarity, there is a lack of standard therapeutic regimens. Patients almost always relapse despite achieving remission, and irrespective of undergoing bone marrow transplantation, despite a recent study reporting on some patients achieving lasting remission following allogeneic hematopoietic stem cell transplantation [15, 17, 45].

T-Cell Prolymphocytic Leukemia

Definition

T-cell prolymphocytic leukemia (T-PLL) is a rare and aggressive T-cell leukemia involving the peripheral blood, bone marrow, lymph nodes, liver, spleen, and skin.

Etiology

Little is known about the etiology of T-PLL which consists of prolymphocytes with a mature, post-thymic T-cell phenotype. The postulated normal counterpart to T-PLL is an unknown T-cell with a mature immunophenotype. Because of the strong expression of CD7, dual CD4 and CD8 positivity, and weak surface CD3 expression, it is proposed that T-PLL originates from a T-cell at an intermediate stage of differentiation between cortical and mature thymocyte.

Epidemiology

T-PLL is rare and accounts for approximately 2% of mature T-cell leukemias in adult patients with an age distribution of 30–94 years (median 65). Besides large granular lymphocyte leukemia, T-PLL represents the only primary T-cell leukemia commonly found in Western countries [46].

Clinical Presentations

The typical clinical presentation includes hepatosplenomegaly and generalized lymphadenopathy. The skin is involved in approximately 20% of patients and cutaneous lesions include a maculopapular rash, nodules, or rarely erythrodermia. Serous effusions, mostly pleural, as well as ascites, although rare, can sometimes be present. The white blood cell count is typically elevated at $>100 \times 10^9/L$, and at $>200 \times 10^9/L$ in 50% of patients, with more than 90% of lymphoid cells featuring prolymphocytic morphology. Anemia and thrombocytopenia are present in approximately 30% of patients secondary to bone marrow failure due to lymphoid infiltration or splenomegaly. Hyperuricemia and elevated lactate dehydrogenase (LDH) level are common, and liver function tests can be mildly altered [46]. Both serology and DNA-based methods have not detected human T-cell leukemia viruses I and II, excluding adult T-cell leukemia/lymphoma [47–49].

Morphology

Microscopic Examination

A well-stained peripheral blood smear is key in the diagnosis of T-PLL and is characterized by small- to medium-sized lymphoid cells with nuclear morphology ranging from oval to markedly irregular, with a centrally located prominent nucleolus and basophilic, non-granular cytoplasm. The small cell variant of T-PLL (25%) features small lymphoid cells with invisible nucleoli, which can lead to misdiagnosis as another mature T-cell lymphoma [49, 50]. A cerebriform nuclear morphology is seen in approximately 5% [49, 51]. A common feature of T-PLL irrespective of nuclear morphology is cytoplasmic protrusions or blebs [49].

Despite diffuse involvement of the bone marrow in T-PLL, the diagnosis is difficult to render by bone marrow histology alone. Hepatic involvement and infiltration of other solid organs demonstrate a sheet-like pattern (Fig. 15.4). When skin involvement is present, it consists of perivascular and periadnexal or diffuse dermal infiltrates of neoplastic cells, and epidermotropism is not seen [46, 52]. Spleen involvement is characterized by a dense neoplastic cell infiltrate in the red pulp and invading the capsule and blood vessels, along with atrophy of the white pulp [53]. Lymph node involvement demonstrates as diffuse infiltration by the neoplastic cells predominantly in the paracortical areas, and prominent high endothelial venules infiltrated by neoplastic cells can be numerous.

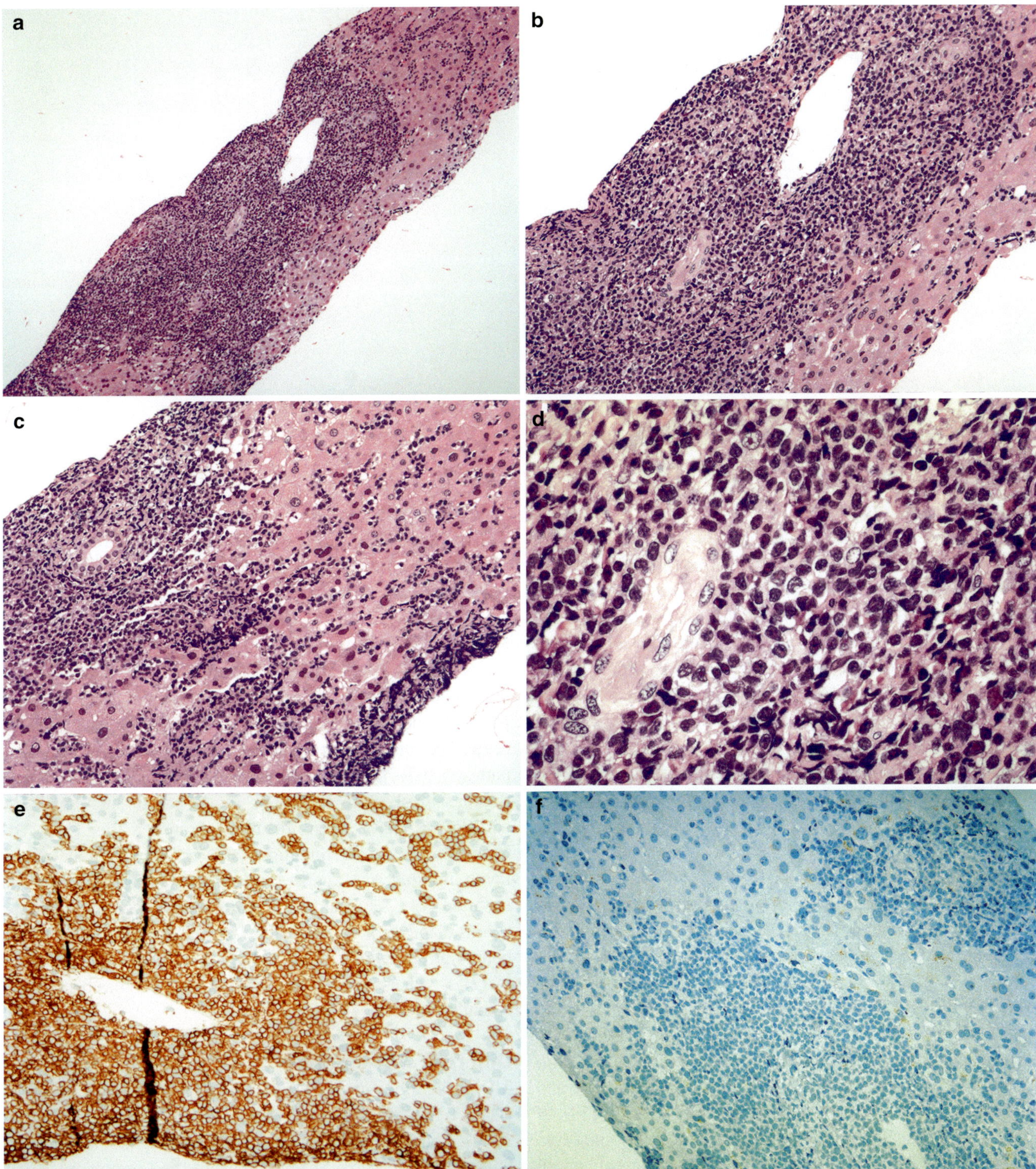

Fig. 15.4 T-cell prolymphocytic leukemia involving the liver. (**a–c**) Neoplastic cells infiltrate hepatic parenchyma in a perivascular, sheet-like pattern (H&E stain, **a** – 100×, **b** – 200×, **c** – 200×). (**d**) High magnification reveals pleomorphic morphology of neoplastic nuclei and scant cytoplasm (H&E stain, 600×). (**e**) Leukemic cells stain uniformly positive for T-cell antigen CD3 (surface) (immunoperoxidase, 200×). (**f**) Neoplastic cells stain negative for B-cell antigen CD20 (immunoperoxidase, 200×). (**g**) Leukemic cells stain uniformly positive for CD4 (immunoperoxidase, 200×). (**h**) Neoplastic cells are negative for EBV-encoded small RNA (in situ hybridization, 200×)

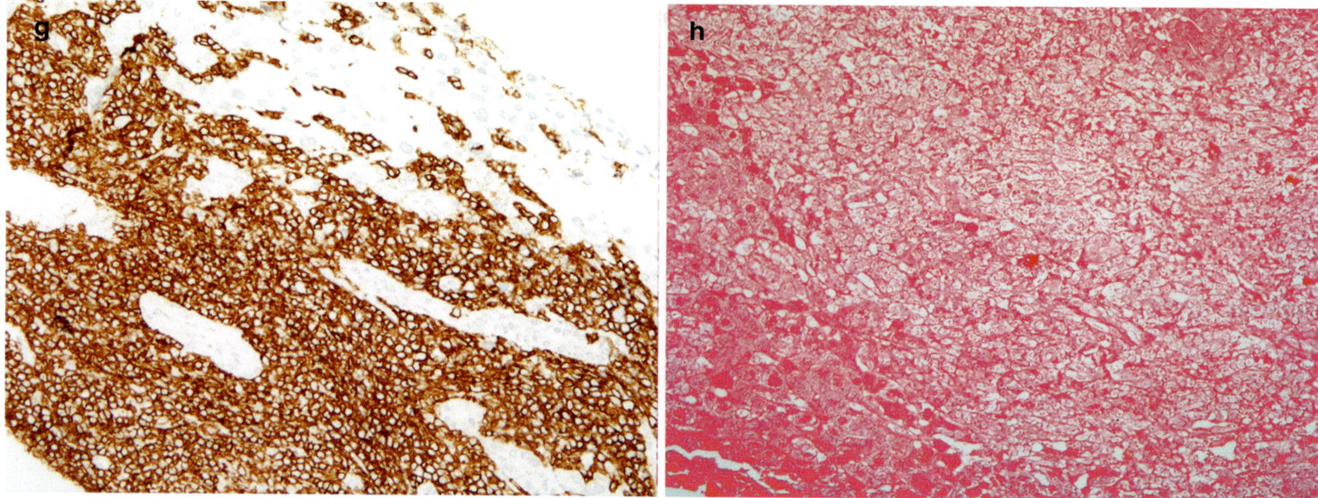

Fig. 15.4 (continued)

Immunophenotyping

Consistent with their stage of differentiation, T-cell prolymphocytes express CD2, CD3, CD5, CD7, and CD52, and are negative for TdT and CD1a [54]. The neoplastic cells are positive for CD4 and negative for CD8 in 60%, positive for CD8 and negative for CD4 in 15%, and co-express CD4 and CD8 in 25% of T-PLL [46, 49]. CD52 expression is typically strong, rendering it a therapeutic target [54]. Furthermore, TCL1 is overexpressed and can be detected by immunohistochemistry and flow cytometry, allowing for initial diagnosis as well as the detection of residual disease following therapy [55]. Of note, S100 expression is present in 30% [56] which could be a diagnostic pitfall without adequate immunophenotyping.

Cytogenetics

Chromosomal abnormalities most commonly reported for T-PLL involve inversion and translocation of chromosome 14. Inversion with breakpoints in the long arm of chromosome 14 at q11.2 and q32.1 is present in 80% of patients, while the translocation involving the identical regions on the long arm is identified in 10% of patients [57, 58]. These translocations juxtapose the *TRA* locus encoding the alpha chain of the T-cell receptor at q11.2 with oncogenes *TCL1A* and *TCL1B* at q32.1 activated through the translocation [59]. A less frequent translocation, t(X;14)(q28;q11.2), also involves the *TRA* locus and *MTCP1* at Xq28, a gene homologous to *TCL1A/B* [60–62]. These oncogenes have been reported to induce T-cell leukemia in a transgenic mouse model, however, rearrangements involving *TCL1A/B* or *MTCP1* are thought to be initiating events but insufficient to drive leukemogenesis. Furthermore, aberrations of chromosome 8, including isodicentric 8p [idic (8)(p11)], as well as translocation t(8;8)(p11–12;q12) and trisomy 8q, have been reported in up to 80% of patients [59], as have occasional gains of the

MYC gene [63]. Chromosomal deletions, including chromosomes 12p13, 22q, and amplification at 5p have also been identified by fluorescence in situ hybridization and/or single nucleotide polymorphism (SNP) array [64–66].

Molecular Findings

Importantly, whole-exome sequencing and targeted sequencing studies have revealed mutations in genes of the JAK/STAT pathway, including *JAK3* (36%), *JAK1* (8%), and *STAT5B* (29%), leading to constitutive activation of the STAT signaling pathway [67–70]. Additionally, mutations of genes encoding proteins involved in epigenetic modification, such as *EZH2* and *BCOR*, have been identified in rare cases [69, 70]. Moreover, missense mutations and chromosomal deletions involving the *ATM* gene (located at 11q22.3) have been reported [71, 72]. Frequent abnormalities involving chromosomes 6 and 17 have also been identified by karyotyping and comparative genomic hybridization [57, 73]. Of note, deletion of *TP53* with associated overexpression of p53 has been occasionally reported [74].

Differential Diagnosis

The differential diagnosis of T-PLL includes several other T-cell lymphomas as well as B-PLL. To distinguish T-PLL from T-cell large granular lymphocytic leukemia, adult T-cell leukemia/lymphoma, Sezary syndrome and peripheral T-cell lymphoma, integration of morphology by peripheral smear analysis, histological features, immunophenotype and cytogenetic and molecular findings is necessary to render the correct diagnosis. Differences in immunophenotype as well as lymph node and skin involvement help distinguish T-PLL from B-PLL. Cutaneous T-PLL can be differentiated from cutaneous T-cell lymphoma/mycosis fungoides by intact CD7 expression, co-expression of CD4/CD8 and inv(14) [75, 49].

Prognosis

T-PLL in general follows an aggressive course with a median survival of 12–24 months, although it can follow a more chronic course; nevertheless, the disease may progress after few years [76]. Immunotherapy with the monoclonal antibody alemtuzumab originally used to treat chronic lymphocytic lymphoma with *TP53* mutations or deletions [77], directed against surface antigen CD52, or CAMPATH-1, has led to response rates of up to 90% as first-line treatment [78, 79]. Additionally, patients achieving remission with immunotherapy should be considered for consolidation therapy by autologous or allogeneic hematopoietic stem cell transplantation [80, 81]. High levels of expression of TCL1 and AKT1 are associated with a poor prognosis, as are mutations of *STAT5B* [70, 82]. Knowledge of activating mutations involving the JAK/STAT pathway may prove useful in developing drugs targeting its individual effectors.

Diagnostic Caveats

- Aggressive natural killer-cell leukemia (ANKL) is a very rare but highly aggressive neoplasm typically associated with the Epstein-Barr (EBV) virus.
- Liver and spleen can be involved by ANKL, yet these two organs are not typically biopsied to render the initial diagnosis.
- ANKL is often complicated by hemophagocytic lymphohistiocytosis and/or multiorgan failure.
- T-cell prolymphocytic leukemia (T-PLL) is a rare and aggressive T-cell leukemia involving the peripheral blood, bone marrow, lymph nodes, liver, spleen, and skin.
- T-PLL typically presents with generalized lymphadenopathy and hepatosplenomegaly.
- Co-expression of CD4 and CD8 is present in ~25% of T-PLL, and is almost exclusive to T-PLL.
- Dense CD52 antigen expression in T-PLL allows for targeted therapy with the anti-CD52 monoclonal antibody alemtuzumab.

References

1. Chan JKCJES, Ko Y-H. Aggressive NK-cell leukemia. In: WHO classification of tumours of the haematopoietic and lymphoid tissues (revised 4th edition). Lyon: WHO Press; 2017. p. 353–4.
2. Chan JKCQ-ML, Ferry JA. Extranodal NK/T-cell lymphoma, nasal type. In: WHO classification of tumours of haematopoietic and lymphoid tissues (revised 4th edition), vol. 4. Lyon: WHO Press; 2017. p. 368–71.
3. Quintanilla-Martinez LKY-H, Kimura H, Jaffe ES. EBV-positive T-cell and NK-cell lymphoproliferative diseases of childhood. In: WHO classification of tumours of haematopoietic and lymphoid tissues (revised 4th edition). Lyon: WHO Press; 2017. p. 355–62.
4. Villamor NMWG, Chan WC, Foucar K. Chronic lymphoproliferative disorder of NK cells. In: WHO classification of tumours of haematopoietic and lymphoid tissues. Lyon: WHO Press; 2017. p. 351–2.
5. Ruskova A, Thula R, Chan G. Aggressive natural killer-cell leukemia: report of five cases and review of the literature. Leuk Lymphoma. 2004;45(12):2427–38.
6. Ishihara S, Ohshima K, Tokura Y, et al. Hypersensitivity to mosquito bites conceals clonal lymphoproliferation of Epstein-Barr viral DNA-positive natural killer cells. Jpn J Cancer Res Gann. 1997;88(1):82–7.
7. Ishihara S, Okada S, Wakiguchi H, Kurashige T, Hirai K, Kawa-Ha K. Clonal lymphoproliferation following chronic active Epstein-Barr virus infection and hypersensitivity to mosquito bites. Am J Hematol. 1997;54(4):276–81.
8. Park S, Ko YH. Epstein-Barr virus-associated T/natural killer-cell lymphoproliferative disorders. J Dermatol. 2014;41(1):29–39.
9. Matsubara A, Matsumoto M, Takada K, et al. Acute transformation of chronic large granular lymphocyte leukemia into an aggressive form associated with preferential organ involvement. Acta Haematol. 1994;91(4):206–10.
10. Ohno Y, Amakawa R, Fukuhara S, et al. Acute transformation of chronic large granular lymphocyte leukemia associated with additional chromosome abnormality. Cancer. 1989;64(1):63–7.
11. Chan JK. Natural killer cell neoplasms. Anat Pathol. 1998;3:77–145.
12. Fernandez LA, Pope B, Lee C, Zayed E. Aggressive natural killer cell leukemia in an adult with establishment of an NK cell line. Blood. 1986;67(4):925–30.
13. Imamura N, Kusunoki Y, Kawa-Ha K, et al. Aggressive natural killer cell leukaemia/lymphoma: report of four cases and review of the literature. Possible existence of a new clinical entity originating from the third lineage of lymphoid cells. Br J Haematol. 1990;75(1):49–59.
14. Ishida F. Recent progress of diagnosis and treatment in NK cell neoplasms. Rinsho ketsueki Jpn J Clin Hematol. 2015;56(6):645–50.
15. Li C, Tian Y, Wang J, et al. Abnormal immunophenotype provides a key diagnostic marker: a report of 29 cases of de novo aggressive natural killer cell leukemia. Transl Res. 2014;163(6):565–77.
16. Song SY, Kim WS, Ko YH, Kim K, Lee MH, Park K. Aggressive natural killer cell leukemia: clinical features and treatment outcome. Haematologica. 2002;87(12):1343–5.
17. Suzuki R, Suzumiya J, Nakamura S, et al. Aggressive natural killer-cell leukemia revisited: large granular lymphocyte leukemia of cytotoxic NK cells. Leukemia. 2004;18(4):763–70.
18. Chan JK, Sin VC, Wong KF, et al. Nonnasal lymphoma expressing the natural killer cell marker CD56: a clinicopathologic study of 49 cases of an uncommon aggressive neoplasm. Blood. 1997;89(12):4501–13.
19. Kwong YL, Chan AC, Liang RH. Natural killer cell lymphoma/leukemia: pathology and treatment. Hematol Oncol. 1997;15(2):71–9.
20. Kwong YL, Wong KF, Chan LC, et al. Large granular lymphocyte leukemia. A study of nine cases in a Chinese population. Am J Clin Pathol. 1995;103(1):76–81.
21. Oshimi K. Lymphoproliferative disorders of natural killer cells. Int J Hematol. 1996;63(4):279–90.
22. Ryder J, Wang X, Bao L, Gross SA, Hua F, Irons RD. Aggressive natural killer cell leukemia: report of a Chinese series and review of the literature. Int J Hematol. 2007;85(1):18–25.
23. Mori N, Yamashita Y, Tsuzuki T, et al. Lymphomatous features of aggressive NK cell leukaemia/lymphoma with massive necrosis, haemophagocytosis and EB virus infection. Histopathology. 2000;37(4):363–71.
24. Okuda T, Sakamoto S, Deguchi T, et al. Hemophagocytic syndrome associated with aggressive natural killer cell leukemia. Am J Hematol. 1991;38(4):321–3.

25. Lima M. Aggressive mature natural killer cell neoplasms: from epidemiology to diagnosis. Orphanet J Rare Dis. 2013;8:95.
26. Oshimi K, Yamada O, Kaneko T, et al. Laboratory findings and clinical courses of 33 patients with granular lymphocyte-proliferative disorders. Leukemia. 1993;7(6):782–8.
27. Kato K, Ohshima K, Ishihara S, Anzai K, Suzumiya J, Kikuchi M. Elevated serum soluble Fas ligand in natural killer cell proliferative disorders. Br J Haematol. 1998;103(4):1164–6.
28. Tanaka M, Suda T, Haze K, et al. Fas ligand in human serum. Nat Med. 1996;2(3):317–22.
29. Tani R, Ozaki S, Kosaka M, et al. Fas ligand-induced apoptosis of hepatocytes in natural killer cell leukaemia. Br J Haematol. 1999;106(3):709–12.
30. Yang CF, Hsu CY, Ho DM. Aggressive natural killer (NK)-cell leukaemia and extranodal NK/T-cell lymphoma are two distinct diseases that differ in their clinical presentation and cytogenetic findings. Histopathology. 2018;72(6):955–64.
31. Guerreiro M, Principe F, Teles MJ, et al. CD56-negative aggressive NK cell leukemia relapsing as multiple cranial nerve palsies: case report and literature review. Case Rep Hematol. 2017;2017:3724017.
32. Gao J, Behdad A, Ji P, Wolniak KL, Frankfurt O, Chen YH. EBV-negative aggressive NK-cell leukemia/lymphoma: a clinical and pathological study from a single institution. Mod Pathol. 2017;30(8):1100–15.
33. Nicolae A, Ganapathi KA, Pham TH, et al. EBV-negative aggressive NK-cell leukemia/lymphoma: clinical, pathologic, and genetic features. Am J Surg Pathol. 2017;41(1):67–74.
34. Wong KF, Chan JK, Kwong YL. Identification of del(6)(q21q25) as a recurring chromosomal abnormality in putative NK cell lymphoma/leukaemia. Br J Haematol. 1997;98(4):922–6.
35. Takahashi E, Ohshima K, Kimura H, et al. Clinicopathological analysis of the age-related differences in patients with Epstein-Barr virus (EBV)-associated extranasal natural killer (NK)/T-cell lymphoma with reference to the relationship with aggressive NK cell leukaemia and chronic active EBV infection-associated lymphoproliferative disorders. Histopathology. 2011;59(4):660–71.
36. Nakashima Y, Tagawa H, Suzuki R, et al. Genome-wide array-based comparative genomic hybridization of natural killer cell lymphoma/leukemia: different genomic alteration patterns of aggressive NK-cell leukemia and extranodal Nk/T-cell lymphoma, nasal type. Genes Chromosomes Cancer. 2005;44(3):247–55.
37. Gao LM, Liu WP, Yang QP, et al. Aggressive natural killer-cell leukemia with jaundice and spontaneous splenic rupture: a case report and review of the literature. Diagn Pathol. 2013;8:43.
38. Ko YH, Park S, Kim K, Kim SJ, Kim WS. Aggressive natural killer cell leukemia: is Epstein-Barr virus negativity an indicator of a favorable prognosis? Acta Haematol. 2008;120(4):199–206.
39. Karube K, Nakagawa M, Tsuzuki S, et al. Identification of FOXO3 and PRDM1 as tumor-suppressor gene candidates in NK-cell neoplasms by genomic and functional analyses. Blood. 2011;118(12):3195–204.
40. Karube K, Tsuzuki S, Yoshida N, et al. Lineage-specific growth inhibition of NK cell lines by FOXO3 in association with Akt activation status. Exp Hematol. 2012;40(12):1005–1015 e1006.
41. Dufva O, Kankainen M, Kelkka T, et al. Aggressive natural killer-cell leukemia mutational landscape and drug profiling highlight JAK-STAT signaling as therapeutic target. Nat Commun. 2018;9(1):1567.
42. Akashi K, Mizuno S. Epstein-Barr virus-infected natural killer cell leukemia. Leuk Lymphoma. 2000;40(1–2):57–66.
43. Nava VE, Jaffe ES. The pathology of NK-cell lymphomas and leukemias. Adv Anat Pathol. 2005;12(1):27–34.
44. Zhang Q, Jing W, Ouyang J, Zeng H, George SK, Liu Z. Six cases of aggressive natural killer-cell leukemia in a Chinese population. Int J Clin Exp Pathol. 2014;7(6):3423–31.
45. Jeong SH, Song HN, Park JS, et al. Allogeneic stem cell transplantation for patients with natural killer/T cell lymphoid malignancy: a multicenter analysis comparing upfront and salvage transplantation. Biol Blood Marrow Transplant. 2018;24:2471–8.
46. Matutes E, Brito-Babapulle V, Swansbury J, et al. Clinical and laboratory features of 78 cases of T-prolymphocytic leukemia. Blood. 1991;78(12):3269–74.
47. Pombo de Oliveira MS, Matutes E, Schulz T, et al. T-cell malignancies in Brazil. Clinico-pathological and molecular studies of HTLV-I-positive and -negative cases. Int J Cancer. 1995;60(6):823–7.
48. Pawson R, Schulz TF, Matutes E, Catovsky D. The human T-cell lymphotropic viruses types I/II are not involved in T prolymphocytic leukemia and large granular lymphocytic leukemia. Leukemia. 1997;11(8):1305–11.
49. Matutes E, Catovsky D, Mueller-Hermelink H. T-cell prolymphocytic leukemia. In: Swerdlow SH, Campo E, Harris NL, et al., editors. WHO classificationof tumors of hematopoietic and lymphoid tissues. Lyon: IARC; 2017. p. 346–7.
50. Matutes E, Garcia Talavera J, O'Brien M, Catovsky D. The morphological spectrum of T-prolymphocytic leukaemia. Br J Haematol. 1986;64(1):111–24.
51. Pawson R, Matutes E, Brito-Babapulle V, et al. Sezary cell leukaemia: a distinct T cell disorder or a variant form of T prolymphocytic leukaemia? Leukemia. 1997;11(7):1009–13.
52. Mallett RB, Matutes E, Catovsky D, Maclennan K, Mortimer PS, Holden CA. Cutaneous infiltration in T-cell prolymphocytic leukaemia. Br J Dermatol. 1995;132(2):263–6.
53. Osuji N, Matutes E, Catovsky D, Lampert I, Wotherspoon A. Histopathology of the spleen in T-cell large granular lymphocyte leukemia and T-cell prolymphocytic leukemia: a comparative review. Am J Surg Pathol. 2005;29(7):935–41.
54. Dearden CE. T-cell prolymphocytic leukemia. Med Oncol. 2006;23(1):17–22.
55. Herling M, Khoury JD, Washington LT, Duvic M, Keating MJ, Jones D. A systematic approach to diagnosis of mature T-cell leukemias reveals heterogeneity among WHO categories. Blood. 2004;104(2):328–35.
56. Aggarwal N, Pongpruttipan T, Patel S, et al. Expression of S100 protein in CD4-positive T-cell lymphomas is often associated with T-cell prolymphocytic leukemia. Am J Surg Pathol. 2015;39(12):1679–87.
57. Brito-Babapulle V, Catovsky D. Inversions and tandem translocations involving chromosome 14q11 and 14q32 in T-prolymphocytic leukemia and T-cell leukemias in patients with ataxia telangiectasia. Cancer Genet Cytogenet. 1991;55(1):1–9.
58. Maljaei SH, Brito-Babapulle V, Hiorns LR, Catovsky D. Abnormalities of chromosomes 8, 11, 14, and X in T-prolymphocytic leukemia studied by fluorescence in situ hybridization. Cancer Genet Cytogenet. 1998;103(2):110–6.
59. Pekarsky Y, Hallas C, Isobe M, Russo G, Croce CM. Abnormalities at 14q32.1 in T cell malignancies involve two oncogenes. Proc Natl Acad Sci U S A. 1999;96(6):2949–51.
60. Stern MH, Soulier J, Rosenzwajg M, et al. MTCP-1: a novel gene on the human chromosome Xq28 translocated to the T cell receptor alpha/delta locus in mature T cell proliferations. Oncogene. 1993;8(9):2475–83.

61. Gritti C, Dastot H, Soulier J, et al. Transgenic mice for MTCP1 develop T-cell prolymphocytic leukemia. Blood. 1998;92(2):368–73.

62. Virgilio L, Lazzeri C, Bichi R, et al. Deregulated expression of TCL1 causes T cell leukemia in mice. Proc Natl Acad Sci U S A. 1998;95(7):3885–9.

63. Hsi AC, Robirds DH, Luo J, Kreisel FH, Frater JL, Nguyen TT. T-cell prolymphocytic leukemia frequently shows cutaneous involvement and is associated with gains of MYC, loss of ATM, and TCL1A rearrangement. Am J Surg Pathol. 2014;38(11): 1468–83.

64. Bug S, Durig J, Oyen F, et al. Recurrent loss, but lack of mutations, of the SMARCB1 tumor suppressor gene in T-cell prolymphocytic leukemia with TCL1A-TCRAD juxtaposition. Cancer Genet Cytogenet. 2009;192(1):44–7.

65. Hetet G, Dastot H, Baens M, et al. Recurrent molecular deletion of the 12p13 region, centromeric to ETV6/TEL, in T-cell prolymphocytic leukemia. Hematol J. 2000;1(1):42–7.

66. Nowak D, Le Toriellec E, Stern MH, et al. Molecular allelokaryotyping of T-cell prolymphocytic leukemia cells with high density single nucleotide polymorphism arrays identifies novel common genomic lesions and acquired uniparental disomy. Haematologica. 2009;94(4):518–27.

67. Bellanger D, Jacquemin V, Chopin M, et al. Recurrent JAK1 and JAK3 somatic mutations in T-cell prolymphocytic leukemia. Leukemia. 2014;28(2):417–9.

68. Bergmann AK, Schneppenheim S, Seifert M, et al. Recurrent mutation of JAK3 in T-cell prolymphocytic leukemia. Genes Chromosomes Cancer. 2014;53(4):309–16.

69. Kiel MJ, Velusamy T, Rolland D, et al. Integrated genomic sequencing reveals mutational landscape of T-cell prolymphocytic leukemia. Blood. 2014;124(9):1460–72.

70. Stengel A, Kern W, Zenger M, et al. Genetic characterization of T-PLL reveals two major biologic subgroups and JAK3 mutations as prognostic marker. Genes Chromosomes Cancer. 2016;55(1):82–94.

71. Stilgenbauer S, Schaffner C, Litterst A, et al. Biallelic mutations in the ATM gene in T-prolymphocytic leukemia. Nat Med. 1997;3(10):1155–9.

72. Vorechovsky I, Luo L, Dyer MJ, et al. Clustering of missense mutations in the ataxia-telangiectasia gene in a sporadic T-cell leukaemia. Nat Genet. 1997;17(1):96–9.

73. Costa D, Queralt R, Aymerich M, et al. High levels of chromosomal imbalances in typical and small-cell variants of T-cell prolymphocytic leukemia. Cancer Genet Cytogenet. 2003;147(1):36–43.

74. Brito-Babapulle V, Hamoudi R, Matutes E, et al. p53 allele deletion and protein accumulation occurs in the absence of p53 gene mutation in T-prolymphocytic leukaemia and Sezary syndrome. Br J Haematol. 2000;110(1):180–7.

75. Magro CM, Morrison CD, Heerema N, Porcu P, Sroa N, Deng AC. T-cell prolymphocytic leukemia: an aggressive T cell malignancy with frequent cutaneous tropism. J Am Acad Dermatol. 2006;55(3):467–77.

76. Garand R, Goasguen J, Brizard A, et al. Indolent course as a relatively frequent presentation in T-prolymphocytic leukaemia. Groupe Francais d'Hematologie Cellulaire. Br J Haematol. 1998;103(2):488–94.

77. Lozanski G, Heerema NA, Flinn IW, et al. Alemtuzumab is an effective therapy for chronic lymphocytic leukemia with p53 mutations and deletions. Blood. 2004;103(9):3278–81.

78. Dearden CE, Matutes E, Cazin B, et al. High remission rate in T-cell prolymphocytic leukemia with CAMPATH-1H. Blood. 2001;98(6):1721–6.

79. Keating MJ, Cazin B, Coutre S, et al. Campath-1H treatment of T-cell prolymphocytic leukemia in patients for whom at least one prior chemotherapy regimen has failed. J Clin Oncol. 2002;20(1):205–13.

80. Guillaume T, Beguin Y, Tabrizi R, et al. Allogeneic hematopoietic stem cell transplantation for T-prolymphocytic leukemia: a report from the French society for stem cell transplantation (SFGM-TC). Eur J Haematol. 2015;94(3):265–9.

81. Krishnan B, Else M, Tjonnfjord GE, et al. Stem cell transplantation after alemtuzumab in T-cell prolymphocytic leukaemia results in longer survival than after alemtuzumab alone: a multicentre retrospective study. Br J Haematol. 2010;149(6):907–10.

82. Herling M, Patel KA, Teitell MA, et al. High TCL1 expression and intact T-cell receptor signaling define a hyperproliferative subset of T-cell prolymphocytic leukemia. Blood. 2008;111(1):328–37.

Elizabeth Margolskee and Attilio Orazi

Introduction

The spleen and, to a lesser extent, the liver may be secondarily involved by myeloid neoplasms. Clinically, the assessment of patients for hepatomegaly and splenomegaly is a routine part of the physical exam. Ultrasound imaging may be helpful for monitoring organ size. Splenic pathology is more commonly documented in chronic myeloid neoplasms, such as chronic myeloid leukemia (CML), primary myelofibrosis (PMF), chronic myelomonocytic leukemia (CMML), and, in a minority of cases, advanced stages of polycythemia vera (PV) or essential thrombocythemia (ET). Rarely, acute myeloid leukemia can involve the spleen, generally with only mild to moderate organomegaly. Less is known about hepatic involvement in myeloid neoplasms. However, hepatomegaly and hepatic dysfunction can be seen in myeloid neoplasms, due either to reactive proliferations of the hepatocytes themselves or infiltration of the liver by hematopoietic cells.

The most common manifestation of myeloid neoplasia in the spleen and liver is extramedullary hematopoiesis (EMH). In addition to myeloid neoplasms, EMH can also occur in non-neoplastic conditions or in association with non-hematopoietic neoplasms. Certain histologic features are more frequently seen in myeloid neoplasm-associated EMH than in reactive EMH, such as increased immature hematopoietic elements which can be identified by immunostaining for CD34 and/or CD117, increased granulocytic cells, and increased megakaryocytes. Immunophenotypically abnormal blasts, cytogenetic abnormalities, and morphologic dys-

plasia also support the presence of neoplastic EMH. Conversely, erythroid-predominant EMH tends to be more closely associated with reactive EMH [1]. A notable exception to this paradigm is G-CSF-induced splenomegaly, in which there is EMH with granulocytic predominance.

Dysregulation of the bone marrow microenvironment and the presence of abnormal clonal hematopoietic progenitor cells result in circulating marrow elements that can localize to the spleen and liver. Although it is well known that splenic hematopoiesis is common in myeloid neoplasms, little is known about the pathogenetic mechanisms involved in this phenomenon. Given the role of the spleen and liver in fetal hematopoiesis, it is likely that the microenvironment of these organs is suited for hematopoiesis. Studies based on loss of heterozygosity and presence of *JAK2* V617F mutation have confirmed that, in the setting of myeloproliferative neoplasms, splenic hematopoietic proliferations are clonal and molecularly identical to neoplastic bone marrow clones, indicating that, in this setting, splenic hematopoiesis is part of a neoplastic process [2]. This chapter will review aspects of splenic and hepatic pathology in AML, myeloproliferative neoplasms (MPN), myelodysplastic syndrome/myeloproliferative neoplasms (MDS/MPN), mastocytosis and blastic plasmacytoid dendritic cell neoplasm.

Myeloproliferative Neoplasms (MPN)

Chronic Myeloid Leukemia, *BCR-ABL1* Positive

Definition

Chronic myeloid leukemia is characterized by a proliferation of granulocytes and their precursors in the peripheral blood and is defined by the presence of the t(9;22) (q34.1;q11.2) translocation, resulting in the Philadelphia (Ph) chromosome. The translocation juxtaposes the *BCR* gene on chromosome 22 with the *ABL1* gene on chromo-

E. Margolskee (✉)
Department of Pathology and Laboratory Medicine, Weill Cornell Medical College/New York Presbyterian Hospital, New York, NY, USA
e-mail: margolskee@email.chop.edu

A. Orazi
Department of Pathology, Texas Tech University Health Sciences Center El Paso, El Paso, Texas, USA

© Springer Nature Switzerland AG 2020
L. Zhang et al. (eds.), *Diagnostic Pathology of Hematopoietic Disorders of Spleen and Liver*,
https://doi.org/10.1007/978-3-030-37708-3_16

some 9, resulting in constitutive activation of the ABL1 tyrosine kinase.

Epidemiology and Etiology

The annual incidence is 1–2 cases per 100,000 people worldwide, with a slight male predominance. The etiology is unknown, although a higher incidence of CML is observed in individuals with acute radiation exposure and in older individuals.

Clinical Presentation

Most patients present in chronic phase. Clinically, up to 50% of cases are found incidentally on routine blood work when the white blood cell (WBC) count is markedly elevated. Other individuals may present with fatigue, weight loss, anemia, or splenomegaly. Approximately 5% of individuals are diagnosed during accelerated or blast phase when the blast count increases over 10% or 20%, respectively. Additional criteria for disease progression in CML are delineated by the 2016 World Health Organization (WHO) classification of hematopoietic and lymphoid neoplasms [3].

Morphology and Immunophenotyping

Splenomegaly is seen in ~75% of CML in chronic phase [4]. In chronic phase, the spleen is enlarged and the cut surface is deep red on gross examination due to the obliteration of normal white pulp structures (Fig. 16.1). Geographic necrosis may be seen due to infarction. Microscopic examination reveals expansion of the red pulp by extramedullary hematopoiesis (EMH) with granulocytic predominance. Erythroid precursors and rare megakaryocytes are present but dwarfed by the increased myeloid elements. Foamy macrophages (pseudo-Gaucher cells) are also present, phagocytosing debris from degenerating granulocytic cells. As the disease progresses to accelerated or blast phase, gross examination of the spleen may show deep red color indicating expanded red pulp or, rarely, discrete tan nodules representing collections of blasts. Microscopic examination shows increased granulopoiesis with left-shifted maturation and increased blasts. These blasts are generally myeloid by cell marker analysis but in up to 25% of cases, lymphoid blast crisis can be seen. Megakaryoblastic or erythroblastic transformation is rare in CML. Immunohistochemical analysis for CD34, CD117, CD68, MPO, CD10, TdT, CD19, CD3, and CD42b may be helpful in characterizing the blast phenotype.

Little is known about hepatic involvement in chronic phase CML as liver biopsies are infrequently performed on these patients in the course of their diagnostic evaluation. Hepatomegaly is seen in ~2% of patients at presentation [4]. Liver biopsy may show a mild periportal infiltrate consisting of myeloid blasts and granulocytic precursors with some extension into the sinusoids. In blast crisis, extreme infiltration of the liver sinusoids by blasts may cause hepatomegaly and elevated alkaline phosphatase (LDH) levels [5].

Cytogenetics and Molecular Findings

All cases of CML harbor the characteristic t(9;22) translocation, which can be detected by routine cytogenetic studies in 90–95% of cases. In the remaining cases, cryptic t(9;22) is present, which can be demonstrated by FISH analysis or RT-PCR. BCR-ABL1 signaling is constitutively active in CML and activates several signaling pathways, resulting in active mitogenic signaling and an antiapoptotic program. The BCR-ABL1 kinase stimulates the MAP kinase cascade, the JAK/STAT pathway, and the PI3K pathway [6]. These alterations allow for growth factor–independent cell growth and survival.

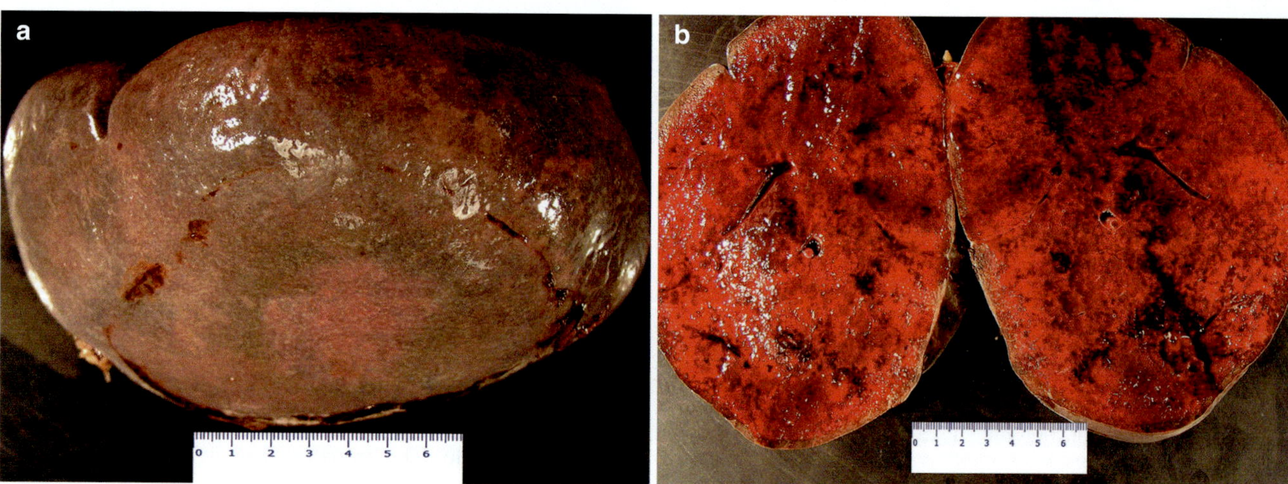

Fig. 16.1 (**a**) The spleen from a patient with CML shows significant enlargement (post splenectomy). (**b**) Cross section of the spleen shows diffuse deep red-tan cut surface associated with focal infarction

Differential Diagnosis

The differential diagnosis includes both reactive and neoplastic conditions. G-CSF effect can cause splenomegaly with granulocytic predominance and foamy macrophages. These lesions are not clonal and will lack *BCR-ABL1* rearrangement. Chronic myelomonocytic leukemia may cause splenomegaly with a prominent myelomonocytic proliferation in the spleen and, less commonly, the liver. Individuals with myelofibrosis or other myelophtheisic processes may have splenomegaly with trilineage hematopoiesis expanding the red pulp. Other rare myeloid disorders, such as atypical CML and chronic neutrophilic leukemia, may involve the spleen secondarily as well with prominent granulopoiesis. Demonstration of *BCR-ABL1* rearrangement by FISH or other methods is critical in establishing the diagnosis of CML.

Prognosis

The prognosis of CML in chronic phase is quite favorable in the era of tyrosine kinase inhibitors (TKI). Treatment with imatinib mesylate, the first-generation TKI, generally results in rapid morphologic and molecular remissions. The size of the spleen is reduced after the TKI therapy. To date, splenectomy is only indicated if it is clinically symptomatic. Patients undergoing prolonged treatment may develop kinase domain mutations resulting in imatinib resistance. Second- and third-generation TKIs such as dasatinib are increasingly used to overcome resistance to earlier TKIs. Blast phase CML is generally a sign of poor prognosis with few therapeutic options available.

Primary Myelofibrosis

Definition

Primary myelofibrosis (PMF) is a chronic myeloproliferative neoplasm marked by a proliferation of granulocytes and atypical megakaryocytes associated in its fully developed stage with myelofibrosis and EMH. Patients generally progress from a prefibrotic stage to a more overt form over the course of several years.

Epidemiology and Etiology

The incidence is 0.5–1.5 cases per 100,000 people [7]. Men and women are affected equally, generally in the sixth or seventh decade of life. The etiology is unknown, although there may be a familial predisposition to the disease as families with increased risk of PMF have been identified [8, 9].

Clinical Presentation

Establishment of the diagnosis requires satisfaction of a combination of major and minor criteria including clinical, laboratory, morphologic, and molecular parameters, as summarized in Table 16.1. Splenomegaly, one of the minor crite-

Table 16.1 Diagnostic criteria for primary myelofibrosis, overt fibrotic stage

Major criteria:	Minor criteria:
Megakaryocytic proliferation and atypia, accompanied by reticulin fibrosis grades 2–3 Exclusion of other myeloid neoplasms Presence of a clonal marker by cytogenetics of molecular testing OR absence of reactive myelofibrosis	Anemia not attributed to comorbid condition Leukocytosis $\geq 11 \times 10^9$/L Palpable splenomegaly Elevated lactate dehydrogenase Leukoerythroblastosis

Diagnosis requires that all three major criteria and one minor criterion are met.

Modified from Thiele et al. [7]

ria, is observed in as many as 90% of patients while hepatomegaly is seen in almost 50% depending on the stage of the disease [10–13].

Morphology

As PMF progresses, the increasingly fibrotic bone marrow drives hematopoietic precursors to establish themselves in other sites of residence, primarily the spleen and, to a lesser extent, the liver. This extramedullary hematopoiesis results in striking splenomegaly and leukoerythroblastosis [14–16]. Extramedullary hematopoiesis, also referred to as myeloid metaplasia, takes place primarily in the splenic red pulp. Grossly, the spleen is enlarged and deep red; white pulp markings are not appreciable. Histologic examination reveals effacement of the white pulp and small foci of extramedullary hematopoiesis based in the sinuses and splenic cords, sometimes accompanied by fibrosis (Fig. 16.2). Areas of ischemic necrosis are common. As in the bone marrow, erythroid cells tend to cluster in sinuses forming colonies or islands. Megakaryocytes show atypical features similar to those seen in the bone marrow of PMF patients, often forming tight clusters with bizarre nuclear atypia. Granulocytic precursors will also be present and can be highlighted by immunohistochemical staining. Evaluation for increased blasts by CD34 and/or CD117 is crucial to assess progression to accelerated or blast phase of the disease.

Morphologically, the differential diagnosis may include other causes of myelophtheisis, such as other chronic myeloproliferative neoplasms, metastasis of carcinoma to the bone marrow or presence of advanced infectious processes in the marrow. In PMF, the megakaryocytes should show atypical features and form tight clusters in the spleen, whereas they would be morphologically normal in other settings. In PMF, trilineage hematopoiesis would be expected in the spleen, while the spleen in CML tends to show granulocytic predominance. Careful correlation with laboratory and molecular parameters may be helpful in confirming a diagnosis of PMF. Table 16.2 shows a comparison of morphologic features of splenic EMH in common myeloproliferative neoplasms.

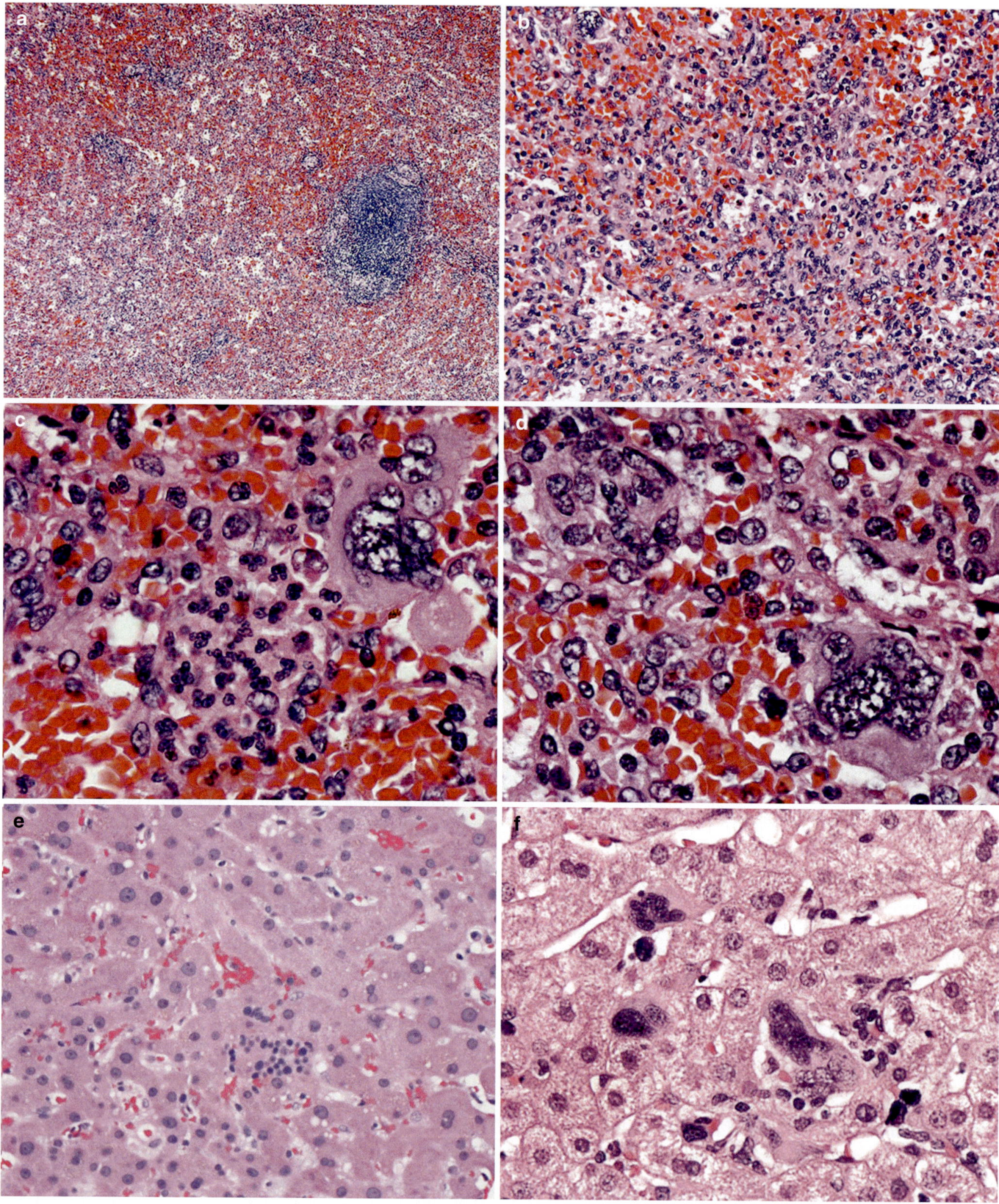

Fig. 16.2 In primary myelofibrosis the red pulp is expanded with partial preservation of the white pulp (**a**). Extramedullary hematopoiesis is present with granulocytic, erythroid, and megakaryocytic precursors. The megakaryocytes may show atypical features frequently seen in the bone marrow of PMF patients including bizarre nuclear morphology (**b–d**). Liver biopsies (**e, f**) will also show EMH (extramedullary hematopoiesis) in the hepatic sinuses

Table 16.2 Comparison of splenic findings in MPN

	CML	ET	PV	PMF
Frequency of splenomegaly	Frequent	Rare	Rare	Frequent
Morphology	Small megakaryocytes Numerous neutrophils, prominent granulopoiesis, rare erythroblasts	Platelet clumps in the cords and sinuses	Congestion of red pulp, increased cordal macrophages	Extensive EMH with abnormal, large megakaryocytes, left-shifted granulopoiesis, few neutrophils, prominent intravascular erythropoiesis
	Less fibrosis			Fibrosis, infarcts

Hepatic pathology is less commonly documented in PMF. In a study of 22 patients with PMF who underwent liver biopsies, all patients had mild to marked myeloid metaplasia in the liver with atypical megakaryocytic forms present (Fig. 16.2) [17, 18]. Approximately half of biopsies also showed widening of the hepatic sinusoids with increased reticulin fibrosis present in 37% [19]. Primary myelofibrosis is also associated with nodular regenerative hyperplasia in the liver, a reactive phenomenon whereby the hepatic parenchyma is transformed into small regenerative nodules, leading to non-cirrhotic portal hypertension [20]. In an autopsy series, 9–18% of PMF patients had clinical features of portal hypertension including esophageal varices and ascites [21]. Microscopically, the liver has nodules of larger hepatocytes with smaller hepatocytes in the intervening areas. These findings can be subtle; a reticulin stain may highlight thickening of the hepatocyte plates within the nodules and compression of the reticulin network in the nodules' periphery (Fig. 16.3).

Cytogenetics and Molecular Findings

There are no specific molecular or cytogenetic alterations in PMF, but most patients have the presence of at least one genetic alteration, most commonly mutations in *JAK2* (50–60%) [22]. Mutations in *CALR* and *MPL* are found in 24% and 8% of cases, respectively. Approximately 12% of cases are "triple-negative" (i.e., lacking mutations in one of these three driver genes) [23]. Targeted next-generation sequencing studies of large cohorts of patients with primary myelofibrosis have found *NRAS*, *TET2*, and *TP53* and *ASXL1* mutation to be associated with adverse prognosis in a multivariable model [24, 25]. Cytogenetic alterations are seen in 30% of cases, the most common being del(20q) and trisomy 1q [26].

Prognosis

In general, the prognosis for individuals with PMF varies by disease stage at the time of diagnosis. In the overt stage, the median overall survival is 3–7 years, while in the prefibrotic stage the median overall survival is greater than 15 years. A subset of patients will progress to blast phase or secondary acute myeloid leukemia, but others suffer from sequela of bone marrow failure, such as anemia and neutropenia.

Polycythemia Vera

Definition

Polycythemia vera (PV) is a chronic myeloproliferative neoplasm characterized by markedly increased red blood cell production, resulting in elevations of hemoglobin, hematocrit, red blood cell count, and red blood cell mass.

Epidemiology and Etiology

The incidence of PV is ~2 per 100,000 individuals and is more common in older individuals [27]. The etiology is unknown.

Clinical Presentation

Most patients present with sequela of erythrocytosis, including hypertension, thrombotic events, or vague physical complaints like aquagenic pruritus, headache, dizziness, and paresthesias. As in PMF, the diagnosis rests on the concurrent presence of major and minor criteria (listed in Table 16.3).

Morphology

Splenomegaly is observed in 44–58% of patients with polycythemia vera at the time of presentation [28]. The degree of splenomegaly is thought to correlate with the duration of the disease. As patients progress through the early erythrocytotic phase, splenomegaly progresses from mild to moderate. More severe splenomegaly is seen in the subset of patients who progress to post-polycythemic myelofibrosis (post-PV MF), in which the marrow cavity is replaced by fibrosis. As in primary myelofibrosis, post-PV MF is associated with leukoerythroblastosis and marked splenomegaly. The spleen in the erythrocytotic phase of PV is only mildly enlarged and shows a deep red color. Histologically, the splenic cords and sinuses appear congested with cordal macrophage hyperplasia and minimal extramedullary hematopoiesis. Splenectomy specimens from patients with post-polycythemic myelofibrosis will show gross and microscopic findings similar to those seen in the advanced stage of primary myelofibrosis, with trilineage extramedullary hematopoiesis expanding the red pulp (Figs. 16.1 and 16.4). Correlation with the clinical picture, bone marrow morphology, and molecular testing may be helpful.

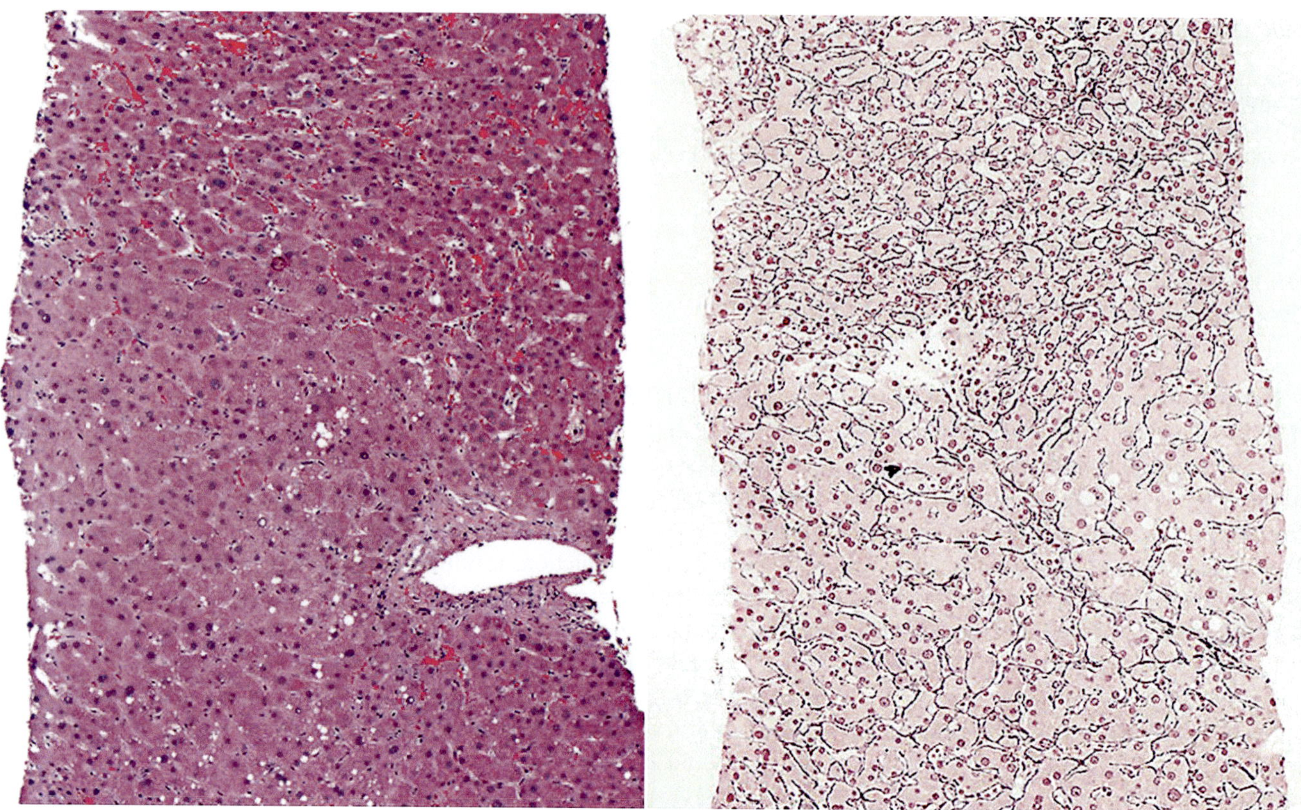

Fig. 16.3 Focal nodular hyperplasia in a liver biopsy in the setting of primary myelofibrosis. Reticulin stain (right) shows thick and thin hepatic cords

Table 16.3 Diagnostic criteria for polycythemia vera

Major criteria:
Elevated hemoglobin concentration (>16.5 g/dL in men; >16 g/dL in women) or elevated hematocrit (>49% in men; >48% women) or elevated red blood cell mass (>25% above mean normal predicted value)
Bone marrow biopsy showing hypercellularity with panmyelosis with pleomorphic megakaryocytes.
Presence of *JAK2* mutation
Minor criterion:
Subnormal erythropoietin level
Diagnosis requires either 3 major criteria or the first 2 major criteria and one minor criterion
Bone marrow biopsy (major criterion 2) may not be necessary in patients with absolute erythrocytosis (hemoglobin >18.5 g/dL in men or >16.5 g/dL in women; hematocrit >55.5% in men, > 49.5% in women) if all other major and minor criteria are met

Modified from Thiele et al. [27]

Little is known about liver biopsy findings in polycythemia vera. Around 5–10% of patients with polycythemia vera may initially present with Budd-Chiari syndrome or portal vein thrombosis [29, 30]. *JAK2*-positive MPN are the most common underlying prothrombotic disorder in patients presenting with abdominal venous thromboses [31]. In Budd-Chiari syndrome, liver biopsy shows sinusoidal dilation, centrilobular necrosis, and perivenular fibrosis (Fig. 16.5).

Long-term injury may result in large regenerative nodules or focal nodular hyperplasia, as seen in PMF (see discussion of histologic features, above) [32].

Cytogenetics and Molecular Findings

The most common genetic abnormality is the somatic gain-of-function *JAK2* V617F mutation, which is present in >95% of cases [33, 34]. A small subset of patients have mutations in exon 12 of *JAK2*. These *JAK2* alterations cause cytokine-independent growth of bone marrow progenitors, resulting in bone marrow hypercellularity and panmyelosis. Mutated JAK2 leads to autophosphorylation and subsequent activation of downstream signaling mediators such as MAPK, PI3K, and STAT proteins. Cytogenetic abnormalities are seen in 20% of patients, most commonly gain of chromosomes 8 or 9, del(20q), del(13q), and del(9p) [27].

Prognosis

The prognosis of polycythemia vera is generally favorable, with recent studies showing median survivals of over 13 years [26, 33]. The rate of progression to blast phase is 20% [35–37]. Thrombotic complications are another major source of morbidity and mortality in patients with polycythemia vera. Progression to post-PV MF is about 20% at 10 years after diagnosis.

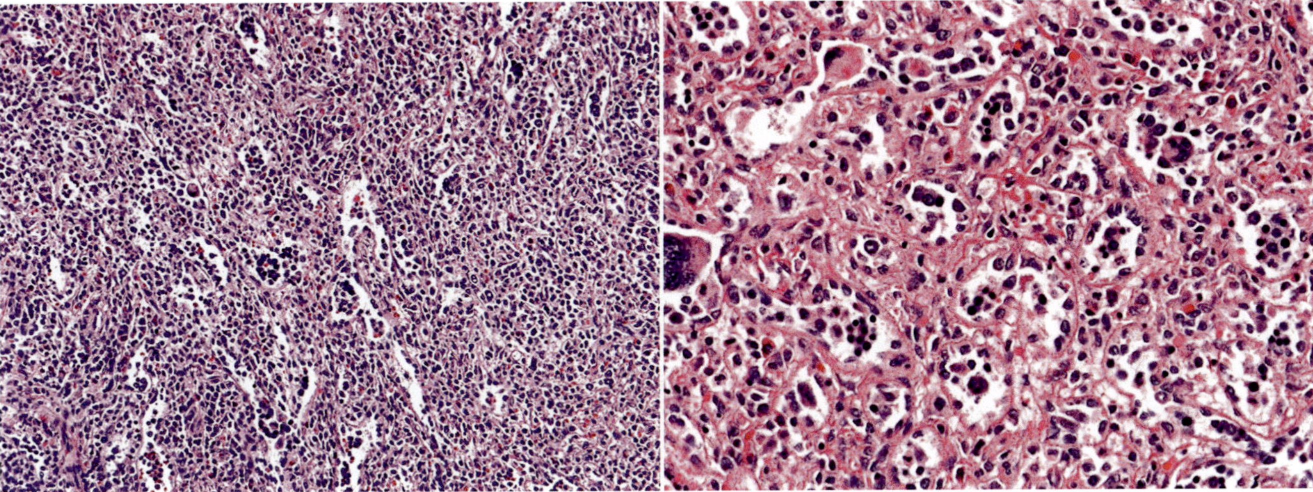

Fig. 16.4 Extramedullary hematopoiesis in polycythemia vera with expanded red pulp and trilineage hematopoiesis

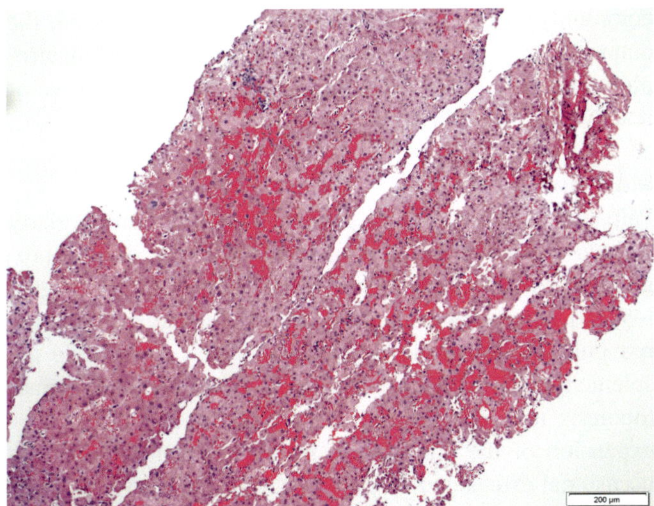

Fig. 16.5 Venous outflow obstruction (Budd-Chiari Syndrome) in a PV patient. There is centrilobular congestion

Essential Thrombocythemia

Definition

Essential thrombocythemia (ET) is a form of myeloproliferative disease that presents with thrombocytosis ($\geq 450 \times 10^9$ /L platelets).

Etiology and Epidemiology

The incidence is difficult to assess as not all patients may obtain a complete evaluation, but it is estimated to be 0.2–2.3 cases per 100,000 individuals [38–40]. There is a slight female predominance; patients present in the sixth and seventh decade of life. The etiology is largely unknown.

Clinical Presentation

Over half of cases are identified incidentally in the course or routine laboratory testing, but a substantial subset of patients present with vascular complications, such as hemorrhage, thrombosis, or microvascular occlusion. In the 2016 WHO, diagnosis of ET requires, in addition to thrombocytosis, the presence of typical bone marrow morphology and exclusion of other causes of reactive thrombocytosis. Demonstration of a clonal marker either via genetic testing or cytogenetic analysis is also essential.

Morphology

Essential thrombocythemia is not usually associated with splenomegaly, and hypersplenism is uncommon. Minor palpable splenomegaly is only present in a minority of patients with ET [41–43]. Little data is available regarding splenic pathology in ET. Rare cases have shown the presence of large aggregates of platelets sequestered in the splenic sinuses and cords of Billroth. In advanced cases, the spleen may appear atrophic and fibrotic with small infarcts due to the presence of these platelet clusters. Extramedullary hematopoiesis is uncommon.

Together with PV, ET is one of the most common causes of splanchnic vein thrombosis, including Budd-Chiari syndrome and portal vein thrombosis. In a cohort study of individuals with abdominal thrombotic disease and myeloproliferative disease, 27% were found to have ET [44]. For a more complete discussion of hepatic pathology in Budd-Chiari, see the section on polycythemia vera, above. Portal vein thrombosis may also be seen in ET, resulting in non-cirrhotic portal hypertension.

Cytogenetic and Molecular Findings

Genetic testing discloses the presence of a driver mutation (*JAK2, CALR, MPL*) in 88% of cases [26, 34, 45, 46]. No molecular alteration is specific for the disease. Only a small subset of ET patients have cytogenetic abnormalities (5–10%) [26].

Prognosis

ET is generally regarded as an indolent myeloproliferative neoplasm with occasional severe complications, both thrombotic and hemorrhagic. Most patients have a life expectancy equivalent to age-matched controls. Progression generally takes one of two forms: either to blast phase, marked by a blast count over 20% in PB or BM, or to post-ET myelofibrosis, where reticulin staining of the bone marrow shows deposition of coarse fibers and collagen. Blast phase is felt to be exceedingly rare in WHO-defined ET, and is seen in approximately <5% of cases [22, 26]. Post-ET myelofibrosis results in a clinical picture similar to that of post-PV MF and PMF, with massive splenomegaly, leukoerythroblastosis, elevated LDH, and extramedullary hematopoiesis. The incidence of post-ET MF is also quite low at about 10% of cases at 10 years after diagnosis in WHO-defined cohorts [26].

Chronic Neutrophilic Leukemia

Definition

Chronic neutrophilic leukemia (CNL) is an exceedingly rare myeloproliferative neoplasm marked by increased, sustained neutrophilia with hepatosplenomegaly. Bone marrow examination shows increased granulopoiesis with complete maturation.

Epidemiology

It affects primarily older adults with a median age at presentation of 66 [47].

Clinical Presentation

Patients often present with leukocytosis discovered incidentally on routine blood work, with a median duration of leukocytosis prior to diagnosis of 12 months [48]. Other patients may present with fatigue, petechiae, or symptomatic splenomegaly.

Diagnosis requires a combination of peripheral blood, bone marrow, and molecular features. Peripheral blood white blood cell count must be $\geq 25 \times 10^9/L$ with 80% bands or neutrophils. Granulocyte precursors must constitute <10% of the remaining white blood cells. Monocytosis and dysgranulocytosis are not permitted. Bone marrow examination must show hypercellular bone marrow with increased granulocytes and <5% myeloblasts. Molecular testing to exclude other MPN must be negative. A plasma cell neoplasm must be excluded, as paraneoplastic neutrophilia can be seen in this setting. Finally, molecular testing frequently will disclose the presence of an activating *CSF3R* mutation, most

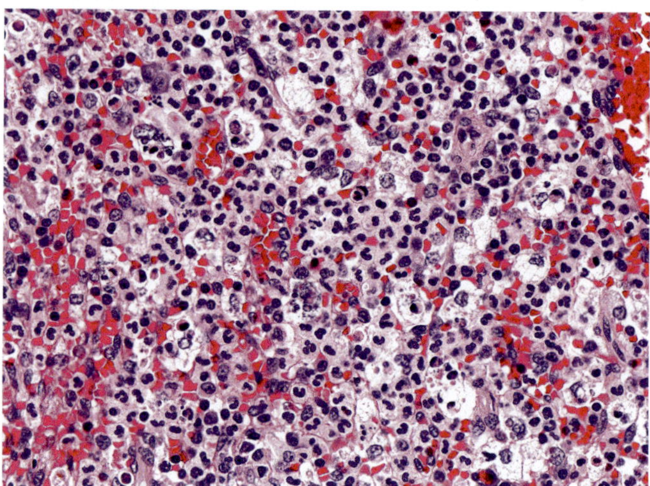

Fig. 16.6 Spleen in chronic neutrophilic leukemia showing expanded red pulp with numerous mature neutrophils

commonly T618I. In the absence of *CSF3R* mutation, the diagnosis may be made in the setting of persistent neutrophilia and splenomegaly, after exclusion of other causes of reactive neutrophilia [49].

Morphology

Palpable splenomegaly is present in 36% of molecularly defined cases of CNL at diagnosis, but as the disease progresses, patients almost invariably develop organomegaly [47, 49]. Microscopically, the spleen shows expansion of the red pulp by numerous neutrophils, which can invade the splenic lymphoid follicles (Fig. 16.6). Extramedullary hematopoiesis may also be seen [50]. Liver biopsy may show expansion of the portal areas by mature neutrophils, with occasional extension to the sinuses. Megakaryocytes, immature myelocytes, and erythroid precursors may also be seen in the liver [50].

Cytogenetic and Molecular Findings

Molecular analysis has greatly informed our ability to identify cases of CNL. Mutations in the gene for the receptor for colony-stimulating actor 3 (*CSF3R*) are strongly associated with CNL [51]. Two classes of *CSF3R* mutation are described. The most common is the activating T618I mutation, which occurs in 80–100% of cases and results in autoactivation of the receptor. The second type of alteration is a truncation mutation resulting in loss of negative-regulatory domain in the C-terminal portion of the protein. This mutation is seen in ~25% of cases in conjunction with the T618I mutation and results in overexpression of the receptor and hypersensitivity to G-CSF [47, 51–53]. Mutations in genes commonly implicated in myeloid neoplasms can also be seen, particularly *SETBP1*, *SRSF2*, and *ASXL1*. *ASXL1* mutations have been associated with poor prognosis [48].

Cytogenetic studies play a limited role in the diagnosis of CNL. Karyotype studies are generally normal at the time of diagnosis, but clonal cytogenetic abnormalities can be acquired as the disease progresses [49, 54].

By definition, *PDGFRA*, *PDGFRB*, *FGFR1*, and *BCR-ABL1* alterations must be excluded to establish the diagnosis.

Differential Diagnosis

The differential diagnosis includes other conditions that can cause granulocyte-predominant infiltrates in the spleen and liver, including G-CSF effect, CML, and CMML. Correlation of clinical, pathologic, and molecular data can help exclude these alternative diagnoses.

Prognosis

The prognosis is variable, ranging from 6 months to over 20 years [49]. Patients generally suffer sequelae of anemia and thrombocytopenia. Rare cases have progressed to blast phase [55, 56].

Myelodysplastic/Myeloproliferative Neoplasms

Chronic Myelomonocytic Leukemia

Chronic myelomonocytic leukemia (CMML) is a myeloid neoplasm with features of both myelodysplastic syndrome and myeloproliferative neoplasms, characterized by persistent peripheral blood monocytosis and dysplastic changes in the bone marrow.

Epidemiology and Etiology

The incidence is 0.4 per 100,000 individuals and is primarily seen in people over the age of 60 [57]. The etiology is unknown.

Clinical Presentation

In the 2016 WHO, CMML is divided into two subtypes: myeloproliferative CMML tends to present with leukocytosis (WBC $\geq$ 13 $\times$ 10^9/L) and constitutional symptoms while myelodysplastic CMML is defined by lower WBC counts and presents with sequela of hematopoietic insufficiency, such as fatigue and infection. Splenomegaly and hepatomegaly can occur in either type but are seen more frequently in individuals with the myeloproliferative subtype [58]. The diagnostic criteria are summarized in Table 16.4.

Morphology and Immunophenotyping

Splenomegaly is seen in 30–40% of individuals with CMML [58, 59]. The spleen generally shows the preservation of

Table 16.4 Diagnostic criteria for CMML

Persistent monocytosis in peripheral blood ($\geq$1 $\times$ 10^9/L) with monocytes accounting for $\geq$10% of WBC
Exclusion of other myeloproliferative neoplasms
Absence of *PDGFRA*, *PDGFRB*, *FGFR1*, and *PCM1-JAK2* rearrangement
<20% blasts in PB and BM
Dysplasia involving 1 or more myeloid lineages Or Molecular or cytogenetic evidence of clonality Or Persistent monocytosis for 3 months or more and exclusion of other causes of monocytosis.

Modified from Orazi et al. [57]

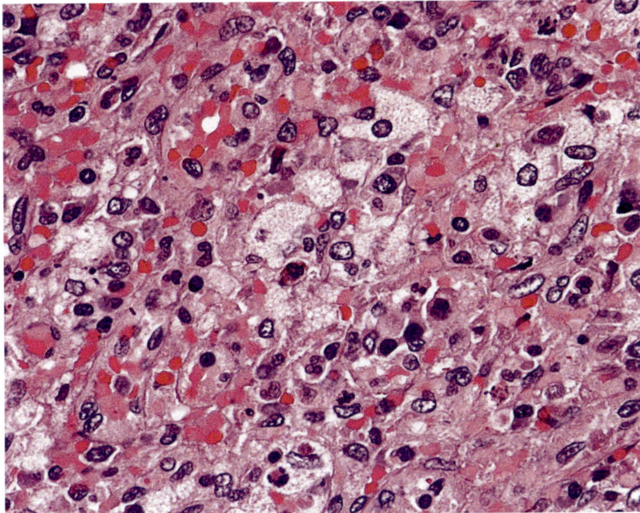

Fig. 16.7 Spleen in chronic myelomonocytic leukemia with foamy macrophage hyperplasia, mimicking those seen in immune-mediated thrombocytopenic purpura

white pulp with mild expansion of the red pulp by a leukemic infiltrate of primarily myelomonocytic cells with complete maturation. A subset of patients may show extramedullary hematopoiesis and nodules of plasmacytoid dendritic cells [60–62]. In patients with progression toward AML, myeloid maturation will be left shifted with an increased proportion of blasts. In some cases, there may be a proliferation of foamy histiocytes in the marginal zone of the splenic white pulp (Fig. 16.7). This pattern is similar to that seen in immune thrombocytopenia [60].

Immunohistochemistry for CD34 and CD117 may be helpful for blast enumeration. Monocytic cells can be highlighted with CD68R (PGM1), CD14, CD163, and HLA-DR. Lysozyme, myeloperoxidase, and CD13 may help identify granulocytic precursors. Plasmacytoid dendritic cell nodules can be identified with CD123, CD4, CD43, and CD303 immunostaining. These accumulations of mature plasmacytoid dendritic cells do not express CD56 and have a low Ki-67 proliferation index.

Differential Diagnosis

The differential diagnosis includes other scenarios which can cause splenomegaly with granulocyte-predominant extramedullary hematopoiesis. This would include CML, BCR-ABL1 positive, CNL, and juvenile myelomonocytic leukemia. Patients receiving G-CSF can also have similar findings on splenectomy samples. Distinguishing acute myeloid leukemia with monocytic or myelomonocytic differentiation from CMML with increased blasts can be challenging as monoblasts generally do not have a distinctive immunophenotypic profile from immature monocytes. Flow cytometric studies may be helpful in separating out monocytes from monocytic precursors as well. Clinical correlation as well as correlation with bone marrow morphology may be helpful.

Although hepatomegaly can be seen in up to 25% of patients with CMML, collective experience with liver biopsy findings is limited to only rare case reports [63].

Cytogenetic and Molecular Findings

Cytogenetic alterations are seen in a minority of patients and none are specific to the disorder [57]. The most common alterations are gain of chromosome 8 and loss of chromosome 7. Genetic alterations are seen in most patients, most commonly *ASXL1*, *TET2*, and *SRSF2*, which are thought to be components of a CMML "signature." However, CMML is genetically quite heterogeneous with mutations seen in various protein families. ASXL1 is a chromatin/histone modulator which, when mutated, results in loss of trimethylation of certain histone residues [64]. It is commonly mutated in myeloid neoplasia (~40–50% of cases of CMML) and is often associated with aggressive disease [65]. *TET2* is an epigenetic regulator that mediates an intermediate step in DNA demethylation, and is mutated in ~60% of CMML [45]. SRSF2 is a spliceosome protein that is mutated in ~50% of cases of CMML [66].

Prognosis

The prognosis is variable, ranging from 1 month to over 10 years with median survival around 20–40 months. Approximately 20% progress to AML, which is best classified as acute myeloid leukemia with myelodysplasia-related changes (AMLMRC). Occasionally they may show myelomonocytic or monocytic differentiation.

Juvenile Myelomonocytic Leukemia

Definition

Juvenile myelomonocytic leukemia (JMML) is a clonal proliferation of mainly the granulocytic and monocytic lineages similar to CMML but it presents in younger individuals and is associated with neurofibromatosis. As it is a hematopoietic stem cell disorder, megakaryocytic and erythroid abnormalities can be seen as well.

Epidemiology

It is relatively rare, with an estimated incidence of 0.13 cases per 100,000 children. It is primarily seen in children under 3 years of age.

Clinical Presentation

Patients generally present with failure to thrive. Neutropenia may result in frequent infection and fever; thrombocytopenia may lead to maculopapular rashes. Dermal neurofibromas, café au lait spots, and other manifestations of neurofibromatosis type 1 may prompt evaluation for JMML as well.

Morphology and Immunophenotyping

Hepatosplenomegaly is almost uniformly present [67, 68]. In a large cohort study, the median size of the spleen and liver was 6.0 cm and 4.0 cm below the costal margin, respectively [69]. In the spleen, myelomonocytic cells infiltrate and expand the splenic sinuses and cords with effacement of the white pulp. Liver biopsy may show a similar myelomonocytic infiltrate, primarily in the sinusoids with extension to the portal tract [67]. A small autopsy series of patients with JMML emphasized the presence of hepatic fibrosis in JMML. They observed portal tract fibrosis with bridging fibrosis between portal tracts imparting a lobular pattern to the liver, distinct from cirrhosis or nodular regenerative hyperplasia. Collagen fibrosis was also present around the central veins and into the sinusoids [70]. However, all patients had received multiple courses of therapy by the time of tissue sampling, which may play a role in the morphologic findings.

The immunophenotype of the myelomonocytic infiltrate is similar to that seen in normal myeloid and monocytes, with no specific immunophenotypic abnormalities. CD34 and CD117 should reveal few, if any, myeloblasts. The monocytes express CD68 (PGM1), CD14, and CD4. The granulocytes express CD15 and MPO.

Molecular and Cytogenetic Findings

Genetic studies have revealed that JMML results from abnormalities in the RAS signaling pathway. Members of the RAS family mediate signaling downstream from the granulocyte-macrophage colony-stimulating factor (GM-CSF) receptor. Somatic or germline mutations involving this pathway are seen in up to 85% of patients with JMML and result in increased RAS signaling. The most common mutation is a heterozygous somatic gain-of-function alteration in *PTPN11*, seen in ~35% of cases [71, 72], and associated with aggressive disease if left untreated. *KRAS* and *NRAS* somatic mutations are seen in 20–25% of patients [71, 73, 74]. These patients generally have aggressive disease, but rare individuals have experienced long-term survival without treatment [74, 75]. Germline variants in *CBL* or *NF1* are present in ~25% of individuals. Patients with *NF1* mutations generally have aggressive disease necessitating early treatment, but *CBL*-mutated JMML often resolves spontaneously. Thus, molecular testing provides crucial prognostic information for children with JMML. Monosomy 7 is the most common karyotypic anomaly, seen in about 25% of patients. The absence of the *BCR-ABL1* translocation is required to establish a diagnosis of JMML.

Differential Diagnosis

The differential diagnosis is limited, especially in very young patients. However, CML, BCR-ABL1-positive, may have similar morphologic findings, as it also tends to have leukocytosis with a granulocytic predominance. Thus, FISH studies to exclude *BCR-ABL1* rearrangement is required to establish a diagnosis of JMML. AML with myelomonocytic differentiation in the spleen may be another diagnostic consideration. In JMML, the infiltrate should show numerous neutrophils and mature monocytes, while the infiltrate in AML will have a preponderance of immature cells. Review of the bone marrow and peripheral blood smear is essential as JMML has less than 20% blasts while AML has 20% or more.

Acute Myeloid Leukemia

Definition

Acute myeloid leukemia (AML) is a clonal proliferation of myeloblasts and is quite heterogenous clinically, morphologically, and genetically. WHO criteria for diagnosis generally require at least 20% myeloblasts or blast equivalents in the bone marrow or peripheral blood, or the presence of myeloid sarcoma in other tissues. AML is then subclassified based on integrated evaluation of the patient's clinical history, molecular/cytogenetic alterations, and histomorphological features.

Etiology and Epidemiology

The incidence of AML is ~3 cases per 100,000 people per year, with a median age of 65 at diagnosis. Although several risk factors have been associated with AML, most cases have no identifiable cause. Individuals with exposure to certain chemicals, radiation, or chemotherapy have an elevated risk of AML and generally have a more aggressive disease course. Myelodysplastic syndrome (MDS) is considered a preleukemic condition with a risk of progression correlated to the percentage of blasts in the bone marrow and peripheral blood. Finally, the 2016 WHO update highlighted myeloid neoplasms with germline predisposition; these include individuals with germline mutations in *CEBPA*, *DDX41*, *RUNX1*, *ANKRD26*, *ETV6*, and *GATA2*, among others. Currently, germline predisposition is thought to play a role in a small fraction of cases of AML, but as awareness of these cases grows, more individuals and cohorts may be identified.

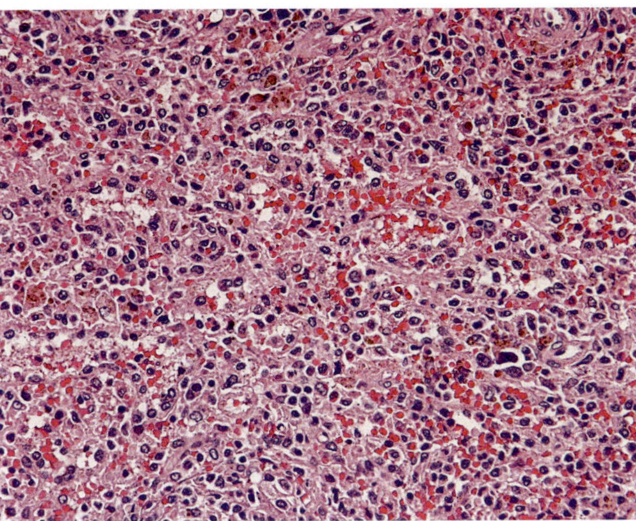

Fig. 16.8 Acute myeloid leukemia in the spleen. Red pulp is expanded with effacement of the red pulp by a proliferation of blasts

Clinical Presentation

Patients generally present either with cytopenias or presence of circulating blasts in the peripheral blood.

Morphology

Splenic involvement is not uncommon in AML. Although most patients with AML have a minimal or only mild splenomegaly, splenomegaly may be seen, particularly in patients with underlying bone marrow fibrosis. On cut section, there is expansion of the red pulp by leukemic blasts. Microscopically, the blasts are medium-sized with a high nucleus-cytoplasmic ratio, fine, dispersed chromatin, and prominent nucleoli (Fig. 16.8). Necrosis may be present. In addition, splenic rupture is a rare and devastating complication of acute myeloid leukemia [76]. Splenic myeloid sarcoma has also been reported as an unusual presentation of acute myeloid leukemia [77].

AML may also involve the liver, although published material on this topic is scarce. In one series, hepatic involvement was seen in 72% of cases of AML. Generally, hepatic involvement is diffuse and non-destructive; discrete masses are uncommon. On microscopic examination, myeloblasts are present in the hepatic sinusoids and in the portal tracts (Fig. 16.9).

Immunophenotyping

The morphologic and immunophenotypic features of the blasts may vary based on the major lineages involved and the degree of maturation. Blasts may be monocytic, erythroid, megakaryoblastic, or show only limited differentiation. Myeloblasts most commonly express CD34, CD117, CD13, CD33, and other myeloid antigens, with cytoplasmic myeloperoxidase (MPO) and aberrant expression of CD7, CD56,

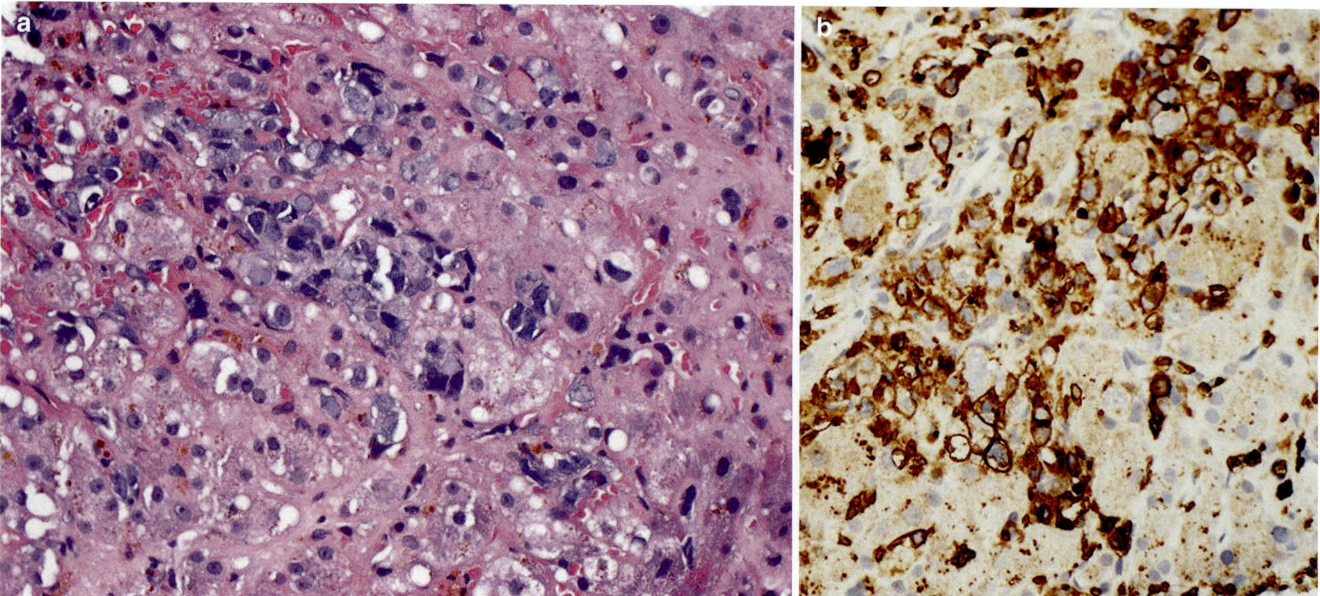

Fig. 16.9 Acute myeloid leukemia in the liver. There is an intrasinusoidal proliferation of blasts with fine chromatin and prominent nucleoli (**a**). Immunostaining for CD34 is positive (**b**)

or TdT. Monoblasts express variable CD14, CD16, and CD64 with cytoplasmic NSE. Megakaryoblasts are generally negative for CD34 and CD117 but are positive for CD42b and CD61. Erythroblastic leukemia is very rare; blasts lack expression of CD34 but express CD117, CD71, and glycophorin A.

Molecular and Cytogenetic Findings

A complete cytogenetic and molecular evaluation is critical in patients with newly diagnosed AML, as certain molecular events are associated with specific therapeutic options, or may provide important prognostic information. A complete review of the molecular landscape of AML is beyond the scope of this chapter, but at a minimum, karyotype studies and evaluation for *NPM1*, *CEBPA*, *RUNX1*, and *FLT3* alterations should be performed in all patients with newly diagnosed AML.

Differential Diagnosis

The differential diagnosis may include extramedullary blast transformation of an underlying myeloproliferative neoplasm, which can be excluded by evaluation of the patient's medical history and a bone marrow examination. The blasts in AML can be morphologically indistinguishable from lymphoblasts or blastic plasmacytoid dendritic cells (BPDCN). A complete immunophenotypic evaluation can resolve this differential, as the lymphoblasts will express CD19 or cytoplasmic CD3, consistent with B or T lineage, respectively. Plasmacytoid dendritic cells express CD4, CD56, and CD123 (see discussion, below). In addition, in the liver, lymphoblasts tend to have a peri-portal growth pattern, expanding

the portal tracts, while myeloblasts tend to diffusely infiltrate the hepatic sinusoids [78].

Systemic Mastocytosis

Definition

Mastocytosis is a clonal proliferation of mast cells which can occur at any age and present as a limited, cutaneous, or systemic disease.

Cutaneous mastocytosis is an indolent disease with only skin involvement and spontaneous regression; there is no involvement of the liver or spleen. Systemic mastocytosis generally falls into one of four major categories: indolent, smoldering, aggressive, or leukemic with a complex scheme for the classification of these patients [79]. Organ involvement, including hepatosplenomegaly, can be seen in smoldering, aggressive, or leukemic disease, but organ damage, including hypersplenism, elevated liver enzymes or ascites, defines the aggressive variants of systemic mastocytosis. These are termed "C" findings in the WHO classification [79]. In view of the frequent co-occurrence of mast cell disease and other clonal hematopoietic neoplasms, such as CMML, myeloproliferative disease, and acute myeloid leukemia, appropriate evaluation for myeloid neoplasia should be pursued in individuals with systemic mastocytosis.

Epidemiology

The incidence of mast cell disease is estimated to be 5–10 patients per 1 million individuals per year [80]. While cutaneous mastocytosis is more common in children, systemic forms of disease are more frequently seen in elderly individuals. Due to the variable extent of disease at presentation, classification requires an extensive clinical, radiologic, and laboratory workup including bone marrow examination, tryptase levels, myeloid mutation panel testing, and baseline PET/CT scans.

Morphology

Mild or moderate splenomegaly is common in systemic mastocytosis. On gross examination, the spleen may have capsular thickening. Early in the course of the disease, the mast cells may be found in the paratrabecular areas or in the white pulp marginal zones, often in association with numerous eosinophils. The mast cells form nodules with or without associated reactive small lymphocytes. Spindle forms are often identified (Fig. 16.10). Under medium to higher magnification, the ensuing fibroblastic

reactions result in a concentric "rimming" of the white pulp and intermingling with mast cells (Fig. 16.11). Case reports have described other morphologic variants including a diffuse infiltration of red pulp and perivascular distribution. The mast cells demonstrate either a round or spindled cytology with pale nuclei and pale cytoplasm. The mast cell granules are inconspicuous on routine hematoxylin and eosin staining. The mast cells in mastocytosis have a characteristic immunophenotype, including bright expression of CD117, mast cell tryptase (Figs. 16.10 and 16.11), and aberrant expression of CD2 and/or CD25.

Liver involvement can also be seen in mastocytosis. Biopsy may show multinodular infiltration of the periportal and sinusoidal parenchyma by spindle cells with dense chromatin and pale cytoplasm. The infiltrate can be somewhat subtle, requiring ancillary staining with tryptase or CD117 to

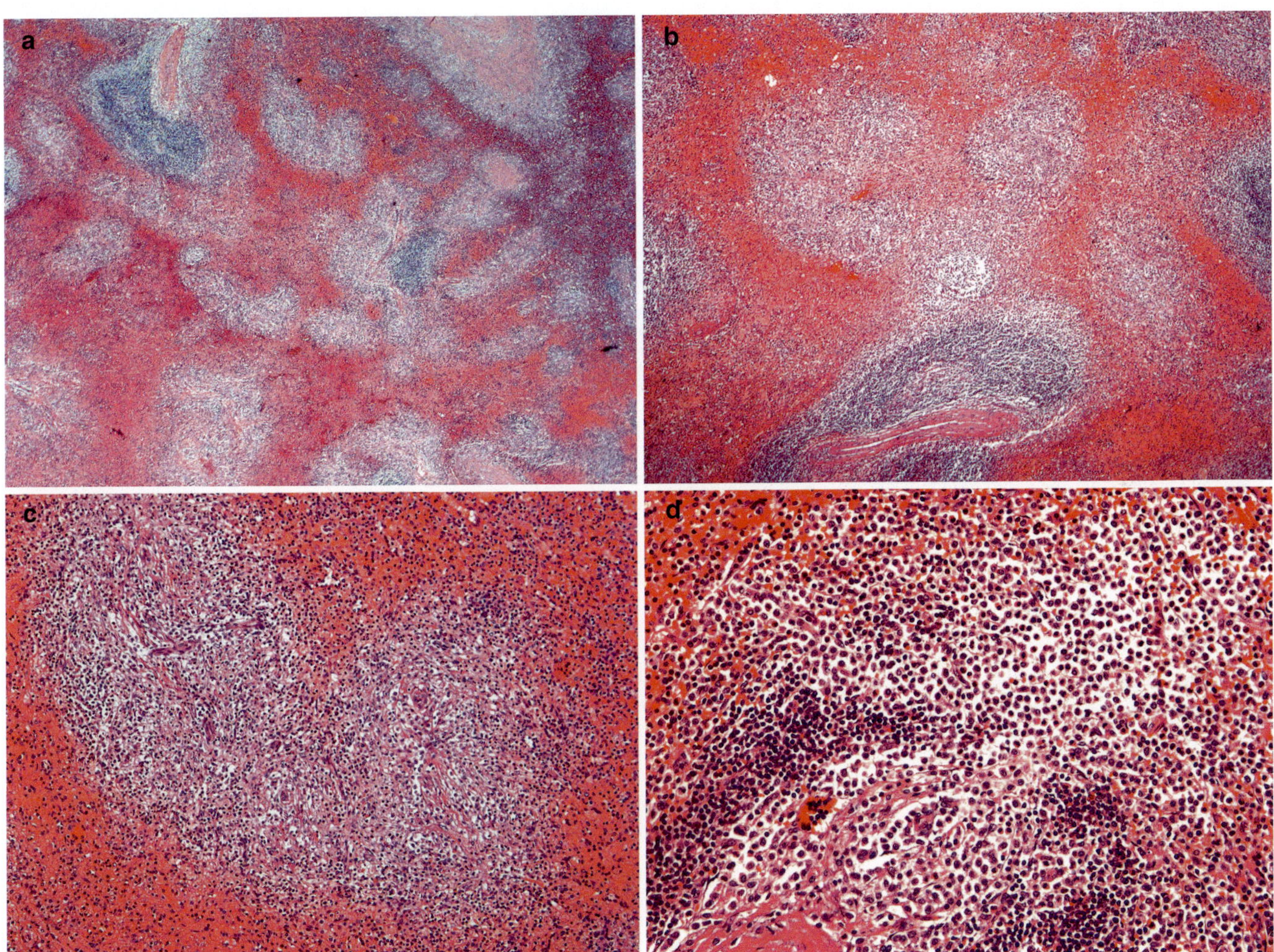

Fig. 16.10 Low power view of systemic mastocytosis involving the spleen. (**a**–**c**) The H&E sections of splenic parenchyma shows multiple nodular proliferation of mast cells, which are round to spindly and focally associated with small lymphocytes in loose aggregates. The background of red pulp congestion is identified (40×, 100×, and 200×, respectively). (**d**) Under higher power of view, the aggregates of mast cells display relatively low N:C ratio and pale cytoplasm, may resemble histiocytes, but show tight relationship with small groups of small lymphocytes (H&E, 600×). (**e**, **f**) Immunohistochemical stains highlight the mast cells to be positive for CD117 (**e**, 600×) and mast cell tryptase (**f**, ×600)

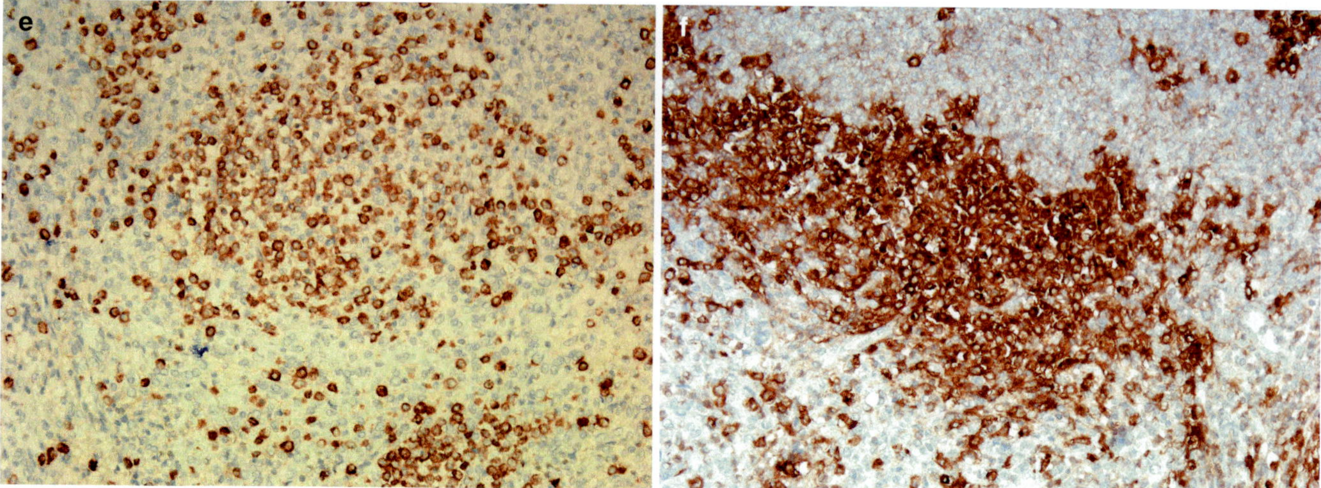

Fig. 16.10 (continued)

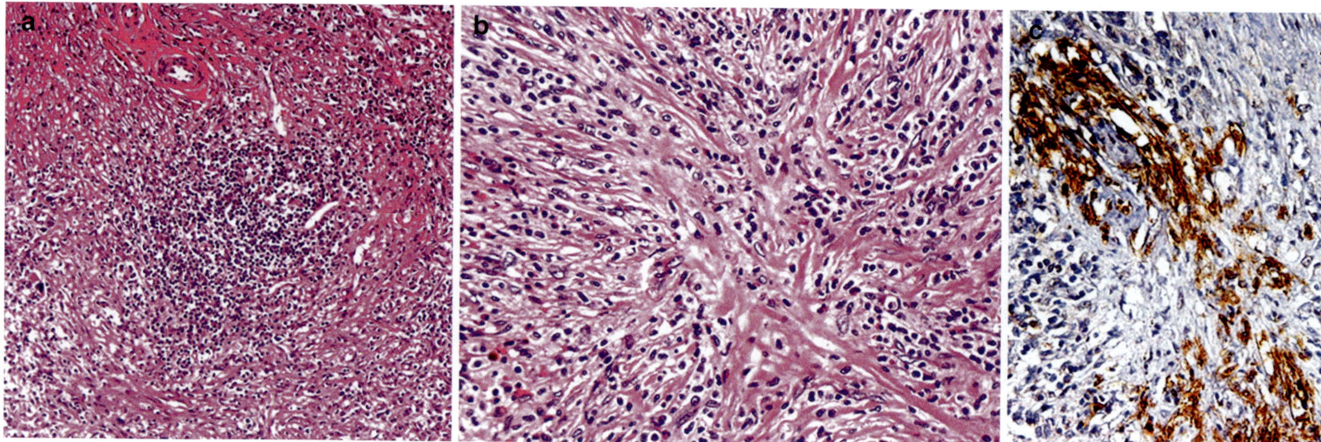

Fig. 16.11 Mastocytosis in the spleen. The spleen may appear nodular with fibrosis rimming residual white pulp (**a**). On higher magnification, increased spindle cells and small mononuclear cells may be embedded in the fibrosis with scattered eosinophils (**b**). Immunostaining for CD117 highlights the increased mast cells (**c**)

identify these cells. A background rich in eosinophils may be a helpful marker to prompt further evaluation. In advanced stages, portal fibrosis can be seen, with rare cases showing extensive, bridging fibrosis. Cirrhosis is uncommon [81]. In aggressive mastocytosis, the degree of liver fibrosis and infiltration by mast cells can result in portal hypertension, ascites, and liver failure. There may also be extramedullary hematopoiesis owing to extensive marrow infiltration, or nodular regenerative hyperplasia [82].

Molecular Findings

The most common genetic alteration, seen in over 93% of cases is the *KIT* D816V mutation, resulting in activation of catalytic domain of KIT [83, 84]. Secondary mutations may also be seen, including *TET2* (29%), *ASXL1* (17%), and *CBL* (11%) [85].

Differential Diagnosis

The differential diagnosis may include T-cell lymphoma, follicular hyperplasia, Kaposi's sarcoma, or granulomatous disease. Bland-appearing mast cells may be confused for hairy cell leukemia. Immunostaining, clinical correlation, flow cytometry, and molecular testing will be essential in resolving this differential.

Blastic Plasmacytoid Dendritic Cell Neoplasm

Definition

Blastic plasmacytoid dendritic cell neoplasm (BPDCN) is a rare, aggressive neoplasm arising from plasmacytoid dendritic cells. Patients are commonly older but pediatric cases have been reported.

Clinical Presentation

They traditionally present with multiple violaceous skin lesions and concurrent bone marrow or peripheral blood involvement.

Morphology and Immunophenotyping

Biopsy of the skin or bone marrow will show the presence of monomorphic infiltrate of blast-like cells with fine chromatin and multiple nucleoli. The diagnosis rests on demonstration of a characteristic immunophenotype with expression of CD4, CD56, and CD123 in the absence of

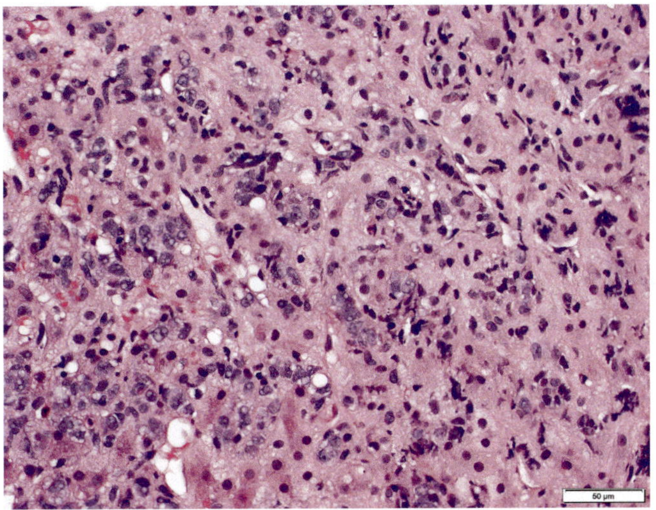

Fig. 16.12 The liver parenchyma is infiltrated by BPDCN cells associated with occasional inflammatory reaction (neutrophils) in the background. These atypical cells are medium in size and display irregular nuclear contour and vesicular chromatin (H&E, 1000×)

other myeloid and lymphoid antigens [86]. Newer antigens, including CD303/BDCA-2 and TCL1, are more sensitive [87].

Although splenomegaly and hepatomegaly are seen in 44% and 42% of patients with BPDCN, respectively, little information is available in the pathology literature [88]. In one case report, the spleen was diffusely infiltrated by lymphoblast-like cells with high mitotic activity. The blasts expressed CD4, CD56, CD123, HLA-DR, CD303, CD10, and CD1a [89]. BPDCN can rarely involve the liver (see Figs. 16.12 and 16.13) and show similar morphology and immunophenotype.

Cytogenetics

Cytogenetic analysis frequently shows a complex karyotype. The most common recurrent abnormality is deletion of 5, followed by losses on 12p, 13q, 6q, 15q, and monosomy 9 [90, 91].

Molecular Findings

Whole exome sequencing studies of BPDCN showed no commonly affected genes across all patients, but frequent mutations in *TET2*, *IKZF3*, and *ZEB2*. Overall, mutations affected DNA methylation or chromatin remodeling pathways [92].

Differential Diagnosis

The differential diagnosis for these cases is generally AML and acute lymphoblastic leukemia. Flow cytometric analysis and appropriate immunohistochemical staining can help resolve this differential. In addition, mature dendritic cell

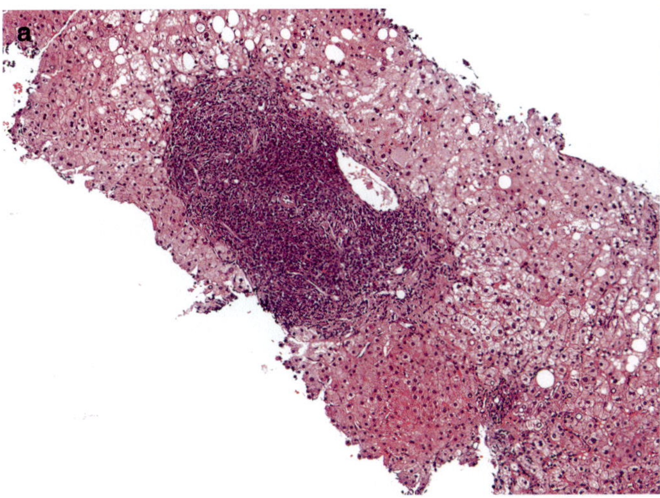
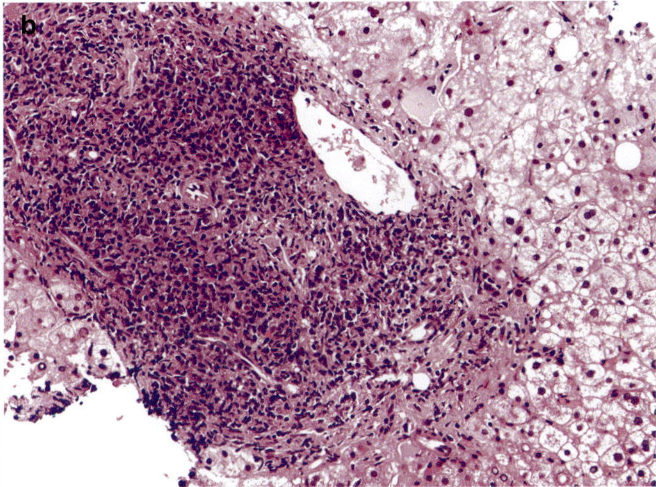

Fig. 16.13 (**a**, **b**) Microscopic examination of the needle core biopsy reveals distinct periportal nodular infiltrate by atypical cells associated with adjacent, relatively normal-appearing hepatocytes (H&E, 100× and 200×, respectively). (**c**) Higher power view of the atypical cells shows they have oval to elongated nuclei, fine chromatin, inconspicu-ous nucleoli, and a certain amount of cytoplasm (H&E, 600×). (**d–h**) A panel of immunohistochemical stains demonstrates characteristic immunophenotype for BPDCN: negative for CD34 (**d**), and positive for CD123 (**e**), CD4 (**f**), and TCL1 (**g**) (immunoperoxidase, 600×, respectively). TdT (**h**) is negative in the case (immunoperoxidase, 600×)

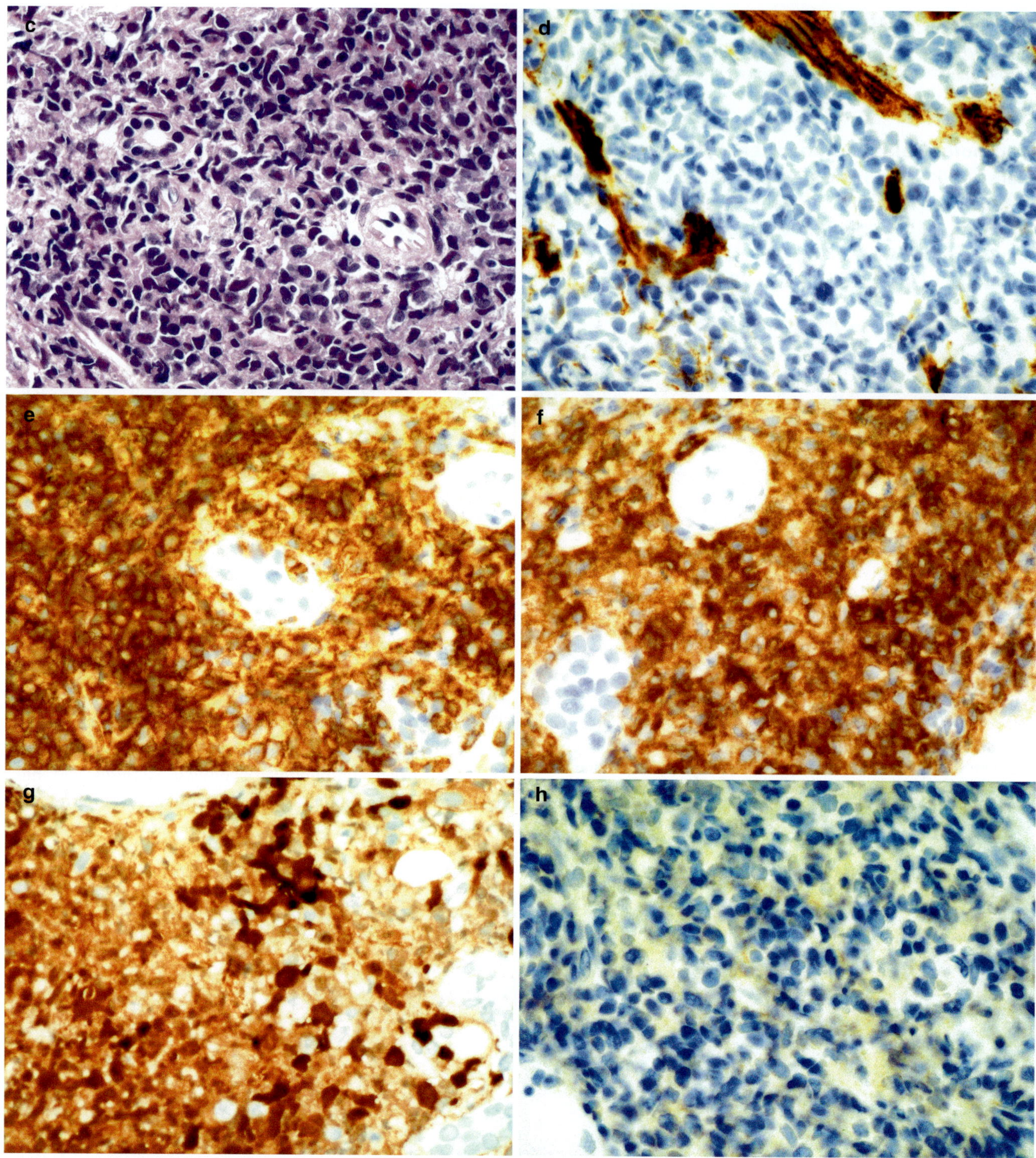

Fig. 16.13 (continued)

proliferations can be present in the spleen, but these are negative for CD56 and have a low Ki-67 proliferation index.

Prognosis

The prognosis for patients with BPDCN is uniformly poor, with a median overall survival of 10–20 months [93].

References

1. O'Malley DP, et al. Morphologic and immunohistochemical evaluation of splenic hematopoietic proliferations in neoplastic and benign disorders. Mod Pathol. 2005;18(12):1550–61.
2. Prakash S, et al. Splenic extramedullary hematopoietic proliferation in Philadelphia chromosome-negative myeloproliferative neo-

plasms: heterogeneous morphology and cytological composition. Mod Pathol. 2012;25(6):815–27.

3. Vardiman JW, Baccarani MJ, Radich JP, Kvasnicka HM. Chronic myeloid leukemia, BCR-ABL1 positive. In: Campo E, Swerdlow SH, Harris NL, Jaffe ES, Pileri SA, Stein H, Thiele J, editors. WHO classification of tumours of haematopoietic and lymphoid tissues. Lyon: IARC; 2017.

4. Savage DG, Szydlo RM, Goldman JM. Clinical features at diagnosis in 430 patients with chronic myeloid leukaemia seen at a referral centre over a 16-year period. Br J Haematol. 1997;96(1):111–6.

5. Ondreyco SM, et al. Monoblastic transformation in chronic myelogenous leukemia: presentation with massive hepatic involvement. Cancer. 1981;48(4):957–63.

6. Deininger MW, Goldman JM, Melo JV. The molecular biology of chronic myeloid leukemia. Blood. 2000;96(10):3343–56.

7. Thiele J, Kvasnicka H, Orazi A, Gianelli U, Barbui T, Barosi G, Tefferi A. Primary myelofibrosis. In: Campo E, Swerdlow SH, Harris NL, Jaffe ES, Pileri SA, Stein H, Thiele J, editors. WHO classification of tumours of haematopoietic and lymphoid tissues. Lyon: IARC; 2017.

8. Rumi E, et al. Familial chronic myeloproliferative disorders: clinical phenotype and evidence of disease anticipation. J Clin Oncol. 2007;25(35):5630–5.

9. Rumi E, et al. LNK mutations in familial myeloproliferative neoplasms. Blood. 2016;128(1):144–5.

10. Cervantes F, Barosi G. Myelofibrosis with myeloid metaplasia: diagnosis, prognostic factors, and staging. Semin Oncol. 2005;32(4):395–402.

11. Cervantes F, et al. Myelofibrosis with myeloid metaplasia in young individuals: disease characteristics, prognostic factors and identification of risk groups. Br J Haematol. 1998;102(3):684–90.

12. Barosi G, Hoffman R. Idiopathic myelofibrosis. Semin Hematol. 2005;42(4):248–58.

13. Tefferi A, Elliott MA, Pardanani A. Atypical myeloproliferative disorders: diagnosis and management. Mayo Clin Proc. 2006;81(4):553–63.

14. Ward HP, Block MH. The natural history of agnogenic myeloid metaplasia (AMM) and a critical evaluation of its relationship with the myeloproliferative syndrome. Medicine (Baltimore). 1971;50(5):357–420.

15. Wolf BC, Neiman RS. Myelofibrosis with myeloid metaplasia: pathophysiologic implications of the correlation between bone marrow changes and progression of splenomegaly. Blood. 1985;65(4):803–9.

16. Thiele J, et al. Idiopathic primary osteo-myelofibrosis: a clinicopathological study on 208 patients with special emphasis on evolution of disease features, differentiation from essential thrombocythemia and variables of prognostic impact. Leuk Lymphoma. 1996;22(3–4):303–17.

17. Cardoso FS, et al. Hepatic nodule: a case of primary myelofibrosis. BMJ Case Rep. 2011;2011:bcr0520114220.

18. Pitcock JA, et al. A clinical and pathological study of seventy cases of myelofibrosis. Ann Intern Med. 1962;57:73–84.

19. Pereira A, et al. Liver involvement at diagnosis of primary myelofibrosis: a clinicopathological study of twenty-two cases. Eur J Haematol. 1988;40(4):355–61.

20. Al-Mukhaizeem KA, Rosenberg A, Sherker AH. Nodular regenerative hyperplasia of the liver: an under-recognized cause of portal hypertension in hematological disorders. Am J Hematol. 2004;75(4):225–30.

21. Wanless IR, et al. Hepatic vascular disease and portal hypertension in polycythemia vera and agnogenic myeloid metaplasia: a clinicopathological study of 145 patients examined at autopsy. Hepatology. 1990;12(5):1166–74.

22. Barbui T, et al. Survival and disease progression in essential thrombocythemia are significantly influenced by accurate morphologic diagnosis: an international study. J Clin Oncol. 2011;29(23):3179–84.

23. Tefferi A, et al. CALR vs JAK2 vs MPL-mutated or triple-negative myelofibrosis: clinical, cytogenetic and molecular comparisons. Leukemia. 2014;28(7):1472–7.

24. Vannucchi AM, et al. Mutations and prognosis in primary myelofibrosis. Leukemia. 2013;27(9):1861–9.

25. Lundberg P, et al. Clonal evolution and clinical correlates of somatic mutations in myeloproliferative neoplasms. Blood. 2014;123(14):2220–8.

26. Tefferi A, et al. Long-term survival and blast transformation in molecularly annotated essential thrombocythemia, polycythemia vera, and myelofibrosis. Blood. 2014;124(16):2507–13; quiz 2615.

27. Thiele J, Kvasnicka H, Orazi A, Tefferi A, Birgegard G, Barbui T. Polycythemia vera. In: Campo E, Swerdlow SH, Harris NL, Jaffe ES, Pileri SA, Stein H, Thiele J, editors. WHO classification of tumours of haematopoietic and lymphoid tissues. Lyon: IARC; 2017.

28. Vannucchi AM, et al. Clinical profile of homozygous JAK2 617V>F mutation in patients with polycythemia vera or essential thrombocythemia. Blood. 2007;110(3):840–6.

29. Anger BR, et al. Budd-Chiari syndrome and thrombosis of other abdominal vessels in the chronic myeloproliferative diseases. Klin Wochenschr. 1989;67(16):818–25.

30. De Stefano V, et al. Recurrent thrombosis in patients with polycythemia vera and essential thrombocythemia: incidence, risk factors, and effect of treatments. Haematologica. 2008;93(3):372–80.

31. Smalberg JH, et al. Myeloproliferative neoplasms in Budd-Chiari syndrome and portal vein thrombosis: a meta-analysis. Blood. 2012;120(25):4921–8.

32. Putra J, et al. Multiple liver lesions in a patient with Budd-Chiari syndrome secondary to polycythemia vera. Ann Hepatol. 2015;14(4):547–9.

33. Tefferi A, et al. Survival and prognosis among 1545 patients with contemporary polycythemia vera: an international study. Leukemia. 2013;27(9):1874–81.

34. Tefferi A. Novel mutations and their functional and clinical relevance in myeloproliferative neoplasms: JAK2, MPL, TET2, ASXL1, CBL, IDH and IKZF1. Leukemia. 2010;24(6):1128–38.

35. Spivak JL. Polycythemia vera: myths, mechanisms, and management. Blood. 2002;100(13):4272–90.

36. Marchioli R, et al. Vascular and neoplastic risk in a large cohort of patients with polycythemia vera. J Clin Oncol. 2005;23(10):2224–32.

37. Polycythemia vera: the natural history of 1213 patients followed for 20 years. Gruppo Italiano Studio Policitemia. Ann Intern Med. 1995;123(9):656–64.

38. Titmarsh GJ, et al. How common are myeloproliferative neoplasms? A systematic review and meta-analysis. Am J Hematol. 2014;89(6):581–7.

39. Moulard O, et al. Epidemiology of myelofibrosis, essential thrombocythemia, and polycythemia vera in the European Union. Eur J Haematol. 2014;92(4):289–97.

40. Mehta J, et al. Epidemiology of myeloproliferative neoplasms in the United States. Leuk Lymphoma. 2014;55(3):595–600.

41. Murphy S, et al. Experience of the Polycythemia Vera Study Group with essential thrombocythemia: a final report on diagnostic criteria, survival, and leukemic transition by treatment. Semin Hematol. 1997;34(1):29–39.

42. Harrison CN, Green AR. Essential thrombocythemia. Hematol Oncol Clin North Am. 2003;17(5):1175–90.. vii

43. Tefferi A, et al. Cytogenetic findings and their clinical relevance in myelofibrosis with myeloid metaplasia. Br J Haematol. 2001;113(3):763–71.

44. Hoekstra J, et al. Long-term follow-up of patients with portal vein thrombosis and myeloproliferative neoplasms. J Thromb Haemost. 2011;9(11):2208–14.

45. Tefferi A, Vainchenker W. Myeloproliferative neoplasms: molecular pathophysiology, essential clinical understanding, and treatment strategies. J Clin Oncol. 2011;29(5):573–82.

46. Tefferi A, et al. Calreticulin mutations and long-term survival in essential thrombocythemia. Leukemia. 2014;28(12):2300–3.

47. Elliott MA, Tefferi A. Chronic neutrophilic leukemia: 2018 update on diagnosis, molecular genetics and management. Am J Hematol. 2018;93(4):578–87.

48. Elliott MA, et al. ASXL1 mutations are frequent and prognostically detrimental in CSF3R-mutated chronic neutrophilic leukemia. Am J Hematol. 2015;90(7):653–6.

49. Bain BJ, Brunning R, Orazi A, Thiele J. Chronic neutrophilic leukemia. In: Campo E, Swerdlow SH, Harris NL, Jaffe ES, Pileri SA, Stein H, Thiele J, editors. WHO classification of tumours of haematopoietic and lymphoid tissues. Lyon: IARC; 2017.

50. You W, Weisbrot IM. Chronic neutrophilic leukemia. Report of two cases and review of the literature. Am J Clin Pathol. 1979;72(2):233–42.

51. Maxson JE, et al. Oncogenic CSF3R mutations in chronic neutrophilic leukemia and atypical CML. N Engl J Med. 2013;368(19):1781–90.

52. Ouyang Y, et al. Clinical significance of CSF3R, SRSF2 and SETBP1 mutations in chronic neutrophilic leukemia and chronic myelomonocytic leukemia. Oncotarget. 2017;8(13):20834–41.

53. Meggendorfer M, et al. Specific molecular mutation patterns delineate chronic neutrophilic leukemia, atypical chronic myeloid leukemia, and chronic myelomonocytic leukemia. Haematologica. 2014;99(12):e244–6.

54. Elliott MA, et al. WHO-defined chronic neutrophilic leukemia: a long-term analysis of 12 cases and a critical review of the literature. Leukemia. 2005;19(2):313–7.

55. Zittoun R, et al. Chronic neutrophilic leukemia. A study of four cases. Ann Hematol. 1994;68(2):55–60.

56. Hasle H, et al. Chronic neutrophil leukaemia in adolescence and young adulthood. Br J Haematol. 1996;94(4):628–30.

57. Orazi A, Brunning J, Germin U, Brunning RD, Bain BJ, Cazzola M, Foucar K, Thiele J. Chronic Myelomonocytic Leukemia. In: Swerdlow SH CE, Harris NL, Jaffe ES, Pileri SA, Stein H, Thiele J, editors. WHO classification of tumours of haematopoietic and lymphoid tissues. Lyon: IARC; 2017.

58. Germing U, et al. Problems in the classification of CMML–dysplastic versus proliferative type. Leuk Res. 1998;22(10):871–8.

59. Onida F, et al. Prognostic factors and scoring systems in chronic myelomonocytic leukemia: a retrospective analysis of 213 patients. Blood. 2002;99(3):840–9.

60. Steensma DP, Tefferi A, Li CY. Splenic histopathological patterns in chronic myelomonocytic leukemia with clinical correlations: reinforcement of the heterogeneity of the syndrome. Leuk Res. 2003;27(9):775–82.

61. Harris NL, Demirjian Z. Plasmacytoid T-zone cell proliferation in a patient with chronic myelomonocytic leukemia. Histologic and immunohistologic characterization. Am J Surg Pathol. 1991;15(1):87–95.

62. Baddoura FK, Hanson C, Chan WC. Plasmacytoid monocyte proliferation associated with myeloproliferative disorders. Cancer. 1992;69(6):1457–67.

63. Boula AM, et al. Veno-occlusive disease of the liver associated with chronic myelomonocytic leukemia treated with vincristine and standard doses of cytarabine. Am J Hematol. 2005;79(3):216–9.

64. Abdel-Wahab O, et al. ASXL1 mutations promote myeloid transformation through loss of PRC2-mediated gene repression. Cancer Cell. 2012;22(2):180–93.

65. Carbuccia N, et al. Mutations of ASXL1 gene in myeloproliferative neoplasms. Leukemia. 2009;23(11):2183–6.

66. Patnaik MM, et al. Spliceosome mutations involving SRSF2, SF3B1, and U2AF35 in chronic myelomonocytic leukemia: prevalence, clinical correlates, and prognostic relevance. Am J Hematol. 2013;88(3):201–6.

67. Case records of the Massachusetts General Hospital. Weekly clinicopathological exercises. Case 37-1994. A newborn boy with petechiae, hepatosplenomegaly, leukocytosis, and thrombocytopenia. N Engl J Med. 1994;331(15):1005–12.

68. Freedman MH, Estrov Z, Chan HS. Juvenile chronic myelogenous leukemia. Am J Pediatr Hematol Oncol. 1988;10(3):261–7.

69. Niemeyer CM, et al. Chronic myelomonocytic leukemia in childhood: a retrospective analysis of 110 cases. European Working Group on Myelodysplastic Syndromes in Childhood (EWOG-MDS). Blood. 1997;89(10):3534–43.

70. Mikel JJ, Owen G, Lewis IJ. Hepatic fibrosis in juvenile chronic granulocytic leukemia: an unusual finding in three cases. Pediatr Pathol. 1990;10(3):385–95.

71. Tartaglia M, et al. Somatic mutations in PTPN11 in juvenile myelomonocytic leukemia, myelodysplastic syndromes and acute myeloid leukemia. Nat Genet. 2003;34(2):148–50.

72. Loh ML, et al. Mutations in PTPN11 implicate the SHP-2 phosphatase in leukemogenesis. Blood. 2004;103(6):2325–31.

73. Sakaguchi H, et al. Exome sequencing identifies secondary mutations of SETBP1 and JAK3 in juvenile myelomonocytic leukemia. Nat Genet. 2013;45(8):937–41.

74. Stieglitz E, et al. The genomic landscape of juvenile myelomonocytic leukemia. Nat Genet. 2015;47(11):1326–33.

75. Locatelli F, Niemeyer CM. How I treat juvenile myelomonocytic leukemia. Blood. 2015;125(7):1083–90.

76. De Santis GC, et al. Pathologic rupture of the spleen in a patient with acute myelogenous leukemia and leukostasis. Rev Bras Hematol Hemoter. 2014;36(4):290–2.

77. Rao Y, et al. Disseminated nonleukemic myeloid sarcoma of the spleen with involvement of the liver in an infant. J Pediatr Hematol Oncol. 2017;39(4):e233–5.

78. Walz-Mattmuller R, et al. Incidence and pattern of liver involvement in haematological malignancies. Pathol Res Pract. 1998;194(11):781–9.

79. Horny HP, Akin C, Arber DA, Peterson LC, Tefferi A, Metcalfe DD, Bennett JM, Bain BJ, Escribano L, Valent P. Mastocytosis. In: Swerdlow SH CE, Harris NL, Jaffe ES, Pileri SA, Stein H, Thiele J, editors. WHO classification of tumours of haematopoietic and lymphoid tissues. Lyon: IARC; 2017.

80. Hartmann K, Henz BM. Mastocytosis: recent advances in defining the disease. Br J Dermatol. 2001;144(4):682–95.

81. Mican JM, et al. Hepatic involvement in mastocytosis: clinicopathologic correlations in 41 cases. Hepatology. 1995;22(4 Pt 1):1163–70.

82. Kyriakou D, et al. Systemic mastocytosis: a rare cause of noncirrhotic portal hypertension simulating autoimmune cholangitis–report of four cases. Am J Gastroenterol. 1998;93(1):106–8.

83. Carter MC, Metcalfe DD, Komarow HD. Mastocytosis. Immunol Allergy Clin N Am. 2014;34(1):181–96.

84. Chatterjee A, Ghosh J, Kapur R. Mastocytosis: a mutated KIT receptor induced myeloproliferative disorder. Oncotarget. 2015;6(21):18250–64.

85. Pardanani A, et al. Next-generation sequencing in systemic mastocytosis: derivation of a mutation-augmented clinical prognostic model for survival. Am J Hematol. 2016;91(9):888–93.

86. Wilson CS, Medeiros LJ. Extramedullary manifestations of myeloid neoplasms. Am J Clin Pathol. 2015;144(2):219–39.

87. Boiocchi L, et al. BDCA-2 (CD303): a highly specific marker for normal and neoplastic plasmacytoid dendritic cells. Blood. 2013;122(2):296–7.

88. Pagano L, et al. Blastic plasmacytoid dendritic cell neoplasm with leukemic presentation: an Italian multicenter study. Haematologica. 2013;98(2):239–46.

89. Borchiellini D, et al. Blastic plasmacytoid dendritic cell neoplasm: a report of four cases and review of the literature. J Eur Acad Dermatol Venereol. 2013;27(9):1176–81.

90. Leroux D, et al. CD4(+), CD56(+) DC2 acute leukemia is characterized by recurrent clonal chromosomal changes affecting 6 major targets: a study of 21 cases by the Groupe Francais de Cytogenetique Hematologique. Blood. 2002;99(11):4154–9.

91. Fu Y, et al. Narrowing down the common deleted region of 5q to 6.0 Mb in blastic plasmacytoid dendritic cell neoplasms. Cancer Genet. 2013;206(7–8):293–8.

92. Menezes J, et al. Exome sequencing reveals novel and recurrent mutations with clinical impact in blastic plasmacytoid dendritic cell neoplasm. Leukemia. 2014;28(4):823–9.

93. Facchetti F, Piccaluga T, Pileri SA. Blastic plasmacytoid dendritic cell neoplasm. In: Campo E, Swerdlow SH, Harris NL, Jaffe ES, Pileri SA, Stein H, Thiele J, editors. WHO classification of tumours of haematopoietic and lymphoid tissues. Lyon: IARC; 2017.

Nukhet Tuzuner

Introduction

The histiocytoses are rare disorders characterized by the accumulation of cells thought to be derived from dendritic cells (DCs) or phagocytes. These hematopoietic-derived cells have long been grouped under the morphological term "histiocytes" (*referring to tissue-resident macrophages*) and their pathologic tissue proliferations termed as "the histiocytoses". DCs, monocytes, and macrophages are members of the mononuclear phagocyte system [1]. Macrophages are large cells that contain numerous cytoplasmic vacuoles, lysosomes, and mitochondria related to the clearance of debris, pathogens, and apoptotic cells. In contrast, DC's are responsible for the initiation of adaptive immune responses. They are starry cells with an irregular surface and numerous projections that contain abundant intracellular structures related to antigen processing.

The first classification of histiocytoses was published in 1987 [2] and followed by several contemporary classifications [3–5]. These classifications were based on biologic behavior, histopathology, and phenotype including "*dendritic cell*" related *[Langerhans cell histiocytosis (LCH), juvenile xanthoranuloma (JXG)]*, "*macrophage*" related *[hemophagocytic syndromes, Rosai-Dorfman disease (RDD)]*, and "*malignant*" disorders (*grouped by their most common morphologic and immunophenotypic counterpart*). World Health Organization (WHO) 2016 proposal has separated Erdheim-Chester disease (ECD) from disseminated juvenile xanthogranuloma (JXG) based on increasing data that this is a distinct disease [4, 5]. Recently, the revised classification scheme has more strongly emphasized the molecular signature of these disorders and pro-poses to lump disparate groups such as LCH and ECD based on common molecular alterations and overlapping clinical presentations. This revised classification system consists of 5 groups of diseases: (1) Langerhans-related (L group), (2) cutaneous and mucocutaneous (C group), (3) malignant histiocytoses (M group), (4) Rosai-Dorfman disease (R group), and (5) hemophagocytic lymphohistiocytosis and macrophage activation syndrome (H group) (Table 17.1) [6].

It is still important to recognize that despite our molecular advances, the diagnosis of many histiocytic neoplasms rests on congruent integration of the pathologic features of cell morphology, immunophenotype, and unique pattern of involvement. Phenotypic markers which are unique for histiocytes and dendritic cells are listed in Table 17.2. For correct diagnosis, pathologists must use an immunohistochemistry (IHC) panel appropriate to a cell in question and exclude other possibilities (e.g., lymphoma, melanoma, carcinoma).

Rosai-Dorfman Disease

Definition

Rosai-Dorfman disease (RDD) is a distinctive, reactive non-Langerhans cell histiocytosis primarily involving lymph nodes and less often involving extranodal sites. First recognized by Rosai and Dorfman in 1969 [7] as a distinctive benign entity characterized by marked, painless lymph node enlargement (*sinus histiocytosis with massive lymphadenopathy*). Extranodal manifestations of RDD with or without lymph node involvement account for approximately 25–43% of all cases [8–10] and can represent a diagnostic challenge because of mimicking neoplastic entities [10–13]. Histologically proven isolated spleen and liver involvement without lymphadenopathy in RDD is extremely rare.

N. Tuzuner (✉)
Department of Pathology, Istanbul University Cerrahpasa Medical Faculty, Fatih-Aksaray, Turkey

© Springer Nature Switzerland AG 2020
L. Zhang et al. (eds.), *Diagnostic Pathology of Hematopoietic Disorders of Spleen and Liver*,
https://doi.org/10.1007/978-3-030-37708-3_17

Table 17.1 Classification of histiocytoses based on histology, phenotype, and molecular alterations

L group histiocytoses
Langerhans cell histiocytosis (LCH)[a]
Indeterminate cell histiocytosis ICH)
Erdheim-Chester disease (ECD)[a]
Mixed LCH/ECD
C group histiocytoses
Cutaneous non-Langerhans cell histiocytoses
Cutaneous non-LCH histiocytoses with a major systemic component
R group histiocytoses
Familial Rosai-Dorfman disease (RDD)
Sporadic RDD
Classic RDD
Extranodal RDD
RDD with neoplasia or immune disease
Unclassified
M Group histiocytoses
Primary malignant histiocytoses
Secondary malignant histiocytoses (following or associated with another hematologic neoplasia)
Subtypes: *Histiocytic, interdigitating, Langerhans, indeterminate cell sarcoma*
H group histiocytoses
Primary HLH: Monogenic inherited conditions leading to HLH
Secondary HLH (non-Mendelian HLH)
HLH of unknown/uncertain origin

Modified from Emile et al. [6]

[a]LCH and ECD have similar frequencies of activating *BRAF*V600E mutations

Etiology and Pathogenesis

The etiology of RDD is unknown and considered an idiopathic histiocytosis. Infectious agents such as Epstein-Barr virus (EBV), human herpesvirus-6 (HHV6), and parvovirus B19 behind RDD have led to conflicting results and remains undetermined [8, 14–17].

The pathogenesis of RDD has also not been defined, but studies suggest that immune-mediated mechanisms and above-mentioned pathogens may be important. These pathogens and immune dysfunction probably act independently or synergistically to initiate the disturbance of homeostasis so as to drive the inflammatory process, which then triggers the recruitment of monocytes [18].

A significant portion of RDD shows features characteristic of IgG4-related disease, indicating these cases of RDD may overlap with IgG4-related disease [19, 20]. However, no clear evidence suggests that these disorders have a common etiopathogenesis.

Epidemiology

Classical head and neck nodal forms are more common in children and young adults though they can affect all ages and typically presents themselves during the second or third decades of life. There is a slight predilection for male patients [9]. The 423 cases in the sinus histiocytosis with

Table 17.2 Immunophenotypic markers in the differential diagnosis of histiocytic and dendritic cell proliferations

Marker	LCH/LCS	FDCS	IDCS	IDCT	HS	RDD	HLH	ECD
CD1a	++	−	−	++	−	−	−	−
S-100	++	+	++	++	+	++	+	+
Langerin	++	−	−	−	−	−	−	−
CD21	−	++	−	−	−	−	−	−
CD35	−	++	−	−	−	−	−	−
CD23	−	+	−	−	−	−	−	−
Clusterin	−	++	−	−	−	−	−	−
CD68	+	+	+/−	+/−	++	++	++	++
CD163	−	−	−	−	++	++	++	++
Lysozyme	−	−	+/−	+/−	++	++	++	++
Fascin	−	−	++	+	+/−	+/−	+/−	+/−
CD45	−	−	+/−	+/−	+/−	−	−	−
CD4	+	+	+	+	+	+	+	+
Ki-67	Variable	1–25%	10–20%	Variable	Variable	Low	Low	Low
EBER		++[a]						
Molecular *BRAF*V600E Mutation	LCH: 35–67% LCS: NA	18%; IPT-like 40%	Rare	Rare	Reported	Absent	Absent	>50%

LCH/LCS Langerhans cell histiocytosis/Langerhans cell sarcoma, *FDCS* follicular dendritic cell sarcoma, *IDCS* interdigitating cell sarcoma, *IDCT* indeterminate cell tumor, *HS* histiocytic sarcoma, *RDD* Rosai-Dorfman disease, *HLH* hemophagocytic lymphohistiocytosis, *EDC*Erdheim-Cesther disease

++: Positive; +:variable positive; +/−: weakly positive

[a]EBV-encoded RNA is positive in inflammatory pseudotumor (IPT) like FDCS by in situ hybridization

massive lymphadenopathy (SHML) registry reflect that people of African descent and the Whites are equally affected and that the disease is less common in the individuals of Asian descent [9]. Occasional familial cases have been reported. Extranodal involvement by sporadic RDD has been documented in 43% of cases with the most frequent sites being skin, nasal cavity, bone, soft tissue, and retro-orbital tissue [21]. In contrast to classic nodal form, there is a marked adult female predominance reported in the literature for the extranodal forms [10].

There were few case reports describing splenic involvement by RDD and in these cases there was also hepatic involvement as well [22, 23]. Isolated splenic involvement is extremely rare [24]. Hepatic involvement rarely occurs and accounts for only 1% of all cases of RDD [9, 25]. Typically, the liver is affected as a part of the systematic spread of RDD with nodal and wide extranodal involvement. Unlike patients with typical RDD, patients with the liver [23, 26–32] and spleen [22–24] involvements tend to be older, in the 5th–7th decades with female predominance.

Clinical Presentation

Patients with nodal RDD typically show bilateral painless cervical lymphadenopathy. The liver and spleen involvement by RDD is either associated with lymphadenopathy or it is an isolated initial manifestation of the disease. In cases without lymphadenopathy, presenting symptoms are usually nonspecific and most patients complain of abdominal pain, hepatomegaly. Laboratory features in RDD are often nonspecific [18]. Leukocytosis, elevated sedimentation rate (ESR), high ferritin levels, anemia, and polyclonal gammopathy have been reported in most patients [8, 9, 14, 33].

Gross Morphology and Radiological Findings

The spleen is enlarged and the cut surface revealed multifocal yellowish-brown or mahogany-colored patchy lesions without well-defined masses [22]. Computed tomography (CT) of few reported cases [22, 23] revealed multiple rounded hypodense splenic nodules measuring up to 2.0–3.0 cm and diffuse enlargement of liver with multiple focal hypodense lesions in both lobes [27, 34].

Microscopic Findings

Nodal RDD is characterized by massive lymphadenopathy with sinus histiocytosis. When involving extranodal sites, RDD shows similar morphologic features to its nodal counterpart. Interstitial or mass-like infiltrates consisting of mononuclear or multinucleated histiocytes with mildly pleomorphic nuclei and abundant pale cytoplasm in a background of lymphocytes, plasma cells, neutrophils, and few eosinophils are seen (Fig. 17.1). The presence of emperipolesis (Fig. 17.2) or the engulfment of lymphocytes and/or neutrophils by histiocytes is characteristic but not pathognomonic [7, 9]. In general, extranodal RDD exhibits more fibrosis, fewer typical histiocytes, and much less emperipolesis than its nodal counterpart. Prominent eosinophils or necrosis are not features of RDD and usually go against the diagnosis.

Immunohistochemical Study

The abnormal histiocytic cells stain for S100 protein, pan-macrophage antigens (CD68, CD163, CD14, CD15, CD68, and CD64), phagocytosis-related antigens (CD64 and IgG

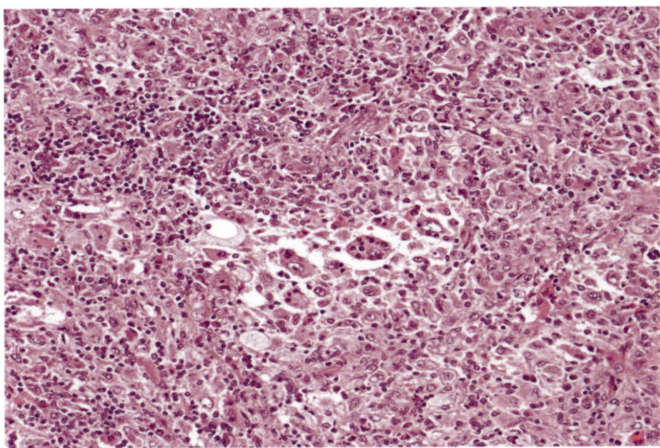

Fig. 17.1 Interstitial infiltrate consists of mononuclear or multinucleated histiocytes with abundant pale cytoplasm in a background of lymphocytes, plasma cells, neutrophils, and few eosinophils (H&E, 200×)

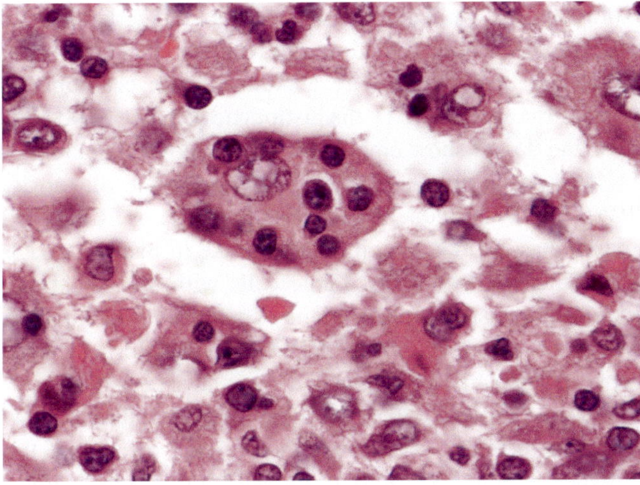

Fig. 17.2 Emperipolesis: the engulfment of lymphocytes and/or neutrophils by histiocytes is a characteristic feature (H&E, 400×)

Fc receptor), and antigens related to the lysosomal activity (lysozyme, α_1-antichymotrypsin). The histiocytic cells do not express CD1a, langerin and the dendritic markers CD21, CD23, and CD35 [8, 35].

Molecular Findings

In contrast to Langerhans cell histiocytosis (LCH) and Erdheim-Chester disease (ECD), no*BRAF*V600E mutations are found in RDD [36, 37]. However, very recently one case has been shown to harbor *BRAF*V600E mutation [38]. On the other hand, mutually exclusive *KRAS* and *MAP2K1* mutations were found in 33% of RDD cases which supports the idea that at least a subset of RDD cases is clonal, expanding the list of histiocytic and non-histiocytic disorders harboring MAPK/ERK pathway mutations [39]. Germline *SLC29A3* mutations (a gene encodes an intracellular equilibrative nucleoside transporter (hENT3) with affinity for adenosine) has been reported in familial Rosai-Dorfman disease [40].

Differential Diagnosis

The histologic differential diagnosis includes LCH, ECD, histiocytic sarcoma (HS), storage disorders, infections caused by *Histoplasma* and *mycobacteria*, monocytic and histiocytic malignancies, peripheral T-cell lymphoma, classic Hodgkin lymphoma, and IgG4-related disease. Identification of the characteristic histiocytic cells, particularly with emperipolesis, in the mixed inflammatory background is essential for distinguishing RDD from these other processes. Emperipolesis is rare or absent in reactive histiocytic proliferations. However, erythrophagocytosis is usually seen in reactive and/or neoplastic histiocytic proliferations. Unlike RDD histiocytes, Langerhans cells have small, usually folded or grooved nuclei that express CD1a and langerin and are associated with eosinophilic micro-abscesses. In ECD, the histiocytic cells are S100 negative and do not show emperipolesis; moreover, the characteristic bone lesions are present to suggest the diagnosis. *BRAF* V600E is frequently identified in LCH or ECD. True granulomas are not seen in RDD, unlike in histiocyte-rich granulomatous infections. Large cells with nuclear atypia and immunohistochemical staining can help to differentiate malignant disorders from RDD. Overlapping features between RDD and IgG4-related disease have been discussed in multiple reports [19, 20]. Most single reproducible discriminant between RDD and IgG4-related disease is the presence of immunoreactivity for S100 protein in lesional histiocytes of RDD [41, 42].

Prognosis

Treatment for the RDD is not recommended unless the disorder becomes life or organ threatening, since the disease will resolve spontaneously in most cases [8]. Complete surgical resection (e.g., splenectomy) is the best option for the treatment of the localized disease. Hematologic deterioration due to hypersplenism, such as hemolytic anemia with reticulocytosis and thrombocytopenia, dramatically improved after splenectomy [22, 24].

The liver is generally affected as a part of the systematic spread of RDD with nodal and wide extranodal involvement of those cases will have a bad prognosis [26, 29]. In a few localized cases, prognosis appears to be good [28]. It is possible to conclude that the prognosis of RDD is mainly dependent on the number of extranodal sites involved by the disease rather than its specific localization. In addition, RDD patients accompanying with immunologic diseases also do poorly than those without such diseases [9].

Diagnostic Caveats

- Rosai-Dorfman disease is not limited in lymph nodes. Extranodal manifestations of RDD with or without lymph node involvement account for approximately 25–43% of all cases.
- Extranodal manifestations of RDD can represent a diagnostic challenge because of mimicking neoplastic entities.
- Spleen and liver are usually affected as a part of the systemic spread of RDD. Histologically proven isolated spleen and/or liver involvement without lymphadenopathy are extremely rare.
- Some cases of RDD may overlap with IgG4-related disease. But, no clear evidence suggests that these disorders have a common etiopathogenesis.
- Engulfment of lymphocytes and/or neutrophils by histiocytes (emperipolesis) is a characteristic but not a pathognomonic feature of RDD.
- The histiocytes of RDD are characteristically S-100 positive as well as pan monocyte/macrophage antigens. They are negative for CD1a, a useful marker to exclude LCH.
- Activating *BRAF*V600E mutations are not seen in RDD.
- It is important to distinguish reactive or malignant histiocytic proliferations from RDD.
- Erythrophagocytosis is seen both in reactive and neoplastic histiocytic proliferations but emperipolesis is rare or absent in reactive histiocytic proliferations.
- Especially in classic nodal form RDD is often a self-limited disease with a good outcome, however, 5–11% of patients may die of their disease.

Langerhans Cell Histiocytosis (LCH)

Definition

Langerhans cell histiocytosis (LCH) is a rare disease characterized by the clonal proliferation of pathogenic Langerhans cells and cytokine overproduction. This leads to inflammation and tissue destruction in different organs of the body [43]. Normal counterpart is presumed to be mature Langerhans cell [44, 45]. In the updated version (WHO-2016), there are 2 types of Langerhans cell tumors: Langerhans cell histiocytosis (LCH) and Langerhans cell sarcoma (LCS). They are separated into either LCH or LCS based on the degree of cytologic atypia and clinical aggressiveness [5, 44].

Etiology and Pathogenesis

The cause of LCH is unknown. Langerhans cell proliferation may be induced by a viral infection, especially human herpesvirus 6(HHV-6) [46, 47], a defect in T cell–macrophage interaction, and/or a cytokine-driven process mediated by tumor necrosis factor (TNF), IL-11, and leukemia inhibitory factor [48]. Smoking may play a role as a chronic irritant in pulmonary LCH.

Although the epidermal Langerhans cell has presumed to be the cell of origin in LCH, it is currently proved that Langerhans cells have the gene expression profile of a myeloid-derived precursor or dendritic cell, not the Langerhans cell in the skin [49]. Therefore, in addition to epidermal Langerhans cells, a variety of other cellular populations may acquire a Langerhans cell phenotype (*expression of langerin and Birbeck granules*) that can be induced by local environmental stimuli [50]. Moreover, *BRAF*V600E mutation arises from somatic mutation of a hematopoietic progenitor in patients who develop high-risk LCH, whereas the mutation arises in tissue-restricted precursor dendritic cells in patients with the low-risk disease [51].

Epidemiology

LCH is generally considered to be a disease of childhood, and adults are rarely affected. The incidence of LCH is estimated to be 1 per 200,000 children [52], and approximately 2–5 cases per million per year for adults [44, 53]. The typical form is more common in females (F/M: 2:1.5) and usually affects children between 1 and 3 years of age [54]. Among adults, the incidence is 10 times less and the mean age for LCH diagnosis is 30 years of age, but the range is wide. In a series of 274 patients from 12 countries, 25% of the patients were older than 43 years old and 10% were over 55 [55]. The adult form is more often observed in males (M/F: 3.7:1). The rate of liver involvement in children is 52% and the majority of the patients were disseminated cases [56].

Clinical Presentation

The clinical presentation may be variable, and can be stratified in two major categories: "single-system" or "multisystem". Single-system is further subdivided into single site (solitary bone, skin, and lung) and multiple sites (multiple bone, skin, liver, spleen, bone marrow, and lymph nodes). Multisystem is defined as the involvement of two or more organs. The liver, spleen, and bone marrow are considered as "risk organs", involvement of any with LCH places patients at higher risk of mortality [57].

The spleen and liver involvements are usually seen as a part of the multisystem disease. LCH confined to the spleen or liver is extremely rare [58, 59]. Evaluation of organ involvement remains difficult, particularly for splenomegaly. Physical exam or imaging are the standard methods for evaluation, but they do not reveal the underlying process causing organ enlargement [60]. LCH in the bone marrow causes pancytopenia, but thrombocytopenia with bleeding and anemia may be exacerbated by an enlarged spleen. Liver disease in LCH has the clinical, histological, and radiological hallmarks of sclerosing cholangitis and may progress rapidly [61].

Morphology

Spleen shows multinodular involvement of red pulp. Radiologically, liver and spleen images reveal nodular hypo-attenuating and irregular lesions [62], MR images with diffuse miliary nodules and no expansion of the intrahepatic bile duct may be misdiagnosed as diffuse liver cancer [63]. It predominantly involves the red pulp in the form of a diffuse infiltrate, or as ill-defined tumor aggregates resembling loosely formed granulomas.

Microscopy

The lesions of LCH, which can be found nearly in any organ with the exception of the kidneys, represent an accumulation of LCH cells admixed with an inflammatory background formed of eosinophils, lymphocyte-activated macrophages, and osteoclast-like multinucleated giant cells [64] (Fig. 17.3). LCH cells are large epithelioid cells with abundant eosinophilic cytoplasm. The nuclei are irregular with prominent folds and grooves, fine chromatin, and indistinct nucleoli (Fig. 17.4). Nuclear atypia is minimal but mitotic activity is variable.

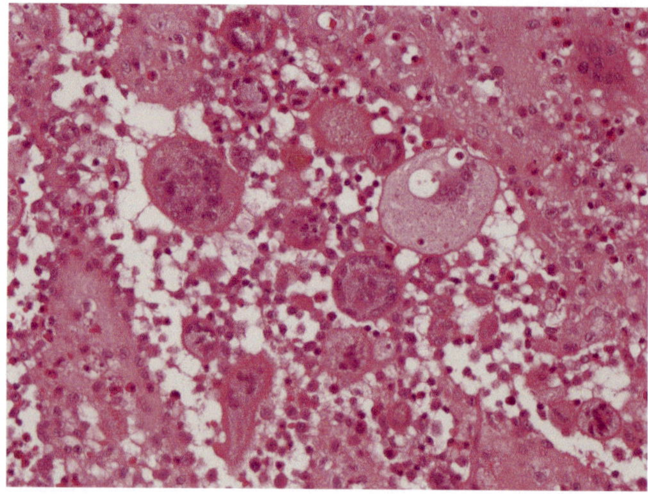

Fig. 17.3 Langerhans cell histiocytosis. LCH cells admixed with an inflammatory background and osteoclast-like multi-nucleated giant cells (H&E, 400×)

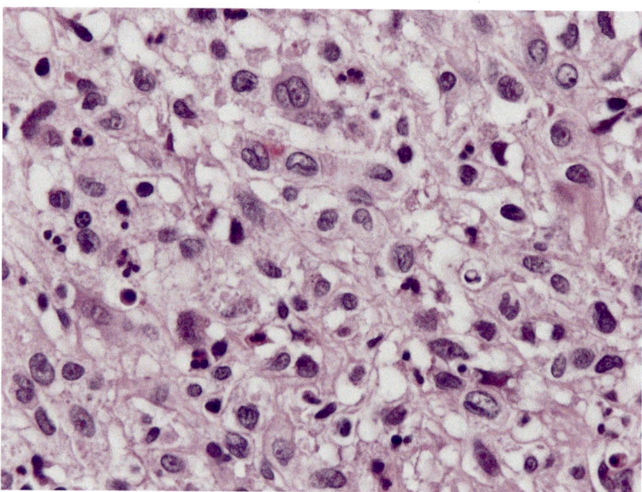

Fig. 17.4 Langerhans cell histiocytosis. The nuclei of LCH cells are irregular with prominent folds and grooves, fine chromatin, and in distinct nucleoli. Nuclear atypia is minimal (H&E, 400×)

In the spleen, the red pulp is preferentially involved as in other myeloid neoplasms. LCH predominantly involves the red pulp in the form of a sinusoidal involvement or ill-defined tumor aggregates resembling loosely formed granulomas [65]. Other abnormalities observed in the spleen include hemorrhages and areas or necrosis and infarction. Two distinct forms of liver involvement is described: (1) nodular Langerhans cell infiltration of the liver due to parenchymal infiltration by Langerhans cells, (2) LCH infiltration centered on bile ducts with little or no histiocytic infiltration, which is associated with chronic fibrosis, progresses to sclerosing cholangitis (SC) [58].

Immunohistochemical Findings

The characteristic immunophenotype of LCH includes expression of langerin (CD207) (Fig. 17.7), CD1a and S100 protein (Fig. 17.5a, b). Expressions of CD68, vimentin, and HLA-Dr are variable. CD207 is a type II transmembrane C-type lectin associated with the formation of Birbeck granules and is highly characteristic for Langerhans cells. Markers for FDC, such as CD21, CD23, and CD35, T-cell and B-cell lineage markers and CD30 are negative [66]. Interdigitating dendritic cells (S100 protein+, CD1a-, CD207-) and indeterminate dendritic cells (S100 protein+, CD1a+, CD207-) are both S100+ and closely related to Langerhans cells; however, they do not express CD207 [66].

Cytogenetics and Molecular Findings

No recurrent chromosomal abnormalities have been reported in LCH. Clonality was established by X-linked androgen receptor gene assay (HUMARA) in early stud-

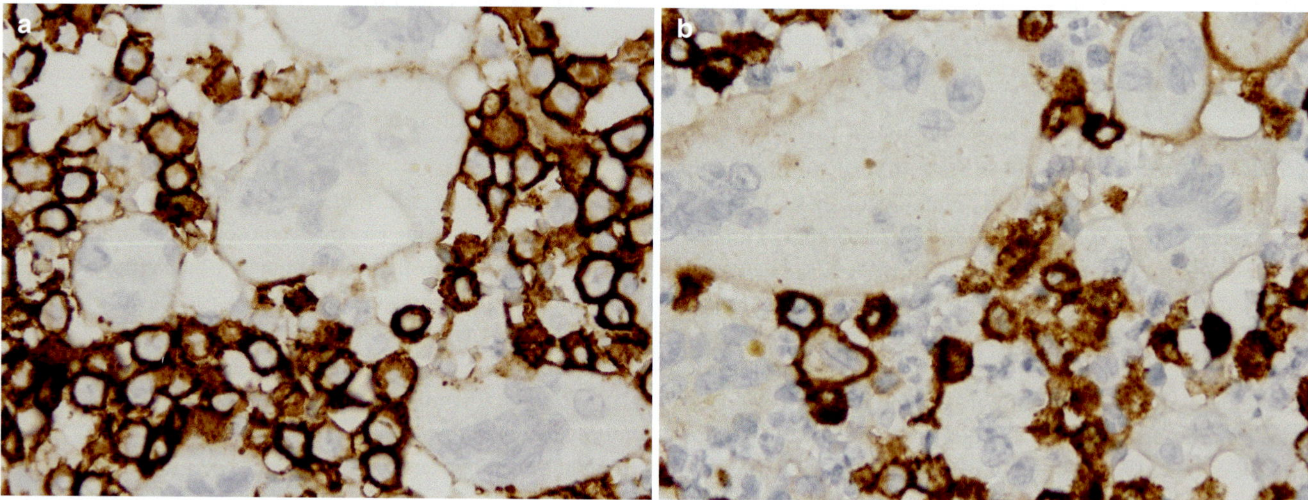

Fig. 17.5 (**a**, **b**) Langerhans cell histiocytosis. Proliferating Langerhans cells are strongly positive for CD1a (**a**) and CD207/Langerin (**b**) Multinucleated histiocytic cells are not stained (Immunoperoxidase stain CD1a & CD207 with hematoxylin counterstain, 1000×, respectively)

ies. However, 71% of pulmonary LCH was found to be non-clonal [66].

LCH and ECD frequently harbor somatic mutations in the *RAS, ARAF, BRAF*, and *MAP2K1* genes, which encode the first three tiers of the canonical RAS-RAF-MEK-ERK pathway [67]. *BRAF*V600E mutation is detected in 38–64% of all cases, including pulmonary LCH [51, 68, 69], while other V600 codon mutations are typically absent [70]. Experiments have suggested that *BRAF* V600E mutation may be mitogenic for dendritic cells [51]. However, *BRAF* V600E mutation is neither lineage nor disease-specific since it has been reported in other dendritic and histiocytic neoplasms and Erdheim-Chester diseases (ECD) as well as LCH. Moreover, it is also seen in melanoma, astrocytic neoplasms, hairy cell leukemia, and carcinomas [66, 71]. The demonstration that LCH cells are clonal, along with the recent discovery of activating *BRAF* mutations in LCH cells, strongly suggests that LCH is a neoplastic disease despite its prominent inflammatory component and occasional benign clinical course [43]. The use of mutation-specific *BRAF*V600E immunohistochemistry (IHC) as a surrogate for molecular testing in LCH is under progress. However, preliminary studies showed that BRAF IHC may not be a reliable surrogate for mutation status in LCH [72, 73].

Differential Diagnosis

Clinical symptoms of the RDD, mastocytosis, and Erdheim-Chester disease (ECD) can be similar to those of LCH. Histologically, LCH has to be differentiated from Langerhans cell hyperplasia, Langerhans cell sarcoma, indeterminate cell histiocytosis, mastocytosis (urticarial pigmentosa), and juvenile xanthogranuloma [74]. Differential diagnosis also includes sinusoidal proliferations of the lymph nodes such as RDD, benign sinusoidal hyperplasia, metastatic carcinoma, and malignant melanoma. Moreover, large numbers of Langerhans cells are present in lymph nodes showing dermatopathic lymphadenopathy. However, in dermatopathic lymphadenopathy, LCs are present in the paracortical areas and are not seen in the sinuses [65].

The distinction of LC hyperplasia from LCH may not be possible by morphology and IHC but can be made by clonality and/or mutation analyses [75]. Adult-onset of LCH can be confused with ECD. Histologically, LCH has been characterized by polymorphic background infiltrate of T lymphocytes, macrophages, multinucleated giant cells and eosinophils mixed with LCs, with or without areas of necrosis. Immunophenotypes of Langerhans cells are CD68+, CD1a+, S100+, and CD207+. Birbeck granules are shown by electron microscopy in the cytoplasm. In contrast, diffuse infiltration dominated by large, foamy histiocytes, rare Touton-like giant cells, fibrosis and lymphocytic aggregates, or xanthogranulomatosis are the characteristic features of

ECD. Histiocytic cells are CD68+, S100-, CD1a-, Langerin-, and lack of Birbeck granules [74].

Rare cases of ECD associated with LCH have been reported suggesting that both proliferations could derive from a common progenitor [67]. Similarly, the co-occurrence of RDD and LCH as a very rare phenomenon has been reported [76, 77]. LCH is a clonal and neoplastic disease usually associated with BRAF mutation [6, 51, 68]. In contrast, RDD is still supposed to be a reactive disease [6]. In reported RDD-LCH cases, RDD appeared secondarily and suggesting that the RDD might be a reactive response to LCH. However, pathophysiology still remains unclear.

Prognosis

The clinical course of LCH depends on the degree of systems or organs involved, with bone marrow, liver, spleen, or pulmonary involvement being listed as poor prognostic factors. More than 99% of LCH patients with single-site involvement are alive [44, 45, 66], while the mortality rate of patients with multisystem involvement is 50–66% [66].

Liver involvement in adult LCH must be searched for not only in multi-organ disease but also in localized LCH forms [78] and it can even be the first manifestation of LCH. It seems very important to diagnose it at an early stage, allowing a better prognosis. Liver biopsy has an important place in the diagnosis and management [58].

Diagnostic Caveats

- Langerhans cells have the gene expression profile of a myeloid-derived precursor or dendritic cell, not the Langerhans cell in the skin.
- LCH is considered to be a disease of childhood, adults are rarely affected.
- Spleen and liver involvement is usually seen part of the multisystem disease and are considered risk organs as well as bone marrow.
- Isolated LCH confined to the spleen or liver is extremely rare.
- Splenic involvement by LHC causes splenomegaly and splenomegaly may be exacerbated to anemia and thrombocytopenia with bleeding.
- Liver involvement by LHC causes sclerosing cholangitis.
- Liver involvement in adult LCH may be seen either in multi-organ disease or in localized disease and it can even be the first manifestation of LCH.
- Diagnosis of liver LCH at an early stage allows a better prognosis. Liver biopsy has an important place in the diagnosis and management.
- Lesions of LCH can be found in any organ with the exception of the kidneys.

- The distinction of LC hyperplasia from LCH may not be possible by morphology and IHC but can be made by clonality and/or mutation analyses.
- Irregular nuclei with prominent folds and grooves are typical morphology for LCs.
- The characteristic immunophenotype of LCs is the expression of langerin (CD207), CD1a, and S100 protein.
- The *BRAF* V600E mutation is detected in 38–64% of all cases.
- Preliminary BRAF IHC may not be a reliable surrogate for mutation status in LCH.

Langerhans Cell Sarcoma

Definition

Langerhans cell sarcoma (LCS) is a rare and aggressive entity, belonging to the family of histiocytic sarcomas (HS) recently reclassified in the M group malignant histiocytoses [6].

Epidemiology

LCS may develop in any age group (median age 41 years), but few cases have been reported in patients aged 10 or younger [79]. LCS is more often observed in females (M/F: 1:2) [80]. In a systemic review of 66 patients with LCS, the most commonly affected sites at diagnosis were lymph nodes (74%) followed by the skin (48.5%), lung (28.8%), liver (16.7%), and spleen (15%). Single site involvement that was seen in 33% and 41% of the cases had disseminated disease [81].

Morphology

The liver and spleen images of LCH such as periportal low density, splenomegaly and multiple low-density lesions on contrast-enhanced CT images may be seen in cases of LCS due to the similar pathophysiology.

Microscopy

The diagnosis of LCS is based on malignant cytological features such as atypia, hyperchromatic nuclei, prominent nucleoli, frequent mitotic figures. However, the diagnosis of borderline lesions remains challenging because precise diagnostic criteria for malignancy are lacking and diagnosis should only be confirmed in patients with rapidly progressing tumors [6].

Immunophenotyping

Although there may be a tendency for lower expression of immune markers in LCS, there is no clear difference in immunophenotypic profiles (*CD1a+, S100+, langerin+, CD68+/−*) between LCH and LCS. In addition, Birbeck granules may be shown by EM in some cases. Histologically, LCS has to be differentiated from other epithelial or mesenchymal malignancies which are mainly based on phenotypic analysis with exclusion of other tumors by negativity for keratins, EMA, Melan-A, HMB45, B and T lymphocyte markers, and follicular DC markers.

Molecular Study

Little is known about molecular alterations in LCS. Whether LCH and LCS could share genetic abnormalities, and whether any mutation could explain the aggressive behavior of LC proliferations and/or could predict the aggressive transformation of LCH into LCS remain unknown [82]. LCS, like other M group histiocytoses occur after or sometimes simultaneously with other hematologic neoplasms such as follicular lymphoma [83], chronic lymphocytic leukemia [82], marginal zone lymphoma [84], and hairy cell leukemia [85]. Clonal relationship between primary lymphoid tumor and LCS has been established. This enigma may be explained, either from anaplastic progression with aberrant expression of some histiocyte and/or DC markers, or from a trans-differentiation of lymphoid tumor into LCS [6, 82, 83]. Complete surgical excision with clear margins is the most effective treatment for local disease control. In disseminated diseases, multi-modality therapy and/or bone marrow transplantation appears to be the most reliable treatment [81].

Diagnostic Caveats

- Langerhans cell sarcoma (LCS) is a rare and aggressive entity, belongs to the family of histiocytic sarcomas.
- Lymph nodes are the commonly affected sites at diagnosis. Most of the patients have disseminated disease.
- The diagnosis of LCS is based on malignant cytological features but the diagnosis of borderline lesions remains challenging.
- No clear difference is found in immunophenotypic profiles between LCH and LCS (*CD1a+, S100+, langerin+, CD68+/−*).
- LCS, like HS may occur after or sometimes simultaneously with another hematologic neoplasm which is clonally related.

Histiocytic Sarcoma (HS)

Definition

Histiocytic sarcoma (HS) is a rare, aggressive hematopoietic neoplasm derived from non-Langerhans histiocytic cells of the monocyte/macrophage system and is not a true sarcoma. Neoplastic cells show morphologic and immunophenotypic features of mature tissue histiocytes. In the 2016 revised classification of histiocytoses and neoplasms of the macrophage-dendritic cell lineages, the term malignant histiocytosis is used to refer to HS [4, 6].

Primary HS of the spleen is exceedingly rare. However, it seems a unique clinical entity; associated with hypo-albuminemia, hypo-γ-globulinemia, and thrombocytopenia [86–89]. Although the liver is the most common site of murine HS [90], primary hepatic HS in humans is very rare.

Etiology

There are no known environmental or hereditary genetic factors predisposing to the development of HS. The pathogenesis of HS is also unclear.

Epidemiology

Histiocytic sarcoma accounts for <1% of all hematolymphoid neoplasms and occurs in all age groups, but is most common in adults. A recent study of 159 cases of HS (99 men, 60 women) from the US Surveillance, Epidemiology, and End Results (SEER) database reported a median age at diagnosis of 63 years (range 18–96 years) and was similar in both sexes. The overall incidence of HS was 0·17 per 1,000,000 individuals [13]. HS may be a sporadic disease or may be related to a synchronous or metachronous hematologic malignancy, such as acute lymphoblastic leukemia or follicular lymphoma. When HS occurs in the context of another hematologic malignancy, the two entities are often clonally related [80, 91, 92]. Solid tumors with morphologic and immunophenotypic features consistent with HS occurring in the context of acute monocytic leukemia are not considered HS.

Clinical Presentation

HS often presents at extranodal sites and followed by lymph nodes. In previous case series the most common primary sites appear to be skin, GI tract, and the lymph nodes [80, 93] with few examples arising in the spleen [80, 86–89, 94, 95], liver [96, 97], or at other extranodal sites. According to the recent SEER database [98],; the most common site of the presentation is skin and soft tissue (35.8%), followed by lymph nodes (17%), respiratory system (8.2%), and nervous system (7.5%). Rarely a more systemic presentation with multiple sites of involvement can be seen. Skin involvement has numerous potential manifestations ranging from solitary tumors to innumerable lesions on the trunk and extremities.

Morphology

Diagnostic imaging findings have not been characterized satisfactorily, but in most reported primary splenic HS cases often show multi-nodular or nodular lesions in the enlarged tissues of the spleen. Gross features of splenectomy specimens are nodular or multinodular lesions with or without fibrous encapsulation, composed of a diffuse proliferation of malignant cells predominantly in a sinusoidal pattern within the red pulp.

Microscopy

The individual neoplastic cells are usually large and round to oval in shape. However, focal areas of spindle features may be present (Fig. 17.6). The cytoplasm is usually abundant and eosinophilic, often foamy, vacuolated, or clear (Fig. 17.7). The nuclei are pleomorphic grooved, indented, convoluted, or irregularly folded and slightly eccentric with moderately dispersed chromatin and one or more prominent nucleoli (Fig. 17.8). Nuclear atypia varies from mild to severe. Multilobated, binucleated, or large multinucleated forms are commonly seen (Fig. 17.9). Necrosis and vascular invasion may be present. A variable number of reactive cells are present, including small lymphocytes, plasma cells, benign histiocytes, and eosinophils.

In the spleen, neoplastic infiltration is mainly within the sinuses and cords of the red pulp. Erythrocytes and leukocytes are occasionally observed in the cytoplasm of the tumor cells. However, hemophagocytosis is more commonly seen in reactive cells than in tumor cells [80].

Immunohistochemistry

On immunohistochemistry, by definition, neoplastic cells express one or more histiocytic markers including CD68 (KP1 and PGM1) and lysozyme (Fig. 17.10a, b), but do not express specific T- and B-cell markers, myeloid cell markers (e.g., CD 33 myeloperoxidase), follicular dendritic cell

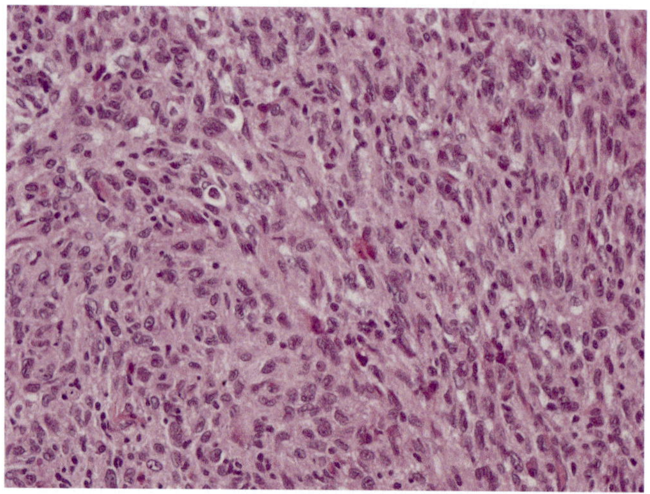

Fig. 17.6 Histiocytic sarcoma. Individual neoplastic cells are usually large and round to oval in shape and focal areas of spindle features are also present. (H&E, 400×)

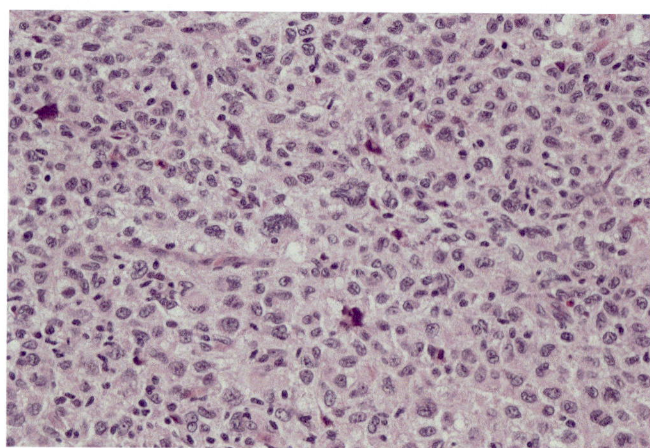

Fig. 17.8 Histiocytic sarcoma. The nuclei are pleomorphic, indented, or irregularly folded with moderately dispersed chromatin and one or more nucleoli (H&E, 400×)

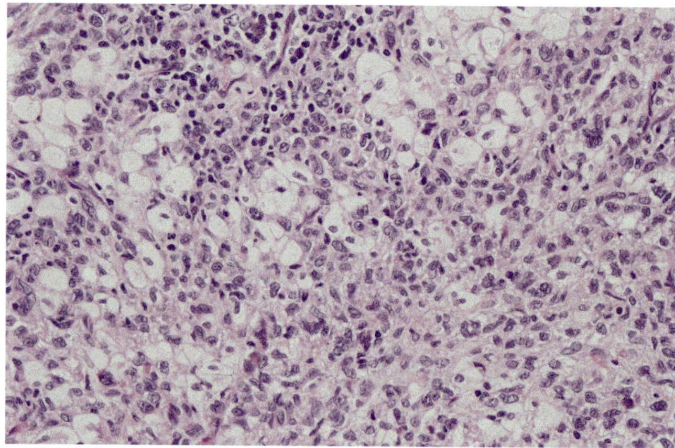

Fig. 17.7 Histiocytic sarcoma. Some of the neoplastic cells have foamy, vacuolated, or clear cytoplasm (H&E, 00×)

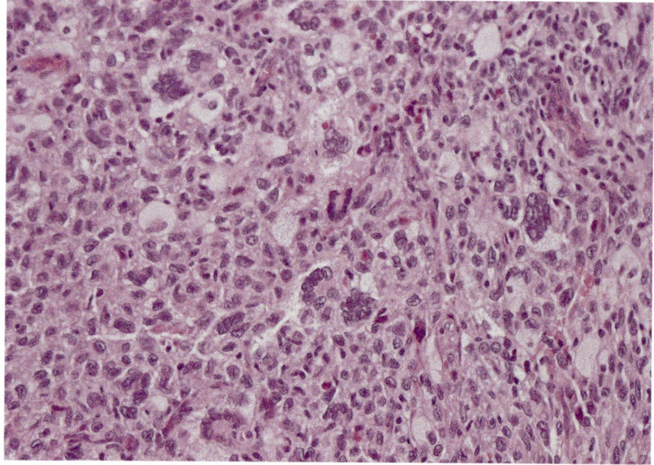

Fig. 17.9 Histiocytic sarcoma. Nuclear atypia varies from mild to severe. Multilobated, binucleated, or large multinucleated forms are present (H&E, 400×)

markers (CD21, CD23, CD35), Langerhans cell markers (CD1a, langerin), or keratins [80, 92, 93, 99]; staining for lysozyme is usually granular with accentuation of the Golgi [80]. Among histiocytic markers CD163 is primarily limited to neoplasms of macrophage/histiocytic derivation, as well as non-neoplastic monocytes, and is more specific than CD68 [100]. Tumor cells are negative for CD30. Some cases can be S-100 protein-positive, but staining is often weak and patchy rather than uniform.

Cytogenetics and Molecular Findings

The 2008 WHO classification no longer required the absence of clonal *IGH* or *TCR* gene rearrangements for the diagnosis

of HS. Although antigen receptor genes are usually germline, clonal rearrangements have been identified in some cases. Indeed, these rare cases of HS are seen in cases that occur subsequent to or concurrent with B- or T-lymphoblastic leukemia aggressive or indolent B-cell lymphoma [92]. However, high frequencies of clonal immunoglobulin receptor gene rearrangements were also detected in sporadic histiocytic sarcomas without either prior or a concordant B-cell lymphoma. It was thought that a large subset of histiocytic/dendritic cell sarcomas might have inherited B-cell genotypes and originally be derived from committed B-cell progenitors [101]. Two main speculations are made about the clonal antigen receptor gene rearrangements in histiocytic

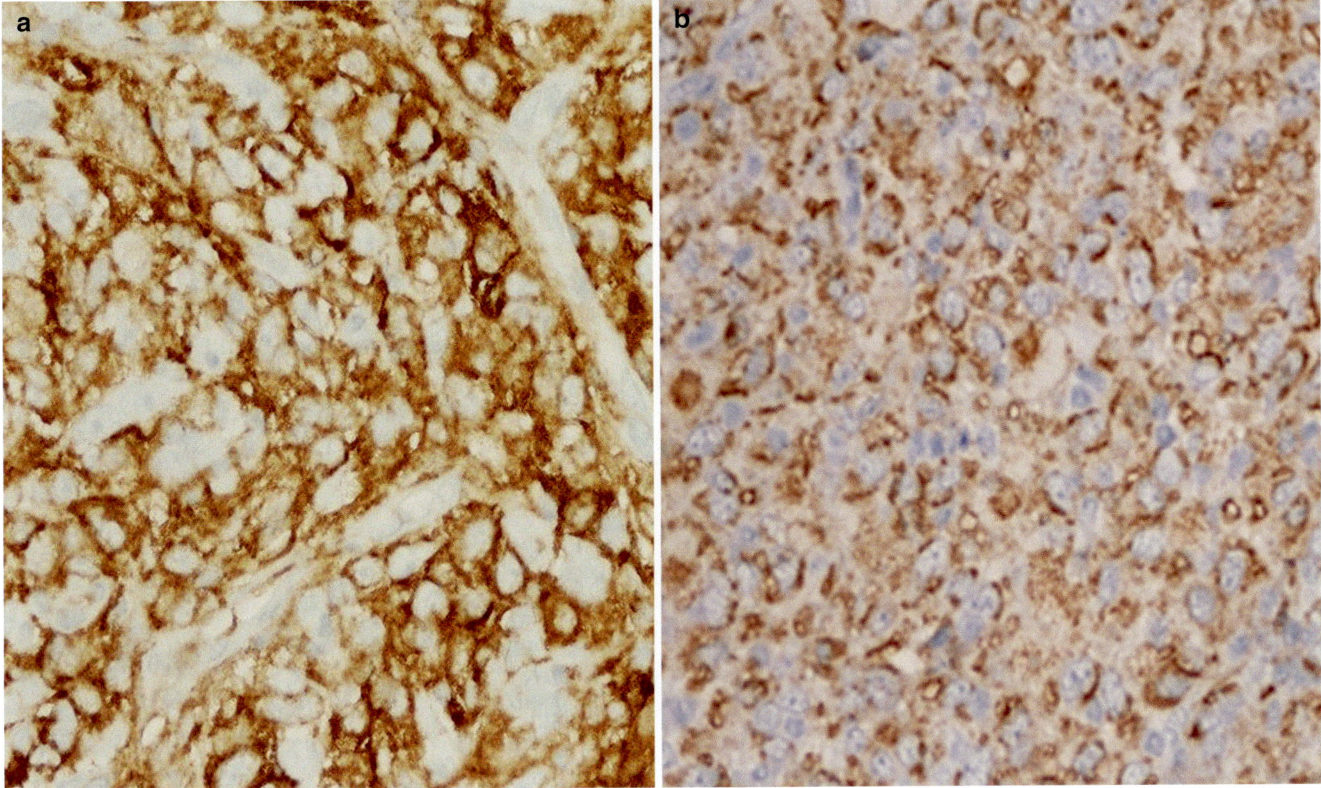

Fig. 17.10 Histiocytic sarcoma. Neoplastic cells are strongly positive both for CD68 (**a**) and CD163 (**b**) (Immunoperoxidase stain CD68 & CD163 with hematoxylin counterstain, 400×)

neoplasms. (1) Tumor lineage switching: in which, one tumor cell might transdifferentiate into another [102, 103]. (2) Two tumor lineages are present, which arises by the malignant transformation of a common stem cell [104].

Recently, the presence of activating *BRAF* V600E mutation in patients with HS is reported more frequently than expected previously, and this suggests that the BRAF pathway may be a common driver in the tumorigenesis of histiocytic sarcoma [105, 106].

Differential Diagnosis

The rarity of HS makes it a difficult diagnosis. Correct diagnosis based on the pathologic evaluation of involved tissue is interpreted within the clinical context [107]. An excisional or incisional biopsy of affected tissue is generally preferred. HS is often confused with other benign and malignant disorders such as reactive histiocytic proliferations, dendritic cell sarcomas, Langerhans cell histiocytosis (LCH), Langerhans cell sarcoma (LCS), and monocytic leukemia due to significant overlap of morphological and immunophenotypical characteristics. HS must also be distinguished from anaplastic large cell lymphoma, diffuse large B-cell lymphoma, malignant melanoma, undifferentiated large cell carcinoma, by way of extensive immunophenotypic analysis.

The first step of the diagnosis relies on the verification of histiocytic lineage and the exclusion of other, poorly differentiated, large cell malignancies [92, 107].

Differential diagnosis between reactive histiocytic proliferations and HS is difficult because they share the expression of histiocyte-associated markers. Therefore, the distinction between these two diseases rests on cytologic features [92]. An important diagnostic problem is the absence of precise diagnostic histologic criteria for malignancy. Prominent mitotic activity with atypical mitoses and cellular atypia is mandatory [6].

Histiocytic sarcoma with a prominent spindle cell component [108] has morphologic similarity with interdigitating dendritic cell sarcoma (IDCS). IDCS consistently expresses S-100 protein and is variably positive for CD68. It should be remembered that both neoplasms may have S-100 protein and CD68-positive cells. Features favoring IDCS include long dendritic cell processes, convoluted nuclei, more diffuse and stronger staining for S-100 protein and variable and often weaker staining for CD68 [92, 107].

Langerhans cell histiocytosis (LCH) and HS are both histiocytic diseases. These two entities can usually be distinguished by morphologic and immunohistochemical evaluation. Unlike LCH, HS tumor cells do not express CD1a or S100 and Birbeck granules are absent in HS.

Monocytic leukemia rarely presents an extramedullary solid tumor without blood and marrow involvement. This rare form of monocytic leukemia may be histologically confused with HS since tumors express CD68 and CD163. However, monocytic leukemia additionally expresses myeloid markers, such as myeloperoxidase, CD33, and CD34, whereas HS does not. Malignant melanoma and HS could be morphologically similar and both tumors may show S-100 protein and CD68 expression. However, HS lacks more specific melanoma markers such as HMB-45, SOX10, and Melan-A, while malignant melanoma lacks the expression of the specific histiocytic marker CD163.

Spleen infiltrations of HS are characteristically intra-sinusoidal and neoplastic cells display intense hemophago-cytosis and these cases must be distinguished from hemophagocytic lymphohistiocytosis (HLH). Gross features and the mass formation in the spleen and the distinct atypia of infiltrating histiocytes are thought to be important features discriminating primary splenic histiocytic sarcoma from HLH. Rare cases of HS may be associated with HLH, in which, malignant histiocytes showing erythrophagocytosis, in addition to numerous reactive histiocytes with a high level of erythrophagocytosis [87].

Prognosis

HS most often presents itself at an advanced clinical stage, with limited response to chemotherapy and high mortality and most patients die of progressive disease within 2 years [109]. Multisystem disease and/or a solitary tumor greater than 3.5 cm seem to carry the worst prognosis [93].

HS of the spleen can also be a potentially lethal condition that might remain asymptomatic or closely related with chronic thrombocytopenia for a long time [86, 89].

The patients of splenic HS have a poor prognosis due to aggressive behavior with liver or bone marrow infiltration, even though a splenectomy might induce temporary remission. The exclusive use of splenectomy does not appear to effectively induce lasting remission in histiocytic sarcoma of the spleen, and postoperative interventions such as chemo-radiotherapy or hematopoietic stem cell transplantation may be necessary to eliminate residual disease after splenectomy.

Diagnostic Caveats

- HS is a rare, aggressive hematopoietic neoplasm derived from histiocytic cells of the monocyte/macrophage system.
- HS is not a true sarcoma.
- Primary HS of the spleen is exceedingly rare. But it seems as a unique clinical entity, associated with hypo-albuminemia, hypo-γ-globulinemia, and thrombocytopenia.
- HS often presents at extranodal sites.
- Splenic HS is characterized by prominent hemophagocytosis by neoplastic cells, which resulted in severe thrombocytopenia and anemia.
- Intra-sinusal infiltrations of splenic HS must be differentiated from HLH when neoplastic histiocytes display hemophagocytosis.
- Neoplastic histiocytes express histiocytic markers as reactive histiocytes.
- HS may harbor clonal antigen receptor gene rearrangements.
- Activating *BRAF* V600E mutations are occasionally present in HS.
- Differential diagnosis is between reactive histiocytic proliferations and HS is difficult when cytologic atypia is absent.
- Solid tumors with morphologic and immunophenotypic features consistent with HS occurring in the context of acute monocytic leukemia (M5) should not be diagnosed as HS. AML M5 is usually associated with overt peripheral blastosis.
- HS does not express myeloid markers such as MPO, CD33, and CD34, which can be used to differentiate from monocytic leukemia.

Follicular Dendritic Cell Sarcoma

Definition

Follicular dendritic cell sarcoma (FDCS) is a rare mesenchymal neoplasm that is characterized by neoplastic proliferation of spindled to ovoid cells with morphologic and immunophenotypic features similar to those of normal follicular dendritic cells. Follicular dendritic cells are present in the germinal centers of lymphoid follicles in the spleen and lymph nodes. In the liver, they are described around portal spaces.

This tumor was first reported in 1986 by Monda et al. [110] and is classified by the World Health Organization (WHO) under histiocytic and dendritic cell neoplasms [4, 111]. Inflammatory pseudotumor-like (IPT-like FDCS) variant of the FDCS is almost exclusively arising from liver and spleen [112–114], shows marked female predilection (female to male ratio, 2.2:1) [115], and is strongly associated with the presence of EBV [113].

Etiology and Pathogenesis

Etiopathogenesis of FDCS remains unclear. Castleman disease, mostly the hyaline vascular variant which is a benign lymphoproliferative disorder, has been suggested as a precursor lesion for this tumor approximately in 10–20% of cases. Some cases of antecedent Castleman disease demonstrate areas of follicular dendritic cell proliferation, and FDCS is hypothesized to arise in these areas [116, 117]. Moreover, EGFR expression in both FDCS and non-neoplastic FDCs of Castleman disease has been shown. This shared feature may promote FDC persistence, allowing subsequent accumulation of mutations that may result in the emergence of this rare sarcoma [118]. Epstein-Barr virus (EBV) is involved in the pathogenesis of a small subset of FDCS cases, but most of them were reported in "inflammatory pseudotumor-like follicular dendritic cell sarcoma" [114]. EBV-encoded RNA is found in almost all neoplastic cells and Southern blot studies have shown that the virus has a monoclonal episomal form [4]. An association between FDCS and autoimmunity such as paraneoplastic pemphigus and myestenia gravis has been reported [119].

Epidemiology

The median age at diagnosis was 50 years (range 9–90 years). Males and females are affected almost equally with no gender predilection (1:1.01). Cases are reported from both Eastern and Western countries. However, the majority of the patients appeared to have an Asian origin when the percent of cases reported from the Far East were concerned [119].

Clinical Presentation

At presentation, most cases of FDCS (58%) occur in extranodal sites. The liver is the most common site and followed by lung, skin, tonsil, spleen, soft tissue, mediastinum, and gastrointestinal tract. One-third of FDCS cases (31%) present with an asymptomatic, slow-growing, cervical or intra-abdominal lymphadenopathy and 10% of cases have both nodal and extranodal involvement. Abdominal pain was the chief manifestation for most patients with abdominal involvement followed in order by systemic symptoms (i.e., fever, weight loss, and fatigue), intestinal obstruction, rectal bleeding, and dyspepsia [119].

The most common initial presentation of the patients with FDCS of the liver is abdominal pain and weight loss [120, 121]. Anemia and fever were also part of the initial presentation in some cases [122]. Some patients with liver and most patients with spleen involvement were asymptomatic and diagnosed incidentally [123–127].

Morphology

Gross Pathology

Follicular dendritic cell sarcomas are characteristically well-circumscribed or even encapsulated, masses that are solid with pink or white to tan-grey cut surfaces. Some tumors may have cystic components. The average size of tumors of all sites has been reported to range from 1.0 to 22.0 cm, largely dependent on the tumor location, with a median size of approximately 7.0 cm. Necrosis was present in 54.1% of the cases [119, 128]. The average size of IPT-like FDCS for hepatic tumors was 11.0 cm whereas the average tumor size of the splenic tumors was 7.1 cm [126] (Fig. 17.11).

Microscopy

Histologically, FDCS is composed of uniform, spindle, and ovoid cells, with eosinophilic cytoplasm and nuclei with a thin nuclear membrane, vesicular or granular chromatin, and small nucleoli. Nuclear pseudo inclusions can occasionally be seen (Fig. 17.12), with frequency increased after radiation therapy [128]. The neoplastic cells are usually arranged in fascicular, somewhat syncytial sheets, with whorled or storiform patterns associated with lymphocyte-

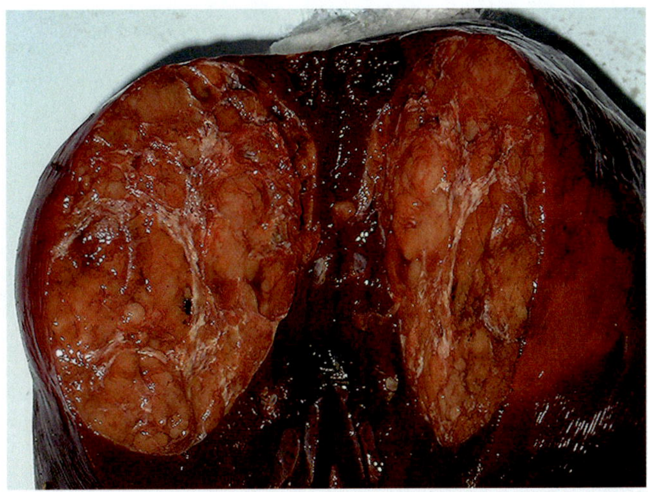

Fig. 17.11 Inflammatory pseudo tumor-like follicular dendritic cell sarcoma. Splenectomy specimen reveal well-demarcated subcapsular solid nodule in the spleen

rich stroma (Figs. 17.13a, b). Epithelioid cells and multi-nucleated giant cells are visible in the lesions (Fig. 17.14a, b). The mitotic rate is usually low. However, cytologic atypia may be seen in some cases with pleomorphic features. Inflammatory pseudotumor-like FDC (IPT-like FDCS) sarcoma is composed of oval to spindle tumor cells, which disperse with a meshwork-like pattern in a background of prominent lymphoplasmacytic infiltrate (Fig. 17.15). The cells have variable nuclear atypia. Hodgkin or Reed-Sternberg-like cells can be occasionally found [114].

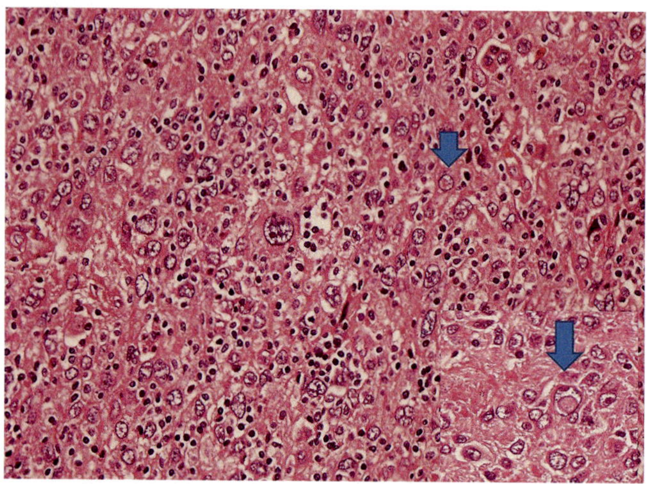

Fig. 17.12 Follicular dendritic cell sarcoma. Nuclear pseudo inclusions (arrow) (H&E, 400×)

Immunohistochemistry

Nodal and extranodal FDCSs have similar immunophenotypes. Follicular dendritic cell sarcomas generally demonstrate the immunophenotype of non-neoplastic follicular dendritic cells and are usually positive for dendritic cell markers CD21 (C3b complement receptor), (Fig. 17.16), CD23, and/or CD35 (C3d complement receptor). The antibody CD23 is of limited utility for diagnosis because of the low positivity rate and only patchy or focal staining [126].

Clusterin is the most sensitive marker when it shows diffuse strong cytoplasmic positivity in FDCS [129]. Podoplanin (D2–40) is another marker shown to have high sensitivity for FDCS with strong membranous staining [130], ɣ-Synuclein is another new helpful marker that strongly stains follicular dendritic cells and may be useful in diagnosis FDCS [131]. Other markers which are usually positive in the tumor are vimentin, S100, CD68, EGFR, fascin, and HLA-DR. But none of these markers are specific for FDCS. Staining for CD1a, lysozyme, myeloperoxidase, CD34, CD3 CD79a, CD30, HMB-45, desmin, and high-molecular weight cytokeratins is negative. Ki-67 labeling ranges from 1% to 25% [4].

The IPT-like variant of FDCS also expressed conventional FDCS markers, including CD21, CD35, CD23, and associated with Epstein-Barr virus (EBV). EBV encoded RNA was found to be positive in 92% of IPT-like FDCS cases by in situ hybridization [126]. (Fig. 17.17).

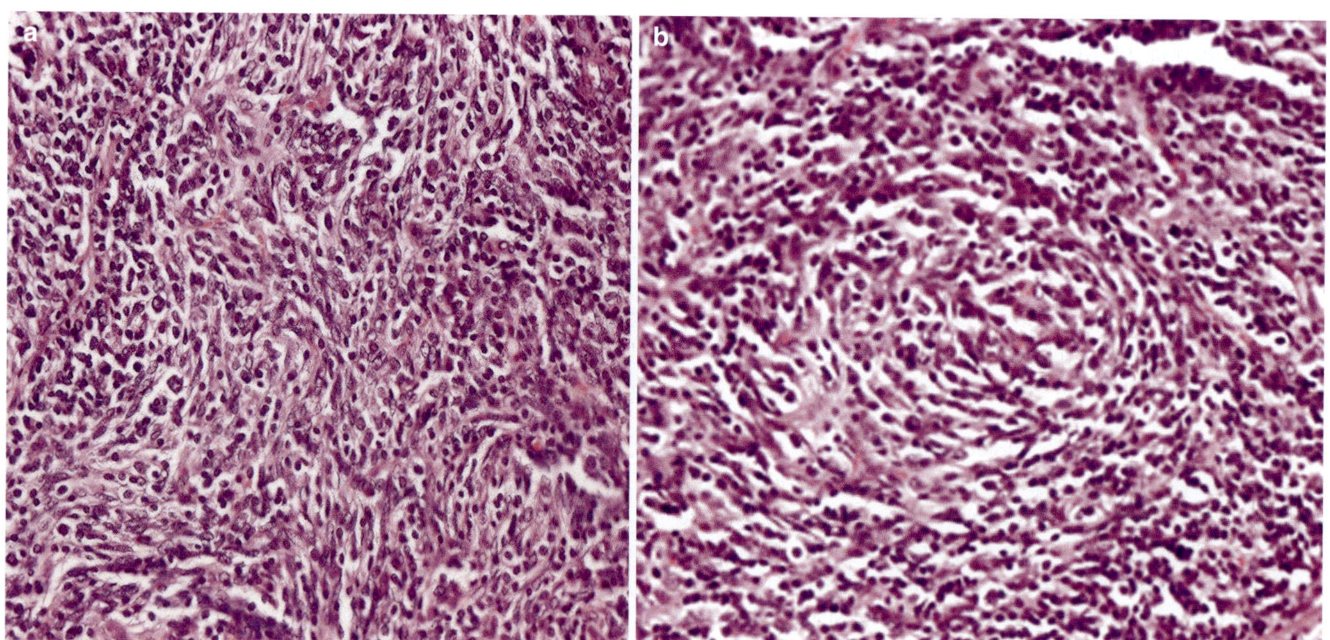

Fig. 17.13 (**a**, **b**) Follicular dendritic cell sarcoma. The neoplastic cells are usually arranged in fascicular, somewhat syncytial sheets with storiform (**a**) or whorled (**b**) patterns associated with lymphocyte-rich stroma (H&E, 200×)

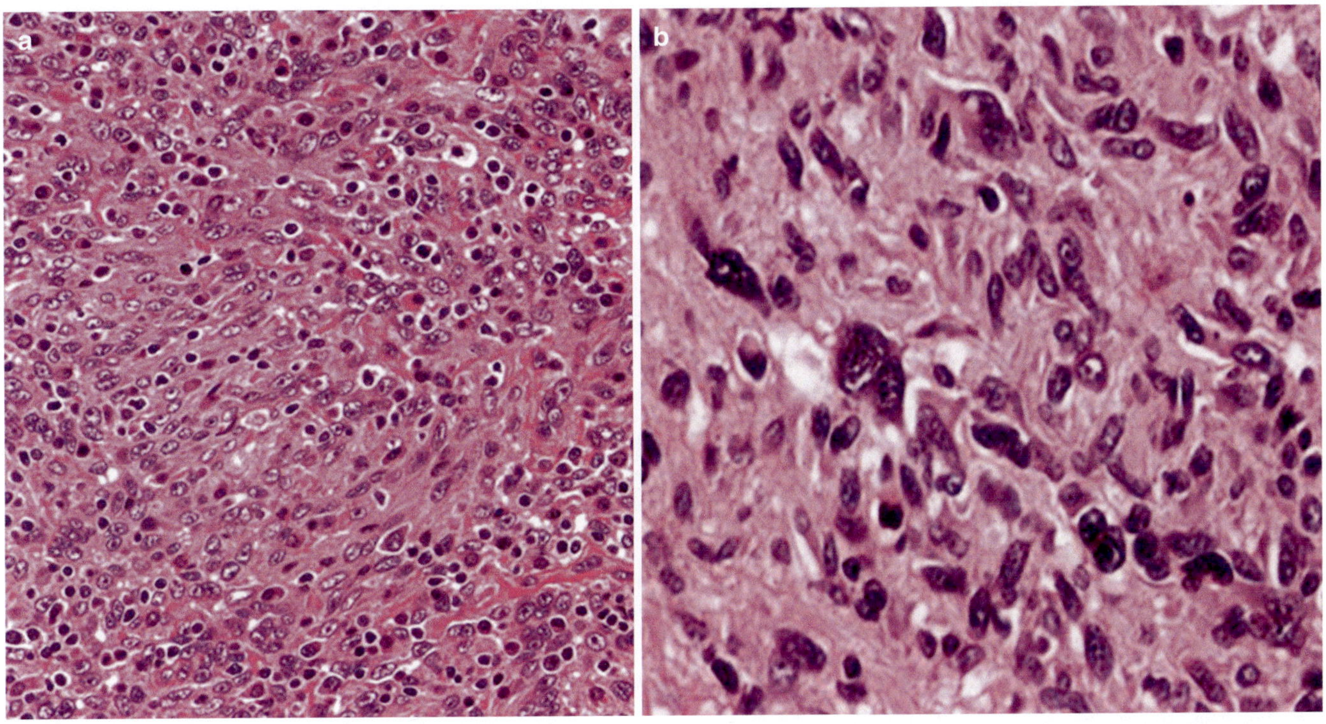

Fig. 17.14 (**a**, **b**) Follicular dendritic cell sarcoma. Epitheloid cells (**a**) and multinucleated giant cells (**b**) are visible in the lesions (H&E, 400×)

Cytogenetics and Molecular Findings

No specific chromosomal aberration has been established in FDCS. Non-recurrent types of complex cytogenetic abnormalities have been documented [132].

Recently, a multicenter study performed by Go et al [105] examined the BRAF pathway and its contribution to the pathogenesis of histiocytic and dendritic cell neoplasms, including FDCS. They showed *BRAF* mutations were present in 18.5% of FDCS and 40% of IPT-like variants of FDCS.

Another study analyzed the somatic alterations in FDCS. They found the recurrent loss of function alterations in tumor suppressor genes which involved in the negative regulation of NF-κB activation and cell cycle progression. Alterations in genes that regulate cell cycle include bi-allelic loss of CDKN2A and RB-1 these findings provide an insight into the genomic landscape of FDCS and suggest shared mechanisms of tumorigenesis with a subset of other tumor types, notably B-cell lymphomas [133].

Differential Diagnosis

A detailed review of all reported cases indicated that at least 18.6% of the patients were diagnosed erroneously at presentation. Entities most commonly confused with FDCS included undifferentiated carcinoma, Hodgkin or non-Hodgkin lymphoma, malignant fibrous histiocytoma, peripheral nerve sheath tumor, ectopic meningioma, inflammatory pseudotumor, granulomatous inflammation, gastrointestinal stromal tumor, and unclassified sarcoma [119]. Although the histological features of FDCS are rather stereotypical, they are likely to be misdiagnosed, as specific FDC markers that are not routinely used in the immunohistochemical study of poorly differentiated malignant tumors. It is important to remember that FDCS has a distinctive immunophenotype and expression of dendritic cell markers is specific. Thus histologically FDCS has to be differentiated from other epithelial or mesenchymal malignancies which is mainly based on immunophenotypic analysis with exclusion of other tumors by negativity for keratins, Melan-A, HMB45, B and T lymphocyte markers, CD30, SMA, desmin, c-KIT, and expression of dendritic cell markers.

Interdigitating dendritic cell sarcoma (IDCS) is a rare entity and usually arises from the lymph nodes and spleen, and may be considered a differential diagnosis for FDCS. IDCS lack the storiform and whorled patterns of FDCS [134]. Unlike FDCS, interdigitating dendritic cell sarcomas are positive for S100, and negative for dendritic cell markers (CD21, CD23, and CD35). Indeterminate cell tumor of the spleen showed some features of dendritic cell lesions, including a focal "whorl-like" pattern, and oval and spindle cells. Tumor cells are strongly positive with CD1a and S-100 and follicular dendritic cell markers are negative [135]. FDCS arising in the gastrointestinal tract may be mistaken for cKIT-negative GIST. GIST is negative for dendritic cell markers and dense lymphocytic infiltrates are uncommon [128]. IPT-like FDCS which arise in the liver and/or spleen morphologically resemble inflammatory myofibroblastic

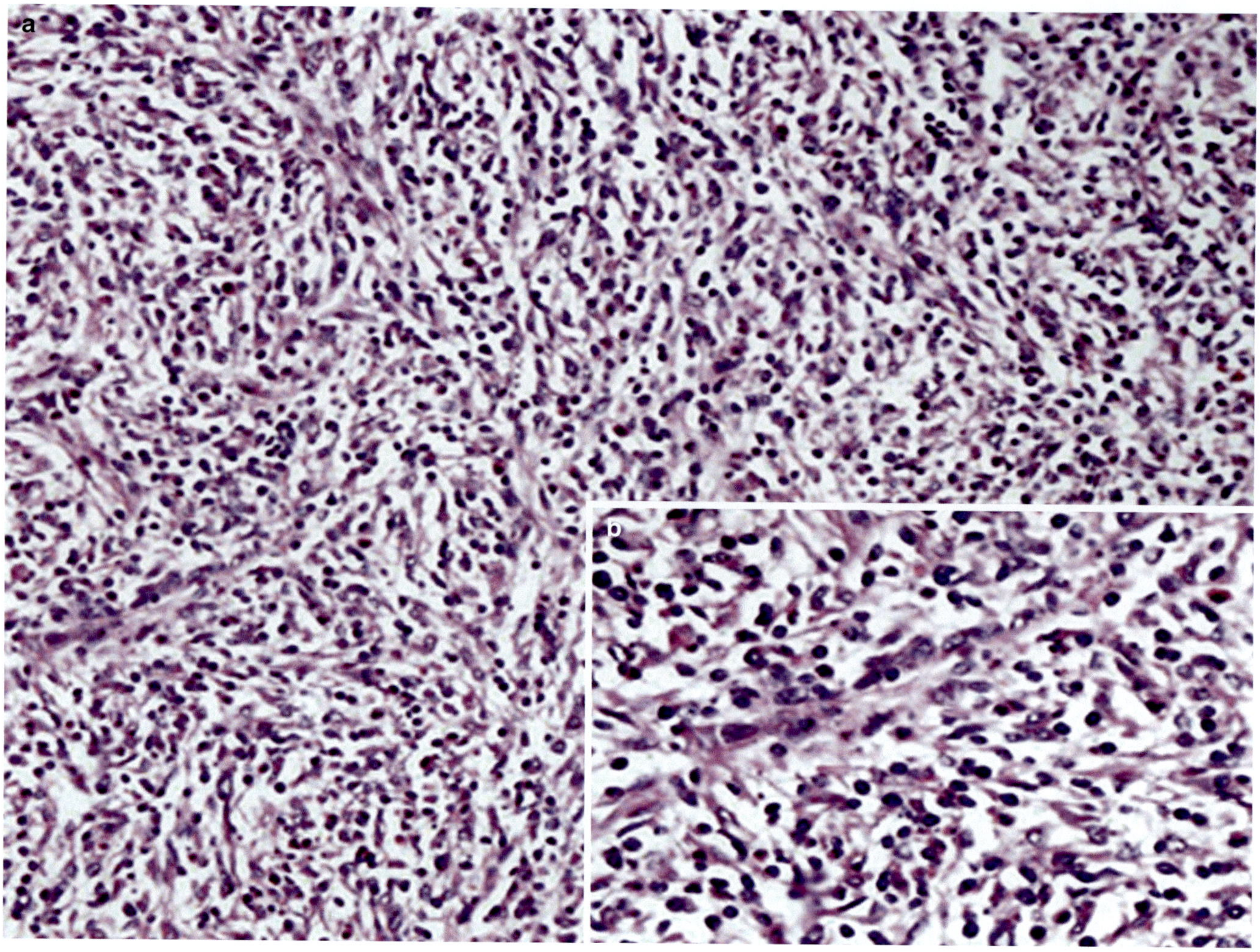

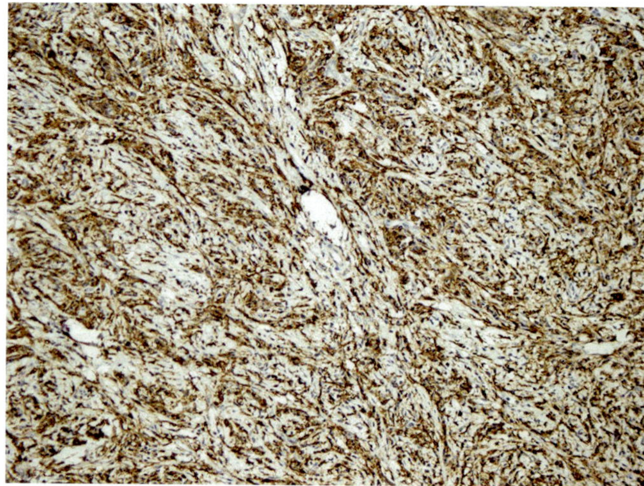

Fig. 17.15 Inflammatory pseudotumor-like follicular dendritic cell sarcoma. Tumor is composed of oval to spindle tumor cells, which disperse with a meshwork-like pattern in a background of prominent lymphoplasmacytic infiltrate infiltrate (**a**) (H&E x200), higher magnifcation (**b**) insert (H&E X400)

Fig. 17.16 Follicular dendritic cell sarcoma. Neoplastic cells strongly stain with CD21. (Immunoperoxidase stain CD21 with hematoxylin counterstain, 200×)

tumor (IMT). IPT-like FDCS may be mixed with reactive myofibroblasts [126, 127] and smooth muscle actin (SMA)-positive myofibroblasts are detected in more than half cases of IPT-like FDCS. However, inflammatory myofibroblastic tumor is not only positive for SMA and may express desmin, but also more than 50% of cases are positive for ALK, with *ALK* gene arrangements [136]. The differential diagnosis of IPT-like FDCS from inflammatory pseudotumor (IPT) of spleen and liver is important. IPT is a non-neoplastic condition of unknown etiology with myofibroblastic or fibrohistiocytic nature. ITP cells did not display pleomorphism and the spindle cells did not express FDC markers. Some of the IPT cases have been reclassified as FDC tumors by using immunohistochemistry.

Age-related EBV-associated lymphoproliferative disorder of the spleen is characterized by the heavy infiltration of lymphocytes, plasma cells, epithelioid granulomas, and numerous EBV-positive cells, which resembles IPT-like

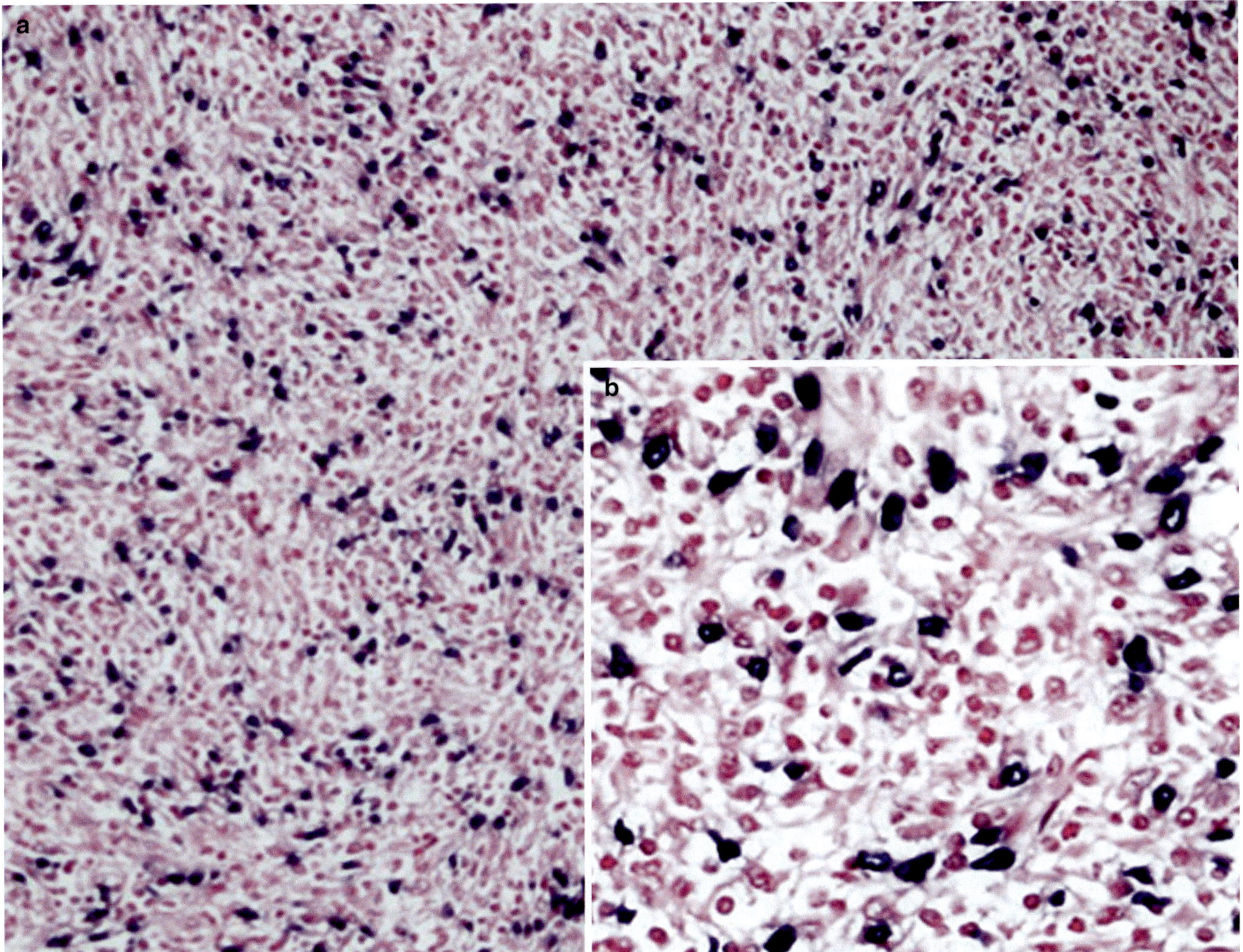

Fig. 17.17 IPT like variant of FDCS are associated with Epstein-Barr virus (EBV). EBV encoded RNA is positive by in situ hybridization (**a**) (EBER 200X) Higher magnification (**b**) (EBER 400X)

FDCS [137]. In such cases, the application of various FDC markers is essential.

Finally, it must be kept in mind that the diagnosis of IPT-like FDC tumors should be very stringent, because not all of the most specific markers are 100% sensitive. All of the FDC markers such as CD21, CD35, CNA42, CD23, clusterin, and podoplanin should be tested in order to rule out the diagnosis of splenic FDC tumors. Detection of ALK protein and EBV using in situ hybridization is also mandatory.

Prognosis

FDCS behaves like an intermediate grade sarcoma with a substantial risk of local recurrence and distant metastasis. Extranodal tumors have a higher risk of metastases than nodal counterparts. Liver, lung, and lymph nodes are common metastatic sites. A review of reported cases limited to extranodal FDCS found the 2 and 5 year recurrence-free survival rates to be 62.3% and 27.4% respectively. Similar to other soft tissue sarcomas, large tumor size ($\geq$6.0 cm), intra-abdominal involvement presence of coagulative necrosis, high mitotic count ($\geq$5 per 10 high-power fields), and significant cytologic atypia were shown to be associated with poor prognosis [115, 119].

No recurrence or metastasis is reported in the splenic cases, while a considerable number of hepatic cases show recurrence or metastasis after initial treatment [126, 138].

Complete surgical excision is the treatment of choice for both primary and recurrent cases. The benefits and advantages of radiotherapy and chemotherapy are not established. In cases with a *BRAF* V600 mutation, BRAF enzyme inhibitors can be a potential choice. EGFR inhibitors can be used in cases that express moderate to strong EGFR.

Diagnostic Caveats

- Follicular dendritic cells (FDCs) are present in the germinal centers of lymphoid follicles in the spleen and lymph nodes and around portal spaces in the liver.
- Some cases of follicular dendritic cell sarcoma (FDCS) are associated with Castleman disease and autoimmune disorders such as paraneoplastic pemphigus and myestenia gravis.
- Most cases of FDCS occur in extranodal sites.
- Most cases of FDCS with spleen involvement were asymptomatic and diagnosed incidentally.
- IPT-like FDCS is almost exclusively arising from the liver and spleen.
- IPT-like FDCS is strongly associated with EBV.
- FDCSs are likely to be misdiagnosed, if specific FDC markers are not routinely used in the immunohistochemical study of poorly differentiated malignant tumors.
- FDCSs generally demonstrate the immunophenotype of non-neoplastic follicular dendritic cells and are usually positive for CD21, CD23, and/or CD35.
- Most sensitive new markers for FDCS are clusterin, podoplanin, and γ-Synuclein
- IPT-like FDCS which arise in the liver and/or spleen morphologically resemble inflammatory myofibroblastic tumor (IMT). Both may be positive for SMA and desmin but IMT does not express FDC markers and half of them express ALK.
- *BRAF*V600E mutations are present in some of the FDCS and most of IPT-like variants of FDCS.
- Large tumor size ($\geq$6.0 cm), intraabdominal involvement, presence of coagulative necrosis, high mitotic count ($\geq$5 per 10 high-power fields), and significant cytologic atypia are associated with poor prognosis.

Hemophagocytic Lymphohistiocytosis

Definition

Hemophagocytic lymphohistiocytosis (HLH) is a rare, often life-threatening syndrome, characterized by overstimulation of the immune system leading to hyper cytokinemia, histiocyte proliferation, and systemic inflammation which can result in end-organ damage and death. Failure to control the immune response leads to increased secretion of inflammatory cytokines and macrophage activation, causing systemic inflammatory symptoms and signs. HLH is simply described as a hyperinflammatory state with a pathologic accumulation and stimulation of monocytes and/or macrophages, resulting in the phagocytosis of blood cells in the bone marrow, liver, and spleen.

Etiology and Pathogenesis

Depending on the etiology, HLH can be divided into genetic (primary) and acquired (secondary) forms [139, 140].

The primary form is caused by genetic mutations impairing the cytotoxic function of natural killer (NK) and cytotoxic T cells and typically present in infancy and childhood. Secondary form tends to occur at older ages in the setting of an associated predisposing condition, such as infection, immunodeficiency, autoimmune disease or malignancy, without an identifiable genetic abnormality [141–143]. Under normal physiologic circumstances, upon encountering a virally infected cell, CD8+ cytotoxic T cells and NK cells release cytolytic granules containing perforin and granzymes that promote cytolytic destruction of the target cell. Disruption of this process via genetic mutations predisposes to the development of primary HLH. The most common and important triggers of secondary HLH are proinflammatory cytokines in lymphomas, high-level cytokine production from proliferating engrafting hematopoietic cells in allogeneic bone marrow transplantation, and macrophage activation syndrome (MAS) in systemic autoimmune disorders. EBV is the most common infectious trigger for both primary and secondary HLH. EBV normally infects B lymphocytes, but can result in EBV-associated HLH via infection of CD8+ cytotoxic T lymphocytes and drives their uncontrolled activation and aberrant activity [144, 145]. The pathogenesis of HLH is not fully understood. However, it is known that the clinical symptoms are the results of excessive polyclonal activation of cytotoxic T lymphocytes (CTLs), NK cells, and macrophages. The inability to clear the antigenic stimulus results in chronic stimulation of CTLs and the release of proinflammatory cytokines including IL-1β, IL-2, IL-6, IL-12, IL-16, IL-18, TNF-α, and IFN-γ. This cytokine storm results in high levels of macrophage activation with resultant hemophagocytosis, tissue damage, and organ failure [144, 146].

Epidemiology

Epidemiologic data on HLH are derived from retrospective analyses that have been published in the literature.

A large retrospective study estimates the prevalence of HLH in Texas at least 1 in 100,000 children, with a median age at diagnosis of 1.8 years [147]. In addition, the incidence of primary HLH varies according to the geographic region. In Sweden, the reported incidence is 1.2 cases per million per year in persons younger than 15 years of age or 1 in 50,000 births and 0.342 in 100,000 in Japan, with an annual incidence of 1 in 800,000 [142].

The congenital form of the disease usually presents in infancy or early childhood. However, the first episode of HLH can occur at any point in a patient's life. Cases of primary HLH were reported in both fetuses and adults [140, 148].

Epidemiological data on the prevalence of HLH among adults are very limited. A single-center retrospective Swedish study reported an incidence of malignancy-associated HLH in adults of 0.9% [149].

Recently, studies from Karolinska University Hospital confirmed that HLH among adults particularly with hematologic malignancies is much more prevalent than previously believed [140]. Both forms of HLH have an equal distribution among males and females.

Clinical Presentation

The clinical presentation of HLH is different in neonates. Fever in this age group is generally absent and hypertriglyceridemia has been reported in only 14% of neonates [150]. Coagulopathy, hepatomegaly, splenomegaly progressive cytopenias, and/or fulminant liver failure should raise suspicion for HLH in this population [141, 142, 151]. Patients may suffer from one or several acute progressive episodes which may be triggered by infection or vaccination. In young children, HLH-like manifestations may also occur in association with primary immune deficiencies, especially with primary T-cell deficiencies [152]. Central nervous syndrome (CNS) symptoms such as seizures, meningitis, encephalopathy, ataxia, hemiplegia, cranial nerve palsies, mental status changes, or simply irritability are seen in up to 75% of pediatric cases [142].

Secondary HLH may occur at any age, and the first clinical symptoms are usually associated with an infectious episode, rheumatic condition, or malignancy [73]. Common symptoms that include some combinations are fever, lymphadenopathy, and hepatomegaly with signs of liver dysfunction splenomegaly, progressive cytopenias, coagulopathy, edema, dermatologic manifestations, and neurologic dysfunctions such as encephalitis, seizures, or coma. However, none of these symptoms are specific, the rapid diagnosis of HLH is difficult. The characteristic laboratory findings are hyperferritinemia, hypertriglyceridemia, hypofibrinogenemia, elevated transaminases and bilirubin, disseminated intravascular coagulation (DIC), hyponatremia, elevated serum lactate dehydrogenase, and hypoproteinemia [140].

When HLH symptoms develop in a patient with an underlying rheumatic disease this condition is called as macrophage activation syndrome (MAS). This particular subset of HLH is recently reclassified under the term of MAS-HLH [6, 152].

Morphology

No specific imaging patterns are diagnostic in HLH. The spleen is usually moderately enlarged, although significant enlargement may occur and shows a firm consistency and a winy color. On the other hand, the liver is markedly enlarged with a smooth external surface. The cut surface shows a lobular pattern and congestion.

Microscopy

The microscopic evidence of hemophagocytosis is one of the HLH-2004 diagnostic criteria [139]. However, hemophagocytosis is the only morphologic criterion. It is neither specific nor sensitive for the diagnosis of HLH. Several studies showed that the presence of hemophagocytosis even in a high amount is not predictive of the diagnosis of HLH in the absence of clinical features concerning the disease [153, 154]. Moreover, hemophagocytosis is often cyclical, and thus a given biopsy specimen may yield negative results at first examination [155]. The histologic features of both forms of HLH are similar, and depend on when the biopsy is obtained in the disease course. Although the most striking findings are present in bone marrow, lymph nodes, spleen, and liver, other organs such as the thymus, CNS, lungs, and subcutaneous tissue may also be involved. In the earlier phases of the disease, involved lymphoid organs may show nonspecific reactive changes, but as the disease progresses, although involved lymphoid organs generally maintain their intact architecture, sinusoids in lymph nodes are filled with numerous histiocytes. However, sinusal distention is not seen. Morphologically, the histiocytes lack cytologic atypia and often show prominent platelet phagocytosis, erythrophagocytosis, and often lymphophagocytosis. The red pulp of spleen shows a proliferation of macrophages, which display prominent hemophagocytosis (Fig. 17.18) most characteris-

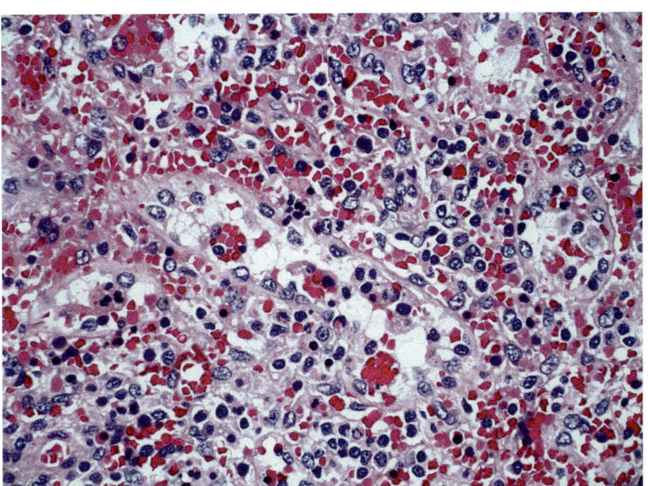

Fig. 17.18 Hemophagocytic lymphohistiocytosis (HLH). Spleen. The red pulp of spleen shows a proliferation of macrophages, which display prominent hemophagocytosis. (H&EX400)

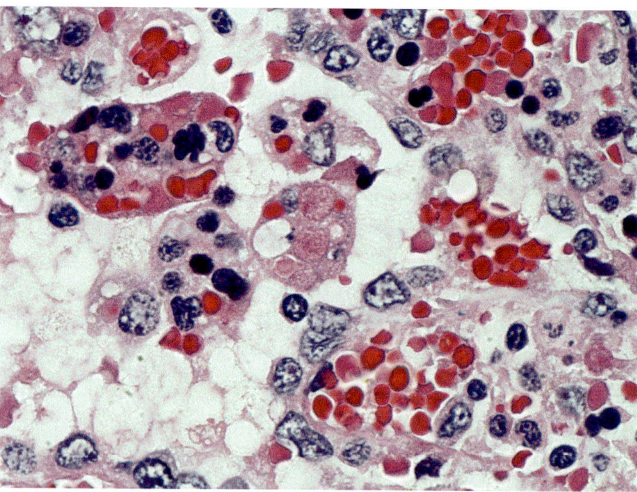

Fig. 17.19 Hemophagocytic lymphohistiocytosis (HLH). Spleen. Hemophagocytosis, characteristically consist of erythrocytes, but granulocytes, lymphocytes, and platelets are also seen (H&E, 1000×)

tically of erythrocytes, but also of granulocytes, lymphocytes, and platelets (Fig. 17.19). Fibrosis, focal ischemic infarctions, and gradual obliteration of the white pulp with B cell depletion are also seen. Hepatic dysfunction often occurs early in the clinical course. Microscopically, there is a portal and sinusoidal cytotoxic T-cell infiltrate admixed with variable hemophagocytic histiocytes. The histologic pattern is commonly described in liver biopsies as similar to chronic persistent hepatitis followed by leukemia-like, histiocytic storage disorder-like, and neonatal giant cell hepatitis-like patterns [156].

Immunohistochemistry

Proliferating macrophages in all sites are CD163 and CD68 (KP-1 or PGM-1) positive. Sinusoidal T cells express cytotoxic phenotype. They stain for CD8, granzyme B, and TIA-1. In patients who have a perforin mutation, the cytotoxic T cells do not stain for perforin [155]. Recent studies explore that perforin and CD107a (Cluster of Differentiation 107a) tests by multicolor flow cytometry are more sensitive for screening genetic HLH [157].

Cytogenetics and Molecular Findings

According to the type of genetic abnormalities, five types of primary HLH have been described [144]. Patients with mutations in these genes result in complete loss of protein function and develop primary HLH in childhood. *Type 1* is due to a genetic abnormality in the 9q21 locus on chromosome 9. The gene defect responsible for this type of HLH remains uncharacterized. *Type 2* results from mutations in

PRF1, which codes for the perforin protein. Perforin is normally contained within cytolytic granules and results in pore formation in the target cell membrane, facilitating the entrance of other cytolytic proteins and promoting osmotic lysis of the cell [158]. *Type 3* results from mutations in *UNC13D*, which codes for the protein Munc-13-4. This protein is normally involved in the regulation of cytolytic granule maturation and exocytosis [159]. *Type 4* results from mutations in *STX11*, which codes for syntaxin 11, a protein responsible for normal transport and exocytosis of cytolytic granules [160]. *Type 5* results from mutations in *STXBP2*, which codes for syntaxin-binding protein 2; this protein normally binds to syntaxin 11 and promotes membrane fusion of and release of cytolytic granules [161]. In young children, HLH-like manifestations may also occur especially, in association with primary T-cell immunodeficiencies. These syndromes are not to be considered as true primary HLH; they are frequently triggered by EBV infection which causes B-cell proliferation [6]. Secondary HLH may trigger malignancy, infection, or autoimmune stimulus in the absence of an identifiable underlying genetic defect.

Diagnosis

HLH-2004 criteria from the Histiocyte Society are widely accepted diagnostic criteria for HLH. The criteria include: (1) fever, (2) splenomegaly, (3) cytopenias (affecting ≥2 lineages) [hemoglobin <9 g/dL, platelet count <100 × 10⁹/L, absolute neutrophil count <1 × 10⁹/L, (4) hypertriglyceridemia (≥265 mg/dL) and/or hypofibrinogenemia (≤150 mg/dL), (5) hemophagocytosis in bone marrow, spleen, or lymph nodes, (6) low or absent NK cell activity, (7) ferritin (≥500 µg/L), (8) serum CD25 (sIL2Rα) (≥2400 U/ml.). Five of the eight criteria are required for diagnosis. In patients with an established above-mentioned genetic abnormalities, diagnosis can be established without meeting the five criteria [162].

Clinically, HLH may simulate a number of common conditions that cause fever, pancytopenia, hepatic abnormalities, and/or neurologic findings. These clinical conditions can be summarized as sepsis, liver disease or liver failure, multiple organ dysfunction syndrome, autoimmune lymphoproliferative syndrome, Kawasaki disease, thrombotic thrombocytopenic purpura, hemolytic uremic syndrome, and transfusion-associated graft-versus-host disease.

It is important both for clinicians and pathologists to be aware that cytologic features of hemophagocytosis should not be considered as the gold standard for the diagnosis of HLH and do not rule out the diagnosis in the absence of cytopathologic evidence of hemophagocytosis.

From a clinical point, differential diagnosis of HLH and sepsis is critically important. Genetic analyses can reveal primary HLH. In adult patients, hyperinflammation, present in both states, gives rise to an overlapping clinical picture. Fever, hemophagocytosis, NK cell activity, and CD25 concentration are not helpful in discriminating HLH from sepsis. However, hyperferritinemia, pronounced cytopenias, hypofibrinogenemia, and low C-reactive protein (CRP) are most helpful parameters [163].

Morphologically, the differential diagnosis of HLH should focus on the distinction of the hematologic neoplasms which involves the sinuses as well as induces secondary reactive hemophagocytosis.

The distinction of hematologic neoplasm is generally based on the cytologic characteristics of the proliferating cells. The histiocytes are cytologically benign in HLH whereas atypia of the proliferating cells should be evident in hematologic malignancies. However, in some cases this distinction may be difficult.

Differential Diagnosis

Hematologic malignancies associated with secondary HLH are often peripheral T-cell or NK/T-cell lymphomas. EBV association of these particular neoplasms is a major risk factor. Thus, HLH is a common complication of extranodal NK/T cell lymphoma, aggressive NK cell leukemia, and systemic EBV-positive lymphoproliferative disease of childhood associated with chronic active EBV infection [164]

Hepatosplenic T-cell lymphoma (HSTCL) is another neoplasm of cytotoxic gamma/delta T cells of the splenic pool. It is a distinct clinical entity characterized by hepatosplenomegaly and sinusoidal tropism of the neoplastic cells. The presenting symptoms include fever, weight loss, hepatosplenomegaly, and variable cytopenias and simulate HLH [165]. Moreover, some cases of HSTCL are associated with a hemophagocytic syndrome [166, 167]. Morphologically, neoplastic T cells admixed with the numerous reactive histiocytes display prominent hemophagocytosis. The diagnosis of background T-cell lymphoma in these cases requires detailed immunohistochemistry and sometimes confirmation of T-cell clonality.

Histiocytic sarcoma of the spleen: Gross features and the mass formation in the spleen and the distinct atypia of infiltrating histiocytes are thought to be important features discriminating primary splenic histiocytic sarcoma from HLH [87]. Spleen infiltrations of histiocytic sarcoma are characteristically intra-sinusal and some of the neoplastic cells display intense hemophagocytosis. Distinct atypia of infiltrating histiocytes and detection of nodular splenic infiltrations (gross or radiology) are thought to be important features discriminating primary splenic histiocytic sarcoma from HLH.

Prognosis

The prognosis of primary HLH without treatment is poor, with a median survival of 1–2 months [142]. However, recent clinical trials have shown an improvement of survival with chemo-immunotherapy followed by allogeneic bone marrow transplantation (alloBMT) in eligible cases [140]. AlloBMT is the only available therapy for cure in patients with primary HLH [168].

Prognosis of adult HLH is not uniform. Overall mortality was reported as 42% in the largest study of 162 patients with all associated HLH conditions [169]. Mortality was lowest in autoimmune disease patients followed by infection-associated and idiopathic HLH patients. Malignancy, particularly T-cell lymphoma-associated HLH, was a prominent adverse prognostic marker correlating with poorer survival in multiple large studies [143, 170]. Treatment of HLH must begin prior to completion of differential diagnosis between the different forms of the disease. It is similar for both forms and directed to control the hyperinflammation and correction of the underlying immune defect.

Diagnostic Caveats

- Primary HLH is typically present in infancy and childhood and caused by genetic mutations impairing the cytotoxic function of natural killer (NK) and cytotoxic T cells.
- Secondary HLH may occur at any age, and the first clinical symptoms are usually associated with an infectious episode, rheumatic condition, or malignancy.
- EBV is the most common infectious trigger for both primary and secondary HLH.
- Hemophagocytosis is the only morphologic criterion. It is neither specific nor sensitive for the diagnosis of HLH.
- Hemophagocytosis is cyclic, and given biopsy specimen may yield negative results at first examination.
- Absence of hemophagocytosis in tissue biopsies does not rule out the diagnosis of HLH.
- In the earlier phases of the disease, involved lymphoid organs may show nonspecific reactive changes.
- For primary HLH patients with perforin mutation, the cytotoxic T cells do not stain for perforin.
- Perforin and CD107a tests by multicolor flow cytometry are more sensitive for screening genetic HLH.
- Clinically, HLH may simulate a number of common conditions that cause fever, pancytopenia, hepatic abnormalities, and/or neurologic findings. Diagnosis is made according to HLH guideline.
- Morphologic differential diagnosis of HLH should focus on the distinction of the hematologic neoplasms which involves the sinuses as well as induces secondary reactive hemophagocytosis.

References

1. Collin M, McGovern N, Haniffa M. Human dendritic cell subsets. Immunology. 2013;140(1):22–30.
2. Histiocytosis syndromes in children. Writing Group of the Histiocyte Society. Lancet. 1987;1(8526):208–9.
3. Favara BE, Feller AC, Pauli M, et al. Contemporary classification of histiocytic disorders. The WHO Committee on Histiocytic/Reticulum Cell Proliferations. Reclassification Working Group of the Histiocyte Society. Med Pediatr Oncol. 1997;29(3):157–66.
4. Chan J, Pileri S, Delsol G, Fletcher C, Weiss LM, Grogg K. Follicular dendritic cell sarcoma. In: Swerdlow SH, Campo H, Harris NL, Jaffe ES, Pileri S, editors. WHO classification of haematopoietic and lymphoid tissues. Lyon: International Agency for Research on Cancer (IARC); 2008. p. 363–4.
5. Swerdlow SH, Campo E, Pileri SA, et al. The 2016 revision of the World Health Organization classification of lymphoid neoplasms. Blood. 2016;127(20):2375–90.
6. Emile JF, Abla O, Fraitag S, et al. Revised classification of histiocytoses and neoplasms of the macrophage-dendritic cell lineages. Blood. 2016;127(22):2672–81.
7. Rosai J, Dorfman RF. Sinus histiocytosis with massive lymphadenopathy. A newly recognized benign clinicopathological entity. Arch Pathol. 1969;87(1):63–70.
8. Dalia S, Shao H, Sagatys E, Cualing H, Sokol L. Dendritic cell and histiocytic neoplasms: biology, diagnosis, and treatment. Cancer Control. 2014;21(4):290–300.
9. Foucar E, Rosai J, Dorfman R. Sinus histiocytosis with massive lymphadenopathy (Rosai-Dorfman disease): review of the entity. Semin Diagn Pathol. 1990;7(1):19–73.
10. Mantilla JG, Goldberg-Stein S, Wang Y. Extranodal Rosai-Dorfman disease: clinicopathologic series of 10 patients with radiologic correlation and review of the literature. Am J Clin Pathol. 2016;145(2):211–21.
11. Sandoval-Sus JD, Sandoval-Leon AC, Chapman JR, et al. Rosai-Dorfman disease of the central nervous system: report of 6 cases and review of the literature. Medicine (Baltimore). 2014;93(3):165–75.
12. Wang CC, Al-Hussain TO, Serrano-Olmo J, Epstein JI. Rosai-Dorfman disease of the genito-urinary tract: analysis of six cases from the testis and kidney. Histopathology. 2014;65(6):908–16.
13. Komaragiri M, Sparber LS, Santos-Zabala ML, Dardik M, Chamberlain RS. Extranodal Rosai-Dorfman disease: a rare soft tissue neoplasm masquerading as a sarcoma. World J Surg Oncol. 2013;11:63.
14. Mehraein Y, Wagner M, Remberger K, et al. Parvovirus B19 detected in Rosai-Dorfman disease in nodal and extranodal manifestations. J Clin Pathol. 2006;59(12):1320–6.
15. Levine PH, Jahan N, Murari P, Manak M, Jaffe ES. Detection of human herpesvirus 6 in tissues involved by sinus histiocytosis with massive lymphadenopathy (Rosai-Dorfman disease). J Infect Dis. 1992;166(2):291–5.
16. Tsang WY, Yip TT, Chan JK. The Rosai-Dorfman disease histiocytes are not infected by Epstein-Barr virus. Histopathology. 1994;25(1):88–90.
17. Luppi M, Barozzi P, Garber R, et al. Expression of human herpesvirus-6 antigens in benign and malignant lymphoproliferative diseases. Am J Pathol. 1998;153(3):815–23.
18. Cai Y, Shi Z, Bai Y. Review of Rosai-Dorfman disease: new insights into the pathogenesis of this rare disorder. Acta Haematol. 2017;138(1):14–23.
19. Liu L, Perry AM, Cao W, et al. Relationship between Rosai-Dorfman disease and IgG4-related disease: study of 32 cases. Am J Clin Pathol. 2013;140(3):395–402.
20. Wimmer DB, Ro JY, Lewis A, et al. Extranodal rosai-dorfman disease associated with increased numbers of immunoglobulin g4 plasma cells involving the colon: case report with literature review. Arch Pathol Lab Med. 2013;137(7):999–1004.
21. Vaiselbuh SR, Bryceson YT, Allen CE, Whitlock JA, Abla O. Updates on histiocytic disorders. Pediatr Blood Cancer. 2014;61(7):1329–35.
22. Ha H, Kim KH, Ahn YJ, Kim JH, Kim JE, Yoon SS. A rare case of Rosai-Dorfman disease without lymphadenopathy. Korean J Intern Med. 2016;31(4):802–4.
23. Karajgikar J, Grimaldi G, Friedman B, Hines J. Abdominal and pelvic manifestations of Rosai-Dorfman disease: a review of four cases. Clin Imaging. 2016;40(6):1291–5.
24. Knox SK, Kurtin PJ, Steensma DP. Isolated splenic sinus histiocytosis (Rosai-Dorfman disease) in association with myelodysplastic syndrome. J Clin Oncol. 2006;24(24):4027–8.
25. Gaitonde S. Multifocal, extranodal sinus histiocytosis with massive lymphadenopathy: an overview. Arch Pathol Lab Med. 2007;131(7):1117–21.
26. Lauwers GY, Perez-Atayde A, Dorfman RF, Rosai J. The digestive system manifestations of Rosai-Dorfman disease (sinus histiocytosis with massive lymphadenopathy): review of 11 cases. Hum Pathol. 2000;31(3):380–5.
27. Maheshwari A, Seth A, Choudhury M, et al. Rosai-Dorfman disease: a case with lymphadenopathy and liver involvement. J Pediatr Hematol Oncol. 2009;31(3):200–2.
28. Di Tommaso L, Rahal D, Bossi P, Roncalli M. Hepatic rosai-dorfman disease with coincidental lymphoma: report of a case. Int J Surg Pathol. 2010;18(6):540–3.
29. Wani J, Quandri IY. Rosai Dorfman disease – case report of a patient with fatal outcome. JK Sci. 2011;13:160–16.
30. Kgomo MK, Elnagar AA, Jeske C, Nagel J. Sinus histiocytosis with massive lymphadenopathy (Rosai-Dorfman disease) and cirrhosis of the liver: a case report and literature review. S Afr Med J. 2016;106(5):48–9.
31. Arabadzhieva E, Yonkov A, Bonev S, et al. Rosai-Dorfman disease involving gallbladder and liver-report of a case. Int J Surg Case Rep. 2015;12:140–2.
32. Mar WA, Yu JH, Knuttinen MG, et al. Rosai-Dorfman disease: manifestations outside of the head and neck. AJR Am J Roentgenol. 2017;208(4):721–32.
33. McClain KL, Natkunam Y, Swerdlow SH. Atypical cellular disorders. Hematology Am Soc Hematol Educ Program. 2004:283–96.
34. Karunanithi S, Singh H, Sharma P, Naswa N, Kumar R. 18F-FDG PET/CT imaging features of Rosai Dorfman disease: a rare cause of massive generalized lymphadenopathy. Clin Nucl Med. 2014;39(3):268–9.
35. Abla O, Jacobsen E, Picarsic J, et al. Consensus recommendations for the diagnosis and clinical management of Rosai-Dorfman-Destombes disease. Blood. 2018;131(26):2877–90.
36. Chakraborty R, Hampton OA, Shen X, et al. Mutually exclusive recurrent somatic mutations in MAP2K1 and BRAF support a central role for ERK activation in LCH pathogenesis. Blood. 2014;124(19):3007–15.
37. Haroche J, Cohen-Aubart F, Rollins BJ, et al. Histiocytoses: emerging neoplasia behind inflammation. Lancet Oncol. 2017;18(2):e113–25.
38. Fatobene G, Haroche J, Helias-Rodzwicz Z, et al. BRAF V600E mutation detected in a case of Rosai-Dorfman disease. Haematologica. 2018;103(8):e377–9.
39. Garces S, Medeiros LJ, Patel KP, et al. Mutually exclusive recurrent KRAS and MAP2K1 mutations in Rosai-Dorfman disease. Mod Pathol. 2017;30(10):1367–77.
40. Morgan NV, Morris MR, Cangul H, et al. Mutations in SLC29A3, encoding an equilibrative nucleoside transporter ENT3, cause a familial histiocytosis syndrome (Faisalabad his-

tiocytosis) and familial Rosai-Dorfman disease. PLoS Genet. 2010;6(2):e1000833.

41. Sato Y, Notohara K, Kojima M, Takata K, Masaki Y, Yoshino T. IgG4-related disease: historical overview and pathology of hematological disorders. Pathol Int. 2010;60(4):247–58.

42. Wick MR, O'Malley DP. Lymphadenopathy associated with IgG4-related disease: diagnosis & differential diagnosis. Semin Diagn Pathol. 2018;35(1):61–6.

43. Badalian-Very G, Vergilio JA, Fleming M, Rollins BJ. Pathogenesis of Langerhans cell histiocytosis. Annu Rev Pathol. 2013;8:1–20.

44. Weiss LM, Jaffe ES, Facchetti F. Tumors derived from Langerhans cell. In: Swerdlow SH, Campo E, Harris NL, et al., editors. WHO classification of tumours of haematopoietic and lymphoid tissues. Lyon: IARC Press; 2017. p. 470–3.

45. Jaffe ES, Weiss LM, Facchetti F. Tumours derived from Langerhans cells. In: Swerdlow SH, Campo E, Harris NL, et al., editors. WHO classification of tumours of haematopoietic and lymphoid tissues. Lyon: IARC Press; 2008. p. 2.

46. Strenger V, Urban C. Chromosomal integration of the HHV-6 genome as a possible cause of persistent HHV-6 detection in a patient with Langerhans cell histiocytosis. Pathol Oncol Res. 2010;16(1):125–6.

47. Csire M, Mikala G, Jako J, et al. Persistent long-term human herpesvirus 6 (HHV-6) infection in a patient with Langerhans cell histiocytosis. Pathol Oncol Res. 2007;13(2):157–60.

48. Andersson By U, Tani E, Andersson U, Henter JI. Tumor necrosis factor, interleukin 11, and leukemia inhibitory factor produced by Langerhans cells in Langerhans cell histiocytosis. J Pediatr Hematol Oncol. 2004;26(11):706–11.

49. Davies H, Bignell GR, Cox C, et al. Mutations of the BRAF gene in human cancer. Nature. 2002;417(6892):949–54.

50. Egeler RM, van Halteren AG, Hogendoorn PC, Laman JD, Leenen PJ. Langerhans cell histiocytosis: fascinating dynamics of the dendritic cell-macrophage lineage. Immunol Rev. 2010;234(1):213–32.

51. Berres ML, Lim KP, Peters T, et al. BRAF-V600E expression in precursor versus differentiated dendritic cells defines clinically distinct LCH risk groups. J Exp Med. 2014;211(4):669–83.

52. Bhatia S, Nesbit ME Jr, Egeler RM, Buckley JD, Mertens A, Robison LL. Epidemiologic study of Langerhans cell histiocytosis in children. J Pediatr. 1997;130(5):774–84.

53. Baumgartner I, von Hochstetter A, Baumert B, Luetolf U, Follath F. Langerhans'-cell histiocytosis in adults. Med Pediatr Oncol. 1997;28(1):9–14.

54. Salotti JA, Nanduri V, Pearce MS, Parker L, Lynn R, Windebank KP. Incidence and clinical features of Langerhans cell histiocytosis in the UK and Ireland. Arch Dis Child. 2009;94(5):376–80.

55. Arico M, Girschikofsky M, Genereau T, et al. Langerhans cell histiocytosis in adults. Report from the International Registry of the Histiocyte Society. Eur J Cancer. 2003;39(16):2341–8.

56. Yi X, Han T, Zai H, Long X, Wang X, Li W. Liver involvement of Langerhans' cell histiocytosis in children. Int J Clin Exp Med. 2015;8(5):7098–106.

57. Abla O, Egeler RM, Weitzman S. Langerhans cell histiocytosis: current concepts and treatments. Cancer Treat Rev. 2010;36(4):354–9.

58. Abdallah M, Genereau T, Donadieu J, et al. Langerhans' cell histiocytosis of the liver in adults. Clin Res Hepatol Gastroenterol. 2011;35(6–7):475–81.

59. Lam KY, Chan AC, Wat MS. Langerhans cell histiocytosis forming an asymptomatic solitary nodule in the spleen. J Clin Pathol. 1996;49(3):262–4.

60. Christiansen EC, Ellwein M, Neglia JP. Splenomegaly unresponsive to standard and salvage chemotherapy in Langerhans cell histiocytosis: a case of extramedullary hematopoiesis. Pediatr Blood Cancer. 2012;58(6):998–9.

61. Griffiths W, Davies S, Gibbs P, Thillainayagam A, Alexander G. Liver transplantation in an adult with sclerosing cholangitis due to Langerhans cell histiocytosis. J Hepatol. 2006;44(4):829–31.

62. Mampaey S, Warson F, Van Hedent E, De Schepper AM. Imaging findings in Langerhans' cell histiocytosis of the liver and the spleen in an adult. Eur Radiol. 1999;9(1):96–8.

63. Ma J, Jiang Y, Chen X, Gong G. Langerhans cell histiocytosis misdiagnosed as liver cancer and pituitary tumor in an adult: a case report and brief review of the literature. Oncol Lett. 2014;7(5):1602–4.

64. da Costa CE, Annels NE, Faaij CM, Forsyth RG, Hogendoorn PC, Egeler RM. Presence of osteoclast-like multinucleated giant cells in the bone and nonostotic lesions of Langerhans cell histiocytosis. J Exp Med. 2005;201(5):687–93.

65. Chank LK, Weisee LM. Histiocytic and dendritic cell proliferations. In: Orazi A, Knowles DM, Foucar K, Weiss LM, editors. Neoplastic hematopathology. Philadelphia: Wolters Kluver/Lippincott Williams & Wilkins; 2014. p. 1175–91.

66. Nakamine H, Yamakawa M, Yoshino T, Fukumoto T, Enomoto Y, Matsumura I. Langerhans cell histiocytosis and Langerhans cell sarcoma: current understanding and differential diagnosis. J Clin Exp Hematop. 2016;56(2):109–18.

67. Hervier B, Haroche J, Arnaud L, et al. Association of both Langerhans cell histiocytosis and Erdheim-Chester disease linked to the BRAFV600E mutation. Blood. 2014;124(7):1119–26.

68. Heritier S, Emile JF, Barkaoui MA, et al. BRAF mutation correlates with high-risk Langerhans cell histiocytosis and increased resistance to first-line therapy. J Clin Oncol. 2016;34(25):3023–30.

69. Harmon CM, Brown N. Langerhans cell histiocytosis: a clinicopathologic review and molecular pathogenetic update. Arch Pathol Lab Med. 2015;139(10):1211–4.

70. Sahm F, Capper D, Preusser M, et al. BRAFV600E mutant protein is expressed in cells of variable maturation in Langerhans cell histiocytosis. Blood. 2012;120(12):e28–34.

71. Kreitman RJ, Arons E. Update on hairy cell leukemia. Clin Adv Hematol Oncol. 2018;16(3):205–15.

72. Ballester LY, Cantu MD, Lim KPH, et al. The use of BRAF V600E mutation-specific immunohistochemistry in pediatric Langerhans cell histiocytosis. Hematol Oncol. 2018;36(1):307–15.

73. Romano RC, Shon W, Jenkins SM, Fritchie KJ. BRAF V600E immunohistochemistry in cutaneous Langerhans cell histiocytosis: an analysis of 20 caess. Int J Path Clin Res. 2016;2(2):1–5.

74. El Demellawy D, Young JL, de Nanassy J, Chernetsova E, Nasr A. Langerhans cell histiocytosis: a comprehensive review. Pathology. 2015;47(4):294–301.

75. Candiago E, Marocolo D, Manganoni MA, Leali C, Facchetti F. Nonlymphoid intraepidermal mononuclear cell collections (pseudo-Pautrier abscesses): a morphologic and immunophenotypical characterization. Am J Dermatopathol. 2000;22(1):1–6.

76. Efared B, Mazti A, Chaibou B, et al. Bone pathologic fracture revealing an unusual association: coexistence of Langerhans cell histiocytosis with Rosai-Dorfman disease. BMC Clin Pathol. 2017;17:5.

77. Litzner BR, Subtil A, Vidal CI. Combined cutaneous Rosai-Dorfman disease and localized cutaneous Langerhans cell histiocytosis within a single subcutaneous nodule. Am J Dermatopathol. 2015;37(12):936–9.

78. Kader NA, Indusarath S, Supriya NK. Solitary Langer hans cell histiocytosis of liver with sclerosing cholangitis in an adult female. Int J Clin Exp Med. 2017;5:2237–9.

79. Chung WD, Im SA, Chung NG, Park GS. Langerhans cell sarcoma in two young children: imaging findings on initial presentation and recurrence. Korean J Radiol. 2013;14(3):520–4.

80. Pileri SA, Grogan TM, Harris NL, et al. Tumours of histiocytes and accessory dendritic cells: an immunohistochemical approach

to classification from the International Lymphoma Study Group based on 61 cases. Histopathology. 2002;41(1):1–29.

81. Howard JE, Dwivedi RC, Masterson L, Jani P. Langerhans cell sarcoma: a systematic review. Cancer Treat Rev. 2015;41(4):320–31.

82. Xerri L, Adelaide J, Popovici C, et al. CDKN2A/B deletion and double-hit mutations of the MAPK pathway underlie the aggressive behavior of Langerhans cell tumors. Am J Surg Pathol. 2018;42(2):150–9.

83. West DS, Dogan A, Quint PS, et al. Clonally related follicular lymphomas and Langerhans cell neoplasms: expanding the spectrum of transdifferentiation. Am J Surg Pathol. 2013;37(7):978–86.

84. Ambrosio MR, De Falco G, Rocca BJ, et al. Langerhans cell sarcoma following marginal zone lymphoma: expanding the knowledge on mature B cell plasticity. Virchows Arch. 2015;467(4):471–80.

85. Furmanczyk PS, Lisle AE, Caldwell RB, et al. Langerhans cell sarcoma in a patient with hairy cell leukemia: common clonal origin indicated by identical immunoglobulin gene rearrangements. J Cutan Pathol. 2012;39(6):644–50.

86. Kimura H, Nasu K, Sakai C, et al. Histiocytic sarcoma of the spleen associated with hypoalbuminemia, hypo gamma-globulinemia and thrombocytopenia as a possibly unique clinical entity–report of three cases. Leuk Lymphoma. 1998;31(1–2):217–24.

87. Audouin J, Vercelli-Retta J, Le Tourneau A, et al. Primary histiocytic sarcoma of the spleen associated with erythrophagocytic histiocytosis. Pathol Res Pract. 2003;199(2):107–12.

88. Kobayashi S, Kimura F, Hama Y, et al. Histiocytic sarcoma of the spleen: case report of asymptomatic onset of thrombocytopenia and complex imaging features. Int J Hematol. 2008;87(1):83–7.

89. Yamada S, Tasaki T, Satoh N, et al. Primary splenic histiocytic sarcoma complicated with prolonged idiopathic thrombocytopenia and secondary bone marrow involvement: a unique surgical case presenting with splenomegaly but non-nodular lesions. Diagn Pathol. 2012;7:143.

90. Ohnishi K, Tanaka S, Oghiso Y, Takeya M. Immunohistochemical detection of possible cellular origin of hepatic histiocytic sarcoma in mice. J Clin Exp Hematop. 2012;52(3):171–7.

91. Feldman AL, Arber DA, Pittaluga S, et al. Clonally related follicular lymphomas and histiocytic/dendritic cell sarcomas: evidence for transdifferentiation of the follicular lymphoma clone. Blood. 2008;111(12):5433–9.

92. Takahashi E, Nakamura S. Histiocytic sarcoma: an updated literature review based on the 2008 WHO classification. J Clin Exp Hematop. 2013;53(1):1–8.

93. Hornick JL, Jaffe ES, Fletcher CD. Extranodal histiocytic sarcoma: clinicopathologic analysis of 14 cases of a rare epithelioid malignancy. Am J Surg Pathol. 2004;28(9):1133–44.

94. Oka K, Nakamine H, Maeda K, et al. Primary histiocytic sarcoma of the spleen associated with hemophagocytosis. Int J Hematol. 2008;87(4):405–9.

95. Paik JH, Jeon KY, Park SS, et al. Histiocytic saroma of spleen-a case report and reivew of the literature. Korean J Pathol. 2005;39:356–9.

96. Llamas-Velasco M, Cannata J, Dominguez I, et al. Coexistence of Langerhans cell histiocytosis, Rosai-Dorfman disease and splenic lymphoma with fatal outcome after rapid development of histiocytic sarcoma of the liver. J Cutan Pathol. 2012;39(12):1125–30.

97. Yang G, Deisch J, Qin H, Zuppan C, Raza AS. Aggressive primary hepatic histiocytic sarcoma: case report and literature review. Hepatoma. 2016;2:300–4.

98. Kommalapati A, Tella SH, Durkin M, Go RS, Goyal G. Histiocytic sarcoma: a population-based analysis of incidence, demographic disparities, and long-term outcomes. Blood. 2018;131(2):265–8.

99. Mikami M, Sadahira Y, Suetsugu Y, Wada H, Sugihara T. Monocyte/macrophage-specific marker CD163+ histiocytic sarcoma: case report with clinical, morphologic, immunohistochemical, and molecular genetic studies. Int J Hematol. 2004;80(4):365–9.

100. Nguyen TT, Schwartz EJ, West RB, Warnke RA, Arber DA, Natkunam Y. Expression of CD163 (hemoglobin scavenger receptor) in normal tissues, lymphomas, carcinomas, and sarcomas is largely restricted to the monocyte/macrophage lineage. Am J Surg Pathol. 2005;29(5):617–24.

101. Chen W, Lau SK, Fong D, et al. High frequency of clonal immunoglobulin receptor gene rearrangements in sporadic histiocytic/dendritic cell sarcomas. Am J Surg Pathol. 2009;33(6):863–73.

102. Grogan TM, Poleri SA, Chan J, Weiss LM, Fletcher C. Histiocytic sarcoma. In: Swerdlow SH, Campo E, Harris NL, Jaffe ES, SA P, editors. World health organization classification of tumours, WHO classification of tumours of haematopoietic and lymphoid tissues. Lyon: IARC; 2008.

103. Shao H, Xi L, Raffeld M, et al. Clonally related histiocytic/dendritic cell sarcoma and chronic lymphocytic leukemia/small lymphocytic lymphoma: a study of seven cases. Mod Pathol. 2011;24(11):1421–32.

104. Huang W, Qiu T, Zeng L, Zheng B, Ying J, Feng X. High frequency of clonal IG and T-cell receptor gene rearrangements in histiocytic and dendritic cell neoplasms. Oncotarget. 2016;7(48):78355–78,362.

105. Go H, Jeon YK, Huh J, et al. Frequent detection of BRAF(V600E) mutations in histiocytic and dendritic cell neoplasms. Histopathology. 2014;65(2):261–72.

106. Ansari J, Naqash AR, Munker R, et al. Histiocytic sarcoma as a secondary malignancy: pathobiology, diagnosis, and treatment. Eur J Haematol. 2016;97(1):9–16.

107. Weiss LM, Pileri SA, Chan J, Fletcher C. Histiocytic sarcma. In: Swerdlow SH, Campa E, Harris NL, editors. WHO classification of tumours of hematopoietic and lymphoid tissues. Lyon, France: IARC Press; 2017. p. 468–70.

108. Alexiev RA, Sailey CJ, McClure SA, Ord RA, Zhao CF, Papadimitriou JC. Primaryhistiocytic sarcoma arising in the head and neck with predominant spindle cell component. Diagn Pathol. 2007;2. http://www.diagnosticpathology.org/content/2/1/7

109. Shimono J, Miyoshi H, Arakawa F, et al. Prognostic factors for histiocytic and dendritic cell neoplasms. Oncotarget. 2017;8(58):98723–32.

110. Monda L, Warnke R, Rosai J. A primary lymph node malignancy with features suggestive of dendritic reticulum cell differentiation. A report of 4 cases. Am J Pathol. 1986;122(3):562–72.

111. chan J, Pileri SA, Fletcher C, Weiss LM, Grogg KL. Follicular dendritic cell sarcoma. In: Swerdlow SH, Campo E, Harris NL, et al., editors. WHO classification of tumours of haematopoietic and lymphoid tissue. Lyon: IARC press; 2017. p. 476–9.

112. Bai LY, Kwang WK, Chiang IP, Chen PM. Follicular dendritic cell tumor of the liver associated with Epstein-Barr virus. Jpn J Clin Oncol. 2006;36(4):249–53.

113. Chen Y, Shi H, Li H, Zhen T, Han A. Clinicopathological features of inflammatory pseudotumour-like follicular dendritic cell tumour of the abdomen. Histopathology. 2016;68(6):858–65.

114. Cheuk W, Chan JK, Shek TW, et al. Inflammatory pseudotumor-like follicular dendritic cell tumor: a distinctive low-grade malignant intra-abdominal neoplasm with consistent Epstein-Barr virus association. Am J Surg Pathol. 2001;25(6):721–31.

115. Shia J, Chen W, Tang LH, et al. Extranodal follicular dendritic cell sarcoma: clinical, pathologic, and histogenetic characteristics of an underrecognized disease entity. Virchows Arch. 2006;449(2):148–58.

116. Pauwels P, Dal Cin P, Vlasveld LT, Aleva RM, van Erp WF, Jones D. A chromosomal abnormality in hyaline vascular Castleman's disease: evidence for clonal proliferation of dysplastic stromal cells. Am J Surg Pathol. 2000;24(6):882–8.

117. Cokelaere K, Debiec-Rychter M, De Wolf-Peeters C, Hagemeijer A, Sciot R. Hyaline vascular Castleman's disease with HMGIC rearrangement in follicular dendritic cells: molecular evidence of mesenchymal tumorigenesis. Am J Surg Pathol. 2002;26(5):662–9.

118. Sun X, Chang KC, Abruzzo LV, Lai R, Younes A, Jones D. Epidermal growth factor receptor expression in follicular dendritic cells: a shared feature of follicular dendritic cell sarcoma and Castleman's disease. Hum Pathol. 2003;34(9):835–40.

119. Saygin C, Uzunaslan D, Ozguroglu M, Senocak M, Tuzuner N. Dendritic cell sarcoma: a pooled analysis including 462 cases with presentation of our case series. Crit Rev Oncol Hematol. 2013;88(2):253–71.

120. Soriano AO, Thompson MA, Admirand JH, et al. Follicular dendritic cell sarcoma: a report of 14 cases and a review of the literature. Am J Hematol. 2007;82(8):725–8.

121. Lee CH, Yen YS, Shan YS, Lin PW. Follicular dendritic cell tumor in liver: a case report and collective review. Gastroenterology Res. 2010;3(3):139–43.

122. Martins PN, Reddy S, Martins AB, Facciuto M. Follicular dendritic cell sarcoma of the liver: unusual presentation of a rare tumor and literature review. Hepatobiliary Pancreat Dis Int. 2011;10(4):443–5.

123. Vardas K, Manganas D, Papadimitriou G, et al. Splenic inflammatory pseudotumor-like follicular dendritic cell tumor. Case Rep Oncol. 2014;7(2):410–6.

124. Wang L, Xu D, Qiao Z, Shen L, Dai H, Ji Y. Follicular dendritic cell sarcoma of the spleen: a case report and review of the literature. Oncol Lett. 2016;12(3):2062–4.

125. Hang JF, Wang LC, Lai CR. Cytological features of inflammatory pseudotumor-like follicular dendritic cell sarcoma of spleen: a case report. Diagn Cytopathol. 2017;45(3):230–4.

126. Ge R, Liu C, Yin X, et al. Clinicopathologic characteristics of inflammatory pseudotumor-like follicular dendritic cell sarcoma. Int J Clin Exp Pathol. 2014;7:2421–9.

127. Choe JY, Go H, Jeon YK, et al. Inflammatory pseudotumor-like follicular dendritic cell sarcoma of the spleen: a report of six cases with increased IgG4-positive plasma cells. Pathol Int. 2013;63(5):245–51.

128. Wu A, Pullarkat S. Follicular dendritic cell sarcoma. Arch Pathol Lab Med. 2016;140(2):186–90.

129. Grogg KL, Macon WR, Kurtin PJ, Nascimento AG. A survey of clusterin and fascin expression in sarcomas and spindle cell neoplasms: strong clusterin immunostaining is highly specific for follicular dendritic cell tumor. Mod Pathol. 2005;18(2):260–6.

130. Yu H, Gibson JA, Pinkus GS, Hornick JL. Podoplanin (D2–40) is a novel marker for follicular dendritic cell tumors. Am J Clin Pathol. 2007;128(5):776–82.

131. Zhang H, Maitta RW, Bhattacharyya PK, et al. gamma-Synuclein is a promising new marker for staining reactive follicular dendritic cells, follicular dendritic cell sarcoma, Kaposi sarcoma, and benign and malignant vascular tumors. Am J Surg Pathol. 2011;35(12):1857–65.

132. Perry AM, Nelson M, Sanger WG, Bridge JA, Greiner TC. Cytogenetic abnormalities in follicular dendritic cell sarcoma: report of two cases and literature review. In Vivo. 2013;27(2):211–4.

133. Griffin GK, Sholl LM, Lindeman NI, Fletcher CD, Hornick JL. Targeted genomic sequencing of follicular dendritic cell sarcoma reveals recurrent alterations in NF-kappaB regulatory genes. Mod Pathol. 2016;29(1):67–74.

134. Hornick JL. Soft tisssue tumors with prominent inflammatory cells. In: Hornick JL, et al., editors. Practical soft tissue pathology: a diagnostic approach. Philadelphia: Elsevier Saunders; 2013. p. 257–61.

135. Chen M, Agrawal R, Nasseri-Nik N, Sloman A, Weiss LM. Indeterminate cell tumor of the spleen. Hum Pathol. 2012;43(2):307–11.

136. Cook JR, Dehner LP, Collins MH, et al. Anaplastic lymphoma kinase (ALK) expression in the inflammatory myofibroblastic tumor: a comparative immunohistochemical study. Am J Surg Pathol. 2001;25(11):1364–71.

137. Dojcinov SD, Venkataraman G, Pittaluga S, et al. Age-related EBV-associated lymphoproliferative disorders in the Western population: a spectrum of reactive lymphoid hyperplasia and lymphoma. Blood. 2011;117(18):4726–35.

138. Chin KM, Ho WY, Lim KHT, Chung YFA, Lee SY. Follicular dendritic cell sarcoma of the liver with metachronous small bowel and splenic metastases: a case report and literature review. Hepatobiliary Surg Nutr. 2017;6(3):179–89.

139. Henter JI, Horne A, Arico M, et al. HLH-2004: diagnostic and therapeutic guidelines for hemophagocytic lymphohistiocytosis. Pediatr Blood Cancer. 2007;48(2):124–31.

140. Malinowska I, Machaczka M, Popko K, Siwicka A, Salamonowicz M, Nasilowska-Adamska B. Hemophagocytic syndrome in children and adults. Arch Immunol Ther Exp (Warsz). 2014;62(5):385–94.

141. Janka GE. Familial and acquired hemophagocytic lymphohistiocytosis. Annu Rev Med. 2012;63:233–46.

142. Rosado FG, Kim AS. Hemophagocytic lymphohistiocytosis: an update on diagnosis and pathogenesis. Am J Clin Pathol. 2013;139(6):713–27.

143. Hayden A, Park S, Giustini D, Lee AY, Chen LY. Hemophagocytic syndromes (HPSs) including hemophagocytic lymphohistiocytosis (HLH) in adults: a systematic scoping review. Blood Rev. 2016;30(6):411–20.

144. Al-Samkari H, Berliner N. Hemophagocytic lymphohistiocytosis. Annu Rev Pathol. 2018;13:27–49.

145. Smith MC, Cohen DN, Greig B, Yenamandra A, Vnencak-Jones C, et al. The ambiguous boundary between EBV related hemophagocytic lymphohistiocytosis and systemic EBV-driven T cell lymphoproliferative disorder. Int J Clin Exp Pathol. 2014;7(9):5738–49.

146. Morimoto A, Nakazawa Y, Ishii E. Hemophagocytic lymphohistiocytosis: pathogenesis, diagnosis, and management. Pediatr Int. 2016;58(9):817–25.

147. Niece JA, Rogers ZR, Ahmad N, Langevin AM, McClain KL. Hemophagocytic lymphohistiocytosis in Texas: observations on ethnicity and race. Pediatr Blood Cancer. 2010;54(3):424–8.

148. Malloy CA, Polinski C, Alkan S, Manera R, Challapalli M. Hemophagocytic lymphohistiocytosis presenting with nonimmune hydrops fetalis. J Perinatol. 2004;24(7):458–60.

149. Machaczka M, Vaktnas J, Klimkowska M, Hagglund H. Malignancy-associated hemophagocytic lymphohistiocytosis in adults: a retrospective population-based analysis from a single center. Leuk Lymphoma. 2011;52(4):613–9.

150. Suzuki N, Morimoto A, Ohga S, et al. Characteristics of hemophagocytic lymphohistiocytosis in neonates: a nationwide survey in Japan. J Pediatr. 2009;155(2):235–238 e231.

151. Freeman HR, Ramanan AV. Review of haemophagocytic lymphohistiocytosis. Arch Dis Child. 2011;96(7):688–93.

152. Emile JF, Charlotte F, Chassagne-Clement C, et al. Histiocytoses: General classification and molecular criteria. Presse Med. 2017;46(1):46–54.

153. Ho C, Yao X, Tian L, Li FY, Podoltsev N, Xu ML. Marrow assessment for hemophagocytic lymphohistiocytosis demonstrates poor correlation with disease probability. Am J Clin Pathol. 2014;141(1):62–71.

154. Gars E, Purington N, Scott G, et al. Bone marrow histomorphological criteria can accurately diagnose hemophagocytic lymphohistiocytosis. Haematologica. 2018;103(10):1635–41.

155. Hsi ED. Hematopathology: a volume in foundations in diagnostic pathology series. London: Churchilln Livingstone; 2007.

156. Chen JH, Fleming MD, Pinkus GS, et al. Pathology of the liver in familial hemophagocytic lymphohistiocytosis. Am J Surg Pathol. 2010;34(6):852–67.

157. Rubin TS, Zhang K, Gifford C, et al. Perforin and CD107a testing is superior to NK cell function testing for screening patients for genetic HLH. Blood. 2017;129(22):2993–9.

158. Goransdotter Ericson K, Fadeel B, Nilsson-Ardnor S, et al. Spectrum of perforin gene mutations in familial hemophagocytic

lymphohistiocytosis. Am J Hum Genet. 2001;68(3): 590–7.

159. Feldmann J, Callebaut I, Raposo G, et al. Munc13–4 is essential for cytolytic granules fusion and is mutated in a form of familial hemophagocytic lymphohistiocytosis (FHL3). Cell. 2003;115(4):461–73.

160. zur Stadt U, Schmidt S, Kasper B, et al. Linkage of familial hemophagocytic lymphohistiocytosis (FHL) type-4 to chromosome 6q24 and identification of mutations in syntaxin 11. Hum Mol Genet. 2005;14(6):827–34.

161. Cote M, Menager MM, Burgess A, et al. Munc18–2 deficiency causes familial hemophagocytic lymphohistiocytosis type 5 and impairs cytotoxic granule exocytosis in patient NK cells. J Clin Invest. 2009;119(12):3765–73.

162. Janka GE, Schneider EM. Modern management of children with haemophagocytic lymphohistiocytosis. Br J Haematol. 2004;124(1):4–14.

163. Machowicz R, Janka G, Wiktor-Jedrzejczak W. Similar but not the same: differential diagnosis of HLH and sepsis. Crit Rev Oncol Hematol. 2017;114:1–12.

164. Quintanilla-Martinez L, Kumar S, Fend F, et al. Fulminant EBV(+) T-cell lymphoproliferative disorder following acute/ chronic EBV infection: a distinct clinicopathologic syndrome. Blood. 2000;96(2):443–51.

165. Maheshwari U, Mahore K, Pereira E, Dhar R. γδ T-cell lymphoma: a rare entity mimicking hemophagocytic syndrome-report of two cases. Int J Res Med Sci. 2017;5:3751–4.

166. Paes VR, de Lima PP, Siqueira SAC. Hemophagocytic lymphohistiocytosis associated with hepatosplenic T-cell lymphoma: case report. Autops Case Rep. 2014;4(4):19–24.

167. Khadanga S, Solomon B, Dittus K. Hemophagocytic Lymphohistiocytosis (HLH) associated with T-cell lymphomas: broadening our differential for fever of unknown origin. N Am J Med Sci. 2014;6(9):484–6.

168. Trottestam H, Horne A, Arico M, et al. Chemoimmunotherapy for hemophagocytic lymphohistiocytosis: long-term results of the HLH-94 treatment protocol. Blood. 2011;118(17):4577–84.

169. Riviere S, Galicier L, Coppo P, et al. Reactive hemophagocytic syndrome in adults: a retrospective analysis of 162 patients. Am J Med. 2014;127(11):1118–25.

170. Otrock ZK, Eby CS. Clinical characteristics, prognostic factors, and outcomes of adult patients with hemophagocytic lymphohistiocytosis. Am J Hematol. 2015;90(3):220–4.

Brent K. Larson and Maha Guindi

Abbreviations

AIH	Autoimmune hepatitis
ALT	Alanine aminotransferase
AMR	Antibody-mediated rejection
AST	Aspartate aminotransferase
CMV	Cytomegalovirus
DILI	Drug-induced liver disease
DSA	Donor-specific antibody
EBER	Epstein-Barr virus-encoded small ribonucleic acids
EBV	Epstein-Barr virus
EBV-LMP1	Epstein-Barr virus latent membrane protein 1
GGT	Gamma-glutamyl transferase
GMS	Grocott methenamine silver
GVHD	Graft-versus-host disease
HBV	Hepatitis B virus
HCV	Hepatitis C virus
HDV	Hepatitis D virus
HEV	Hepatitis E virus
HHV6	Human herpesvirus-6
HIV	Human immunodeficiency virus
HLH	Hemophagocytic lymphohistiocytosis
HSV	Herpes simplex virus
NK	Natural killer
PAS D	Periodic-acid Schiff with diastase predigestion
PAS	Periodic-acid Schiff
PBC	Primary biliary cholangitis
PSC	Primary sclerosing cholangitis
PTLD	Post-transplant lymphoproliferative disorder
RAI	Rejection activity index
RNA	Ribonucleic acid
SOS	Sinusoidal obstruction syndrome
TCMR	T cell-mediated rejection

B. K. Larson (✉) · M. Guindi
Department of Pathology and Laboratory Medicine, Cedars-Sinai
Medical Center, Los Angeles, CA, USA
e-mail: brent.larson@cshs.org

Introduction

Many previous resources have been published addressing the topic of the post-transplant liver and of the native liver in patients after transplantation of other organs and tissue. But few, if any, single sources concisely discuss the histopathology of the liver across all of transplantation in a single source. Post-transplant-related splenic changes are rare as splenectomy is not performed in these patients. In addition, the risk of splenic biopsy procedure is high. It is assumed that the histomorphologic changes found in the post-transplant spleen are similar to those occurring in the liver. Given the various types of transplantation, this chapter will discuss transplant-related liver damage and reactive response, this chapter will address five main concerns: (1) issues that affect the liver across all transplantation settings; (2) issues unique to hematopoietic stem cell transplantation; (3) problems of liver allografts after liver transplantation; (4) problems that arise in the native liver after non-liver solid organ transplantation; and (5) new and evolving topics, such as hepatitis C treatment and antibody-mediated rejection. Special attention is devoted to findings that may differ in the post-transplant setting from those of identical etiologies in the non-transplanted patient.

Of note, indications for liver biopsy vary with the organ or tissue transplanted [1–3]. However, virtually all post-transplant patients undergo monitoring of liver enzymes for a variety of reasons. Serum elevations of liver enzymes indicating hepatic injury (e.g., aminotransferases) or impaired hepatic function (e.g., alkaline phosphatase or bilirubin) during routine monitoring are often the first sign of hepatic complications and may prompt a liver biopsy. Liver biopsy is considered the gold standard for diagnosis of acute rejection in transplant patients and is able to disclose other liver disease, interpret the severity of disease and monitor treatment response regardless of status (pre- or post-transplant) [4–6].

Post-transplant liver biopsies should undergo similar processing to other liver biopsies. Particular comment should be

© Springer Nature Switzerland AG 2020
L. Zhang et al. (eds.), *Diagnostic Pathology of Hematopoietic Disorders of Spleen and Liver*,
https://doi.org/10.1007/978-3-030-37708-3_18

made regarding overall adequacy of the biopsy. Cores should have a total length of ≥2.0 cm and contain ≥11 portal areas [7]. Limitations regarding any of these parameters and biopsy fragmentation may lead to less representative sampling.

Multiple hematoxylin-and-eosin-stained sections should be viewed, as diagnostic foci for many conditions may be very rare. While no single panel of stains is widely considered definitive, there is a wide consensus that, at minimum, a collagen stain, such as Masson trichrome, should be ordered along with routine hematoxylin-and-eosin-stained sections. Periodic-acid Schiff with diastase pre-digestion (PAS D) and iron stains to screen for alpha-1-antitrypsin deficiency and hemochromatosis, respectively, are also recommended, at least in the initial liver biopsy, as these disorders may be clinically unsuspected and diagnosed in both transplanted and non-transplanted patients.

All of the aforementioned topics and many more are discussed in this chapter's comprehensive and concise review of liver allograft pathology and pathology of the native liver after other organ or tissue transplantation. For a discussion of post-transplant lymphoproliferative disorders involving the liver, refer to the chapter on lymphoproliferative disorders.

Issues Common Across Transplant Settings

The liver in the transplanted patient is susceptible to all of the same attacks as the liver of non-transplanted patients, including viral hepatitis, autoimmune liver disease, and fatty liver disease, among many other insults. However, the post-transplant patient has some unique issues, and some of the most common occur regardless of the organ or tissue transplanted. In addition, immunosuppressive medications themselves may contribute to hepatic dysfunction.

Opportunistic Infections

As a result of chronic immunosuppression, opportunistic infections, both hepatotropic and systemic, may affect the liver. Non-hepatotropic (non-hepatitis A-E) viruses may infect immunocompetent patients, but one's threshold should be considerably lowered when assessing a liver biopsy from a post-transplant patient.

Viral Infections

Cytomegalovirus (CMV)

Cytomegalovirus (CMV) lies latent in infected B cells in a majority of Americans. Post-transplantation, infection in the liver can lead to clinically significant hepatitis. CMV hepatitis may arise from CMV transmission from a seropositive donor organ to a seronegative recipient, reactivation of a latent infection, or primary infection in a seronegative transplant patient [8–10]. Patients typically present weeks to months post-transplant with nonspecific gastrointestinal

symptoms like nausea and abdominal pain; systematic symptoms like myalgia, arthralgias, and fever; and/or hepatic symptoms like jaundice and hepatosplenomegaly [9]. Polymerase chain reaction (PCR) may demonstrate copies of viral DNA in plasma, though PCR positivity does not correlate well with liver infection [11]. The characteristic finding is the large, brightly eosinophilic nuclear inclusions. However, these are frequently not present, so a low threshold for ordering a CMV immunostain is encouraged. Although immunohistochemical staining is more sensitive and very specific when compared to microscopic examination, false negativity due to only focal presence of CMV infection can occur [12, 13]. Histological features of infection include lobular neutrophilic microabscesses, mixed lobular inflammation, mild-moderate portal lymphocytic infiltrate, mild duct injury/cholangitis, and Kupffer cell hyperplasia (Fig. 18.1a&b). Less common findings include mild portal venulitis, cholestasis, sinusoidal lymphocytosis, and granulomatous hepatitis. These findings are not specific. Neutrophilic microabscesses merit special mention, as they gained acclaim as a feature of CMV hepatitis, though they are neither specific nor sensitive for this diagnosis. In one study, microabscesses were found in only 17% of liver allograft biopsies done for graft dysfunction and of these 17%, only 19% proved to have CMV [14]. Microabscesses can be seen in other conditions, such as other infections (bacterial, viral, and fungal), and biliary obstruction. Antiviral agents (such as ganciclovir and foscarnet) are the mainstays of treatment for CMV hepatitis, in combination with reduced immunosuppression. Rarely, patients may develop biliary complications years after acute infection.

Epstein-Barr Virus (EBV)

Epstein-Barr virus (EBV) can (1) cause EBV hepatitis, (2) drive post-transplant lymphoproliferative disorders (PTLD), and (3) stimulate hemophagocytic lymphohistiocytosis (HLH). PTLD is covered extensively elsewhere in this text, and HLH is covered in a separate section below. In this section, EBV hepatitis is described. EBV infects B lymphocytes and reaches the liver in the circulation, which invokes a vigorous T cell response. Hepatocytes and ductal epithelium are not infected, and therefore no viral cytopathic effect is observed. The liver typically shows a moderate to marked mixed, but lymphocyte-predominant, portal infiltrate. Scattered large, activated lymphoid cells may be seen, and the portal changes are accompanied by sinusoids packed by a linear arrangement of lymphocytes (Fig. 18.1c). The portal infiltrate is frequently accompanied by mild spillover into the periportal parenchyma. Hepatocellular injury is minimal or absent compared to the degree of inflammation, and lymphocytes that spill into the periportal parenchyma do not destroy hepatocytes at the interface. Small epithelioid lobular granulomas may occasionally be present. The lymphoid infiltrate may be so dense that, together with an atypical

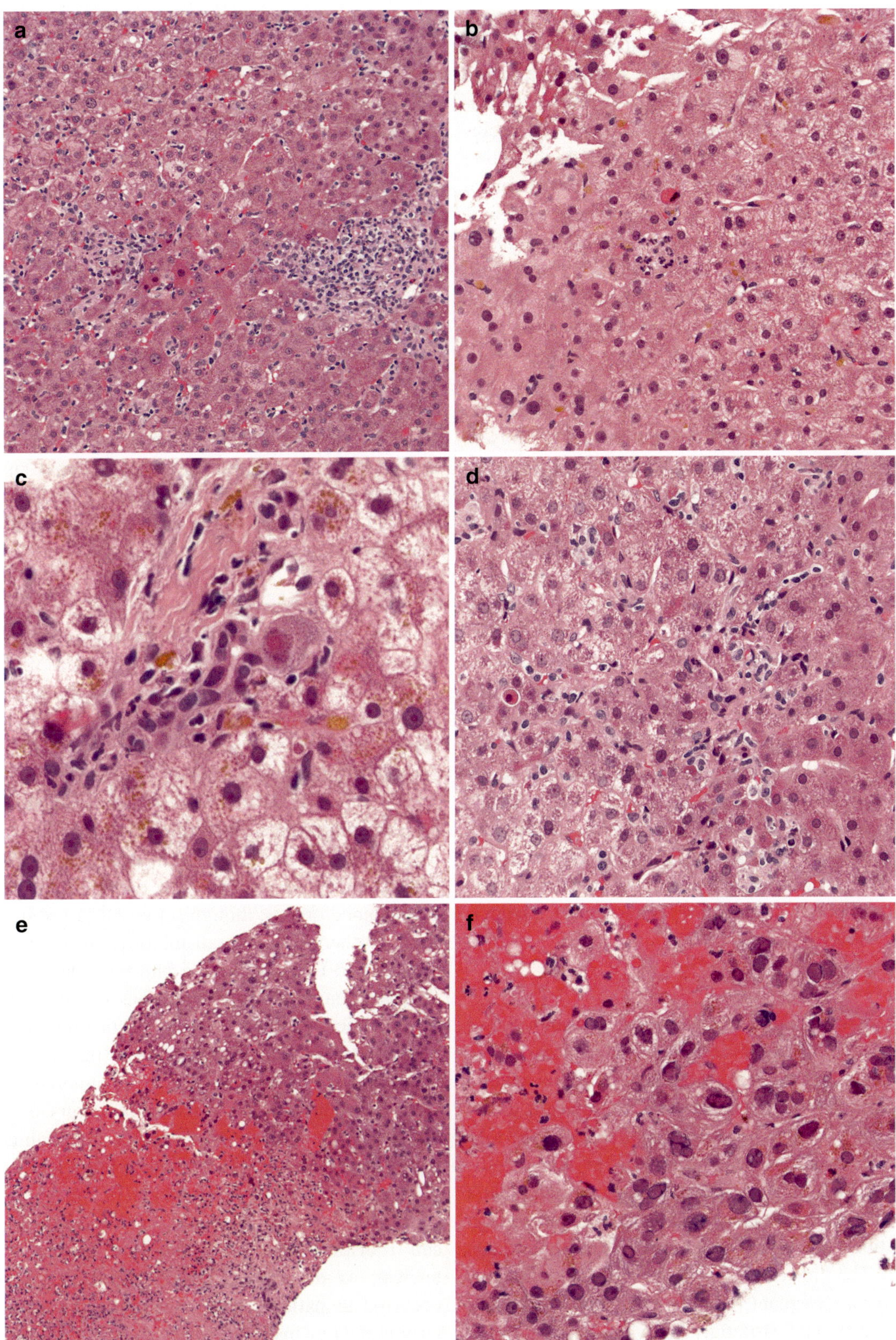

Fig. 18.1 Examples of non-hepatotropic viral hepatitides. (**a**) Portal and lobular inflammation in CMV hepatitis (H&E stain, 200× original magnification). (**b**) Lobular cholestasis, rare acidophil bodies, and a neutrophilic microabscess in CMV hepatitis (H&E stain, 400× original magnification). (**c**) Rare viral inclusion in CMV hepatitis (H&E stain, 400× original magnification). (**d**) Lobular hepatitis with acidophil bod- ies and lymphocytes lined up single file in sinusoids of EBV hepatitis (H&E stain, 400× original magnification). (**e**) Geographic necrosis in HSV hepatitis (H&E stain, 100× original magnification). (**f**) Viral inclu- sions at the border of necrotic and viable parenchyma in HSV hepatitis (H&E stain, 400× original magnification)

appearance of the lymphocytes, it can be concerning for leukemic infiltrate, especially considering that EBV can also drive PTLD [15]. In these situations, a formal lymphoma work up may be needed to exclude PTLD. In situ hybridization for Epstein-Barr virus-encoded small ribonucleic acids (EBER) is helpful to confirm the diagnosis by highlighting infected cells, which may be rare. Immunohistochemical staining for Epstein-Barr virus latent membrane protein 1 (EBV-LMP1) is typically negative and of no use in making the diagnosis. Clinically, EBV hepatitis may present with elevations in aminotransferases, bilirubin, and/or alkaline phosphatase. Treatment is primarily symptomatic.

Herpes Simplex Virus (HSV)

Herpes simplex virus (HSV) hepatitis is uncommon, but the great majority of cases occur in the immunocompromised. Patients frequently present with an acute, even fulminant, hepatitis with markedly elevated aminotransferases (frequently >1000 U/L) and fever. HSV hepatitis is typically an early post-transplant event, usually occurring from 5 to 46 days post-transplant [16]. Acyclovir is the mainstay of treatment, and a significant number of patients may require liver transplantation. Histologically, infection is characterized by pauci-inflammatory azonal and geographic coagulative necrosis. Amphophilic ground-glass nuclear inclusions and multinucleation are most typically seen in the hepatocytes at the interface between necrotic and viable tissue (Fig. 18.1d–f). Less commonly, brightly eosinophilic nuclear inclusions with a surrounding clear halo (Cowdry A type inclusions) may be seen. Viral inclusions may be inconspicuous, and immunohistochemistry for HSV1 and HSV2 should be used to differentiate the azonal necrotic pattern from toxic liver injury (most notably, acetaminophen toxicity), adenovirus, and acute ischemic injury.

Adenovirus

Like HSV hepatitis, adenovirus hepatitis typically shows azonal coagulative necrosis with minimal inflammation. Smudgy amphophilic nuclear inclusions with basophilic marginated chromatin are typically present adjacent to the necrosis, though they may be sprinkled throughout the lobules, and may appear more eosinophilic in some cells. Patients post orthotopic liver transplant or hematopoietic stem cell transplant are most commonly affected, though rare presentations after other solid organ transplants have been reported. The time of presentation ranges from 20 days up to 1 year post-transplant [17]. Patients most commonly present with fever and strikingly high aminotransferases (>1000 U/L), with AST typically double or triple ALT. Abdominal imaging studies may uncommonly show what appear to be mass lesions, which actually represent particularly necrotic foci. Infection may be detected by serum PCR, though definitive diagnosis of liver involvement can only be confirmed with tissue sampling. Most patients treated successfully have responded to antivirals and/or a reduction in immunosuppression, though survival is poor overall with 75% patients dying in 9 days, on average [17]. The most common adenovirus serotypes causing hepatitis are 2 and 5, though >25% of infections are of neither of these serotypes [18]. This is especially important to recognize when working up a case by immunohistochemistry, as different commercially available immunostains contain antibodies against different serotypes.

Hepatitis E (HEV)

Hepatitis E (HEV) can cause both acute and chronic hepatitis in solid organ transplant patients. This is a recent departure recognized as of 2008 from the previous typical association of HEV with sporadic or epidemic cases [19]. The infections have a high risk of causing chronic disease and have been reported to cause accelerated fibrosis [20]. The liver biopsy shows mild and nonspecific lobular and portal inflammation, with or without mild cholestasis.

Human Herpesvirus-6 (HHV6)

Human herpesvirus-6 (HHV6) is a ubiquitous virus in the herpesviridae family closely related to CMV, which infects over 95% of humans. It can cause primary infection or reactivate from latency. Most reactivations, even in the immunosuppressed population, are mild febrile illnesses or are entirely asymptomatic. HHV6 reactivation is diagnosed by testing for viral DNA in the plasma or whole blood, by presence of antigenemia, or demonstration of virus-specific proteins in tissue biopsies. Serum testing by PCR can be of limited utility, as virus may be harbored and reactivated in transplanted organs, though serum DNA testing is undetectable. Furthermore, a small minority of the population harbors HHV6 DNA integrated into the host genome that will give copy numbers in the millions on serum testing, even when clinically silent, whereas reactivation most commonly causes copy number elevations into the tens of thousands. Liver biopsy to demonstrate histopathological effects of HHV6 remains the gold standard for diagnosis of end-organ disease to show tissue effects, since infection can be localized in an organ without significant DNA levels in the blood [21]. While it is recognized that HHV6 may cause clinically significant hepatitis after solid organ and hematopoietic stem cell transplantation, the histologic pattern is somewhat unclear, as descriptions of HHV6-related hepatitis have occurred in patients with concomitant infections (particularly CMV) or histologically typical T cell-mediated rejection. The most commonly described injury pattern is a lymphocytic portal inflammation with interface activity and periportal necrosis. Other cases show a nonspecific mild to moderate lobular hepatitis. Very rare cases show hepatocyte giant cell transformation. Viral inclusions are not identified.

Immunohistochemical staining for HHV6 typically reveals positivity in portal or periportal inflammatory cells, with only rare staining in hepatocytes, including multinucleated giant hepatocytes. According to recent published guidelines from the American Society of Transplantation Infectious Disease Community of Practice, given that the majority of infections are asymptomatic, it is not recommended to have routine screening for HHV6 or HHV7 DNAemia [22]. While there is no standard treatment for HHV6, antivirals used for CMV treatment and prophylaxis (ganciclovir, valganciclovir, cidofovir, and foscarnet) may be used in combination with a reduction in immunosuppression.

It is of note that some of the described viral infections may show mild duct injury and phlebitis that do not necessarily signify the presence of acute cellular rejection. However, because treatment of viral infection includes lowering immunosuppression in addition to antiviral agents, repeat biopsies after treatment for monitoring persistent or worsening liver tests may show that T cell-mediated rejection (TCMR) has developed secondary to the lowering of immunosuppression.

Bacterial and Fungal Infections

Bacterial and fungal infections affecting the liver take two forms: abscesses and invasive disease. Abscesses are not typically biopsied, as laboratory and imaging studies are frequently diagnostic. Invasive infections in the liver are typically the result of disseminated disease, and are also not frequently biopsied, as combined clinical, imaging, and laboratory findings frequently signal the diagnosis.

When biopsied, abscesses typically show the dense fibrous tissue that composes the wall. Features may vary from densely collagenized to highly cellular with abundant fibroblasts and mixed inflammatory cells. Ductular reaction may be pronounced. If the biopsy needle passes through the cavity, the core may predominantly show necrotic or purulent debris or bile. Adjacent parenchyma sampled may show mixed or neutrophil-rich inflammation. Though it is unlikely to pinpoint a causative organism, special stains can be helpful in identifying sparse organisms, and acid-fast, periodic acid-Schiff (PAS), and Grocott methenamine silver (GMS) should be performed to identify acid-fast bacilli or fungal organisms that may take weeks to culture. The main differential diagnostic consideration for an infectious abscess is a necrotic tumor.

For disseminated infections, the findings are frequently those of sepsis, namely ductular reaction and cholestasis, with or without lobular mixed or neutrophil-rich inflammation. Other reactive changes may include Kupffer cell hyperplasia and hepatocyte necrosis. Differential diagnostic considerations for this pattern include drug reactions and large duct obstruction. Granulomas may be seen with fungal infections, and should prompt an acid-fast and PAS or GMS stain. As an exception, cryptococcosis may present with minimal inflammation other than portal and lobular histiocytes containing organisms. Liver transplantation has the highest rate of fungal infection, at approximately 10% [23]. The majority of infections occur in the first month post transplantation, with *Candida* being the most common infection. *Cryptococcus*, while rare, is more common as a late infection.

Hemophagocytic Lymphohistiocytosis (Hemophagocytic Syndrome) (also refer to Chaps. 17 and 21)

Hemophagocytic lymphohistiocytosis (HLH) is a syndrome characterized by dysregulation of natural killer (NK) cell function causing marked and ineffective activation of the immune system with multi-organ damage and deficient function of cytotoxic granules. HLH is classically recognized as being either primary (usually in children) or secondary (more commonly in adults). It is diagnosed in one of two situations: (1) molecular studies demonstrating a mutation in a gene known to be associated with HLH (e.g., *PRF*, *UNC13D*, or *STX11*), or (2) at least five findings from the following constellation: fever; splenomegaly; cytopenias in at least two cell lineages (<90 g/L hemoglobin, $<100 \times 10^9$ platelets/L, or $<1.0 \times 10^9$ neutrophils/L); hypertriglyceridemia (≥ 265 mg/dL) and/or hypofibrinogenemia (≤ 1.5 g/L); elevated ferritin (≥ 500 µg/L); elevated soluble CD25 (≥ 2400 U/mL); low/absent NK-cell activity; or evidence of hemophagocytosis on tissue sampling, with no evidence of malignancy [24]. The associations of secondary HLH with underlying etiologies are numerous and include infection, malignancy, and immune suppression, with an increasing awareness in recent years of the development of HLH after solid, tubular, and stem cell transplantation.

Although tissue sampling is only one of the above-mentioned criteria, the liver biopsy can provide evidence of HLH in the appropriate clinical setting. Liver biopsies obtained with HLH in the clinical differential are typically urgent, not only for confirmation of HLH, but also for the possibility of identifying an underlying, treatable etiology. In fact, in half of all patients in one study, the liver biopsy demonstrated the underlying pathology, including hematopoietic malignancies, viral infection, and mycobacteria [25]. Microscopic examination of the affected liver shows sinusoidal dilatation, Kupffer cell hyperplasia with variable degrees of hemosiderin deposition, hemophagocytosis (activated macrophages containing platelets, leukocytes, and red cells), and variable cholestasis, though the findings are not specific as to etiology (Fig. 18.2). The same study found a variety of histologic features in fewer patients, including hepatocyte necrosis (56%), steatosis (56%), portal congestion (52%), siderosis (44%), and lobular granulomas (24%) [25]. Portal infiltrates were also noted in all 25 biopsies, though in 24% the portal inflammation was due to involvement by a hematopoietic malignancy [25].

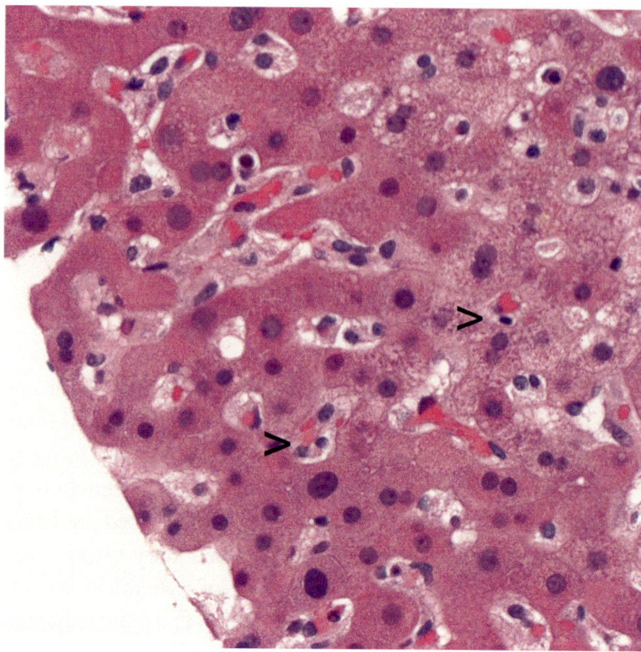

Fig. 18.2 Prominent Kupffer cell hyperplasia in the setting of hemophagocytic lymphohistiocytosis (HLH). Red blood cells are readily identified within abundant pink cytoplasm of Kupffer cells. Less frequently, lymphoid cells are identified in close proximity to Kupffer cell nuclei, indicating phagocytosis of lymphoid cells (arrowheads) (H&E stain, 400× original magnification). These findings may be very subtle and need additional immunohistochemical stains (e.g., CD68) to highlight them (image not included)

Medication Effects

Most drug-induced liver disease (DILI) occurring post-transplant shows a similar pattern to that seen in the non-transplant setting. Generally, the most common histologic pattern associated with DILI is lobular cholestasis without significant accompanying inflammation ("bland lobular cholestasis") (Fig. 18.3a). Many other patterns may be seen, including autoimmune-like reactions and chronic hepatitis-like patterns, and a careful medication history should be correlated with post-transplant biopsies. A few patterns and situations somewhat peculiar to post-transplant patients are worth noting, however.

Tacrolimus

Tacrolimus is a common immunosuppressant in post-transplant patients, and a typical first-line medication after liver transplantation, in particular. While drug-induced liver injury from tacrolimus is rare, two different patterns have been reported. Clinically, the reactions resemble cholestatic liver disease with elevated bilirubin and alkaline phosphatase. In a series of pediatric liver transplant recipients, 5.4% had lobular cholestasis with ductular reaction [26]. Similar serum findings have been reported in lung and kidney transplant patients, though without biopsy confirmation. Tacrolimus has also been associated with sinusoidal obstruction syndrome (SOS). Early biopsy-proven

cases of SOS in kidney transplant patients showed classical histology of SOS (see below), though identification of tacrolimus as the cause was obscured due to the possibility of confounding effects of concomitant medications.

Azathioprine

Azathioprine is a common component of anti-rejection regimens after renal transplantation and is a well-documented cause of SOS. Rare reports of azathioprine-related SOS have also been reported after other solid-organ transplants, where it is less commonly used as antirejection treatment.

Pseudoground-glass Inclusions

Pseudoground-glass inclusions, named for their resemblance to the ground-glass inclusions of hepatitis B viral infection, are palely eosinophilic cytoplasmic inclusions composed of glycogen, sometimes with a clear "halo" surrounding them (Fig. 18.3b). Their presence can be confirmed by paired PAS and PAS D stains, with which the inclusions will stain fuchsinophilic (deep magenta) on PAS and negatively on PAS D due to the diastase predigestion of the glycogen. In most cases, inclusions are concentrated in zone 1 hepatocytes with fewer cases showing a panacinar distribution. They are uncommon findings, but have been demonstrated in immunosuppressed patients and other patients on many medications, including those with prior kidney, liver, and hematopoietic stem cell transplants. In most cases, liver biopsy is prompted by mild elevation in AST, ALT, and/or alkaline phosphatase, and biopsy also shows mild portal and/or mild lobular inflammation in addition to the inclusions. Pseudoground-glass inclusions may also be seen as a bystander effect in biopsies performed for marked enzyme abnormalities due to other processes like acute T cell-mediated rejection and graft-versus-host disease. When these inclusions are noted, hepatitis B infection must be excluded, and immunostains for hepatitis B surface and core antigens should be performed. Similar inclusions may be seen in type IV glycogen storage disease and Lafora's disease, though these are typically diseases of childhood and present with neuromuscular symptoms. Retained fibrinogen globules in afibrinogenemia or dysfibrinogenemia may look similar and occur in childhood (for congenital forms) or severely injured adult livers (acquired dysfibrinogenemia). Fibrinogen globules are PAS-negative, and can be confirmed by immunohistochemistry, if necessary. While pseudoground-glass inclusions are associated with polypharmacy, specific drugs may cause similar inclusions and should be excluded by careful review of the clinical history, including disulfiram, cyanamide, chlorpromazine, and barbiturates.

Glycogenic hepatopathy

Glycogenic hepatopathy is classically described in patients with poorly controlled type I diabetes mellitus, less com-

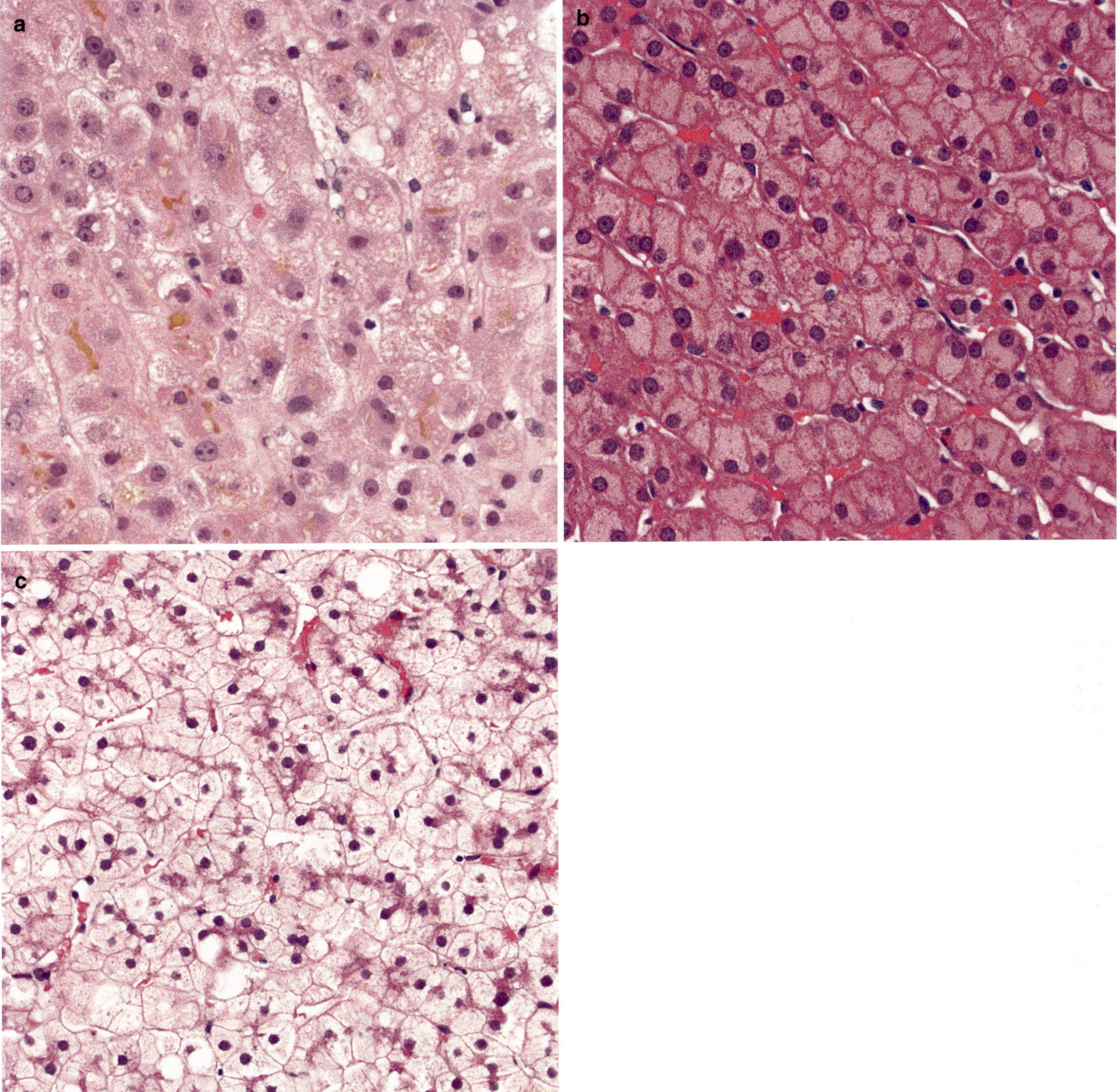

Fig. 18.3 Examples of drug-induced liver injury patterns. (**a**) Marked canalicular cholestasis without significant inflammation ("bland lobular cholestasis") (H&E stain, 400× original magnification) (**b**) Glassy cyto- plasm of pseudoground-glass inclusions (H&E stain, 400× original magnification). (**c**) Hepatocytes with abundant clear cytoplasm of gly- cogenic hepatopathy (H&E stain, 400× original magnification)

monly with poorly controlled adult onset/type II diabetes mellitus, and very rarely in non-diabetic patients after high-dose glucocorticoid administration and other immune-deficient states. The underlying mechanism is the same: altered glycogen metabolism leads to swollen hepatocytes with cytoplasmic clearing, glycogenated nuclei, and scat- tered megamitochondria with no or minimal inflammatory infiltrate (Fig. 18.3c). While classically described in diabetic patients, a population prone to conventional fatty liver dis-

ease, typical features of fatty liver disease such as steatosis and ballooned hepatocytes are usually minimal or absent in glycogenic hepatopathy. Patients typically present with hep- atomegaly and aminotransferase and/or alkaline phosphatase elevations that can range from minimally to markedly ele- vated. Glycogenic hepatopathy has been very rarely reported after orthotopic liver transplantation in response to steroid treatment, and should be considered when the characteristic diffuse cytoplasmic clearing is observed. Differential diagnostic considerations include glycogen storage diseases (excluded by clinical history), microvesicular steatosis, and smooth endoplasmic reticulum buildup seen in some drug reactions (both of which can be excluded by demonstrating positivity on PAS staining and negativity with PAS D). Glycogen accumulation may regress once glycemic control is reestablished.

Post-transplant Lymphoproliferative Disorder (PTLD)

Post-transplant lymphoproliferative disorders (PTLDs) may be nodal or extranodal in presentation. Hepatic or splenic involvement can occur. A detailed overview is beyond the scope of this chapter, and may be found in other chapters of this text.

According to the 2016 World Health Organization classification of tumors of hematopoietic and lymphoid tissues, PTLDs are subcategorized into the following: (1) non-destructive PTLDs (plasmacytoid hyperplasia, infectious mononucleosis, florid follicular hyperplasia); (2) polymorphic PTLDs; (3) monomorphic PTLDs (B and T/NK cell types); and (4) classic Hodgkin lymphoma PTLD [27, 28].

The non-destructive PTLDs resemble reactive lymphoid hyperplasia or pseudolymphoma in the liver (Fig. 18.4). The common B cell lymphomas under monomorphic PTLDs are diffuse large B cell lymphoma (Fig. 18.5), Burkitt lymphoma, plasma cell myeloma and plasmacytoma, while the common T cell PTLDs are peripheral T cell lymphoma, not otherwise specified (NOS), and hepatosplenic T cell lymphoma [27].

Most PTLDs are associated with EBV. The infection leads to clonal proliferation of B or T cell proliferation or, less frequently, causes a polyclonal B cell reaction [28–31]. EBV can be detected by using immunohistochemical staining (EBV LMP1) or in situ hybridization (EBER). A recent study of PTLDs after solid organ (61 patients) and allogeneic hematopoietic stem cell transplant (allo-HSCT) (21

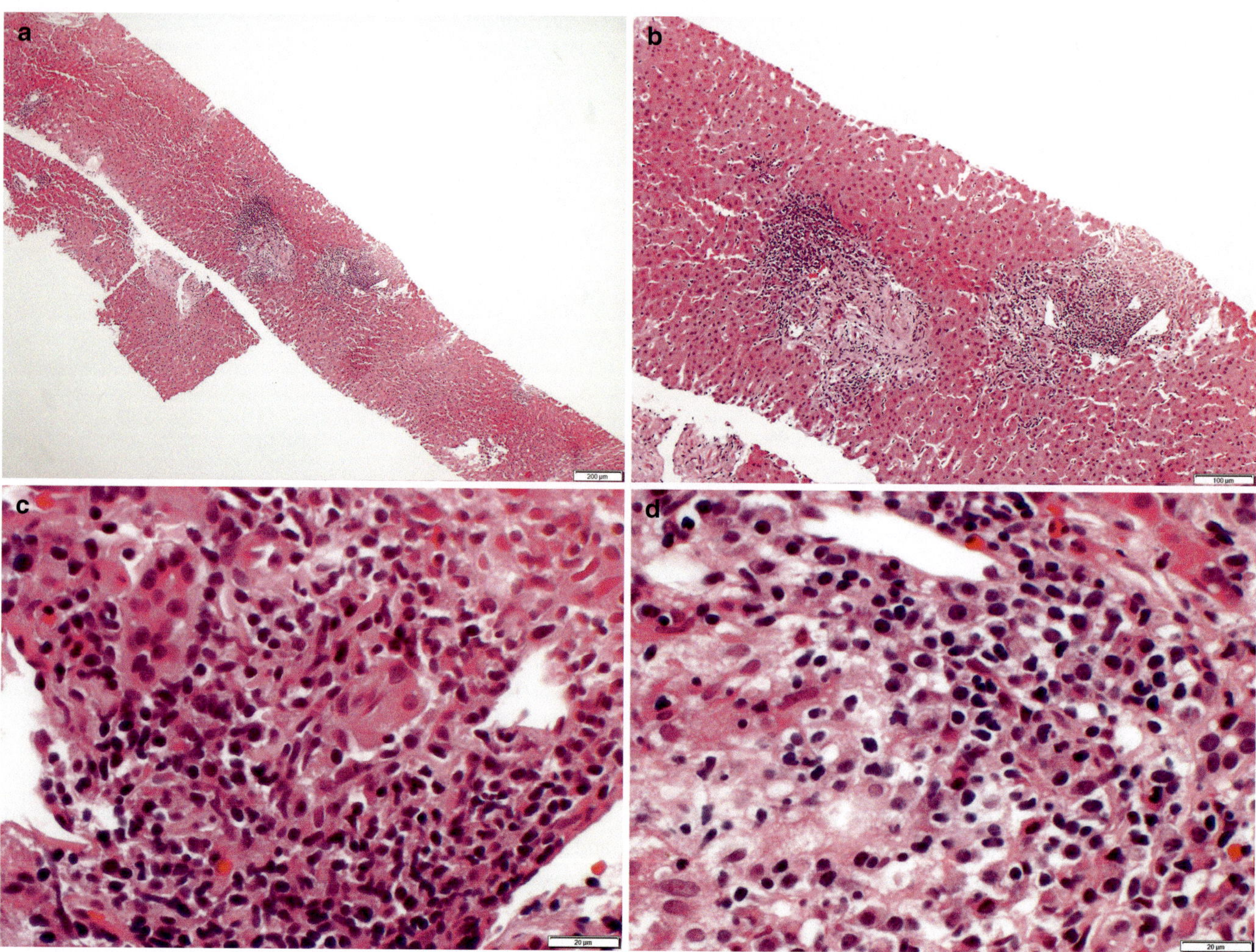

Fig. 18.4 Post-transplant lymphoproliferative disorder, polymorphic subtype, involving the liver as atypical lymphoid hyperplasia, mostly restricted in portal areas with focal fibrosis. The cellularity is composed of small mature lymphoid cells, some with plasmacytoid differentiation, and occasional lymphoblasts. (H&E, **a**: 40×, **b**: 100×, **c**: 600×, and **d**: 600×, respectively). (The above images are provided by Dr. Kung Jiang, MD, PhD, Department of Pathology, Moffitt Cancer Center)

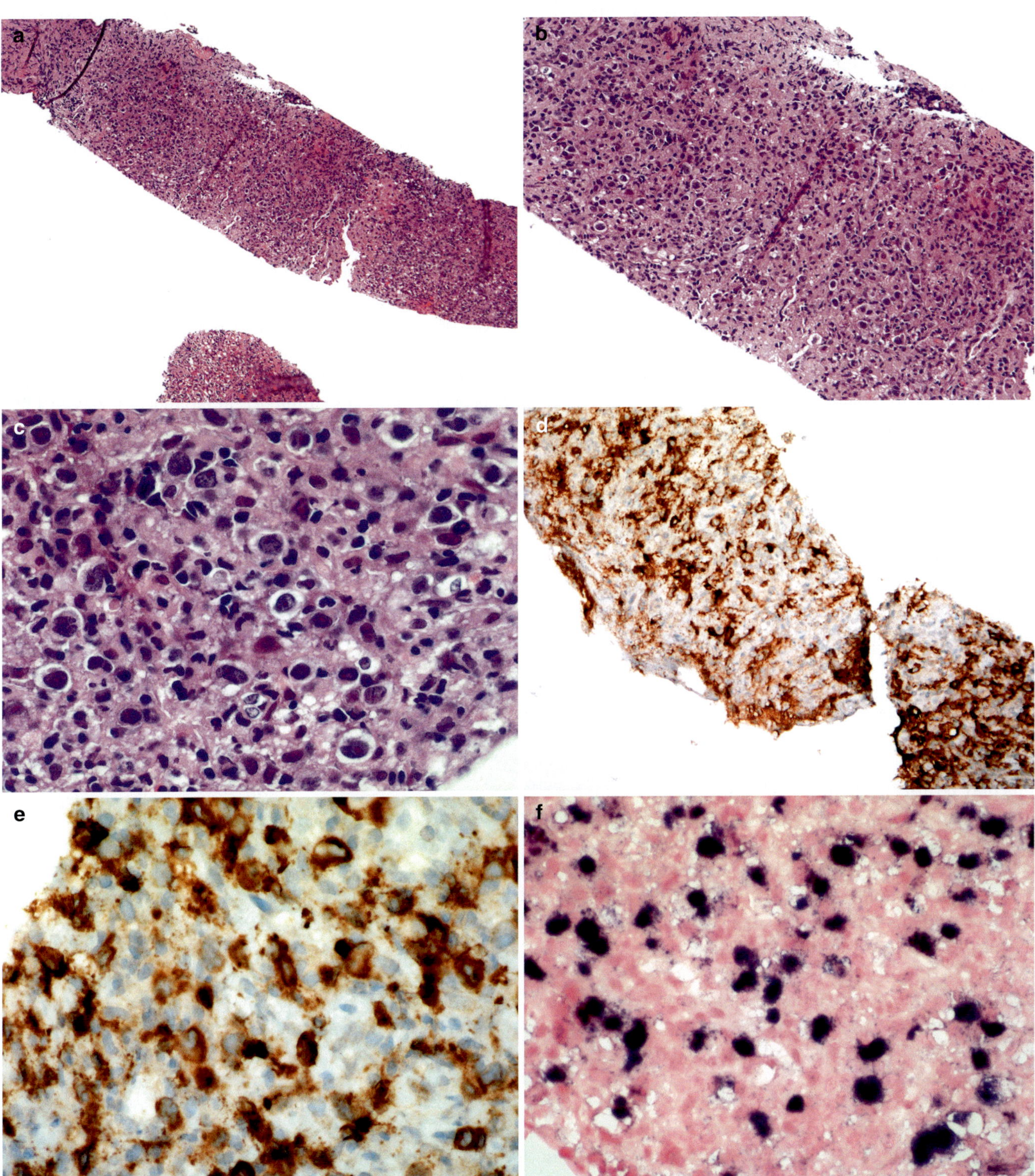

Fig. 18.5 Post-transplant lymphoproliferative disorder, monomorphic subtype, EBV-positive. (**a, b**) The needle core biopsy shows a diffuse cellular infiltrate of small to large lymphoid cells associated with focally identifiable hepatocytes (H&E, 100× and 200×, respectively). (**c–f**) Higher power view of these cells reveals the large atypical lymphoid cells with hyperchromatic to vesicular nuclei, irregular nuclear contours and some prominent nucleoli (**c**: H&E, 600×) which are positive for B cell markers: CD20 (**d**: immunoperioxidase, 200×), CD79a (**e**: immunoperioxidase, 600×), and EBER (**f**: in situ hybridization, 600×), consistent with post-transplant EBV-driven lymphoproliferative disorder

patients) showed 100% EBV positivity in post allo-HSCT while EBV infection/reactivation was only identified in a half of patients (47%) post solid organ transplant [32]. In a large cohort study, the data also showed the patients post allo-HSCT more often presented with B symptoms, advanced stage, and involvement of the liver, spleen, Waldeyer ring, and central nervous system (CNS) when compared with the patients post solid organ transplantation [32]. EBV-negative PTLDs have also been reported in 20–40% of cases, approximately two-thirds of which fell into the T cell PTLD category [27, 30, 33, 34]. HHV8-associated PTLDs (e.g., primary effusion lymphoma or Kaposi lymphoma) have also been documented [35, 36].

As B or T cell lymphomas, plasma cell myeloma/plasmacytoma, and classic Hodgkin lymphoma show no morphological differences from the lymphomas in patients who do not undergo transplantation and phenotypically they are also similar, the details of PTLD lymphomas will not be further discussed in this section (please refer to the corresponding lymphoma sections in different chapters).

Epstein-Barr Virus-Associated Post-transplant Smooth Muscle Tumor

Epstein-Barr virus (EBV)-associated smooth muscle tumors are rare neoplasms that may develop in the setting of chronic immunosuppression, including post-transplantation. The liver is the most common location for these tumors to arise in the post-transplant setting, whether native or allograft (accounting for 56% of cases). Kidney transplantation is the most commonly associated transplantation procedure (60% of reported cases of this tumor), though this may be affected by the much larger absolute number of kidney transplants performed than other organ transplants [37]. These tumors are a relatively late complication, occurring at a median of 48 months post-transplant, with only 4% occurring within 1 year [37]. A minority (18–31%) of patients with EBV-associated smooth muscle tumors will have a preceding post-transplant lymphoproliferative disorder (PTLD), also an EBV-driven process, and EBV-associated smooth muscle tumors appear to preferentially occur in patients that are EBV seronegative pre-transplant with later seroconversion, a known risk factor for PTLD development [37, 38].

Despite these similarities to PTLD, the pathophysiology of EBV-associated post-transplant smooth muscle tumors is less well understood. The tumors appear to arise predominantly from the smooth muscle of vascular walls, possibly explaining how they develop in organs like the liver that are typically devoid of significant smooth muscle. Though the liver is the most common organ affected, tumors have been reported in a wide variety of sites and are frequently multifocal, typically the result of multifocal infection rather than

metastasis [39]. The development of EBV-associated smooth muscle tumors appears independent of the immunosuppressive regimen. Tumor size ranges from 0.8 to 15.0 cm, with an average tumor size of 3.7 cm [40].

These tumors are characterized histologically by intersecting fascicles of spindle cells with abundant eosinophilic cytoplasm and spindled nuclei. There is also frequently a sparse to moderate T cell infiltrate, and a subset of these tumors shows a primitive round cell component. Smooth muscle actin is nearly universally positive by immunohistochemistry, with fewer tumors showing desmin positivity. EBV is demonstrated by diffuse EBER in situ hybridization positivity, while EBV-LMP immunostaining is negative, focal, or weak. These tumors may rarely show marked atypia, sarcoma-like fascicles, tumor necrosis, or elevated mitotic rates (>5 per high-power field), though these features do not appear to confer any difference in biological behavior [38]. These features are most important to keep in mind when considering the differential diagnosis, which includes: leiomyoma, leiomyosarcoma, smooth muscle tumor of uncertain malignant potential, and angiomyolipoma/perivascular epithelioid cell tumor, though the history and demonstration of EBV infection are definitional for post-transplant EBV-associated smooth muscle tumor.

The clinical course is typically favorable for these tumors, with only very rare instances of death from the disease. Reduction in immunosuppression and/or surgical resection is the treatment of choice, though scattered cases of treatment with sirolimus have been reported, and overall treatment experience is limited due to the rarity of this tumor.

Issues Primarily Arising in the Setting of Hematopoietic Stem Cell Transplantation

Graft-Versus-Host Disease

Graft-versus-host disease (GVHD) is the immune-mediated damage inflicted by donor-derived lymphocytes on host tissues. In the native liver, this is primarily manifested as infiltration of biliary epithelium by lymphocytes and resultant bile duct damage, including hypereosinophilic cytoplasm, nuclear membrane irregularities, cytoplasmic vacuolization, and incomplete lumens. The earliest change in the first 35 days post-transplant is the presence of lobular apoptotic bodies, which is highly nonspecific as to etiology [41]. More chronic damage may lead to portal fibrosis, lobular cholestasis, and duct loss (including ductopenia) (Fig. 18.6). Unlike in other organ systems, apoptosis is not a prominent feature of hepatic GVHD. Immunostains for cytokeratins 7 and 19 highlight biliary epithelium and can be helpful to identify remaining bile ducts. GVHD is frequently diagnosed based on elevated alkaline phosphatase and direct

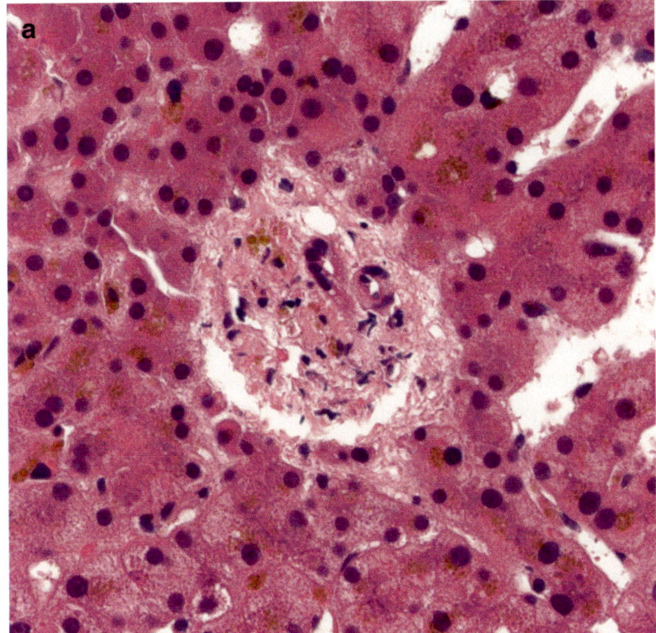

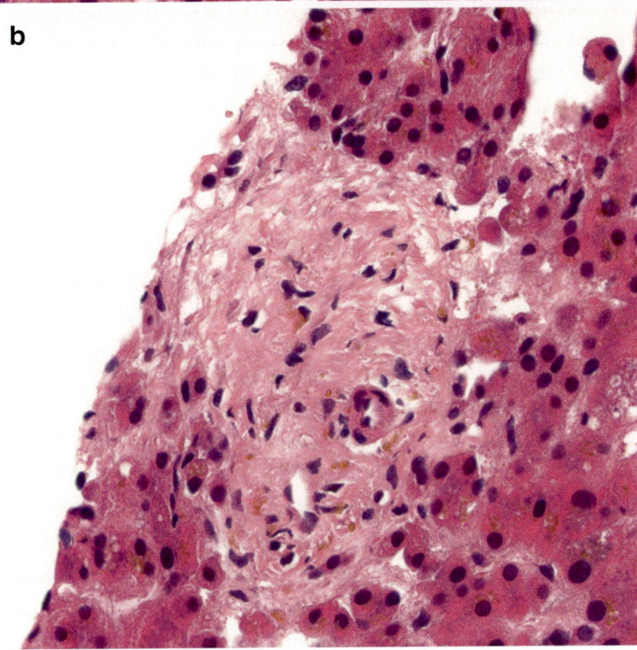

Fig. 18.6 Histological changes in graft-versus-host disease. (**a**) A damaged bile duct showing hypereosinophilic cytoplasm and nuclear disarray (H&E stain, 400× original magnification). (**b**) A portal tract without a bile duct (duct loss) and with mild expansion by fibrosis (H&E stain, 400× original magnification)

bilirubin and treated with immunosuppressants without a biopsy. Biopsy may be performed if the clinical diagnosis is unclear or in an attempt to quantify the degree of bile duct loss or fibrosis (though a single biopsy may not be representative, and the effects of GVHD may be reversible). If the biopsy occurs after the initiation of therapy, the lymphocytic

infiltrate may be reduced, though the characteristic features of duct damage remain.

Differential diagnostic considerations include drug-induced liver disease, sepsis, and infection. While drug reactions are frequently cholestatic, bile duct damage is not typically prominent. Sepsis most commonly shows ductular reaction, which is not typically prominent in GVHD. Most viral infections present with greater lobular inflammation and a hepatitic pattern of enzyme elevation, though in immunosuppressed patients the typical inflammation may be reduced. A careful search for viral inclusions and a low threshold for ancillary stains are recommended. Because histological features of GVHD may significantly overlap with other entities in the differential diagnosis, it is recommended that biopsy to assess for GVHD be reported in one of three categories: (1) "no GVHD" when no histological features are present; (2) "possible GVHD" when histological features of GVHD are present, but there are confounding histological or clinical features, such as the presence of viral inclusions or clinical features strongly suggesting a drug reaction; or (3) "likely GVHD" when histological features of GVHD are present without an obvious alternative cause of injury [42].

A few unusual situations should be kept in mind regarding GVHD. A hepatitic injury pattern has been rarely described, in which bile duct injury is mild and the prominent feature is a T cell-dominant lobular hepatitis. This variant presents with AST and ALT elevations greater than ten-fold the upper limits of normal. Hepatitic GVHD most commonly occurs after donor lymphocyte infusion for the treatment of relapsed leukemia, with a median time to liver dysfunction of 35 days post-infusion [43]. While GVHD is overwhelmingly a disease of the post-hematopoietic stem cell transplant setting, rare cases of GVHD have been reported after solid organ and intestinal transplantation, with transplanted liver (alone or as a multi-visceral transplant) having the highest rate of occurrence.

Sinusoidal Obstruction Syndrome

Sinusoidal obstruction syndrome (SOS, also previously referred to as veno-occlusive disease) is a hepatic injury pattern with many associations, but it is particularly common and severe in the setting of hematopoietic stem cell transplantation. In this setting, it is a side effect of myeloablative regimens based on cyclophosphamide, with increased incidence with the addition of busulfan and total body irradiation. GVHD prophylactic agents, such as sirolimus and methotrexate, have also been implicated in the post-transplant setting. SOS is the result of toxic damage to sinusoidal endothelial cells leading to sinusoidal congestion, extravasation of red blood cells into the space of Disse, and parenchymal collapse, with chronic injury resulting in zone 3 perisinusoi-

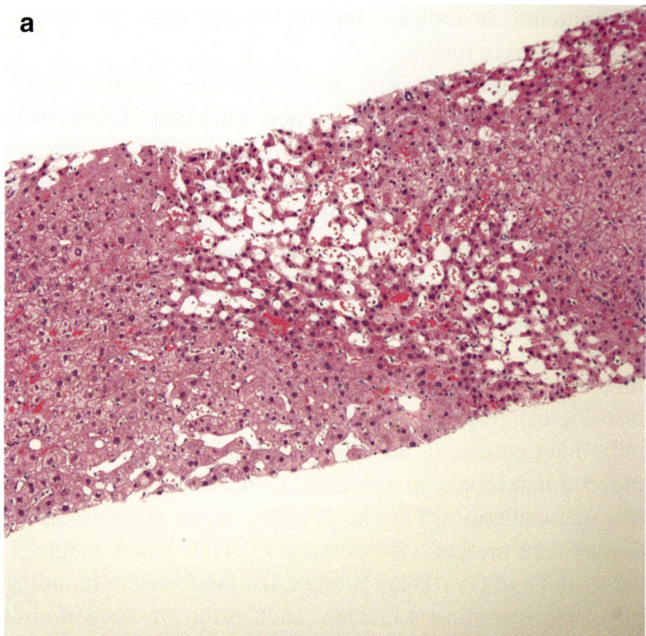

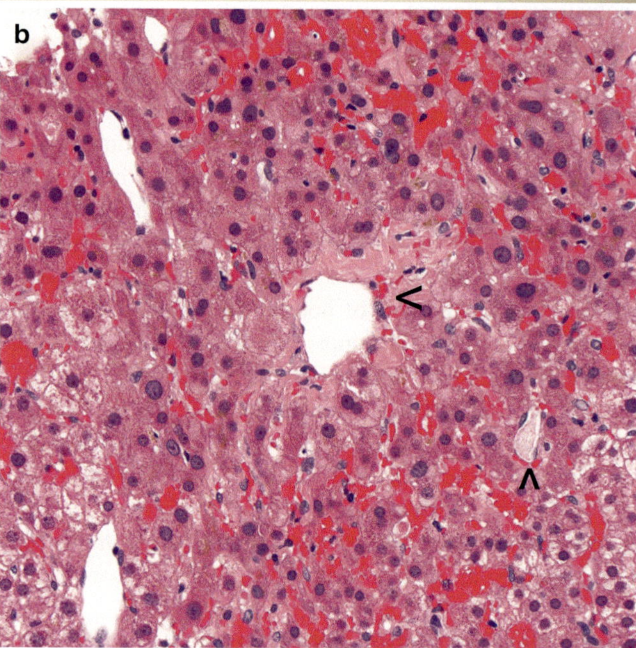

Fig. 18.7 Sinusoidal obstruction syndrome. (**a**) Prominent sinusoidal dilatation, predominantly in zone 3, with sinusoidal congestion (H&E stain, 100× original magnification). (**b**) Prominent sinusoidal congestion with extravasated red blood cells directly adjacent to endothelial cells in the space of Disse (arrowheads) (H&E stain, 400× original magnification)

dal fibrosis and loss of small hepatic veins that are replaced by a dense collagenous knot (Fig. 18.7). SOS is frequently diagnosed clinically with identification of a bilirubin of 2 mg/dL or higher and at least two of the following three criteria: (1) ascites, (2) painful hepatomegaly, and (3) weight gain of >5% [44]. Biopsy, however, may be used as supporting evidence. SOS can be treated with the novel agent defib-

rotide that is thought to protect the endothelial cells from the toxic damage that causes SOS.

Issues Primarily Arising in the Setting of Liver Transplantation

These can be classified in a variety of ways and encompass (1) liver disease/injury specific to the post-liver transplant setting, such as rejection; (2) recurrence of underlying chronic liver disease, such as recurrent hepatitis C; and (3) liver disease as may occur in the general population, such as primary hepatitis A infection.

Donor Liver

Steatosis

Steatosis of donor livers is associated with several problems post-transplant and is one of the primary indications for frozen section evaluation of donor livers before orthotopic liver transplantation. In general, steatosis is divided into macrovesicular and microvesicular steatosis. Macrovesicular steatosis is divided into large and small droplet types. Small droplet macrovascular steatosis should not be confused with microvesicular steatosis. The latter is separately addressed at the end of this section, as it has a different differential diagnosis. Microvesicular steatosis typically develops in certain serious clinical situations and not in livers considered for donation.

Large droplet macrovesicular steatosis describes a single lipid droplet occupying more than half of the cytoplasm and displacing the nucleus. Small droplet macrovesicular steatosis is characterized by multiple, typically two to five, lipid droplets, none of which take up more than half of the total cytoplasmic area and that do not typically indent the nucleus. Large droplet macrovesicular steatosis is best measured at low power, 4× ocular magnification, as a percentage of total parenchymal area occupied by lipid droplets. Small droplet macrovesicular steatosis can then be assessed at higher power, 20× ocular magnification, as a percentage of the remaining parenchyma occupied by small lipid droplets. Strictly applying these definitions and this system can help minimize interpretative errors, such as overestimating the quantity of macrovesicular steatosis, due to examination at high power or insufficient distinction between large droplet, small droplet, and microvesicular steatosis.

Lipopeliosis is a rare lesion that may occur in the immediate post-transplant period if the transplanted liver contained significant large droplet steatosis. Perfusion injury causes hepatocyte necrosis, but also the release of lipid vacuoles that become lodged in the sinusoids and/or spaces of Disse, most commonly in a centrilobular distribution, that can cause further ischemia and hepatocyte necrosis (Fig. 18.8). Lipopeliosis can lead to prolonged post-transplant cholestasis, graft dys-

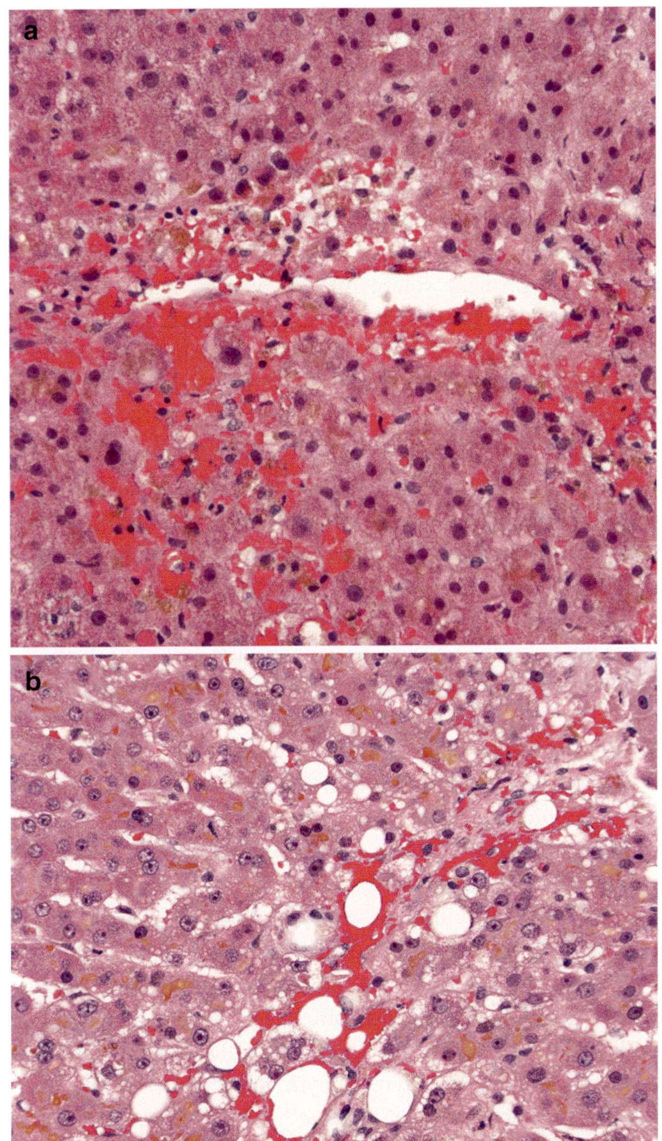

Fig. 18.8 Ischemic changes. (**a**) Severe preservation injury showing zone 3 coagulation necrosis with rare apoptotic bodies (H&E stain, 200× original magnification). (**b**) Lipid vacuoles in the sinusoids with associated sinusoidal dilatation and congestion in lipopeliosis, in this example associated with preservation injury (H&E stain, 400× original magnification)

function, and graft loss. Even in organs that recover, the injury may lead to zone 3 fibrosis [45]. Steatosis in the allograft liver resolves post-transplant, and only a minority of even significantly steatotic livers will undergo lipopeliosis.

Even aside from lipopeliosis, large amounts of steatosis are associated with primary graft non-function or dysfunction. Livers that are grossly steatotic, being yellow or having a greasy consistency, are typically rejected by the surgeon before implantation. Upon microscopic examination, >60% large droplet steatosis is almost universally agreed upon as grounds for rejecting the organ for transplantation. With transplantable organs in short supply, numerous studies have examined the suitability of livers with more moderate amounts (typically 20–50%) of large droplet and/or total steatosis. These borderline steatotic livers may have more early complications, such as prolonged cholestasis and intensive care unit stays, but long-term graft function appears to be comparable to grafts without significant steatosis. Even severely steatotic livers (>60%) have been successfully transplanted in some situations with low rates of graft non-function or dysfunction.

The impact of allograft steatosis other than large droplet macrovesicular steatosis on graft function is less clear. In many studies, it is not clear whether the strict definitions of steatosis described above were used, likely contributing to the heterogeneity of results. True microvesicular steatosis, as strictly defined above, is an uncommonly seen histologic pattern, and its limitation to a few clinical situations means that it only very rarely appears in donor liver evaluations. One recent study that followed a strict definition of small droplet macrovesicular steatosis indicated there was no adverse patient survival in recipients of these livers, but that there were higher rates of T cell-mediated rejection and bile duct loss [46]. The full effect of microvesicular and small droplet macrovesicular steatosis on graft function remains to be seen.

Frozen section analysis of either a core or wedge biopsy from the donor liver pre-implantation is a reliable way to assess for steatosis. The most common error in this setting is overestimating the degree of macrovesicular steatosis, due to artifacts introduced by the freezing process. Another important caveat is that wedge biopsy or pre-reperfusion fluid flushing through the liver may lead to artificial dilatation of the sinusoids that should not be overinterpreted as outflow obstruction or nodular regenerative hyperplasia. In addition to providing a valuable real-time assessment, frozen tissue also makes available the option for using an oil red O stain to assess for microvesicular steatosis (see below) if the clinical situation is suspicious for any of the associated disorders or if the possibility is raised by cytoplasmic vacuolization seen on the initial hematoxylin and eosin-stained examination. However, oil red O is not recommended for routine assessment of steatosis, as it tends to exacerbate the preexisting risk of overestimating large droplet steatosis, which could lead to a valuable organ being discarded.

Microvesicular steatosis usually results from mitochondrial toxicity. The hepatocyte cytoplasm acquires a vacuolated appearance, as it is filled with innumerable small droplets of fat, each smaller than the size of the hepatocyte nucleus. A detailed discussion of the various causes of microvesicular steatosis is beyond the scope of this chapter. In the post-transplant setting, relevant causes include alcoholic foamy degeneration, an unusual form of alcohol-related liver disease [47] (may be seen in recidivism after liver transplantation for alcohol-related liver disease), and drug effects, such as with nucleoside analog reverse transcriptase inhibitors used in human immunodeficiency virus (HIV) treatment [48].

Vascular and Biliary Injury

Circulatory and biliary injury are closely related in allograft livers, in that one frequently leads to the other, and both may be the result of surgical complications. Vascular injury can occur at the level of the portal, arterial, or sinusoidal vasculature.

Ischemic injury may be seen in allograft livers after prolonged cold or warm ischemic time. The damage is typically precipitated upon reperfusion of the liver. Biopsies obtained in the first week post-transplant may show scattered apoptotic bodies, mild hepatocellular ballooning, cholestasis, and increased mitoses (Fig. 18.8). With more severe ischemia, zone 3 hepatocyte dropout or bridging necrosis may be seen.

Small-for-size syndrome is related to portal hyperperfusion when the volume of the transplanted liver is less than 30% of that which is ideal for the recipient or <0.8% of recipient body weight [49]. Portal hyperperfusion is thought to lead to hepatic artery constriction by decreasing levels of adenosine, a vasodilator, in the hepatic circulation. The histologic changes can develop early, are subtle and nonspecific, and require a high degree of suspicion. They include denudation of portal vein and sinusoidal endothelium, portal hemorrhages, and eventually fibrointimal hyperplasia, and luminal obstruction.

Hepatic artery thrombosis in the immediate post-transplant phase is most typically diagnosed via clinical and imaging findings. Findings on peripheral liver biopsies may be unrevealing, as the most frequently affected structures are the large vessels and bile ducts of the hilum that are exclusively supplied by arterial blood (Fig. 18.9). Histological findings vary, but may include prominent lobular acidophil bodies; cholestasis; and zone 3 sinusoidal dilatation, hepatocyte atrophy, or coagulative necrosis.

Biliary strictures occur in approximately 5–15% of liver allografts, with rates even higher in partial/living donor allografts [50]. Bile duct strictures usually occur 6–12 months post-transplant. With regard to etiology, biliary strictures may be anastomotic or non-anastomotic. Anastomotic strictures develop at the site of biliary anastomosis and are related to technical aspects or suboptimal healing at the anastomotic line. Non-anastomotic strictures are not located at the anastomotic site, but are present in a wider distribution including away from anastomosis sites. They are related to ischemic injury, including hepatic artery thrombosis (ischemic cholangiopathy) [51]. Both etiologies produce typical findings of biliary obstruction (similar to those in native livers), includ-

ing ductular proliferation, degenerative bile duct changes, and lobular cholestasis. True cholangitis, neutrophilic infiltrate of the interlobular bile ducts, may be seen intermittently, and may be seen with large duct obstruction. Of note, multiple post-transplant biliary strictures have variable etiologies that include ischemia and CMV among others, and can cause a secondary sclerosing cholangitis pattern. This can be difficult to distinguish radiologically and histologically from primary sclerosing cholangitis that is recurrent post-transplant. In these instances, correlation with the time of onset and other factors, such as graft cold ischemic time (see cold ischemic injury below), is important to make the distinction.

Cold ischemic injury may particularly damage the biliary epithelium so that it sloughs into the lumens, forming the "sludge" of biliary sludge syndrome. Biliary sludge syndrome shows features similar to duct obstruction, including ductular reaction, portal fibrosis, duct injury, and duct loss (Fig. 18.9). Increasing duct loss, portal fibrosis, and mural fibrosis of the large ducts leads to progressive cholestasis and graft dysfunction. Patients may also have repeated bouts of cholangitis.

T Cell-Mediated Rejection

T cell-mediated rejection (TCMR), previously referred to as acute cellular rejection, is the immune-mediated reaction to the allograft liver by the recipient immune system with the potential to cause graft dysfunction or failure. Clinically, TCMR is often divided into early (within 6 months of transplantation) and late (after 6 months from transplantation). TCMR is characterized and graded based on three components: portal inflammation, bile duct damage, and venous endothelial inflammation. The portal inflammatory infiltrate typically begins as a lymphocytic infiltrate with the later addition of activated or "blastic" forms, neutrophils, and eosinophils. Injury to the bile ducts is seen as subepithelial or epithelial infiltration of inflammatory cells; mild reactive changes, such as increased nucleus-to-cytoplasm ratios; or more marked degenerative changes, such as disordered nuclear polarity, cytoplasmic vacuolization, nuclear pleomorphism, and luminal disruption. Venous endothelial inflammation includes inflammation of both the portal and central venules (Fig. 18.10). To confidently identify venous endotheliitis, inflammatory cells should be directly beneath the endothelial cells, and the endothelium should have an "activated" appearance, including a prominent appearance with a slight bulging out into the lumen. The histological features and grading scheme for TCMR are detailed in Table 18.1. At least two of the three features should be present to diagnose TCMR, while one feature may be characterized as "indeterminate" for TCMR. It is recommended to provide both a global, semi-quantitative assessment of the severity of TCMR, and a formal numerical score (the rejection activity index, RAI) [52].

Patients typically present with a sudden onset hepatitic or mixed hepatitic and cholestatic enzyme elevation. If serum levels of immunosuppressive medications are available, levels of one or more drugs may be below the typically accepted trough, though they may also be within the acceptable range. Treatment of TCMR includes modification of the immuno-suppressive regimen with or without a short course of high dose corticosteroids. Understanding the timing of when the biopsy was taken in relation to the presentation and treatment is important, as steroid administration can reduce the mononuclear infiltrate, the number of eosinophils, and the degree of venous endothelial inflammation, and the intensity

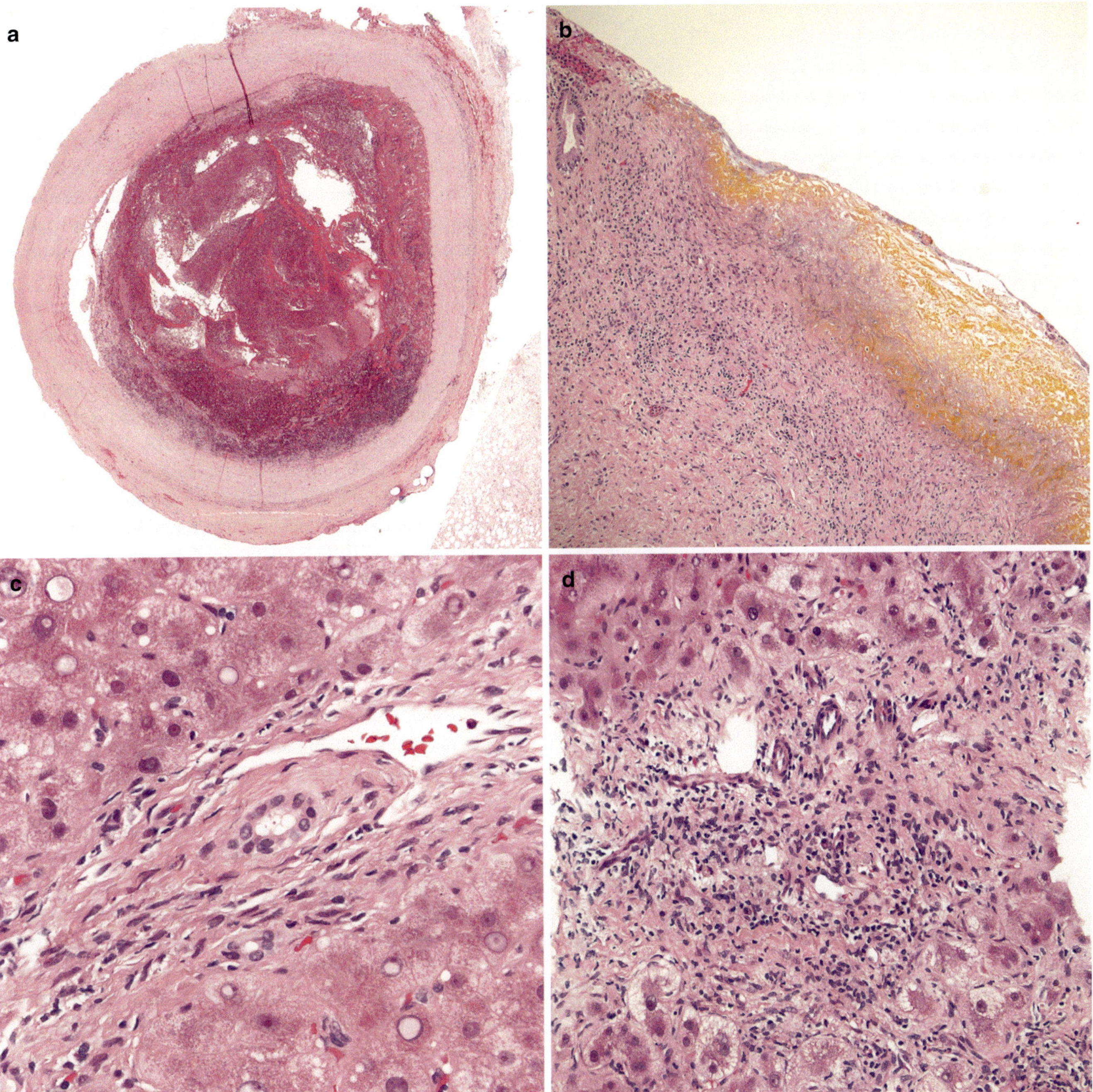

Fig. 18.9 Examples of histological findings in vascular and biliary abnormalities. (**a**) A thrombosed hepatic artery from a resection speci-men (H&E stain, 20× original magnification. (**b**) Infarction of a large hilar bile duct from a resection specimen with hepatic artery thrombosis (H&E stain, original magnification 100×). (**c**) A damaged bile duct showing cytoplasmic hypereosinophilia and nuclear disarray in a patient with biliary strictures (H&E stain, 400× original magnification). (**d**). Irregular portal fibrosis and duct loss in a patient with ischemic cholangiopathy (H&E stain, 200× original magnification). (**e**) Irregular portal fibrosis with marked ductular reaction in a patient with biliary sludge syndrome (H&E stain, 200× original magnification)

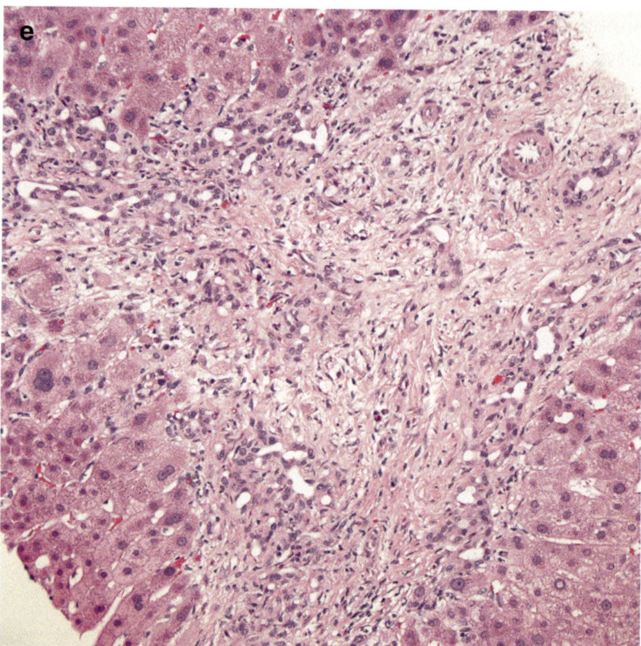

Fig. 18.9 (continued)

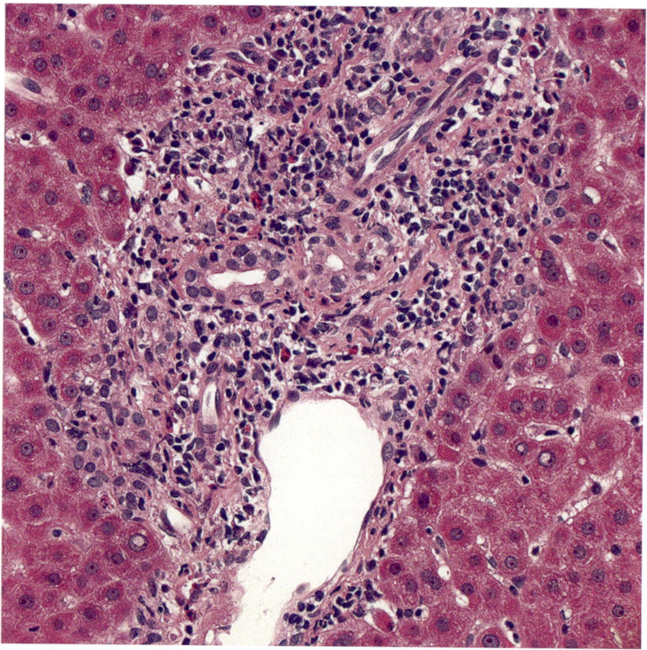

Fig. 18.10 T cell-mediated rejection. The image demonstrates portal expansion by mixed inflammation and bile duct injury, including epithelial infiltration by lymphocytes, irregular nuclear spacing, and cytoplasmic vacuolization. Portal vein phlebitis with activated endothelial cells is also present (H&E stain, 400× original magnification)

of all the findings may be reduced if days or weeks elapse between the peak injury and the biopsy.

The histopathological differential is wide and varies depending on which histological findings of TCMR are most prominent. Biliary anastomotic strictures can lead to small bile duct damage like that seen in TCMR, and the neutrophils of mild ductular reaction may be mistaken for mixed portal infiltrate. Treatment of TCMR prior to the biopsy could minimize the lymphocytic component of the portal infiltrate, leaving neutrophils that can mimic duct obstruction changes. Venous endothelial damage and the presence of more mixed inflammation composed of not only neutrophils, but also activated lymphocytes and eosinophils favor TCMR. Ductular reaction is also not a component of TCMR.

Hepatic vein anastomotic strictures can lead to zone 3 sinusoidal dilatation and congestion with perivenular hepatocyte necrosis, which may be seen in TCMR. However, in TCMR, the destruction of central veins and zone 3 hepatocytes is immune-mediated, with prominent lymphoplasmacytic infiltrate. With hepatic venous outflow obstruction, the destruction is pauci-immune. Extravasated red blood cells in the space of Disse also provide a clue that the damage is due to pressurized backflow.

CMV, EBV, and HHV6 typically have portal inflammation and possibly concomitant bile duct and venous inflammation, as in TCMR. These viral infections commonly have more lobular inflammation than TCMR, and may have lesser bile duct and venous injury than would be expected for the degree of portal inflammation attributable to TCMR. Viral inclusions may be rare in CMV and are not typically seen in EBV and HHV6 infections, so a low threshold for the addition of ancillary stains (immunohistochemistry for CMV and in-situ hybridization for EBER) is encouraged.

Among possible recurrences of pre-transplant pathology, the most frequent mimic of TCMR is recurrent viral hepatitis and autoimmune hepatitis (AIH). Post-transplant recurrences of hepatitis B and C tend to have more lobular inflammation than pre-transplant manifestations, though they will also frequently show portal inflammation. Bile duct damage and venous endothelial inflammation favor TCMR over viral hepatitis, though severely active viral hepatitis is frequently associated with some degree of venous and biliary inflammation. One or two occasions of biliary or venous inflammation in such cases are insufficient to establish the pattern of TCMR, but rather the pace/repetition of such lesions in the biopsy is the clue. Activated lymphocytes and plasma cells may be prominent in both TCMR and viral hepatitis, though well-developed lymphoid aggregates and germinal centers favor viral hepatitis over TCMR. In the setting of severe inflammation, admixed neutrophils and eosinophils favor TCMR.

Chronic Rejection

Chronic rejection encompasses the loss of bile ducts, small hepatic artery branches, and terminal central venules. It is the result of a combination of direct immune-mediated damage and damage secondary to ischemia. The effects of chronic rejection are potentially irreversible, leading to graft loss in some patients. Patients typically present with a chole-

Table 18.1 Summarized assessment of T cell-mediated rejection and chronic rejection in liver allografts

T cell-mediated rejection (TCMR), global assessment[a]

Grade	Histological features
Indeterminate	Minimal portal infiltrate insufficient for diagnosis of TCMR[a]
Mild	Mild mononuclear or mixed inflammatory infiltrate in a minority of portal or perivenular areas without significant periportal infiltrate or confluent necrosis/hepatocyte dropout
Moderate	Mixed inflammatory infiltrate expanding most portal areas and/or confluent necrosis/hepatocyte dropout affecting a minority of perivenular areas
Severe	Mixed inflammatory infiltrate expanding most portal areas with periportal infiltration and/or moderate to severe perivenular inflammation with extension into the lobules and perivenular confluent necrosis/hepatocyte dropout affecting most perivenular areas

TCMR, Rejection Activity Index (RAI)[a]

	Score	Histological features
Portal inflammation	1	Predominantly lymphocytic inflammation involving, but not significantly expanding, a minority of portal areas
	2	Expansion of most or all of the portal areas by a mixed inflammatory infiltrate composed of lymphocytes with occasional activated forms, neutrophils, and eosinophils[b]
	3	Marked expansion by most or all of the portal areas by a mixed inflammatory infiltrate containing lymphocytes with activated forms and eosinophils with periportal infiltration
Bile duct inflammation damage	1	A minority of the ducts are cuffed and infiltrated by inflammatory cells and showing only mild reactive changes
	2	Most or all of the ducts are infiltrated by inflammatory cells with significant degenerative changes
	3	Most or all of the ducts are infiltrated by inflammatory cells with a majority of the ducts showing significant degenerative changes or luminal disruption
Venous endothelial inflammation	1	Subendothelial lymphocytic inflammatory infiltrate of a minority of the portal and/or central venules
	2	Subendothelial inflammatory infiltrate of most or all of the portal and/or central venules, with/without confluent necrosis/hepatocyte dropout involving a minority of perivenular areas
	3	Subendothelial inflammatory infiltrate of most or all of the portal and/or central venules with moderate to severe perivenular inflammation extending into the perivenular parenchyma and confluent necrosis/hepatocyte dropout involving a majority of perivenular areas

Chronic rejection[c]

Type	Structure	Histological features
Early	Small bile ducts	Degenerative changes involving the majority of ducts; <50% duct loss
	Portal hepatic arterioles	Lost in <25% of portal areas
	Central veins	Perivenular mononuclear inflammation; zone 3 hepatocyte dropout, mild perivenular fibrosis
	Large perihilar hepatic artery branches	Intimal inflammation; focal foamy macrophage deposition without luminal obstruction
	Large perihilar bile ducts	Inflammation and focal foamy macrophage deposition
	Other	Spotty lobular hepatocyte necrosis
Late	Small bile ducts	>50% duct loss (ductopenia); degenerative changes involving the remaining ducts
	Portal hepatic arterioles	Lost in >25% portal areas
	Central veins	Variable inflammation; focal obliteration; moderate to severe fibrosis
	Large perihilar hepatic artery branches	Luminal narrowing by foamy macrophage deposition; fibrointimal hyperplasia
	Large perihilar bile ducts	Mural fibrosis
	Other	Cholestasis and sinusoidal accumulation of foamy macrophages

Adapted from Demetris et al. [7]

[a]At least two of three histological features are necessary to diagnose TCMR

[b]If eosinophils are prominent and accompanied by edema and portal vein and capillary endothelial cell hypertrophy, antibody-mediated rejection should be considered

[c]At least two features should be present to diagnose either early or late chronic rejection

static pattern with persistently elevated alkaline phosphatase, gamma glutamyl transferase (GGT), and total bilirubin, or, if presenting with mixed chronic rejection and TCMR, a mixed cholestatic and hepatitic pattern.

The term "chronic" here refers primarily to the possible irreversibility of the effects, rather than the timeframe in which the process occurs. Affected patients frequently begin showing effects of chronic rejection within the first year post-transplant with graft failure at approximately 1 year. Chronic rejection most commonly occurs as a sequela of ongoing unresolved TCMR or by repeated bouts of TCMR. Less commonly, chronic rejection may result from an insidious process without previously documented TCMR that only becomes apparent after more than 1 year post-transplant (late-onset rejection).

As with TCMR, a global assessment should be made to diagnose chronic rejection before attempting to further classify. Changes should be seen in at least two of the five examined compartments, including the small bile ducts, small hepatic arteries, central veins, large hepatic artery branches, and large perihilar bile ducts (see Table 18.1).

Bile ducts will develop degenerative changes, including cytoplasmic eosinophilia, nucleomegaly, uneven nuclear spacing, hyperchromasia, syncytia formation, and incomplete duct structures without complete epithelial lining (Fig. 18.11). Eventually, these changes may be accompanied by duct loss, with duct profiles in <80% of portal tracts considered loss, and in <50% of portal tracts considered ductopenia. Arterial changes in chronic rejection are primarily seen in the large hepatic artery branches not typically sampled by peripheral liver biopsies. These large arteries show lymphocytic inflammation and accumulation of foamy macrophages in the subintimal, medial, and adventitial compartments of the arteries. Accumulation of these foamy macrophages may eventually lead to fibrosis and luminal occlusion. This then causes ischemia to the small downstream arterioles and the bile ducts, which are supplied exclusively by arterial blood. Large ducts may show similar occlusion by foamy macrophages and fibrosis. The terminal central hepatic venules show mononuclear endotheliitis with perivenular hepatocyte dropout. Later stages may develop perivenular and subsequent bridging fibrosis (though true well-developed cirrhosis is rare) and/or fibrous obliteration. The lobules may show scattered acidophil bodies, canalicular cholestasis, and sinusoidal foamy macrophages.

Differential diagnostic considerations for chronic rejection include various biliary processes. Strictures, other forms of obstruction, ischemic or infectious cholangiopathies, or recurrent biliary disease, such as primary biliary cholangitis (PBC) and primary sclerosing cholangitis (PSC), may lead to similar reactive duct changes and duct loss. The combination of imaging studies and clinical presentation can exclude most processes affecting the large ducts. The perivenular

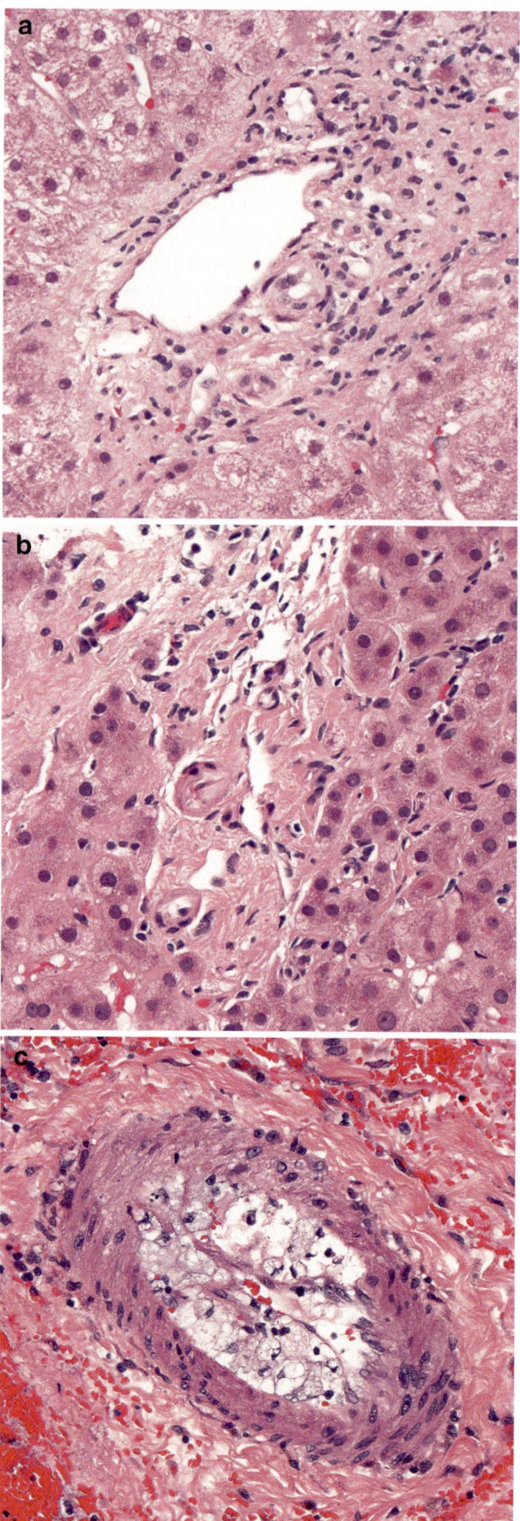

Fig. 18.11 Chronic rejection. (**a**) Bile duct damage, including cytoplasmic hypereosinophilia, irregular nuclear spacing, and cytoplasmic vacuolization (H&E stain, 400× original magnification). (**b**) Portal area with duct loss (H&E stain, 400× original magnification). (**c**). Obliterative arteriopathy in a resection specimen, composed of foamy histiocytes infiltrating the intima and occluding the lumen (H&E stain, 400× original magnification)

inflammation and zone 3 fibrosis of chronic rejection would be uncommon for either recurrent PBC or PSC.

Antibody-Mediated Rejection

Antibody-mediated rejection (AMR) is characterized by antibody-mediated damage to vascular and sinusoidal endothelium, with or without complement activation, and subsequent ischemic changes. AMR is less frequent in liver allografts than in other transplanted organs, due to the liver's large surface area of endothelial cells, its innate regenerative capabilities, and its resident immune system (Kupffer cells) capable of removing immune complexes.

ABO blood group-incompatible transplants are the classic cause of "hyper-acute" AMR, in which pre-formed antibodies attack the new graft and may cause graft failure within minutes. Even in ABO-incompatible transplants, such occurrences are now rare, thanks to pre-transplant reduction of circulating antibodies via plasmapheresis and careful post-transplant monitoring.

Acute AMR is characterized by rapid production of antibodies against the liver allograft in highly sensitized patients. Injury typically occurs in the first weeks following transplant, and may manifest as graft dysfunction, persistent hyperbilirubinemia, disproportionately elevated transaminases, low serum complement and thrombocytopenia, circulating immune complexes, and persistent donor-specific antibodies (DSAs).

Histological features of acute AMR are variable. Portal changes include portal edema, portal vein and capillary endothelial hypertrophy, leukocyte margination, and lymphocytic arteritis and fibrinoid necrosis of small hepatic arteriole branches. Interface and periportal changes include periportal coagulative necrosis and ductular reaction. In the lobules and perivenular regions, there may be sinusoidal congestion and hemorrhage with extravasation of red blood cells into the space of Disse, patchy acidophil bodies, canalicular cholestasis, zone 3 hepatocyte swelling, and central vein obliteration reminiscent of SOS. Based on histology alone, differential diagnostic considerations for these changes are wide, and AMR frequently occurs coincidentally with TCMR.

The presence of DSAs and/or C4d endothelial staining may be helpful in patients with the appropriate histology and clinical setting. Cutoffs for clinically relevant DSAs vary between laboratories, but ≥5000 mean fluorescence intensity is broadly considered indicative of acute AMR. The optimal testing methodology for C4d is also not entirely settled: immunohistochemical staining is widely available, though the evaluation of frozen tissue by immunofluorescence is more sensitive. Granular or linear staining of portal vein and/or capillary endothelium constitutes positive C4d staining. Care should be taken, as portal venous and capillary endothelial staining may be seen in a wide variety of other conditions, and must be interpreted within the context of the histology (see Table 18.2). Other nonspecific C4d staining patterns include staining of portal stroma, sinusoidal endo-

thelial cells, central veins, periductal stroma, lymphoid aggregates, and elastic lamina of veins and arteries.

Chronic or late-onset acute AMR is less well-defined. Injury associated with the late post-transplant de novo appearance of DSAs has been attributed to chronic AMR. Proposed chronic AMR lesions include mild portal and lymphocytic or lymphoplasmacytic inflammation with mild interface activity, portal capillary dilatation, endothelial hypertrophy, and leukocyte margination. Endothelial C4d deposition may be seen, though it is frequently less diffuse than in acute AMR. The histological features frequently overlap with late-onset TCMR, and a component of AMR should be suspected if there is a poor response to steroid treatment.

Plasma Cell-Rich Rejection

Plasma cell-rich rejection is an uncommon pattern of rejection characterized by a plasma-cell rich infiltrate histologically resembling autoimmune hepatitis (AIH), previously referred to as plasma cell hepatitis or de novo AIH. Proposed minimal diagnostic criteria include two of the following three features: (1) a plasma cell-rich infiltrate involving a majority of portal areas and/or central veins, with plasma cells constituting at least one-third of the inflammatory infiltrate (Fig. 18.12); (2) the original liver disease was something other than AIH; and (3) there is a component of lymphocytic bile duct injury [7].

Plasma cell-rich rejection shares some features of TCMR, AMR, and AIH. Although a predominantly zone 3 process, there is typically still marked bile duct inflammation and damage, like TCMR. In a study by Fiel et al., almost all the patients with plasma cell-rich rejection had low titer autoantibodies, and some had autoantibody titers of 1:40 or greater. Most cases were associated with suboptimal or recent lowering of immune suppression, suggesting that plasma cell-rich rejection is a form of acute rejection. These patients also had a high incidence of TCMR before developing plasma cell-rich rejection, indicating a propensity for rejection [53].

Portal vasculature may show significant endothelial C4d deposition, as in AMR. *De novo* DSAs are demonstrated in over half of patients. Unlike AIH of the native liver, plasma cell-rich rejection contains a preponderance of IgG4-positive plasma cells. It typically appears late (>6 months posttransplant), and may be treated with high dose corticosteroids, though it may be difficult to manage without continuous steroid treatment. Differential diagnostic considerations include viral hepatitis. If available, explanted livers should be examined to exclude indications of pre-transplant AIH.

Recurrent Liver Disease

For many indications, liver transplantation is curative. Hereditary hemochromatosis, alpha-1-antitrypsin deficiency, Wilson disease, glycogen storage disease, progressive familial intrahepatic cholestasis, biliary atresia, Alagille syndrome, and tyrosinemia, are all primary hepatobiliary disorders, in which transplantation removes the metabolic or

Table 18.2 Summarized assessment of acute antibody-mediated rejection

Criterion	Histological features
Lesion component scoring for acute antibody-mediated rejection	
Histopathology score	
1	Portal venous, portal capillary, and inlet venules with endothelial hypertrophy involving a majority of portal tracts Generally mild portal venous, portal capillary, and inlet venule dilation 3–4 marginated monocytes, neutrophils, or eosinophils in the maximally involved capillary
2	Prominent portal venous, portal capillary, inlet venule, and/or sinusoidal endothelial cell hypertrophy involving a majority of portal tracts Variable, but noticeable, portal capillary and inlet venule dilatation with variable portal edema 5–10 marginated monocytes, neutrophils, or eosinophils in the maximally involved capillary
3	Prominent portal venous, portal capillary, inlet venule, and/or sinusoidal endothelial cell hypertrophy involving a majority of portal tracts Marked portal capillary and inlet venule dilatation with portal edema ≥10 marginated monocytes, neutrophils, or eosinophils in the maximally involved capillary with at least focal luminal disruption, fibrin deposition, and extravasation of red blood cells into the portal stroma and/or space of Disse
C4d score[a]	
0	No C4d deposition in portal venous or capillary endothelium
1	C4d deposition in >50% of the circumference of portal venous or capillary endothelium involving <10% of portal tracts
2	C4d deposition in >50% of the circumference of portal venous or capillary endothelium involving 10–50% of portal tracts (predominantly not involving periportal sinusoids)
3	C4d deposition in >50% of the circumference of portal venous or capillary endothelium involving >50% of portal tracts (may have frequent extension into inlet venules and periportal sinusoids)
Criteria for establishing the diagnosis of acute antibody-mediated rejection in liver allografts	
Definite acute antibody-mediated rejection (all 4 criteria required)	
1	Histopathologic pattern of injury consistent with acute antibody-mediated rejection, typically including: Portal venous or portal capillary endothelial cell hypertrophy Portal capillary or inlet venule dilatation Monocytic, eosinophilic, and neutrophilic margination Portal edema Ductular reaction Cholestasis (variable) Periportal hepatocyte edema and dropout (variable) Lymphocytic and/or necrotizing hepatic arteritis (variable)
2	Positive testing for serum donor-specific antibodies
3	C4d score of 3 on formalin-fixed, paraffin-embedded tissue in ABO-compatible allografts or Portal stromal C4d deposition in ABO-incompatible allografts
4	Reasonable exclusion of other etiologies of a similar injury pattern
Suspicious for acute antibody-mediated rejection (both criteria required)	
1	Positive for serum donor-specific antibodies
2	Histopathology score ≥1 and a combined histopathology score plus C4d score of 3–4
Indeterminate for acute antibody-mediated rejection (both criteria 1 and 2 are required, plus either criterion 3 or 4)	
1	Combined histopathology score plus C4d score of ≥2
2	Serum donor-specific antibody results equivocal, negative, or not available
3	C4d staining equivocal, negative, or not available
4	Coexisting etiology may be contributing to the injury

Adapted from Demetris et al. [7]

[a]Applicable to immunohistochemical staining on formalin-fixed, paraffin-embedded tissue

structural defect. Liver transplantation is also indicated for a number of tumoral conditions, including hepatocellular carcinoma, hepatocellular adenomatosis, select cases of cholangiocarcinoma, and metastatic neuroendocrine tumors. Malignant tumors may recur in the liver or as extrahepatic metastases. Alcohol- and drug-induced liver disorders recur with similar histologic patterns after transplantation if the offending agent is reintroduced. PSC, PBC, and AIH may also recur, showing features typical of the disease in the native liver. However, hepatitis B and C infections, two of the most common indications for liver transplantation, may recur in allograft livers with different histopathological patterns than in native livers.

Recurrent Hepatitis C

Untreated hepatitis C virus (HCV) nearly inevitably recurs in transplanted livers, with the majority of patients progressing from viremia to clinical hepatitis. Recurrent HCV frequently progresses to advanced fibrosis and liver failure at a more rapid pace than in native livers.

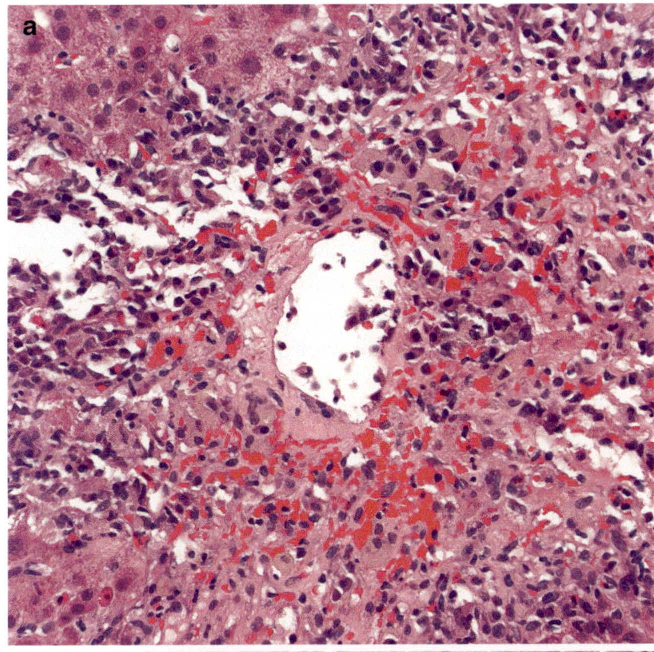

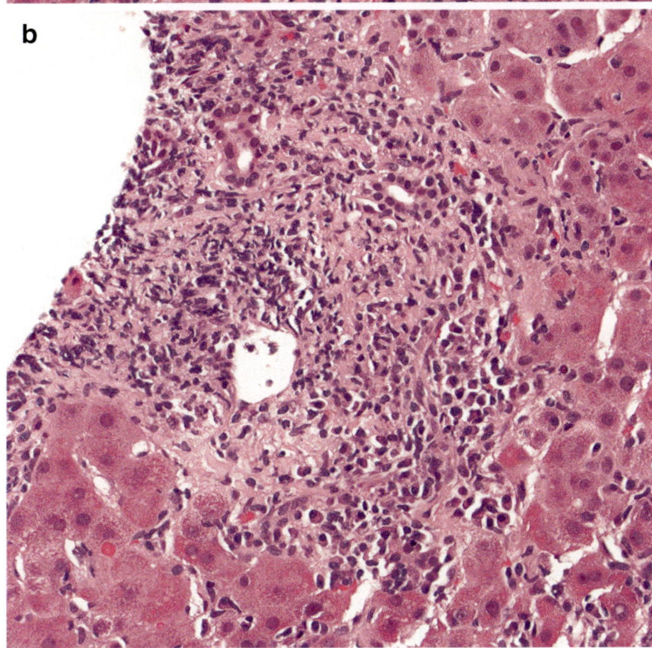

Fig. 18.12 Plasma cell-rich rejection. (**a**) Severe lobular hepatitis with central venulitis, zone 3 necrosis, and prominent plasma cells (H&E stain, 400× original magnification). (**b**) Severe portal and interface hepatitis with portal venulitis and prominent plasma cells (H&E stain, 400× original magnification)

While not an entirely specific histologic feature, macrovesicular steatosis accumulation in the allograft liver is associated with HCV reinfection, unrelated to obesity or metabolic syndrome. It is most commonly associated with HCV genotype 3. Steatotic change may herald an increased rate of post-transplant fibrosis.

Unlike HCV hepatitis in the native liver, the initial manifestations of recurrent HCV are found in the allograft's lobules. Early features of recurrence include the presence of acidophil bodies, increased sinusoidal lymphocytes, Kupffer cell hyperplasia, lobular hepatocyte disarray, and mild ballooning changes (Fig. 18.13). Mild lymphocytic portal and interface inflammation may be seen, but typically becomes more prominent in the later phases of infection. Portal lymphoid aggregates with well-formed germinal centers may be seen, though are less frequent than in HCV hepatitis of the native liver. The differential diagnosis of recurrent HCV in the allograft includes multiple entities, but distinction from TCMR is likely the most significant differential diagnosis. An erroneous diagnosis of TCMR could lead to increased immunosuppression, which would be detrimental to recurrent HCV. Less common features of recurrent HCV include a plasma-cell rich infiltrate, mimicking plasma cell-rich rejection; bile duct injury, raising the possibility of TCMR; lobular cholestasis, raising the possibility of drug-induced liver disease or biliary complications; and ductular reaction, also mimicking duct obstruction. It should be noted that prominent ductular reaction has been reported in HCV pre-transplant, with strong correlation with portal fibrosis [54] and post-transplant, associated with aggressive HCV recurrence [55].

However, the predominant pattern should be kept in mind when any of these features are seen. Prominent venulitis or out-of-proportion bile duct injury favors TCMR. Prominent cholestasis or ductular reaction in the absence of the other features described argues against recurrent HCV as the cause of injury. As always, careful correlation with clinical, laboratory, and imaging information is necessary, including suggesting additional studies in the report, if other causes of liver injury have not been investigated clinically.

Fibrosing cholestatic HCV is a particular pattern of injury associated with an aggressive clinical course independent of fibrosis. It is associated with massive viremia and overimmunosuppression, and is thought to be due to direct viral cytopathic effect, as only minimal inflammation is present. Recent studies with strong clinical correlation have proposed utilizing at least three out of four histological features for proposing a diagnosis of fibrosing cholestatic HCV, including prominent ductular reaction, hepatocyte ballooning, cholestasis, and perisinusoidal fibrosis [56]. Clinical features frequently associated with fibrosing cholestatic HCV include GGT ≥150 U/L, serum total bilirubin ≥2.0 mg/dL, AST ≥70 U/L, older donor age, recent bouts of moderate or severe TCMR, and the exclusion of biliary obstruction or hepatic artery thrombosis [57]. This unique histological pattern leads to differential diagnostic considerations that include alcoholic and non-alcoholic steatohepatitis, biliary obstruction, and chronic rejection, though strict application of the criteria and correlation with imaging findings can exclude these. While most commonly associated with HCV reinfection in liver allografts, fibrosing cholestatic HCV may also occur in native livers after solid organ or hematopoietic stem cell transplantation. Fibrosing cholestatic HCV is an aggressive disease typically portending graft loss, though reduced immunosuppression may lead to long-term graft survival.

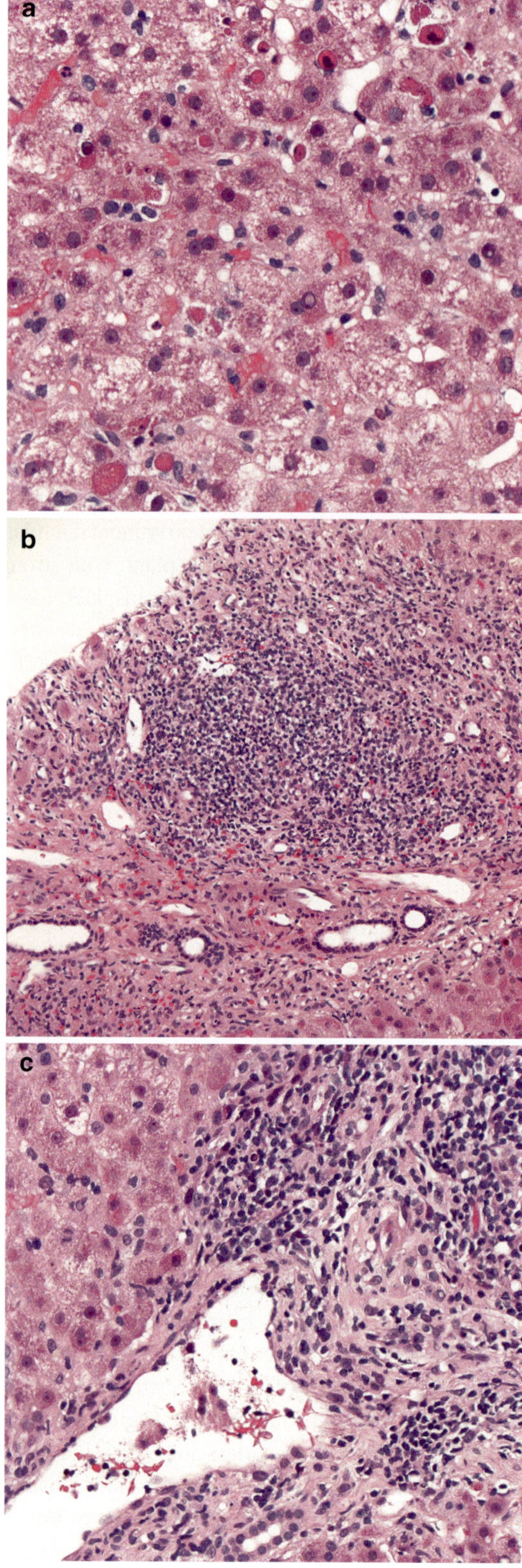

Fig. 18.13 Recurrent hepatitis C. (**a**) Prominent lobular apoptotic bodies in early recurrence (H&E stain, 400× original magnification). (**b**) Prominent portal lymphoid infiltrate, including a lymphoid aggregate (H&E stain, 200× original magnification). (**c**) Venulitis in a case with marked lymphoplasmacytic infiltrate (H&E stain, 400× original magnification)

The recent advent of direct-acting antiviral agents for the treatment of HCV has drastically improved the rate of achieved sustained viral response in patients with HCV. In some patients with undetectable virus in the serum, HCV RNA can still be demonstrated via PCR from liver tissues, even after liver transplantation. Some of these patients have abnormal aminotransferases, suggesting that HCV may persist even after "cure" [58]. Other patients show histological findings similar to active hepatitis, even after achieving sustained viral response and liver transplantation, despite no detectable HCV in serum or liver tissue. These changes may persist for years, and some patients may even have progressive fibrosis [59]. These findings suggest that, even after viral eradication, abnormal immune system activation may persist and damage the liver. While direct-acting antivirals hold great promise for the treatment of HCV, studies with long-term follow-up of treated and transplanted patients are still needed to understand the full range of liver changes post-treatment and post-transplantation.

Recurrent Hepatitis B

Hepatitis B virus (HBV) may be encountered in liver allografts in several settings. Like HCV, clinically apparent hepatitis may recur after transplantation in patients with HBV. Using current pre- and post-transplant antiviral regimens, liver reinfection rates may be as low as 2%, though reinfection may occur years after transplant [60]. Donor livers may also harbor HBV infection: some centers have begun transplanting previously HBV-infected livers (i.e., livers from donors with positive HBV core antibodies and negative HBV surface antibodies) into HBV-negative recipients in an effort to expand the donor pool, given the critical shortage of available donor livers and good management of HBV in compliant transplanted patients on current antiviral regimens. Lastly, HBV may be encountered in post-transplant patients transplanted for other causes that acquire new HBV infection (e.g., by sexual transmission). Viral reinfection of a liver allograft may be detected by immunohistochemical stains for HBV surface and core antigens before clinical hepatitis occurs. Typical recurrences show features similar to infection of the native liver, including mild portal inflammation with interface activity. Lobular changes, including acidophil bodies, hepatocyte disarray, and cholestasis may also be present. As HBV progresses, greater portal inflammation and interface activity may be seen, and the characteristic cytoplasmic ground-glass inclusions may be seen in hepatocytes. The main differential diagnostic considerations include TCMR, AIH, or other viral hepatitides. Prominent venous endotheliitis suggests either TCMR or AIH, and prominent bile duct damage favors TCMR. It is also noteworthy that clinical HBV hepatitis does not typically occur before 2 months post-transplantation, whereas TCMR typically occurs within this time period [61].

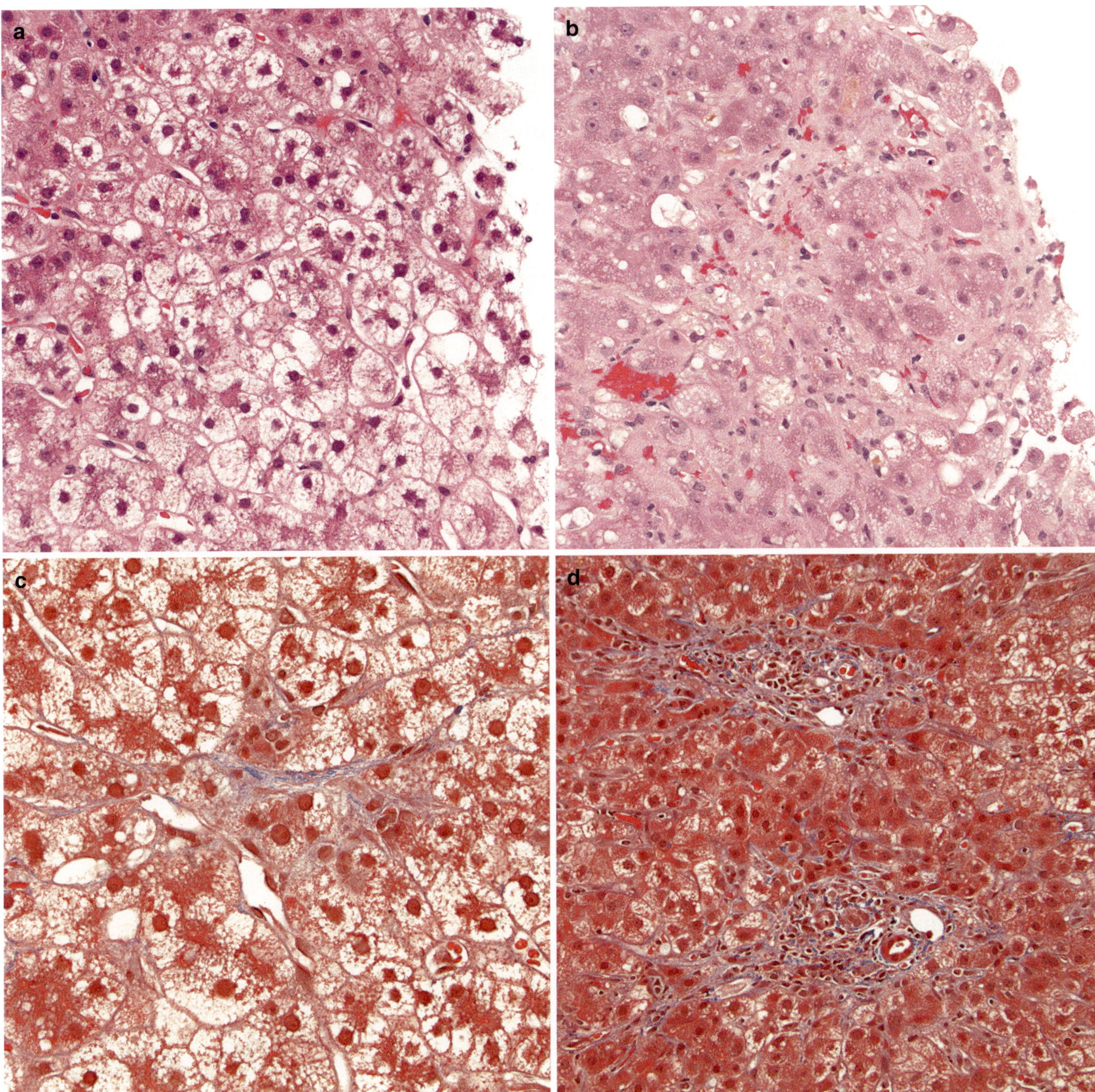

Fig. 18.14 Fibrosing cholestatic hepatitis. (**a**) Prominent hepatocellular ballooning with minimal inflammation (H&E stain, 400× original magnification). (**b**) Hepatocellular ballooning with lobular cholestasis and minimal inflammation (H&E stain, 400× original magnification). (**c**) Delicate sinusoidal fibrosis (Masson trichrome, 400× original magnification). (**d**) Periportal fibrosis (Masson trichrome, 200× original magnification)

Ancillary stains and correlation with serum testing can help to exclude other viral hepatitides, such as EBV, CMV, or HCV. HBV-infected patients or HBV-naïve patients receiving HBV-infected livers may receive HBV antiviral prophylaxis, typically consisting of lamivudine. HBV immune globulin or other antivirals, such as tenofovir or adefovir for HBV infections with lamivudine resistance mutations, may be added for the treatment of recurrent HBV hepatitis.

Like HCV, HBV can also manifest in the highly aggressive fibrosing cholestatic pattern, associated with high levels of HBV DNA replication and due to direct viral cytopathic effects. It is histologically characterized by prominent hepatocellular ballooning and periportal fibrosis (Fig. 18.14). Inflammation is minimal. Both ballooning and fibrosis may rapidly progress with increasing liver dysfunction. Some cases show cholestasis and ductular reaction. Immunohistochemical expression of HBV core and surface antigens is typically marked, including cytoplasmic expression of HBV core antigen. Fibrosing cholestatic HBV is not unique to allograft livers, and has been documented in native livers after other solid organ transplants and after hematopoietic stem cell transplantation.

Special note must be made of HBV reactivation. Strictly speaking, a liver from an uninfected donor into a HBV-infected recipient undergoes reinfection of HBV. Reactivation is the sudden increase in viral replication in a patient with inactive or "resolved" HBV (as measured by a circulating HBV DNA, conversion from HBV E antigen negativity to positivity, or conversion from HBV surface antigen negativity to positivity). The induction of immune suppression during solid organ or hematopoietic stem cell transplantation may induce reactivation of HBV and with histological features of recurrence, as previously described. However, a minority of patients present with acute, and even fulminant, hepatitis (Fig. 18.15). Most fulminant cases of HBV reactivation present not in the setting of transplantation, but with intensive chemotherapy for hematopoietic malignancies. However, the intensive myeloablative regimens involving pre-hematopoietic stem cell transplantation may lead to fulminant HBV reactivation post-transplantation.

Hepatitis D virus (HDV) is an RNA virus that requires HBV coinfection to replicate in native hepatocytes. After transplantation, HDV may reinfect allograft hepatocytes even before HBV reinfection. Hepatitis typically does not occur until coinfection with HBV, at which point the typical histological findings follow those described above for post-transplant HBV infection. Pre-transplantation, HDV superinfection may lead to a severe acute hepatitis. In the post-transplant setting, HDV coinfection actually tempers HBV infection, reducing viral replication and histological inflammation compared to HBV infection alone. Allograft livers with HDV coinfection also typically show fewer or no ground-glass inclusions.

Diagnostic Caveats

1. For transplant-related diseases involving the liver and spleen, the liver is addressed as the biopsy is the gold standard of liver investigation, and there is no indication for performing splenic biopsy. The lesions involving the liver are representative.
2. The issues that affect the liver across all transplantation settings include opportunistic infections, HLH, medication effects, and Epstein-Barr virus-associated post-transplant smooth muscle tumor.
3. The issues unique to hematopoietic stem cell transplantation include GVHD and sinusoidal obstruction syndrome.

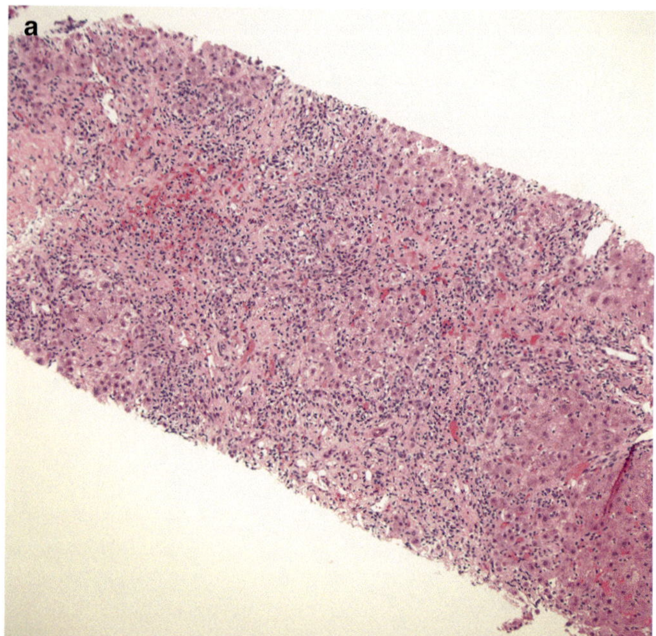

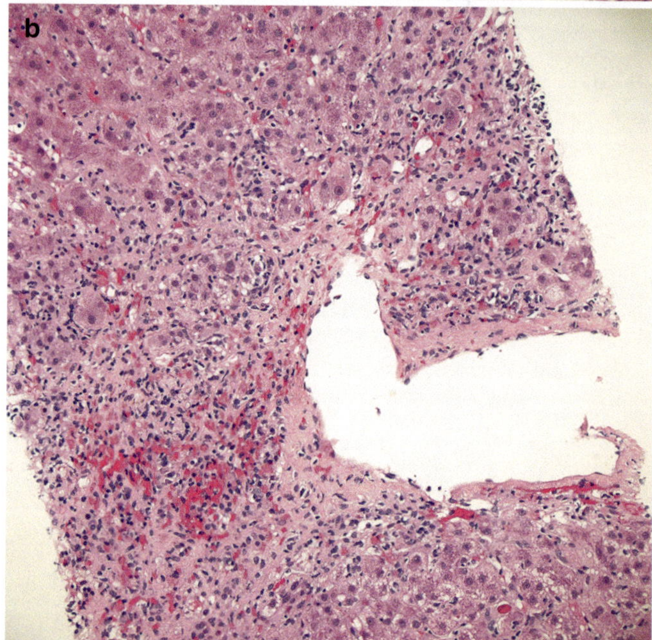

Fig. 18.15 Reactivation of hepatitis B. (**a**) Severe lobular hepatitis with bridging necrosis (H&E stain, 100× original magnification). (**b**) Severe lobular hepatitis with zone 3 necrosis (H&E stain, 200× original magnification)

4. Attention should also be paid to the recurrence of the primary liver diseases or hepatic involvement by systemic diseases, infectious or non-infectious, during the assessment of transplant-related disease.
5. Post-transplant lymphoproliferative disorders show similar morphological and phenotypical features to those in the non-transplant that are under the umbrella of other chapters.

References

1. Van Ha TG. Liver biopsy in liver transplant recipients. Semin Intervent Radiol. 2004;21(4):271–4.
2. Ozgun G, Ozdemir BH, Tunca MZ, Borcek P, Haberal M. Importance of liver biopsy findings on prognosis of kidney transplant patients. Exp Clin Transplant. 2016;14(Suppl 3):37–41.
3. Chahal P, Levy C, Litzow MR, Lindor KD. Utility of liver biopsy in bone marrow transplant patients. J Gastroenterol Hepatol. 2008;23(2):222–5.
4. Spycher C, Zimmermann A, Reichen J. The diagnostic value of liver biopsy. BMC Gastroenterol. 2001;1:12.
5. Colonna JO 2nd, Brems JJ, Goldstein LI, et al. The importance of percutaneous liver biopsy in the management of the liver transplant recipient. Transplant Proc. 1988;20(1 Suppl 1):682–4.
6. Hultcrantz R, Gabrielsson N. Patients with persistent elevation of aminotransferases: investigation with ultrasonography, radionuclide imaging and liver biopsy. J Intern Med. 1993;233(1):7–12.
7. Demetris AJ, Bellamy C, Hubscher SG, et al. Comprehensive update of the Banff Working Group on liver allograft pathology: introduction of antibody-mediated rejection. Am J Transplant. 2016;16(10):2816–35.
8. Staras SA, Dollard SC, Radford KW, Flanders WD, Pass RF, Cannon MJ. Seroprevalence of cytomegalovirus infection in the United States, 1988–1994. Clin Infect Dis. 2006;43(9):1143–51.
9. Gandhi MK, Khanna R. Human cytomegalovirus: clinical aspects, immune regulation, and emerging treatments. Lancet Infect Dis. 2004;4(12):725–38.
10. Boeckh M, Geballe AP. Cytomegalovirus: pathogen, paradigm, and puzzle. J Clin Invest. 2011;121(5):1673–80.
11. Ross SA, Novak Z, Pati S, Boppana SB. Overview of the diagnosis of cytomegalovirus infection. Infect Disord Drug Targets. 2011;11(5):466–74.
12. Paya CV, Holley KE, Wiesner RH, et al. Early diagnosis of cytomegalovirus hepatitis in liver transplant recipients: role of immunostaining, DNA hybridization and culture of hepatic tissue. Hepatology. 1990;12(1):119–26.
13. Colina F, Juca NT, Moreno E, et al. Histological diagnosis of cytomegalovirus hepatitis in liver allografts. J Clin Pathol. 1995;48(4):351–7.
14. Lamps LW, Pinson CW, Raiford DS, Shyr Y, Scott MA, Washington MK. The significance of microabscesses in liver transplant biopsies: a clinicopathological study. Hepatology. 1998;28(6):1532–7.
15. Parker A, Bowles K, Bradley JA, et al. Diagnosis of post-transplant lymphoproliferative disorder in solid organ transplant recipients – BCSH and BTS guidelines. Br J Haematol. 2010;149(5):675–92.
16. Kusne S, Schwartz M, Breinig MK, et al. Herpes simplex virus hepatitis after solid organ transplantation in adults. J Infect Dis. 1991;163(5):1001–7.
17. Schaberg KB, Kambham N, Sibley RK, Higgins JPT. Adenovirus hepatitis: clinicopathologic analysis of 12 consecutive cases from a single institution. Am J Surg Pathol. 2017;41(6):810–9.
18. Ronan BA, Agrwal N, Carey EJ, et al. Fulminant hepatitis due to human adenovirus. Infection. 2014;42(1):105–11.
19. Kamar N, Selves J, Mansuy JM, et al. Hepatitis E virus and chronic hepatitis in organ-transplant recipients. N Engl J Med. 2008;358(8):811–7.
20. Unzueta A, Rakela J. Hepatitis E infection in liver transplant recipients. Liver Transpl. 2014;20(1):15–24.
21. Phan TL, Lautenschlager I, Razonable RR, Munoz FM. HHV-6 in liver transplantation: a literature review. Liver Int. 2018;38(2):210–23.
22. Madan R, Hand J. Human herpesvirus 6, 7, and 8 in solid organ transplantation: guidelines from the American Society of Transplantation Infectious Diseases Community of Practice. Clin Transplant. 2019;33:e13518.
23. Fung JJ. Fungal infection in liver transplantation. Transpl Infect Dis. 2002;4(Suppl 3):18–23.
24. Henter JI, Horne A, Arico M, et al. HLH-2004: diagnostic and therapeutic guidelines for hemophagocytic lymphohistiocytosis. Pediatr Blood Cancer. 2007;48(2):124–31.
25. de Kerguenec C, Hillaire S, Molinie V, et al. Hepatic manifestations of hemophagocytic syndrome: a study of 30 cases. Am J Gastroenterol. 2001;96(3):852–7.
26. Ganschow R, Albani J, Grabhorn E, Richter A, Burdelski M. Tacrolimus-induced cholestatic syndrome following pediatric liver transplantation and steroid-resistant graft rejection. Pediatr Transplant. 2006;10(2):220–4.
27. Swerdlow S, Webber S, Chardburn A, Ferry J. Post-transplant lymphoproliferative disorders. In: Press W, editor. WHO classification of tumors of haematopoietic and lymphoid tissues. Lyon: IARC; 2017. p. 453.
28. Swerdlow SH. T-cell and NK-cell posttransplantation lymphoproliferative disorders. Am J Clin Pathol. 2007;127(6):887–95.
29. Cleary ML, Warnke R, Sklar J. Monoclonality of lymphoproliferative lesions in cardiac-transplant recipients. Clonal analysis based on immunoglobulin-gene rearrangements. N Engl J Med. 1984;310(8):477–82.
30. Ferry JA, Jacobson JO, Conti D, Delmonico F, Harris NL. Lymphoproliferative disorders and hematologic malignancies following organ transplantation. Mod Pathol. 1989;2(6):583–92.
31. Knowles DM, Cesarman E, Chadburn A, et al. Correlative morphologic and molecular genetic analysis demonstrates three distinct categories of posttransplantation lymphoproliferative disorders. Blood. 1995;85(2):552–65.
32. Romero S, Montoro J, Guinot M, et al. Post-transplant lymphoproliferative disorders after solid organ and hematopoietic stem cell transplantation. Leuk Lymphoma. 2019;60(1):142–50.
33. Al-Mansour Z, Nelson BP, Evens AM. Post-transplant lymphoproliferative disease (PTLD): risk factors, diagnosis, and current treatment strategies. Curr Hematol Malig Rep. 2013;8(3):173–83.
34. Leblond V, Davi F, Charlotte F, et al. Posttransplant lymphoproliferative disorders not associated with Epstein-Barr virus: a distinct entity? J Clin Oncol. 1998;16(6):2052–9.
35. Dotti G, Fiocchi R, Motta T, et al. Primary effusion lymphoma after heart transplantation: a new entity associated with human herpesvirus-8. Leukemia. 1999;13(5):664–70.
36. Matsushima AY, Strauchen JA, Lee G, et al. Posttransplantation plasmacytic proliferations related to Kaposi's sarcoma-associated herpesvirus. Am J Surg Pathol. 1999;23(11):1393–400.
37. Jonigk D, Laenger F, Maegel L, et al. Molecular and clinicopathological analysis of Epstein-Barr virus-associated posttransplant smooth muscle tumors. Am J Transplant. 2012;12(7):1908–17.
38. Jossen J, Chu J, Hotchkiss H, et al. Epstein-Barr virus-associated smooth muscle tumors in children following solid organ transplantation: a review. Pediatr Transplant. 2015;19(2):235–43.
39. Deyrup AT, Lee VK, Hill CE, et al. Epstein-Barr virus-associated smooth muscle tumors are distinctive mesenchymal tumors reflecting multiple infection events: a clinicopathologic and molecular analysis of 29 tumors from 19 patients. Am J Surg Pathol. 2006;30(1):75–82.
40. Hussein K, Rath B, Ludewig B, Kreipe H, Jonigk D. Clinicopathological characteristics of different types of immunodeficiency-associated smooth muscle tumours. Eur J Cancer. 2014;50(14):2417–24.
41. Shulman HM, Sharma P, Amos D, Fenster LF, McDonald GB. A coded histologic study of hepatic graft-versus-host disease after human bone marrow transplantation. Hepatology. 1988;8(3):463–70.
42. Shulman HM, Cardona DM, Greenson JK, et al. NIH consensus development project on criteria for clinical trials in chronic graft-

versus-host disease: II. The 2014 pathology working group report. Biol Blood Marrow Transplant. 2015;21(4):589–603.

43. Akpek G, Boitnott JK, Lee LA, et al. Hepatitic variant of graft-versus-host disease after donor lymphocyte infusion. Blood. 2002;100(12):3903–7.

44. Mohty M, Malard F, Abecassis M, et al. Revised diagnosis and severity criteria for sinusoidal obstruction syndrome/veno-occlusive disease in adult patients: a new classification from the European Society for Blood and Marrow Transplantation. Bone Marrow Transplant. 2016;51(7):906–12.

45. Cha I, Bass N, Ferrell LD. Lipopeliosis. An immunohistochemical and clinicopathologic study of five cases. Am J Surg Pathol. 1994;18(8):789–95.

46. Choi WT, Jen KY, Wang D, Tavakol M, Roberts JP, Gill RM. Donor liver small droplet macrovesicular steatosis is associated with increased risk for recipient allograft rejection. Am J Surg Pathol. 2017;41(3):365–73.

47. Uchida T, Kao H, Quispe-Sjogren M, Peters RL. Alcoholic foamy degeneration--a pattern of acute alcoholic injury of the liver. Gastroenterology. 1983;84(4):683–92.

48. Coghlan ME, Sommadossi JP, Jhala NC, Many WJ, Saag MS, Johnson VA. Symptomatic lactic acidosis in hospitalized antiretroviral-treated patients with human immunodeficiency virus infection: a report of 12 cases. Clin Infect Dis. 2001;33(11):1914–21.

49. Demetris AJ, Kelly DM, Eghtesad B, et al. Pathophysiologic observations and histopathologic recognition of the portal hyperperfusion or small-for-size syndrome. Am J Surg Pathol. 2006;30(8):986–93.

50. Kochhar G, Parungao JM, Hanouneh IA, Parsi MA. Biliary complications following liver transplantation. World J Gastroenterol. 2013;19(19):2841–6.

51. Sharma S, Gurakar A, Jabbour N. Biliary strictures following liver transplantation: past, present and preventive strategies. Liver Transpl. 2008;14(6):759–69.

52. Demetris AJ, Batts KP, Dhillon AP, et al. Banff schema for grading liver allograft rejection: an international consensus document. Hepatology. 1997;25(3):658–63.

53. Fiel MI, Agarwal K, Stanca C, et al. Posttransplant plasma cell hepatitis (de novo autoimmune hepatitis) is a variant of rejection and may lead to a negative outcome in patients with hepatitis C virus. Liver Transpl. 2008;14(6):861–71.

54. Clouston AD, Powell EE, Walsh MJ, Richardson MM, Demetris AJ, Jonsson JR. Fibrosis correlates with a ductular reaction in hepatitis C: roles of impaired replication, progenitor cells and steatosis. Hepatology. 2005;41(4):809–18.

55. Taga SA, Washington MK, Terrault N, Wright TL, Somberg KA, Ferrell LD. Cholestatic hepatitis C in liver allografts. Liver Transpl Surg. 1998;4(4):304–10.

56. Moreira RK, Salomao M, Verna EC, Brown RS Jr, Lefkowitch JH. The Hepatitis Aggressiveness Score (HAS): a novel classification system for post-liver transplantation recurrent hepatitis C. Am J Surg Pathol. 2013;37(1):104–13.

57. Verna EC, Abdelmessih R, Salomao MA, Lefkowitch J, Moreira RK, Brown RS Jr. Cholestatic hepatitis C following liver transplantation: an outcome-based histological definition, clinical predictors, and prognosis. Liver Transpl. 2013;19(1):78–88.

58. Elmasry S, Wadhwa S, Bang BR, et al. Detection of occult hepatitis C virus infection in patients who achieved a sustained virologic response to direct-acting antiviral agents for recurrent infection after liver transplantation. Gastroenterology. 2017;152(3):550–553. e558.

59. Whitcomb E, Choi WT, Jerome KR, et al. Biopsy specimens from allograft liver contain histologic features of hepatitis C virus infection after virus eradication. Clin Gastroenterol Hepatol. 2017;15(8):1279–85.

60. Zhang D, Jiao Z, Han J, Cao H. Clinicopathological features of hepatitis B virus recurrence after liver transplantation: eleven-year experience. Int J Clin Exp Pathol. 2014;7(7):4057–66.

61. Demetris AJ, Todo S, Van Thiel DH, et al. Evolution of hepatitis B virus liver disease after hepatic replacement. Practical and theoretical considerations. Am J Pathol. 1990;137(3):667–76.

Xiaohui Zhang

Immune Thrombocytopenia (ITP)

Definition

Immune thrombocytopenia is an acronym for primary immune thrombocytopenia, previously referred to as idiopathic thrombocytopenic purpura. ITP is an acquired autoimmune disorder characterized by isolated thrombocytopenia in the absence of conditions known to cause thrombocytopenia, such as infections, other autoimmune disorders, drugs, malignancy, etc.

Introduction

Immune thrombocytopenia (ITP), previously known as idiopathic thrombocytopenic purpura and immune thrombocytopenic purpura, is a syndrome characterized by isolated thrombocytopenia that is caused by antibody-mediated platelet destruction and variably reduced platelet production. Characteristic clinical manifestation is purpuric rash and an increased tendency to bleed. However, many patients remain asymptomatic until the platelet count is very low.

A normal platelet count is considered to be in the range of 150–450×10^9/L of blood for most healthy individuals, and a platelet count of $<150 \times 10^9$/L has been traditionally considered as thrombocytopenia. In 2009, an International Working Group (IWG) recommended the platelet count threshold for the definition of ITP set at 100×10^9/L, recognizing that the majority of patients with borderline thrombocytopenia maintain stable platelet count and are asymptomatic [1]. The IWG classified ITP into primary ITP, in which no predisposing condition is identified, and secondary ITP, which may be associated with broader autoimmune conditions, inherited or acquired immune deficiency, or certain infections [2]. They further classified the disease into "newly diagnosed ITP" (0–3 months), "persistent ITP" (3–12 months), and "chronic ITP" (>12 months) [3].

Secondary ITP refers to autoimmune thrombocytopenia mainly associated with infections (human immunodeficiency virus (HIV), hepatitis C virus (HCV), Epstein-Barr virus (EBV), cytomegalovirus (CMV), Helicobacter pylori, other autoimmune disorders (AID) (such as systemic lupus erythematosus (SLE), Evans syndrome, Sjögren's syndrome, antiphospholipid syndrome), hematologic malignancies (mainly non-Hodgkin lymphoma, particularly chronic lymphocytic leukemia(CLL)) or primary immune deficiency (common variable immune deficiency (CVID), autoimmune lymphoproliferative syndrome (ALPS)). Diagnosis of ITP requires exclusion of thrombocytopenia secondary to medications (including heparin-induced thrombocytopenia), disseminated intravascular coagulation (DIC), vitamins B9 (folic acid) and B12 deficiency, congenital thrombocytopenia, spleen sequestration, portal hypertension, and bone marrow disorders such as myelodysplastic syndromes [4].

Splenectomy is an effective therapy for steroid-refractory or steroid-dependent ITP cases. With the advent of medical alternatives such as rituximab and thrombopoietin receptor agonists, the use of splenectomy has declined and is generally reserved for patients that fail multiple medical therapies.

Etiology/Pathogenesis

ITP is an autoimmune disease most often caused by autoantibodies against several platelet surface antigens that accelerate platelet clearance and impair platelet production to a variable extent. Autoantibody against platelets usually directs against glycoproteins (GPs) or GP complexes (especially GPIIb/IIIa and GPIb/IX/V, and less commonly GPIa/IIa, IV, or VI) [5, 6]. Antiplatelet autoantibodies can be detected in approximately 75% of the ITP patients [7].

X. Zhang (✉)
Department of Pathology, H. Lee Moffitt Cancer Center and Research Institute, Tampa, FL, USA
e-mail: Xiaohui.zhang@moffitt.org

© Springer Nature Switzerland AG 2020
L. Zhang et al. (eds.), *Diagnostic Pathology of Hematopoietic Disorders of Spleen and Liver*,
https://doi.org/10.1007/978-3-030-37708-3_19

There are two aspects in the pathogenesis of ITP: (1) platelet peripheral destruction and (2) impaired bone marrow platelet production. Antiplatelet autoantibody is produced by the plasma cells differentiated from autoreactive B cells in the spleen, the bone marrow, or other niches. The production involves splenic macrophages, follicular dendritic cells, autoreactive T cells and B cells. The antiplatelet autoantibodies are most often IgG but can be IgA and IgM that usually associate with IgG [5]. As a consequence, the antiplatelet autoantibodies in the circulation can coat platelets and render them susceptible to opsonizaiton and phagocytosis by splenic macrophages, as well by Kupffer cells in the liver [8]. Besides increased platelet destruction, the production of platelets is impaired as well. The megakaryocytes can be damaged by the antiplatelet autoantibodies via antibody-dependent cellular cytotoxicity by macrophages surrounding the megakaryocytes, although this mechanism is believed to contribute only slightly to the platelet decrease [4]. Impaired production of the thrombopoietin (TPO), the major growth factor of megakaryocytes, is also believed to be a contributing factor to the decreased platelet production.

The primary triggering factor for ITP is largely unknown, although infections can act as a starter for the antiplatelet autoimmune process. Molecular mimicry between infectious components and platelet glycoproteins has been demonstrated [9, 10]. Genetic predisposing factors involving both the innate and the adaptive immune system are believed to be associated with the pathogenesis [4].

Epidemiology

The annual incidence of ITP is estimated at 10 in 100,000 in the general population in the United States, and around 2.5 per 100,000 persons in Northern Europe [11]. About half of the affected population are children [12]. The overall male to female ratio varies from 1:1.2 to 1:1.7. The median age of adults at the diagnosis is 56–60 years [13]. It is noted that the incidence of ITP increases with age [14].

Clinical Presentations

Generally, patients with ITP present with petechiae, purpura, or ecchymoses, especially on the extremities, gingival bleeding, epistaxis, menorrhagia, hematuria, and less commonly, melena. The signs can develop when the platelet counts drop to 10–20 × 10^9/L. Spontaneous bruising or hematoma formation in the mouth or other mucosal sites can occur when the platelet count is very low (<10 × 10^9/L). Rarely, fatal subarachnoid or intracranial hemorrhage or bleeding at other internal sites can occur when the platelets drop to an extremely low level (<5 × 10^9/L). Patients with a platelet count above 50 × 10^9/L may be asymptomatic and are likely discovered incidentally, although chronic fatigue, inability to focus, and similar protean complaints may be presented.

Clinically, the presentation can be acute or chronic. The acute ITP generally lasts less than 6 months, mainly occurs in children, and often follows a viral infection. Chronic ITP mainly affects adults, persists longer than 6 months, and has an unclear etiology. If splenomegaly or lymphadenopathy is present, an underlying illness that causes secondary thrombocytopenia may be indicated.

Morphology

Gross or Radiological Findings

The spleen is normal or slightly to moderately enlarged [15]. Prominence of the Malpighian corpuscles may be seen in some cases.

Microscopic Examination

Microscopically, lymphoid hyperplasia with variably developed germinal centers can be seen in white pulp [16]. Histiocytes and neutrophils can be found in the red pulp [17]. Diffuse proliferation of foamy histiocytes can be seen in the red pulp (Fig. 19.1a, b). Foamy histiocytes can also form aggregates, resembling lipogranulomas (Fig. 19.1c). Variable amounts of neutrophils can be seen in the red pulp, infiltrating diffusely throughout the cords, or surrounding the lymphoid tissue. Extramedullary hematopoiesis may be present, ranging from mild form with limited to occasional megakaryocytes or early myeloid cells, to more extensive form mimicking spleen in patients with myeloproliferative neoplasm. Variable numbers of plasma cells in marginal zone, foamy, or ceroid laden macrophages can be present in the red pulp. Periarterial fibrosis can be seen in some cases [18]. It has been reported that steroid treatment can diminish the prominence of follicles [19]. Although these morphological findings are considered to be pathologic features of the spleen in ITP patients, they are not specific or diagnostic.

In the liver, hepatic fibrosis has been described in patients with ITP [20]. Electronic microscopy demonstrated phagocytic activity in Kupffer cells [8, 20].

In peripheral blood, platelet count is moderately to significantly decreased. Large to giant platelets are present. In the bone marrow, megakaryocytes are hyperplastic with evenly distributed pattern. At the same time, there are increased immature forms and may be some scattered, small, and pyknotic-appearing megakaryocytes [21]. These megakaryocytes have been shown to have structural abnormality, including defects in the platelet-forming membranes of maturing megakaryocytes, and evidence of apoptosis and phagocytic engulfment by macrophages, suggesting an impaired thrombopoiesis besides the peripheral destruction of platelets [22, 23].

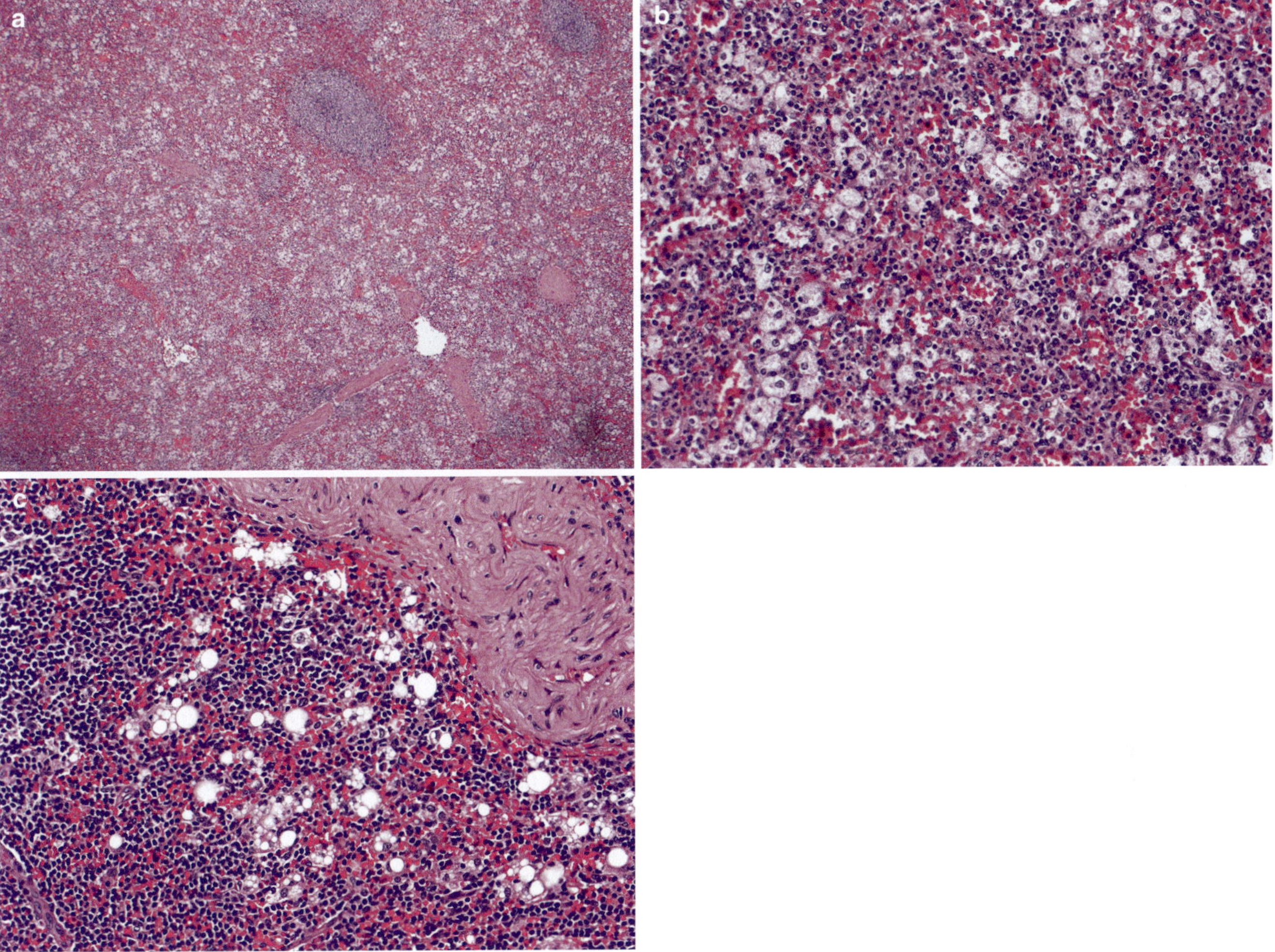

Fig. 19.1 In ITP, there is a diffuse proliferation of foamy histiocytes in the red pulp (**a, b**) (H&E, 100× and 200×, respectively). Foamy histiocytes can also form focal aggregates, resembling lipogranulomas (**c**) (H&E, 200×)

Molecular Study

Predisposing genetic changes for ITP have been reported. The major histocompatibility complex (MHC), Fcγ receptor (FcγR), transcription factors, regulatory proteins such as phosphatase PTPN22, chemokines and their receptors display polymorphisms [4]. Specific epitopes on human platelet antigens (HPA) have also been linked to ITP [24]. Variations in the level of some microRNAs, non-coding RNAs that lead to dysregulation of cytokines involved in the immune response, have also been reported. However, most of the molecular data were from small cohort studies, and further validation is needed.

Immunophenotyping

The infiltrating foamy histiocytes are positive for histiocytic markers (CD68, lysozyme, and CD163), and abundant plate-

let origin cellular debris in the histiocytes can be stained with CD41. B-cell markers (CD20, PAX5) can show the expansion of B-cell compartments including follicle germinal centers and marginal zones. T-cell markers (CD2, CD3, CD5, CD7, CD4, and CD8) usually show no significant abnormalities with a normal CD4 to CD8 ratio [25].

Cytogenetics

N/A

Differential Diagnosis

ITP is largely a clinical diagnosis of exclusion. There may be secondary causes of ITP including systemic lupus erythematosus (SLE), lymphoproliferative disorder, and HIV infection. Other diseases that can cause non-immune-related thrombocytopenia also need to be excluded. These conditions include inherited thrombocytopenia, drug-induced thrombocytopenia, hypersplenism, hematological disorders such as myelodysplastic syndrome, leukemia, aplastic anemia, thrombotic thrombocytopenic purpura/hemolytic uremic syndrome (TTP/HUS), disseminated intravascular coagulation (DIC), etc.

The morphological findings in the spleen, liver, and bone marrow are nonspecific, and a pathological diagnosis requires close clinicopathological correlation.

Prognosis

ITP is a benign disease with a good long-term outcome. Spontaneous remissions have been observed in a significant percentage of untreated patients (about 9%). With treatment such as splenectomy, the majority of patients can achieve a complete remission and reach a stable, safe platelet count for many years [26]. There are risks to develop fatal hemorrhage from thrombocytopenia or infection in the setting of therapies that cause immunosuppression; however, the mortality rate of ITP is similar to or only marginally higher than the age-matched population. Patients with ITP are more likely to die of conditions unrelated to ITP [27, 28].

Diagnostic Caveats

- ITP is a clinical diagnosis of exclusion.
- Histological findings in the spleen, liver, and bone marrow are nonspecific.
- The findings include histiocyte and neutrophil infiltrate in the splenic red pulp, extramedullary hematopoiesis in the spleen, phagocytic activity by reticulocytes in the liver and spleen, and megakaryocytes hyperplasia in the bone marrow.
- Megakaryocytes have also been shown to have structural abnormality.

Thrombotic Thrombocytopenic Purpura (TTP)

Definition

Thrombotic thrombocytopenic purpura (TTP) is a thrombotic microangiopathy caused by severely reduced activity of the von Willebrand factor-cleaving protease ADAMTS13 (a disintegrin and metalloproteinase with a thrombospondin type 1 motif, member 13). It is characterized by formation of platelet-rich thrombi in small vessels, which cause thrombocytopenia, microangiopathic hemolytic anemia with red blood cell fragmentation, and sometimes organ damage due to disturbed microcirculation, often involving kidneys, heart, and brain.

Etiology/Pathogenesis

TTP is caused by severe deficiency of ADAMTS13, either by genetic abnormalities (congenital TTP) or by autoantibodies inhibiting the enzyme ADAMTS13 (acquired autoimmune TTP). ADAMTS13 is a metalloprotease responsible for cleaving large multimers of von Willebrand factor (vWF) into smaller units [29]. Deficiency of ADAMTS13 causes an increase in circulating ultra-large vWF multimers, which in turn enhance platelet aggregation and platelet adhesion to areas with injured endothelial cells in small arterioles (platelet-rich microthrombi formation). The platelets are consumed in the formation of thrombi, which can in turn cause life-threatening bleeds. Red blood cells are subject to shear stress when passing the microscopic clots and can be ruptured, causing anemia and schistocyte formation. The thrombi affect the blood flow in the microcirculation and cause organ damage [30–32].

Congenital TTP is rare, comprising ~2% of all TTP cases. This recessively inherited disease is also known as Upshaw–Schulman syndrome [33, 34]. It is caused by biallelic mutations of the *ADAMTS13* gene [35], and numerous mutations have been identified [36], mainly causing quantitative ADAMTS13 defects [37].

The majority of TTP cases are acquired form caused by ADAMTS13 deficiency due to autoantibodies [38]. The autoantibodies can inhibit the proteolytic activity of the enzyme, and increase the formation of circulating ADAMTS13 immune complexes. Several conditions can trigger this autoimmune process (non-idiopathic TTP which comprises ~50% of all TTP), such as viral infections (EBV, CMV, HIV, etc.), bacterial infections, malignancy, certain drugs, other concomitant autoimmune diseases (SLE, antiphospholipid syndrome, Gougerot-Srogren syndrome), pregnancy, drugs (mitomycin C, cyclosporine, quinine, clopidogrel, ticlopidine), pancreatitis, cancers, organ transplantation, etc. [29, 39–41]. However, there are many cases without identifiable associated clinical conditions (idiopathic TTP) [42, 43]. Risk factors of TTP include female gender, black ethnicity, HLA-DRB1∗11, and obesity [39].

Epidemiology

TTP is a rare hematological disorder with an annual prevalence of about 10 per million people and an annual incidence of about 1 new case per million people [44]. Onset is typically in adulthood (~90% of all TTP cases) but about 10% of cases begin in childhood or adolescence [39]. Female is more often affected in adult-onset form.

Clinical Presentations

Historically, clinical pentad of fever, thrombocytopenia, microangiopathic hemolytic anemia, neurological symptoms, and renal insufficiency were used to define TTP. However, more clinical studies demonstrated that these five symptoms were only present in less than 10% of TTP patients [39, 45, 46]. The key clinical symptoms of TTP constantly found in the patients are severe thrombocytopenia, usually less than $30 \times 10^9/L$, and microangiopathic hemolytic anemia, characterized by schistocytes on the peripheral blood smear. Corresponding symptoms and signs associated with consumption of platelets and disturbance of microcirculation such as skin and mucosal hemorrhage, weakness, and dyspnea may develop. Hypoperfusion and anemia can impact organs including brain, heart, and kidneys, causing neurological symptoms, cardiac failure, and renal insufficiency [44]. Other organs that may be involved include lungs, pancreas, stomach, and others [47].

Splenectomy was used to treat TTP prior to the era of effective treatment with plasma exchange, and the need for splenectomy has been greatly diminished. It is only rarely considered in stable patients who are refractory to other therapies including rituximab.

Morphology

Gross or Radiological Findings

The spleen can be normal in size or enlarged. Grossly, the spleen may be unremarkable or show Malpighian corpuscles and occasionally infarct [15].

Microscopic Examination

The main histological finding is micro-thrombi formation in arteries and arterioles without inflammation. A pre-thrombus change, periodic acid-Schiff (PAS)-positive diastase-resistant hyaline subendothelial deposits (SEDs) can be seen in all cases, and some arterioles may show a transition between thrombi and SEDs [15]. In addition, the spleen can show some nonspecific findings, including germinal center hyperplasia, vascular endothelial cell proliferation, periarteriolar concentric fibrosis ("onion-skinning"), prominent iron deposits, and hemophagocytosis in histiocytes. Extramedullary hematopoiesis is present in nearly half of the cases [15, 48].

Immunophenotyping

The presence of platelets or platelet-related material in SEDs and thrombi can be shown by factor VIII immunohistochemical staining. Otherwise, there are no specific immunophenotypic findings. Assays to measure ADAMTS13 activity and ADAMTS13 antibodies can establish the correct diagnosis.

Cytogenetics

N/A

Molecular Findings

Biallelic mutations or compound heterozygous mutations of the *ADAMTS13* gene can be detected in congenital TTP or Upshaw-Schulman syndrome (USS) [35, 49]. Numerous mutations have been documented [36, 50], and it is found that child-onset and adult-onset TTP cases have different sequence variations [50].

Differential Diagnosis

Clinically, the differential diagnosis for TTP is other thrombotic microangiopathies. The main differential diagnosis is hemolytic uremic syndrome (HUS), which is associated with *Escherichia coli* infection or abnormalities of proteins of the alternative complement pathway (atypical HUS) [51]. The histological changes in the spleen are similar among these conditions.

Prognosis

Without treatment, 95% of the TTP patients succumb to the disease, however, with proper treatment, such as therapeutic plasma exchange for acquired TTP and immunosuppression, and replacement of ADAMTS13 by plasma infusion for congenital TTP, the average survival rate from a first episode of TTP is 80–90% [52, 53]. Among these patients, 40% will relapse due to persistence or recurrence of anti-ADAMTS13 antibodies [40, 54].

Diagnostic Caveats

- TTP is a clinical diagnosis.
- Histological findings in the spleen include micro-thrombi formation in arteries and arterioles without inflammation, and hyaline subendothelial deposits.
- Other nonspecific changes include germinal center hyperplasia, periarteriolar concentric fibrosis, prominent iron deposits and hemophagocytosis in histiocytes and extramedullary hematopoiesis.

RBC Membrane Disorders: Congenital Spherocytosis, Elliptocytosis, and Others

Definition

Red blood cell membrane disorders are inherited diseases resulting from mutations in genes encoding various red blood cell membrane or skeletal proteins, including hereditary spherocytosis, hereditary elliptocytosis, hereditary ovalocytosis, and hereditary stomatocytosis. Hereditary spherocytosis (HS) and hereditary elliptocytosis (HE) are the two most common inherited red cell membrane disorders. The disorders cause decreased red cell life span as a result of splenic sequestration of red blood cells. The affected patients manifest as hereditary hemolytic anemia, splenomegaly, and increased free bilirubin levels. Hereditary spherocytosis is characterized by spheroid red blood cells with increased osmotic fragility, hemolytic anemia, and splenomegaly. Hereditary elliptocytosis is characterized by elliptically shaped red blood cells and anemia in some patients. Other red blood cell membrane disorders include hereditary pyropoikilocytosis (HPP), hereditary stomatocytosis, hereditary ovalocytosis, etc.

Etiology/Pathogenesis

Red blood cell membrane has a unique feature of flexibility and mechanical stability, which depends on the membrane structure that is composed of phospholipid bilayer, spectrin-based membrane skeleton, and protein complexes linking the two. Defects in any of the proteins involved in the membrane structure result in loss of structural and functional integrity of the membrane, and lead to red blood cell membrane disorders [55].

There are two critical types of linkages in the membrane structure: vertical linkages between the membrane skeleton and the phospholipid bilayer, and horizontal linkages among components that form the membrane skeleton meshwork. Weakening or loss of vertical linkages leads to membrane vesiculation and surface area loss, and the resultant hereditary spherocytosis. Disruption of horizontal linkages causes decreased red blood cell membrane mechanical stability, and results in hereditary elliptocytosis.

The vertical linkages involve band 3, RhAG, ankyrin, protein 4.2, and spectrin. The most common cause of hereditary spherocytosis is ankyrin deficiency due to ankyrin gene mutation (50–60% of the cases, both autosomal dominant and recessive forms of inheritance) [56], spectrin deficiency due to mutations in either α-spectrin or β-spectrin (20% of the cases) [56], quantitative band 3 deficiency due to band 3 gene mutation (15–20% of the cases) [57, 58], homozygous mutations in protein 4.2 gene (most common cause in Japanese population, recessive inheritance) [59], and Rh-null or markedly reduced RhAG

expression [60]. Less than 1% of the cases are due to Rh deficiency. Etiologies in approximately 10% of the cases are not clear [61].

The horizontal linkages are between spectrin-spectrin dimers, and between spectrin, actin, and protein 4.1R in the junctional complex in the spectrin-based membrane skeleton. Mutations in gene encoding for α-spectrin, β-spectrin, or protein 4.1R can cause autosomal dominant hereditary elliptocytosis. The most common cause of hereditary elliptocytosis is mutations in α-spectrin (65% of the cases), β-spectrin (30% of the cases), and protein 4.1R (5% of the cases) [62].

Hereditary pyropoikilocytosis (HPP) is a subset of hereditary elliptocytosis that is caused by severe disruption of spectrin dimers due to homozygous or compound heterozygous mutations in the α-spectrin gene [62].

Hereditary stomatocytosis is an autosomal dominant disorder characterized by large numbers of stomatocytes on peripheral blood smears in association with anemia [55]. The red blood cell change can be due to marked increase of intracellular sodium, which is caused by the inability of the cells to regulate the cation homeostasis (overhydrated hereditary stomatocytosis). Two mutations in RhAG (Ile61Arg and Ser65Phe) are associated with overhydrated hereditary stomatocytosis [63]. It can also be caused by decreased intracellular potassium and loss of cell water (dyhydrated stomatocytosis). The genetic basis of dehydrated hereditary stomatocytosis is still unclear [64].

Hereditary ovalocytosis is characterized by oval-shaped red blood cells, which are due to decreased membrane deformability. A genomic 27-bp deletion encoding amino acids 400–408 of band 3 has been identified [55].

Epidemiology

Hereditary spherocytosis is the most common inherited red cell membrane disorder, with an estimated prevalence ranging from 1:2000 to 1:5000 [65]. It is reported in all countries, although more often diagnosed in Europe and North America. The inheritance is dominant in 75% of cases [66]. Hereditary elliptocytosis is more common in malaria-endemic regions in West Africa with a prevalence of 2% [55]. Prevalence has been estimated at approximately 1 in 2000 to 1 in 4000 worldwide [67]. Hereditary ovalocytosis is common in Southeast Asia with a prevalence of 2–25% [55]. Hereditary stomatocytosis is very rare, and the estimated incidences for dehydrated type and overhydrated type are 1 in 10,000 and 1 per one million births, respectively [68].

Clinical Presentations

Patients with red blood cell membrane disorders can present with hemolytic anemia. Common complications include jaundice, splenomegaly, and cholelithiasis. Additional complications related to hemolytic anemia may include pigmenturia, vaso-occlusion, thrombosis, etc. Hereditary spherocytosis patients can have these symptoms at any age and with any severity [57, 69, 70]. The clinical presentation of hereditary elliptocytosis and hereditary stomatocytosis is also highly variable, ranging from clinically asymptomatic to severe hemolytic anemia [67, 68].

Splenectomy can be performed in these patients after taking into account the severity of hemolysis, age of the patient, and the complications of the procedure.

Morphology

Gross or Radiological Findings

The spleen is usually moderately to markedly enlarged with red-tan cut surface in congenital spherocytosis with hemolytic anemia patients (Fig. 19.2) [71].

Microscopic Examination

The red blood cells with membrane disorders are vulnerable to trapping by the spleen. There is a secondary hypersplenic state with the stagnation of the red blood cells and macrophage hyperplasia [72]. In hereditary spherocytosis, the described morphologic features of the spleen include massive red pulp congestion with spherocytic red blood cells (the spherocytic nature of the red cells may not be readily apparent on H&E stained slides), pronounced widening of the splenic cords, lack or scarcity of the cells in the cords, hyperplasia of the sinus lining endothelium, presence of erythropoiesis, moderate to marked hemosiderosis, diminished lymphoid follicles, occasional infarcts, etc. [71–73].

Immunophenotyping

N/A

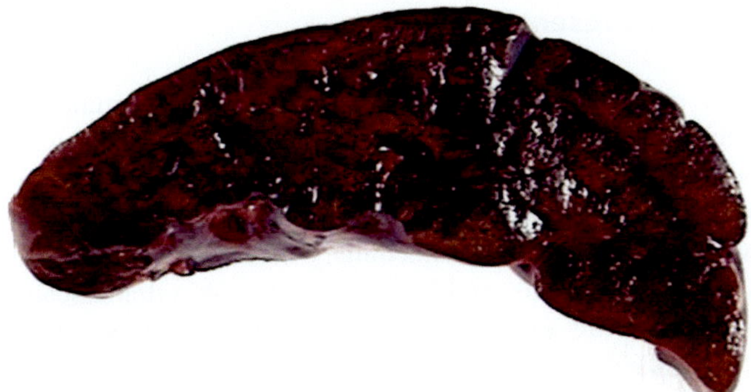

Fig. 19.2 Gross picture of a spleen from a patient with congenital spherocytosis

Cytogenetics

N/A

Molecular Findings

Germline mutations of corresponding genes can be identified in different diseases (see section "Etiology"), although genes involved in a small subset of the cases remain unknown.

Differential Diagnosis

Patients with red blood cell membrane disorders present with variable degrees of anemia and hemolysis that can also be found in red blood cell enzyme disorders including glucose-6-phosphate dehydrogenase (G6PD) deficiency, pyruvate kinase (PK) deficiency, and other metabolic disorders, hemolytic disease of the fetus and newborn (HDFN), autoimmune hemolytic anemia, etc. [74–76]. The diagnosis of each disorder relies on family history, clinical presentation, peripheral blood smear findings, lab tests such as negative Coomb's test to exclude other causes, and other more specialized tests such as acid glycerol lysis time test (AGLT), eosin-5'-maleimide (EMA) binding, or osmotic fragility for hereditary spherocytosis. Blood cell membrane disorders have distinctive morphologies on the blood smear, such as hereditary spherocytosis which is characterized by spherocytosis as the predominant morphology. Typically, at least 15% of the RBCs show the abnormal morphology, although there may be exceptions such as a recent episode of severe hemolysis. It should be noted that hereditary spherocytosis and hereditary stomatocytosis must be distinguished since the two are treated differently (splenectomy helpful in hereditary spherocytosis but should be undertaken with extreme caution in the hereditary stomatocytosis). Analysis of RBC membrane proteins and genetic testing are not required for the clinical diagnosis but may be helpful when there is diagnostic uncertainty, or a need for genetic counseling or prenatal diagnosis.

Prognosis

RBC membrane disorders are benign diseases with variable clinical presentation requiring different clinical treatments. The treatment is directed at preventing or minimizing complications of chronic hemolysis and anemia and there are no specific treatments directed at the underlying red blood cell membrane defect. Splenectomy is curative in almost all patients with the typical form of hereditary spherocytosis. Most symptomatic patients with hereditary elliptocytosis benefit from splenectomy too. In hereditary stomatocytosis, splenectomy can improve but not fully correct the hemolysis, but in some cases, it can be deleterious or even contraindicated [77].

Diagnostic Caveats

- Histology findings in the spleen include red pulp congestion with red blood cells that show characteristic morphologic features (more obvious in peripheral blood smear), and other nonspecific findings related to red cell trapping.

Hemoglobinopathy, Including Sickle Cell Disease

Definition

Hemoglobinopathy is a group of disorders with genetic defect that results in abnormal hemoglobin with defects in the structure of the globin chain. In contrast, reduced or absent synthesis of the hemoglobin chain causes thalassemias.

There are more than one thousand different hemoglobin variants identified (1331 hemoglobin variants registered on Global Gene Server as of 2018 [78, 79]). Common hemoglobinopathies include hemoglobin S (sickle cell disease), C, E, and D. Hemoglobinopathy may cause anemia such as the well-known sickle cell disease. Many hemoglobin variants do not cause anemia or diseases. In contrast to the above qualitative hemoglobinopathies, thalassemias are quantitative hemoglobinopathies, with reduced or absent synthesis of one or more of the globin chains of hemoglobin. The major types of thalassemias are α and β thalassemias.

Etiology/Pathogenesis

The normal hemoglobin molecule is a tetramer consisting of two dimers, which contain an α-like globin (including α and ζ globins) and a β-like globin (including β, γ, δ, and ε globins). The majority of structural hemoglobin variants are due to single amino acid substitution, and the remaining 10% are frameshift, insertion, deletion, nonsense mutations, or fused or hybrid chains [80]. Hemoglobin S (HbS) is the abnormal hemoglobin with the glutamic acid in the sixth position on the β chain replaced by valine (β6 Glu > Val). HbS is responsible for sickle cell trait (HbAS) and sickle cell disease (HbSS). The mutated HbS gene provides protection against the clinical consequences of *Plasmodium*

falciparum infestation, thus is prevalent in the tropical African population.

Thalassemias are autosomal inheritable diseases resulting from decreased production of respective globin chains (α, β, γ, δ) in different thalassemias. Alpha thalassemia is a result of decreased or absent production of α globins due to deletion of α chain gene, and β thalassemia is a result of decreased or absent production of β globins due to mutated β globin chain gene [81, 82].

Epidemiology

Hemoglobin gene variants are present at low prevalence (carriers 1–1.5/1000 people) in all sizeable populations [83]. It is estimated that 7% of the world's population are carriers. Hemoglobinopathies are most common in populations from Africa, the Mediterranean basin, and Southeast Asia. The HbS gene is distributed primarily in populations of native tropical African origin, with an incidence as high as 40% in some African populations. The incidence is 8% in African-Americans. The gene is found with less frequency in peoples of India and Middle East. Rare cases have been reported in Caucasians of Mediterranean descent. One in every 600 African-Americans has sickle cell anemia [84].

Thalassemia is the most common hemoglobinopathy, with the highest prevalence in historically malaria-endemic areas, including sub-Saharan Africa, the Mediterranean, the Asian-Indian subcontinent, and Southeast Asia, affecting approximately 4.4 of every 10,000 live births throughout the world. An estimated 5% of the world's population have at least one thalassemia variant allele [85, 86]. Alpha thalassemia is common among populations of Southeast Asian descent, and there are a high number of carriers in Sub-Saharan Africa and Western Pacific regions. The β thalassemia is particularly prevalent among Mediterranean people [87]. It is most common among populations of Mediterranean, African, and South Asian ancestry.

Clinical Presentations

The clinical manifestation of the hemoglobinopathies is highly variable, ranging from asymptomatic carriers, mild anemia, to severe, transfusion-dependent anemia with multiorgan involvement. In severe forms, the patients can present with severe anemia, extramedullary hematopoiesis, skeletal and growth deficits, and iron overload, with a dramatically shortened life expectancy without appropriate treatment [88]. Take thalassemia as example, the severity of the anemia correlates well with genotype (e.g., β^0 thalassemia), which determines the reduction rate in functional globin chains produced. In α thalassemia, the severity of clinical presentation increases with loss of one, two, three, or four functioning alpha globin alleles. In β thalassemia, the severity of the disease correlates with the amount of normal beta globin production, which is affected by different mutations in β globin gene. Some mutations result in reduced expression (β^+thalassemia) and others result in the complete absence of expression (β^0 thalassemia).

Sickle cell trait is a benign carrier condition, and individuals with sickle cell trait are usually asymptomatic. However, they may be at risk for certain conditions under certain circumstances, such as splenic infarction due to vaso-occlusive phenomena and splenic sequestration described as splenic sequestration crisis [89].

Sickle cell disease can manifest as hemolytic anemia and vaso-occlusion, which can lead to acute and chronic pain and tissue ischemia or infarction. The spleen can be infarcted in early life leading to functional hyposplenism, which in turn increases the risk of infection. Life-threatening complication in which multiple organ systems are affected by ischemia and/or infarction can be typically seen in the setting of an acute painful episode [90].

For patients with sickle cell disease, complete or partial splenectomy may be performed to prevent further spleen sequestration or reduce the recurrence of acute splenic sequestration crisis. Splenectomy may be performed in patients with thalassemia (typically β-thalassemia) who show severe anemia, increased transfusion requirement, growth retardation, cytopenias, splenic infarction, etc.

Morphology

Gross or Radiological Findings

In the first decade of the life of the patients with sickle cell disease, moderate splenomegaly (1.0–2.0 cm below the costal margin) is the classic finding. Hypersplenism may occur and prolonged hypersplenism with excessive destruction of red blood cells can lead to subsequent growth impairment and bone marrow hyperplasia [91]. Surgical splenectomy is the solution to this clinical problem.

Splenic infarctions secondary to vaso-occlusion are common, and repetitive massive infarction leads to progressively smaller spleen (atrophic) and dysfunctional spleen (autosplenectomy) [92–94]. Autosplenectomy occurs in ~6% of the sickle cell disease patients in one study [91].

Microscopic Examination

In those patients with hemoglobinopathy who present with hemolytic anemia (not all individuals with hemoglobin variants have hemolytic anemia), the anemia can be mild or severe, and the hemolysis can be intravascular or extravascu-

lar. The unstable hemoglobin variants can form Heinz bodies, which reduce the RBC's deformity, and cause the RBCs to be trapped in the spleen. Heinz bodies can cause adjacent RBC membrane to be excised in the spleen, forming "bite" or "blister" cells [95]. When the patient is anemic, the involved spleen usually is dysfunctional [96]. In such cases, the spleen is usually enlarged [97, 98].

In sickle cell disease, the spleen is central in three complications: splenic sequestration crisis, vaso-occlusive crisis, and aplastic crisis. A sequestration crisis is a sudden pooling of blood and rapid enlargement of the spleen, followed by hypovolemic shock. Acute splenic sequestration is an early life complication that occurs at the median age at first episode of 1.4 years (0.1–7 years) in a study of 190 cases [99] and rarely occurs after 6 years [100]. Vaso-occlusive crisis occurs due to the plugging of small blood vessels by masses of sickled cells, causing debilitating episodes of abdominal and bone or joint pain. Vaso-occlusive complications have been associated with asplenia. Aplastic crisis occurs when there is a serious fall in hemoglobin concentration due to the temporary failure of red cell production.

Microscopically, the enlarged spleen shows expanded red pulp congested with sickled red blood cells. When the spleen is atrophic, there are hemorrhages and infarctions, and eventually replaced by fibrous tissue. Nodules composed of fibrous tissue and elastic fibers with deposition of iron and calcium salts can be seen [101].

Immunophenotyping

N/A

Cytogenetics

N/A

Molecular Findings

Hemoglobinopathies including sickle cell disease show respective gene mutation (see above).

Differential Diagnosis

Hemoglobinopathies and sickle cell disease are diagnosed clinically based on the patient's clinical presentation, laboratory findings, and genetic testing results. The spleen morphological changes are nonspecific, but usually sickled red blood cells can be seen in the sinusoids of the spleen.

Prognosis

The prognosis is variable ranging from asymptomatic to life-threatening without appropriate clinical treatment.

Diagnostic Caveats

- Hemoglobinopathy is a group of disorders with genetic defect that results in abnormal hemoglobin. Common hemoglobinopathies include hemoglobin S (sickle cell disease), C, E, D, and α and β thalassemias.
- The spleen plays important roles in sickle cell disease pathophysiology such as splenic sequestration crisis, vaso-occlusive crisis, and aplastic crisis.
- In early life of the patients with sickle cell disease, there is usually splenomegaly, and the enlarged spleen shows expanded red pulp congested with sickled red blood cells.
- Later in life of the patients with sickle cell disease, splenic infarctions can occur and lead to splenic atrophy or auto-splenectomy, and eventually replacement by fibrous tissue can be seen.

Autoimmune Hemolytic Anemia

Definition

Autoimmune hemolytic anemia (AIHA) occurs when a patient's immune system produces antibodies against self-antigen on the red blood cells and causes hemolysis resulting in anemia. The red blood cell lifespan is shortened. There are three types of AIHA: warm autoimmune hemolytic anemia (WAIHA), cold agglutinin disease, and paroxysmal cold hemoglobinuria (PCH) [102]. WAIHA is caused by warm autoantibodies binding to RBCs at 37 °C; cold agglutinins in cold agglutinin disease are almost always IgM and cause aggregation of RBCs at cold temperature and occasionally lead to hemolysis; PCH is mediated by Donath-Landsteiner antibody that binds to RBC membranes after cold exposure and activates the complement-mediated intravascular hemolysis when the cells are warmed to 37 °C [102, 103].

Etiology/Pathogenesis

In AIHA, the autoantibodies coat RBCs and lead to their premature destruction or removal. The red cell removal predominantly takes place in the liver and spleen, in which the macrophages recognize and bind to the antibodies. The etiology of AIHA is poorly understood. The disease may be idiopathic (primary AIHA, 50% of cases), or secondary to other conditions, such as lymphoproliferative disorders such as chronic lymphocytic leukemia and other lymphomas, autoimmune disorders such as systemic lupus erythematosus, rheumatoid arthritis, scleroderma, Crohn's disease, and ulcerative colitis, other neoplasms, and infection [104, 105]. Cold agglutinin disease can be caused by lymphoproliferative disorders and infection, especially by mycoplasma, viral pneumonia, infectious mononucleosis, and other respiratory infections. AIHA can also be caused by medication (drug-induced AIHA). The hallmark feature of PCH is the formation of polyclonal IgG autoantibody against the red blood cell P antigen and the exact etiology is unclear [106].

Epidemiology

The incidence of AIHA is approximately 1 in 100,000 in adults and less than 0.2 in 100,000 in children [102]. In teenagers and adults, it is more common in women than in men. The peak incidence is in preschool-age children, and in children, it affects boys more often than girls.

Clinical Presentations

Clinical presentation of primary WAIHA is variable with different degrees of anemia, which is determined by the rate of hemolysis and the body's ability to compensate. The onset of symptoms can be insidious over months, but can occur acutely with rapidly developing anemia. The clinical presentation of cold agglutinin disease is usually stable moderate anemia, and attacks of acrocyanosis precipitated by exposure to cold, which is intraarteriolar agglutination of red blood cells in the tips of fingers, feet, earlobes, and nose. In PCH, patients experience paroxysmal hemoglobinuria after exposure to cold. Constitutional symptoms such as fever and pain follow. Post viral PCH is characterized by constitutional symptoms due to fulminant intravascular hemolysis and associated signs including hematuria [102].

Splenectomy has been advised as the most effective second-line treatment for WAIHA following the use of glucocorticoids. In contrast, splenectomy is not an effective therapy in the majority of patients with cold agglutinin disease. Splenectomy is not indicated in PCH.

Morphology

Gross or Radiological Findings

Splenomegaly is present in many AIHA cases [107, 108]. The weight of the spleen varies from 100 to 1000 grams [109].

Microscopic Examination

Splenic cord congestion and extramedullary hematopoiesis are the main histopathological findings in the spleen of the patients with autoimmune hemolytic anemia [107]. Besides mild to marked congestion, erythrophagocytosis, neutrophil infiltrate, increased deposition of hemosiderin can be seen [108]. Localized reactive follicular hyperplasia maybe present [110]. In cases of AIHA with lymphoproliferative disorder, the primary disease can be present in the spleen [111]. The spleen infarction is observed in rare cases [112].

Immunophenotyping

N/A

Cytogenetics

N/A

Molecular Findings

N/A

Differential Diagnosis

AIHA is a clinical diagnosis based on clinical presentation and laboratory findings. The autoantibodies can be confirmed by direct antiglobulin test (DAT) and indirect antiglobulin test (IAT). If intravascular hemolysis is present, schistocytes, microspherocytes, and elliptocytes are observed in the peripheral blood smear.

Prognosis

AIHA may develop gradually, or have a fulminant onset with life-threatening anemia [113].

Diagnostic Caveats

- AIHA is a clinical diagnosis.
- In the spleen, cord congestion and extramedullary hematopoiesis are the main histopathological findings.
- The other findings include erythrophagocytosis, neutrophil infiltrate, increased deposition of hemosiderin, and localized reactive follicular hyperplasia. Infarction is observed in rare cases.

References

1. Stasi R, et al. Long-term outcome of otherwise healthy individuals with incidentally discovered borderline thrombocytopenia. PLoS Med. 2006;3(3):e24.
2. Cines DB, et al. The ITP syndrome: pathogenic and clinical diversity. Blood. 2009;113(26):6511–21.
3. Rodeghiero F, et al. Treatment practices in adults with chronic immune thrombocytopenia – a European perspective. Eur J Haematol. 2010;84(2):160–8.
4. Audia S, et al. Pathogenesis of immune thrombocytopenia. Autoimmun Rev. 2017;16(6):620–32.
5. He R, et al. Spectrum of Ig classes, specificities, and titers of serum antiglycoproteins in chronic idiopathic thrombocytopenic purpura. Blood. 1994;83(4):1024–32.
6. van Leeuwen EF, et al. Specificity of autoantibodies in autoimmune thrombocytopenia. Blood. 1982;59(1):23–6.
7. McMillan R. Autoantibodies and autoantigens in chronic immune thrombocytopenic purpura. Semin Hematol. 2000;37(3):239–48.
8. Coopamah MD, et al. Cellular immune mechanisms in autoimmune thrombocytopenic purpura: an update. Transfus Med Rev. 2003;17(1):69–80.
9. Bettaieb A, et al. Cross-reactive antibodies between HIV-gp120 and platelet gpIIIa (CD61) in HIV-related immune thrombocytopenic purpura. Clin Exp Immunol. 1996;103(1):19–23.
10. Zhang W, et al. Role of molecular mimicry of hepatitis C virus protein with platelet GPIIIa in hepatitis C-related immunologic thrombocytopenia. Blood. 2009;113(17):4086–93.
11. Michel M. Immune thrombocytopenic purpura: epidemiology and implications for patients. Eur J Haematol Suppl. 2009;71:3–7.
12. Burrows RF, Kelton JG. Fetal thrombocytopenia and its relation to maternal thrombocytopenia. N Engl J Med. 1993;329(20):1463–6.
13. Cines DB, Bussel JB. How I treat idiopathic thrombocytopenic purpura (ITP). Blood. 2005;106(7):2244–51.
14. Diagnosis and treatment of idiopathic thrombocytopenic purpura: recommendations of the American Society of Hematology. The American Society of Hematology ITP practice guideline panel. Ann Intern Med. 1997;126(4):319–26.
15. Saracco SM, Farhi DC. Splenic pathology in thrombotic thrombocytopenic purpura. Am J Surg Pathol. 1990;14(3):223–9.
16. Tavassoli M, McMillan R. Structure of the spleen in idiopathic thrombocytopenic purpura. Am J Clin Pathol. 1975;64(2):180–91.
17. Hayes MM, et al. Splenic pathology in immune thrombocytopenia. J Clin Pathol. 1985;38(9):985–8.
18. Berendt HL, Mant MJ, Jewell LD. Periarterial fibrosis in the spleen in idiopathic thrombocytopenic purpura. Arch Pathol Lab Med. 1986;110(12):1152–4.
19. Hassan NM, Neiman RS. The pathology of the spleen in steroid-treated immune thrombocytopenic purpura. Am J Clin Pathol. 1985;84(4):433–8.
20. Lafon ME, Bioulac-Sage P, Balabaud C. Hepatic fibrosis in patients with idiopathic thrombocytopenic purpura. Liver. 1988;8(1):24–7.
21. Foucar K, Reichard K, Czuchlewski D. Bone marrow pathology, vol. 1. 3rd ed. Chicago: American Society for Clinical Pathology; 2010.
22. Houwerzijl EJ, et al. Ultrastructural study shows morphologic features of apoptosis and para-apoptosis in megakaryocytes from patients with idiopathic thrombocytopenic purpura. Blood. 2004;103(2):500–6.
23. Houwerzijl EJ, et al. Megakaryocytic dysfunction in myelodysplastic syndromes and idiopathic thrombocytopenic purpura is in part due to different forms of cell death. Leukemia. 2006;20(11):1937–42.
24. Castro V, et al. The human platelet alloantigen 5 polymorphism as a risk for the development of acute idiopathic thrombocytopenia purpura. Thromb Haemost. 2000;84(2):360–1.

25. Jiang DY, Li CY. Immunohistochemical study of the spleen in chronic immune thrombocytopenic purpura. With special reference to hyperplastic follicles and foamy macrophages. Arch Pathol Lab Med. 1995;119(6):533–7.

26. Stasi R, et al. Long-term observation of 208 adults with chronic idiopathic thrombocytopenic purpura. Am J Med. 1995;98(5):436–42.

27. Bourgeois E, et al. Long-term follow-up of chronic autoimmune thrombocytopenic purpura refractory to splenectomy: a prospective analysis. Br J Haematol. 2003;120(6):1079–88.

28. Portielje JE, et al. Morbidity and mortality in adults with idiopathic thrombocytopenic purpura. Blood. 2001;97(9):2549–54.

29. Knobl P. Thrombotic thrombocytopenic purpura. Memo. 2018;11(3):220–6.

30. Chapman K, Seldon M, Richards R. Thrombotic microangiopathies, thrombotic thrombocytopenic purpura, and ADAMTS-13. Semin Thromb Hemost. 2012;38(1):47–54.

31. Moake JL. Thrombotic microangiopathies. N Engl J Med. 2002;347(8):589–600.

32. Moake JL. von Willebrand factor, ADAMTS-13, and thrombotic thrombocytopenic purpura. Semin Hematol. 2004;41(1):4–14.

33. Schulman I, et al. Studies on thrombopoiesis. I. A factor in normal human plasma required for platelet production; chronic thrombocytopenia due to its deficiency. Blood. 1960;16:943–57.

34. Upshaw JD Jr. Congenital deficiency of a factor in normal plasma that reverses microangiopathic hemolysis and thrombocytopenia. N Engl J Med. 1978;298(24):1350–2.

35. Levy GG, et al. Mutations in a member of the ADAMTS gene family cause thrombotic thrombocytopenic purpura. Nature. 2001;413(6855):488–94.

36. Lotta LA, et al. ADAMTS13 mutations and polymorphisms in congenital thrombotic thrombocytopenic purpura. Hum Mutat. 2010;31(1):11–9.

37. Hanby HA, Zheng XL. Current status in diagnosis and treatment of hereditary thrombotic thrombocytopenic purpura. Hereditary Genet. 2014;3(1):e108.

38. Joly BS, et al. Child-onset and adolescent-onset acquired thrombotic thrombocytopenic purpura with severe ADAMTS13 deficiency: a cohort study of the French national registry for thrombotic microangiopathy. Lancet Haematol. 2016;3(11):e537–46.

39. Joly BS, Coppo P, Veyradier A. Thrombotic thrombocytopenic purpura. Blood. 2017;129(21):2836–46.

40. Kremer Hovinga JA, et al. Survival and relapse in patients with thrombotic thrombocytopenic purpura. Blood. 2010;115(8):1500–11; quiz 1662.

41. Deford CC, et al. Multiple major morbidities and increased mortality during long-term follow-up after recovery from thrombotic thrombocytopenic purpura. Blood. 2013;122(12):2023–9; quiz 2142.

42. Jang MJ, et al. Clinical features of severe acquired ADAMTS13 deficiency in thrombotic thrombocytopenic purpura: the Korean TTP registry experience. Int J Hematol. 2011;93(2):163–9.

43. Blombery P, et al. Diagnosis and management of thrombotic thrombocytopenic purpura (TTP) in Australia: findings from the first 5 years of the Australian TTP/thrombotic microangiopathy registry. Intern Med J. 2016;46(1):71–9.

44. Mariotte E, et al. Epidemiology and pathophysiology of adulthood-onset thrombotic microangiopathy with severe ADAMTS13 deficiency (thrombotic thrombocytopenic purpura): a cross-sectional analysis of the French national registry for thrombotic microangiopathy. Lancet Haematol. 2016;3(5):e237–45.

45. Scully M, et al. Regional UK TTP registry: correlation with laboratory ADAMTS 13 analysis and clinical features. Br J Haematol. 2008;142(5):819–26.

46. Fujimura Y, Matsumoto M. Registry of 919 patients with thrombotic microangiopathies across Japan: database of Nara Medical University during 1998–2008. Intern Med. 2010;49(1):7–15.

47. Knobl P. Inherited and acquired thrombotic thrombocytopenic purpura (TTP) in adults. Semin Thromb Hemost. 2014;40(4):493–502.

48. Kass L, Schnitzer B. Extramedullary haematopoiesis in thrombotic thrombocytopenic purpura. Folia Haematol Int Mag Klin Morphol Blutforsch. 1979;106(1):32–6.

49. Hassenpflug WA, et al. Genetic and functional characterization of ADAMTS13 variants in a patient cohort with Upshaw-Schulman syndrome investigated in Germany. Thromb Haemost. 2018;118(4):709–22.

50. Joly BS, et al. ADAMTS13 gene mutations influence ADAMTS13 conformation and disease age-onset in the French cohort of Upshaw-Schulman syndrome. Thromb Haemost. 2018;118(11):1902–17.

51. Noris M, Remuzzi G. Atypical hemolytic-uremic syndrome. N Engl J Med. 2009;361(17):1676–87.

52. Zheng XL, et al. Effect of plasma exchange on plasma ADAMTS13 metalloprotease activity, inhibitor level, and clinical outcome in patients with idiopathic and nonidiopathic thrombotic thrombocytopenic purpura. Blood. 2004;103(11):4043–9.

53. Vesely SK, et al. ADAMTS13 activity in thrombotic thrombocytopenic purpura-hemolytic uremic syndrome: relation to presenting features and clinical outcomes in a prospective cohort of 142 patients. Blood. 2003;102(1):60–8.

54. Ferrari S, et al. Prognostic value of anti-ADAMTS 13 antibody features (Ig isotype, titer, and inhibitory effect) in a cohort of 35 adult French patients undergoing a first episode of thrombotic microangiopathy with undetectable ADAMTS 13 activity. Blood. 2007;109(7):2815–22.

55. Mohandas N, Gallagher PG. Red cell membrane: past, present, and future. Blood. 2008;112(10):3939–48.

56. Eber S, Lux SE. Hereditary spherocytosis--defects in proteins that connect the membrane skeleton to the lipid bilayer. Semin Hematol. 2004;41(2):118–41.

57. Perrotta S, Gallagher PG, Mohandas N. Hereditary spherocytosis. Lancet. 2008;372(9647):1411–26.

58. Jarolim P, et al. Characterization of 13 novel band 3 gene defects in hereditary spherocytosis with band 3 deficiency. Blood. 1996;88(11):4366–74.

59. Yawata Y, et al. Characteristic features of the genotype and phenotype of hereditary spherocytosis in the Japanese population. Int J Hematol. 2000;71(2):118–35.

60. Ballas SK, et al. Red cell membrane and cation deficiency in Rh null syndrome. Blood. 1984;63(5):1046–55.

61. Narla J, Mohandas N. Red cell membrane disorders. Int J Lab Hematol. 2017;39(Suppl 1):47–52.

62. Gallagher PG. Hereditary elliptocytosis: spectrin and protein 4.1R. Semin Hematol. 2004;41(2):142–64.

63. Bruce LJ, et al. The monovalent cation leak in overhydrated stomatocytic red blood cells results from amino acid substitutions in the Rh-associated glycoprotein. Blood. 2009;113(6):1350–7.

64. Bruce LJ. Hereditary stomatocytosis and cation-leaky red cells--recent developments. Blood Cells Mol Dis. 2009;42(3):216–22.

65. Barcellini W, et al. Hereditary red cell membrane defects: diagnostic and clinical aspects. Blood Transfus. 2011;9(3):274–7.

66. Da Costa L, et al. Hereditary spherocytosis, elliptocytosis, and other red cell membrane disorders. Blood Rev. 2013;27(4):167–78.

67. Gallagher PG. Red cell membrane disorders. Hematology Am Soc Hematol Educ Program. 2005;2005:13–8.

68. King MJ, et al. ICSH guidelines for the laboratory diagnosis of nonimmune hereditary red cell membrane disorders. Int J Lab Hematol. 2015;37(3):304–25.

69. Eber SW, Armbrust R, Schroter W. Variable clinical severity of hereditary spherocytosis: relation to erythrocytic spectrin concentration, osmotic fragility, and autohemolysis. J Pediatr. 1990;117(3):409–16.

70. Friedman EW, Williams JC, Van Hook L. Hereditary spherocytosis in the elderly. Am J Med. 1988;84(3 Pt 1):513–6.

71. Wiland OK, Smith EB. The morphology of the spleen in congenital hemolytic anemia (hereditary spherocytosis). Am J Clin Pathol. 1956;26(6):619–29.

72. Molnar Z, Rappaport H. Fine structure of the red pulp of the spleen in hereditary spherocytosis. Blood. 1972;39(1):81–98.

73. Shneidman D, et al. Red pulp of the spleen in hereditary elliptocytosis. Virchows Arch A Pathol Anat Histol. 1977;372(4):337–42.

74. Mentzer WC. Hereditary spherocytosis. [cited 2018 November 8th]. Available from: https://www.uptodate.com/contents/hereditary-spherocytosis?search=hereditary%20spherocytosis&source=search_result&selectedTitle=1~89&usage_type=default&display_rank=1#H15480873.

75. Mentzer WC. Hereditary elliptocytosis and related disorders. [cited 2018 November 8th]. Available from: https://www.uptodate.com/contents/hereditary-elliptocytosis-and-related-disorders?topicRef=7079&source=see_link.

76. Brugnara C. Stomatocytosis and xerocytosis. [cited 2018 November 8th]. Available from: https://www.uptodate.com/contents/stomatocytosis-and-xerocytosis?sectionName=HSt%20AND%20HX&topicRef=7079&anchor=H1905393114&source=see_link#H1905393114.

77. Gallagher PG, Jarolim P. Red blood cell membrane disorders. In: Hoffman R, et al., editors. Hematology: basic principles and practice. Philadelphia: Elsevier; 2008. p. 623–43.

78. Patrinos GP, et al. Improvements in the HbVar database of human hemoglobin variants and thalassemia mutations for population and sequence variation studies. Nucleic Acids Res. 2004;32(Database issue):D537–41.

79. Huisman THJ, MFH C, Efremov GD. A syllabus of human hemoglobin variants. 2nd ed. Augusta: The Sickle Cell Anemia Foundation; 1998.

80. Elghetany MT, Banki K. Erythrocytic disorders. In: McPherson R, Pincus MR, editors. Henry's clinical diagnosis and management by laboratory methods. Philadelphia: Saunders Elsevier; 2007. p. 504–44.

81. Taher AT, Weatherall DJ, Cappellini MD. Thalassaemia. Lancet. 2018;391(10116):155–67.

82. Higgs DR, Engel JD, Stamatoyannopoulos G. Thalassaemia. Lancet. 2012;379(9813):373–83.

83. Modell B, et al. Epidemiology of haemoglobin disorders in Europe: an overview. Scand J Clin Lab Invest. 2007;67(1):39–69.

84. Steinberg MH. Management of sickle cell disease. N Engl J Med. 1999;340(13):1021–30.

85. Martin A, Thompson AA. Thalassemias. Pediatr Clin North Am. 2013;60(6):1383–91.

86. Weatherall DJ. The definition and epidemiology of non-transfusion-dependent thalassemia. Blood Rev. 2012;26(Suppl 1):S3–6.

87. Galanello R, Origa R. Beta-thalassemia. Orphanet J Rare Dis. 2010;5:11.

88. Forget BG. Thalassemia syndromes. In: Hoffman R, et al., editors. Hematology: basic principles and practice. New York: Churchill Livingstone; 2000. p. 485.

89. Vichinsky EP. Sickle cell trait. [cited 2018 December 14]. Available from: https://www.uptodate.com/contents/sickle-cell-trait?search=sickle%20cell%20traits&source=search_result&selectedTitle=1~109&usage_type=default&display_rank=1.

90. Vichinsky EP. Overview of the clinical manifestations of sickle cell disease. [cited 2018 December 14]. Available from: https://www.uptodate.com/contents/overview-of-the-clinical-manifestations-of-sickle-cell-disease?search=sickle%20cell%20disease&source=search_result&selectedTitle=2~150&usage_type=default&display_rank=2.

91. Brousse V, Buffet P, Rees D. The spleen and sickle cell disease: the sick(led) spleen. Br J Haematol. 2014;166(2):165–76.

92. Al-Salem AH. Splenic complications of sickle cell anemia and the role of splenectomy. ISRN Hematol. 2011;2011:864257.

93. Pearson HA, Spencer RP, Cornelius EA. Functional asplenia in sickle-cell anemia. N Engl J Med. 1969;281(17):923–6.

94. William BM, et al. Hyposplenism: a comprehensive review. Part II: clinical manifestations, diagnosis, and management. Hematology. 2007;12(2):89–98.

95. Greenberg MS. Heinz body hemolytic animea. "Bite cells" -a clue to diagnosis. Arch Intern Med. 1976;136(2):153–5.

96. Grover R, Wethers DL. Spleen dysfunction in hemoglobinopathies determined by pitted red cells. Am J Pediatr Hematol Oncol. 1988;10(4):340–3.

97. Karpathios T, et al. Spleen size changes in children with homozygous beta-thalassaemia in relation to blood transfusion. Scand J Haematol. 1982;28(3):220–6.

98. Tassiopoulos T, et al. Spleen size in beta-thalassaemia heterozygotes. Haematologia (Budap). 1995;26(4):205–9.

99. Airede AI. Acute splenic sequestration in a five-week-old infant with sickle cell disease. J Pediatr. 1992;120(1):160.

100. Emond AM, et al. Acute splenic sequestration in homozygous sickle cell disease: natural history and management. J Pediatr. 1985;107(2):201–6.

101. Khatib R, Rabah R, Sarnaik SA. The spleen in the sickling disorders: an update. Pediatr Radiol. 2009;39(1):17–22.

102. Powers A, Silberstein LE. Autoimmune hemolytic anemia. In: Hoffman R, et al., editors. Hematology basic principles and practice. Philadelphia: Churchill Livingstone Elsevier; 2008.

103. Dacie JV. Autoimmune hemolytic anemia. Arch Intern Med. 1975;135(10):1293–300.

104. Hill A, Hill QA. Autoimmune hemolytic anemia. Hematology Am Soc Hematol Educ Program. 2018;2018(1):382–9.

105. Schreiber AD. Autoimmune hemolytic anemia. Pediatr Clin North Am. 1980;27(2):253–67.

106. Shanbhag S, Spivak J. Paroxysmal cold hemoglobinuria. Hematol Oncol Clin North Am. 2015;29(3):473–8.

107. Anguiano-Alvarez VM, et al. Splenic myeloid metaplasia in warm autoimmune hemolytic anemia (wAIHA): a retrospective study. Blood Res. 2018;53(1):35–40.

108. Chang CS, et al. Clinical features and splenic pathologic changes in patients with autoimmune hemolytic anemia and congenital hemolytic anemia. Mayo Clin Proc. 1993;68(8):757–62.

109. Mansouri J. Hemolytic anemia. 2018 [cited 2018 Dec 20th]. Available from: http://www.pathologyoutlines.com/topic/spleen-hemolyticanemia.html.

110. Burke JS, Osborne BM. Localized reactive lymphoid hyperplasia of the spleen simulating malignant lymphoma. A report of seven cases. Am J Surg Pathol. 1983;7(4):373–80.

111. Breitfeld V, Lee RE. Pathology of the spleen in hematologic disease. Surg Clin North Am. 1975;55(2):233–51.

112. Park MY, et al. Splenic infarction in a patient with autoimmune hemolytic anemia and protein C deficiency. Korean J Hematol. 2011;46(4):274–8.

113. Zanella A, Barcellini W. Treatment of autoimmune hemolytic anemias. Haematologica. 2014;99(10):1547–54.

Benign Hematologic Disorders Involving the Liver and Spleen

Haipeng Shao and Deniz Peker

Ectopic or Accessory Spleen

Definition

Ectopic spleen refers to splenic tissue located at ectopic sites. Ectopic spleen (ES) can be found in two forms: accessory spleen (AS) and splenosis. The Accessory spleen is a congenital anomaly and arises from the left side of dorsal mesogastrium, while splenosis is an acquired condition and occurs as a result of intraabdominal autoimplantation [1].

Etiology

Accessory spleen often occurs as a failure of fusion of the primordial splenic buds in the dorsal mesogastrium during embryologic development [2, 3]. Autoimplantation during splenectomy or after a physical trauma causes foci of splenic tissue displaced in the abdomen or, if the diaphragm is not intact, the thorax and results in splenosis [4, 5].

Epidemiology

Accessory spleen is a relatively rare condition and found in estimated 10–30% of the population [6]. Splenosis, on the other hand, has been reported in up to 70% of patients with a history of splenic trauma and is often found in men [7].

H. Shao (✉)
Department of Pathology, H. Lee Moffitt Cancer Center and
Research Institute, Tampa, FL, USA
e-mail: Haipeng.shao@moffitt.org

D. Peker
Department of Pathology and Laboratory Medicine, Emory
University, Atlanta, GA, USA
e-mail: Deniz.peker@emory.edu

However, these lesions are often incidental findings during surgery or imaging and the actual incidence is unknown.

Clinical Presentation

Accessory spleen is usually single but can rarely be more than one in a single patient. The most common location for AS is the splenic hilum followed by the pancreatic tail but can be found in other body sites including greater omentum, stomach, intestine, and pelvic cavity. Splenosis can be found in any part of the abdominal cavity and also thoracic cavity if the diaphragm is not intact.

Accessory spleen and splenosis are usually asymptomatic and detected incidentally. The imaging using ultrasonography (USG), contrast-enhanced USG, computed tomography, magnetic resonance imaging, and scintigraphy can help to accurately diagnose ES [8].

Morphology and Immunophenotyping

Accessory spleen is often situated in splenic hilum or adjacent to the pancreatic tail (Fig. 20.1). AS is usually up to 1.0 cm in diameter and, both macroscopically and on radiologic imaging, resembles a lymph node with round to oval appearance [9]. AS displays features of normal spleen with well-formed capsule and hilum and receives blood supply from the branch of splenic artery [7].

Splenic implants in splenosis can be solid gray or multiple and are usually small in size (<3.0 cm), as they do not have proper blood supply [10]. On macroscopy and imaging, the nodules can be round, oval or multinodular and often have irregular architecture with a poorly formed capsule and no hilum [7].

On microscopic examination, both AS and splenic implants may exhibit red and white pulp similar to normal splenic parenchyma (Fig. 20.2) as well as normal CD8-positivity in sinusoids.

© Springer Nature Switzerland AG 2020

L. Zhang et al. (eds.), *Diagnostic Pathology of Hematopoietic Disorders of Spleen and Liver*,
https://doi.org/10.1007/978-3-030-37708-3_20

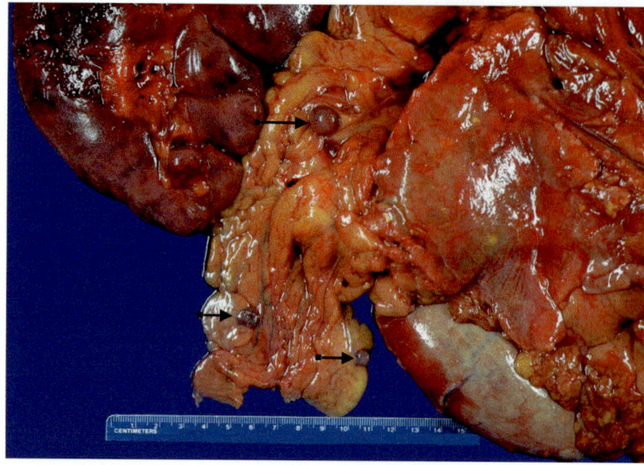

Fig. 20.1 Gross image of accessory spleens in the pancreatic fat and splenic hilum (arrows) all measuring less than 1.0 cm. (Photo credit to Drs. Ona Faye-Peterson and Dr. Oraine Snaith at the University of Alabama at Birmingham)

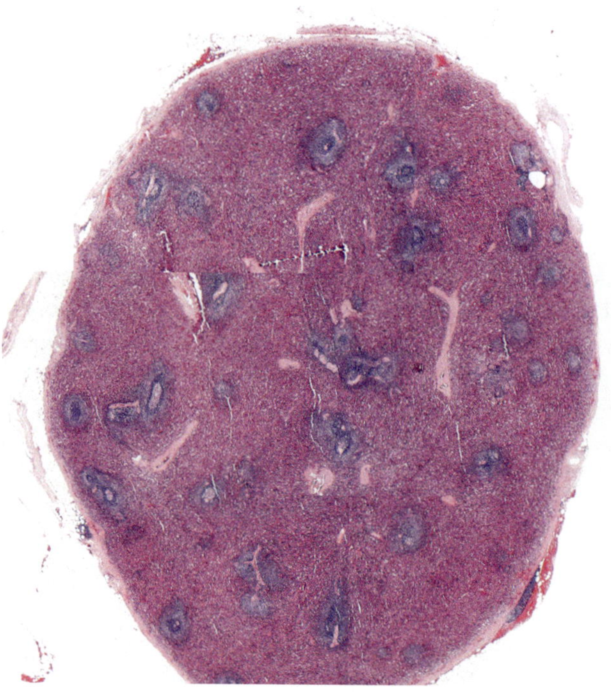

Fig. 20.2 Microscopic image of an accessory spleen with unremarkable white and red pulps surrounded by an intact capsule

Prognosis and Differential Diagnosis

Ectopic spleen is usually not a life-threatening condition. However, they can pose a clinical challenge in various medical conditions. Identification and removal of ectopic splenic tissue is important in patients with refractory hypersplenism, i.e., immune thrombocytopenia [11].

ES may mimic malignant tumors or metastatic lymph nodes in patients with malignancy. Therefore, it is crucial to recognize this anomaly using imaging or during surgical procedures. ES usually does not require surgical resection, however due to the high vascularization of splenic parenchyma, traumatic or spontaneous laceration and rupture of ectopic splenic tissue it can result in bleeding. Recognition and management of ES is important due to the clinical significance of this ectopic organ.

Benign Extramedullary Hematopoiesis

Definition

Blood cells play a fundamental role in oxygen transportation, cellular and humoral immunity, and hemostasis and coagulation. Therefore, appropriate production and proliferation of the hematopoietic cells is crucial. Hematopoiesis takes place in the bone marrow in adult life. In intrauterine life, extramedullary organs including the yolk sac, liver, and spleen home hematopoiesis.

Extramedullary hematopoiesis (EMH) is defined by the production of hematopoietic cells outside of the bone marrow. EMH can involve any body site, including the spleen, liver, lymph nodes, skin, bone, heart, and other visceral organs [12].

Etiology

EMH can be divided into two categories (1) active EMH and (2) passive EMH [13]. Active EMH can be seen in intrauterine development as a part of normal hematopoiesis in the yolk sac, liver, and spleen. It also includes EMH that occurs in the liver and spleen, i.e., as a response to immune activation following infections. The passive EMH often occurs as a result of bone marrow failure [13]. Rarely, EMH can develop spontaneously without clinical symptoms or diagnostic implications [14, 15]. The most common hematologic causes of EMH are summarized in Table 20.1.

Table 20.1. Causes of extramedullary hematopoiesis (EMH)

Physiological EMH
Fetal development
Pathological EMH
Infections
Immune responses
Hemolytic anemia (i.e., thalassemia)
Myeloproliferative neoplasms (MPN)
Chronic myelogenous leukemia
Primary myelofibrosis
Other end (fibrotic)-stage MPNs
Radiation-induced marrow fibrosis
Idiopathic marrow fibrosis

The spleen is a common site of EMH in the postnatal stage in spite of its microenvironment that is inhospitable for hematopoietic stem cells (HSC) [15]. Recent data suggest that splenic EMH occurs in red pulp and the expression of CXCL12 in splenic sinus endothelial cells may facilitate the homing of HSC within the splenic parenchyma forming bone-marrow niche-like regions [16]. EMH in the spleen is a common finding in patients with myeloproliferative neoplasms (MPN) including chronic myelogenous leukemia and ongoing hemolysis, i.e., thalassemia. EMH in the spleen in the context of MPN is associated with abnormal clonal proliferation of hematopoietic stem cells. It has been shown that splenomegaly due to EMH in MPN with *JAK2V617F* mutation is a clonal process and the hematopoietic cells proliferating in the spleen are derived from the clonal progenitor in the bone marrow [17, 18].

Additionally, EMH is a characteristic finding in hepatoblastoma and the molecular mechanism of this association is unknown [19]. Epithelial hepatoblastoma cells can express cytokines and hormones, including erythropoietin, stem cell factor, and IL-1β, which can stimulate stromal cell production of other hematopoietic cytokines including IL-6, G-CSF, GM-CSF, M-CSF, and leukemia inhibitory factor resulting in EMH in these cases [20].

Epidemiology

Extramedullary hematopoiesis is a compensatory phenomenon and has been reported in approximately 15% of patients with thalassemia as well as myelofibrosis and other anemic conditions [21, 22].

Clinical Presentations

Extramedullary hematopoiesis can occur in any organ and body site such as the liver, spleen, other abdominal organs, lymph nodes, endocrine glands, thymus, kidneys, gastrointestinal tract, and paraspinal regions [21]. Splenomegaly is the most common presentation of EMH.

Hepatic EMH is often seen in benign and malignant hematologic diseases along with splenomegaly. Isolated intrahepatic EMH is extremely rare and reported only in sporadic cases [23]. It can present as a single nodule or multiple nodules and create diagnostic challenge.

Morphology and Immunophenotyping

The imaging studies and tissue biopsy are crucial to diagnose this entity in the liver to avoid a misdiagnosis of primary or metastatic tumor. The imaging studies with CT often reveal a fat containing lesion or multiple lesions.

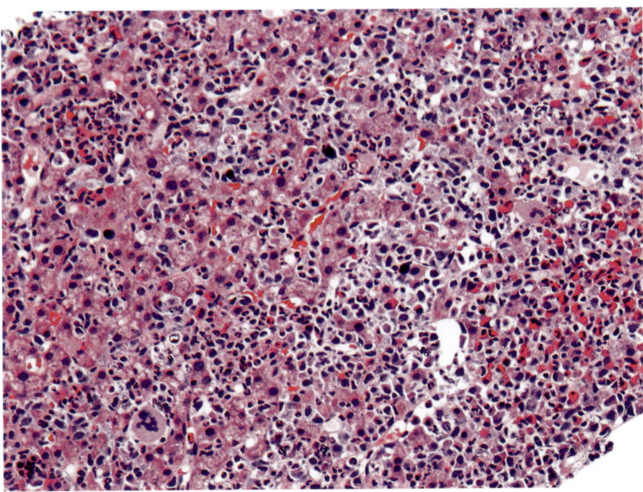

Fig. 20.3 Microscopic image of extramedullary hematopoiesis in the liver. All three hematopoietic cell lines including megakaryocytic, myeloid, and erythroid cells are easily identifiable

Microscopically, the involved parenchyma shows infiltration of hematopoietic precursors including megakaryocytes, nucleated erythroid precursors, and myeloid cells in various maturation stages (Fig. 20.3).

EMH is a common finding in hepatoblastoma, particularly in ones with epithelial morphology.

In most cases, immunophenotyping is not necessary as the process can easily be recognized on hematoxylin and eosin-stained sections. The megakaryocytic cells can be highlighted by stains including CD41 and CD61; MPO and CD117 can be used to determine the myeloid components; and CD71, hemoglobin A, and spectrin are often used for erythroid cells.

Cytogenetics and Molecular Findings

There are no cytogenetic abnormalities directly linked to EMH; however, cytogenetic/molecular abnormalities can be detected due to the underlying disease, i.e., *Philadelphia chromosome* in CML and *JAK2* or *Calreticulin* mutations in primary myelofibrosis.

Differential Diagnosis

EMH is a manifestation of hematologic and non-hematologic diseases and can present only in splenomegaly form depending on the underlying disease, i.e., CML or hemolytic anemia. The differential diagnosis includes other causes of splenomegaly including infections such as infectious mononucleosis, hypersplenism, involvement of the spleen by other malignant diseases such as classic Hodgkin's lymphoma or chronic lymphocytic leukemia, autoimmune disorders, metabolic diseases (i.e., Gaucher's disease), and congenital diseases (i.e., G6PD deficiency).

When in single or multiple-nodular pattern, EMH should be accurately differentiated from benign and malignant diseases using imaging studies and preferably by biopsy. EMH should be considered in the differential diagnosis along with other lipomatous proliferations including lipoma, angiolipoma, adenoma, liposarcoma, hepatocellular carcinoma with fatty component, and malignant teratoma containing adipose tissue [24, 25].

Prognosis

EMH is often a benign proliferation of hematopoietic cells outside of the bone marrow stroma due to various underlying conditions and the prognosis depends on the causative disease.

Diagnostic Caveats

Myelolipoma and EMH are both benign processes with sometimes indistinguishable imaging and histomorphologic features creating a diagnostic pitfall [26]. Myelolipoma is almost always associated with normal bone marrow without an underlying hematopoietic disorder, while passive EMH is commonly a manifestation of a hematologic disorder or malignancy.

Splenic Reactive Lymphoid Hyperplasia

Definition

Reactive lymphoid hyperplasia is the benign and reversible enlargement of the lymph node due to hyperplasia of lymphoid follicles in response to antigen stimulus.

Etiology

Reactive follicular hyperplasia is commonly seen in the splenic white pulp in response to a variety of stimuli. There are many etiologic factors including bacteria, virus, fungi, environmental agents and chemicals, a variety of medicines such as phenytoin, quinidine, etc., autoimmune disorders, and inflammation. In most cases, the specific etiology factor for lymphoid hyperplasia in the spleen cannot be identified.

Clinical Presentations

The spleen may be normal in size or variably enlarged depending on the extent and level of lymphoid hyperplasia. There are no specific symptoms associated with reactive lymphoid hyperplasia.

Morphology and Differential Diagnosis

Follicular hyperplasia is the most common type of reactive lymphoid hyperplasia in the spleen. In follicular hyperplasia, the germinal centers are hyperplastic with scattered tingible body macrophages and show polarization with dark and light zones. The dark zones are composed predominantly of centroblasts with high proliferation rate, and the light zones are composed mostly of centrocytes with lower proliferation. The mantle zones of the hyperplastic follicles also show polarization and sharply delineated from the germinal centers. The reactive hyperplastic follicles are positive for B-cell markers (CD20, CD79a, PAX5), CD10, and BCL6, and negative for BCL2. IgD highlights the mantle zones. Ki-67 shows a very high proliferation rate of the follicles and helps the identification of polarization of the germinal centers. The main differential diagnosis is follicular lymphoma. In contrast to the well-separated follicles of follicular hyperplasia, the follicular lymphoma shows densely packed follicles. The atypical lymphoid follicles of follicular lymphoma are ill-defined, monotonous with mixture of centrocytes and centroblasts, and lack polarization. The germinal centers of these atypical follicles are usually positive for BCL2. The absence of polarization by Ki-67 immunostain can help the diagnosis of difficult cases of follicular lymphoma, especially the BCL2-negative cases.

An unusual lymphoid hyperplasia, "localized reactive lymphoid hyperplasia of the spleen", is rarely seen and closely mimics malignant lymphoma grossly [27]. Macroscopically, localized reactive lymphoid hyperplasia manifests as isolated and solitary nodules in the spleen. Histologically, it shows two patterns. In one pattern, the nodules are formed by local aggregation of reactive hyperplastic germinal centers. In the other pattern, the nodules show localized proliferation of lymphocytes, including immunoblasts and plasma cells. The etiology is unknown.

The marginal zone is typically present in the lymphoid follicles of the spleen. Splenic marginal zone hyperplasia shows thickening of the marginal zones around reactive germinal centers. It may be associated with autoimmune disorders, such as systemic lupus erythematosus and autoimmune thrombocytopenic purpura. Grossly, the spleen may show more prominent white pulp miliary nodules. The main differential diagnosis is splenic marginal zone lymphoma. In contrast to splenic marginal zone lymphoma, splenic marginal zone hyperplasia shows no infiltrate of B cells into the red pulp and the marginal zone B cells are negative for IgD. In difficult cases, flow cytometry and PCR for B-cell gene rearrangement can be used to confirm the diagnosis.

Infectious Mononucleosis

Definition

Infectious mononucleosis, also called mono or "kissing disease", is an infectious disease caused by Epstein-Barr virus (EBV) characterized clinically by fever, fatigue, pharyngitis, and lymphadenopathy (also refer to other chapters).

Etiology

The etiology agent is Epstein-Barr virus (EBV). Most people are exposed to EBV during childhood. The EBV is primarily transmitted through saliva by kissing, but also by coughing, sneezing or sharing drinks or utensils. The EBV first replicates in the nasopharynx and infects B lymphocytes. After primary infection, EBV remains in the body for life and primarily in B lymphocytes.

Epidemiology

EBV infection is ubiquitous with over 90% of adults seropositive for EBV. Infectious mononucleosis occurs at all ages, but most commonly in adolescents and young adults between 15 and 25 years old [28].

Clinical Presentation

In young children, the primary EBV infection is usually asymptomatic. The typical symptoms of infectious mononucleosis occur in adolescents and young adults. Most patients present with a characteristic triad of fever, pharyngitis, and lymphadenopathy. The fever usually lasts 2 weeks with temperature of around 39.5 °C. The pharyngitis is usually severe in the first 5 days and gradually resolves in 1–2 weeks. The pharyngitis can be painful and exudative and mimic strep throat. The swollen adenopathy typically involves posterior cervical lymph nodes. Fatigue is common and usually most severe in the first couple of weeks. Splenomegaly is present in approximately 50% of patients with infectious mononucleosis, and is maximal in the second and third weeks. The spleen may occasionally rupture with physical activity or spontan-

ously. The splenic rupture is accompanied by sudden sharp pain in the left upper abdomen.

Morphology and Immunophenotyping

Spleen is usually not biopsied in patients with infectious mononucleosis, and splenic biopsy is not required for the diagnosis of infectious mononucleosis. The histology of infectious mononucleosis in the spleen is revealed in the splenectomy specimen after splenic rupture [29]. The spleen shows red pulp expansion by variably activated immunoblasts. The infiltrate is polymorphous and shows large numbers of cytotoxic T cells. The immunoblasts include both B-immunoblasts and T-immunoblasts, and scattered large lymphocytes with both T- and B-cell markers. Some of the immunoblasts may resemble Reed-Sternberg cells. In situ hybridization for EBER shows numerous EBV-positive cells. Clonal T-cell gene rearrangement can be seen in the majority of cases.

Differential Diagnosis

The main differential diagnosis of infectious mononucleosis is large-cell lymphoma. In patients suspected for infectious mononucleosis, biopsy of lymphoid tissue including spleen is usually avoided by clinicians due to the risk of misdiagnosis of malignant lymphoma. The diagnosis of infectious mononucleosis can be made by typical clinical features and positive heterophile antibody test (monospot test). In patients with atypical presentation, biopsy of lymphoid tissue, such as tonsil or lymph node, may be performed. In contrast to malignant lymphoma, infectious mononucleosis does not efface underlying lymphoid architecture. A positive monospot test will help the diagnosis of infectious mononucleosis.

Prognosis

Infectious mononucleosis is usually self-limiting and requires only supportive care. It is important to avoid splenic rupture by limiting physical activity, especially contact sports for at least the first month of the disease.

Autoimmune Lymphoproliferative Syndrome

Definition

Autoimmune lymphoproliferative syndrome (ALPS) is a rare genetic disorder characterized by dysregulation of immune system to regulate lymphocyte homeostasis through apoptosis, which results in proliferation of lymphocytes in lymphoid tissues, including lymph nodes, spleen, and liver.

Etiology

ALPS is caused by inherited or acquired mutations of the *FAS* gene, or rarely *FASLG* gene or caspase 10 [30]. *FAS* mutation results in defective FAS/FAS ligand-induced apoptosis of lymphocytes, with subsequent expansion of lymphocytes. The self-antigen-specific lymphocytes are normally removed from the body through FAS-induced apoptosis. In ALPS, the expansion of such lymphocytes leads to autoimmunity.

Epidemiology

The incidence and prevalence of ALPS is unknown, due to variable expression of the disease, and many patients are misdiagnosed or undiagnosed. There are approximately 500 patients in more than 300 families with hereditary ALPS worldwide. There is a male predominance in affected patients with a male to female ratio of 1.6–2.2 [31, 32].

Clinical Presentation

The clinical manifestation of ALPS typically occurs during the first couple years of life, with a median age of 2.7–3 years. Clinically, ALPS is characterized by chronic lymphadenopathy, splenomegaly, and hepatomegaly often in an asymptomatic child that are incidentally found during routine physical examination. Patients with ALPS can have chronic autoimmune cytopenia, including hemolytic anemia and thrombocytopenia, more severe in early childhood. The patients may show symptoms of cytopenia, such as fatigue, pallor, icterus, bruising, and mucocutaneous bleeding.

Morphology and Immunophenotyping

In ALPS, the spleen is markedly enlarged. The white pulps are moderately expanded and show follicular hyperplasia with some expansion of the marginal zones. The red pulps are greatly expanded and infiltrated by lymphocytes in varying stages of immunoblastic transformation mixed with small mature lymphocytes and numerous polyclonal plasma cells. The lymphocytes are medium-sized to large in size with round to oval nuclei and moderate amounts of clear to pale eosinophilic cytoplasm. There are frequent mitotic figures.

The lymphocytes are positive for CD3, and double negative for CD4 and CD8. They are positive for CD43, CD57, TIA01, perforin, and CD45RA, and negative for CD25, CD45RO, CD16, or CD56. The T cells show a high proliferation rate by Ki-67 immunostain. PCR studies show no clonal B- or T-cell gene rearrangements.

The histology of ALPS in the liver is less well studied. The liver may show mild periportal fibrosis and extramedullary hematopoiesis, or chronic active hepatitis. There is mild lymphocytic infiltrate by mostly CD3[+] T cells, with more than 50% CD4/CD8 double-negative T cells [33].

Differential Diagnosis

The main differential diagnosis by histology is peripheral T-cell lymphoma, NOS. The increased immunoblasts, high proliferation rate, and predominance of double CD4/CD8-negative T cells may simulate a peripheral T-cell lymphoma. However, the largely uneffaced architecture with the presence of white pulp germinal centers, negative clonal T-cell gene rearrangement by PCR study, and typical clinical presentation of ALPS should point to the right diagnosis.

Prognosis

The prognosis of ALPS is good, with only few patients died of postsplenectomy sepsis and progressive malignancy. There is an increased risk of development of Hodgkin and non-Hodgkin lymphomas later in life. While many patients respond to conventional short-term immunosuppression, some require chronic long-term immunosuppression for cytopenias and other end-organ damage.

Epstein-Barr Virus-Associated Inflammatory Pseudotumor of the Spleen

Definition

Epstein-Barr virus-associated inflammatory pseudotumor of the spleen is a mass lesion of the spleen composed of EBV-positive spindle cells and numerous polymorphous inflammatory cells.

Etiology

The etiology of EBV-associated inflammatory pseudotumor of the spleen is unknown. EBV infection is postulated to play an important role in the pathogenesis.

Epidemiology

The EBV-associated inflammatory pseudotumor of the spleen is very rare, accounting for <1% of primary splenic tumors [34]. It occurs in adults with age ranging from 24 to 87 years (median: 66 years).

Clinical Presentation

The most common symptom is left upper abdominal or epigastric pain. Some patients show systemic symptoms including fatigue, fever, and weight loss. Approximately half of the patients are asymptomatic with lesion identified incidentally during imaging study for other indications.

Morphology and Immunophenotyping

Grossly, the EBV-associated inflammatory pseudotumor of the spleen presents as a solitary well-circumscribed tan or yellow mass. Areas of necrosis, hemorrhage, or fibrosis can be seen. Microscopically, the EBV-associated inflammatory pseudotumor of the spleen shows loose aggregates or scattered spindle cells in a mixed background of inflammatory cells including abundant small mature lymphocytes, plasma cells, and histiocytes. The spindle cells have oval to spindle nuclei, thin nuclear membrane, vesicular chromatin, small nucleoli, and moderate amount of pale or weakly eosinophilic cytoplasm. Fascicles and storiform spindle cell proliferation are uncommon. Multinucleated giant cells and granuloma composed of epithelioid histiocytes are common. Eosinophils and neutrophils can be seen focally in some cases. The spindle cells are positive for vimentin, SMA and/or CD68, and EBV by EBV-encoded small RNA (EBER) in situ hybridization (ISH). The lymphocytes are negative for EBV by EBER. The plasma cells are polyclonal for kappa and lambda light chains.

The expression of vimentin, SMA, and/or CD68 suggests fibroblastic, myofibroblastic, or histiocytic differentiation. Some of the cases with identical morphology show expression of follicular dendritic cell (FDC) markers including CD21, CD23, CD35, and clusterin. Such cases are diagnosed of EBV-associated inflammatory pseudotumor-like follicular dendritic cell tumors [35, 36].

Differential Diagnosis

The differential diagnosis of the EBV-associated inflammatory pseudotumor of the spleen includes a variety of reactive disorders and lymphomas. Inflammatory and infectious conditions include mycobacterial spindle cell pseudotumor and granulomatous inflammation. Mycobacterial spindle cell pseudotumor rarely occurs in immunocompromised patients with AIDS or post solid organ transplant. The spindle cells are histiocytes with expression of CD68, and filled with acid fast bacilli by AFB stain, and are negative for EBV.

The main differential diagnosis is an inflammatory myofibroblastic tumor (IMT), which shows similar histologic features. However, approximately half of the cases of IMT are positive for ALK, and IMT is consistently negative for EBV. Interdigitating dendritic cell sarcoma and conventional follicular dendritic cell (FDC) sarcoma are characterized by the proliferation of spindle cells. In contrast to EBV-associated inflammatory pseudotumor of the spleen, both interdigitating dendritic cell sarcoma and conventional FDC sarcoma show more abundant spindle cells with only minor component of inflammatory cells, and are always negative for EBV.

Classical Hodgkin lymphoma (CHL) can be included in the differential diagnosis in rare cases of EBV-associated inflammatory pseudotumor of the spleen with Reed-Sternberg-like cells and CD30$^+$ immunoblasts. The Reed-Sternberg cells in CHL are positive for CD30, PAX5 (weak), MUM1, and CD15 (in most cases). CHL can be positive for EBV, but the EBV-positive cells are large Reed-Sternberg cells, and in EBV-associated inflammatory pseudotumor of the spleen, the EBV-positive cells are spindle cells.

Prognosis

EBV-associated inflammatory pseudotumor of the spleen is benign and patients have an excellent prognosis. In contrast to conventional FDC sarcoma with aggressive clinical course, inflammatory pseudotumor-like follicular dendritic cell tumor is considered a low-grade malignant lesion and has the potential for metastasis [37, 38]. The inflammatory pseudotumor-like follicular dendritic cell tumor and EBV-associated inflammatory pseudotumor of the spleen are most likely of same entity with different phenotypes.

Castleman Disease

Definition

Castleman disease (CD) is a rare heterogeneous group of lymphoproliferative disorders involving lymph nodes and can present with variable clinical symptoms and findings. The first classification of CD is based on the number of lymph node regions involved and includes unicentric CD (UCD) and multicentric CD (MCD). UCD involves a single lymph node region and often presents without systemic symptoms, whereas MCD involves more than one lymph node regions and frequently accompanied by systemic symptoms [39].

MCD is subclassified based on human herpesvirus 8 (HHV8) status. MCD that is not associated with HHV8 is further divided into idiopathic MCD (iMCD) and POEMS (polyneuropathy, organomegaly, endocrinopathy, monoclonal gammopathy, and skin changes)-associated MCD [40].

Etiology

The etiology of UCD is unknown. Although the clonal neoplastic transformation of stromal cells such as follicular dendritic cells is thought to be an underlying process, this has not been fully confirmed [41]. MCD is strongly associated with Kaposi sarcoma-associated virus (KHSV), particularly in immunocompromised patients [42] and less than half of the patients are HHV8-negative and not immunocompromised; this group has been recently classified as idiopathic MCD (iMCD) [43].

Epidemiology

Castleman disease is a rare disease with an estimated 7000 new cases diagnosed each year in the United States. Approximately 25% of these cases are MCD while the rest is of UCD type [44]. The disease can affect individuals of all ages. HHV8-positive MCD affects men more often than women and is more frequent in HIV-infected individuals [45]. HHV8-negative MCD is also slightly more prevalent in men. There are no known risk factors playing a role in the etiology of UCD or HHV8-negative MCD.

Clinical Presentation

UCD is often an asymptomatic disease and may present with localized lymphadenopathy. Systemic symptoms in UCD are uncommon. The most common site of CD is lymph nodes and extranodal disease in the spleen and liver is extremely rare. Splenic CD is reported only in a few cases in the literature and all four cases were UCD type with hyaline-vascular morphology [46–49] except for one case in which both the spleen and the accessory spleen were involved as a part of systemic disease in a HHV8-positive MCD case [50].

HHV8-positive MCD involves multiple lymph nodes with frequent systemic manifestations including fever, night sweats, weight loss, loss of appetite, fatigue, shortness of breath, nausea, vomiting, neuropathy, extremity edema, skin rashes, and Kaposi sarcoma.

Many patients with HHV8-negative iMCD presents with a unique clinicopathologic picture characterized by thrombocytopenia, ascites (anasarca), myelofibrosis, renal dysfunction, and organomegaly (TAFRO syndrome) also known as Castleman-Kojima disease [51].

HHV8-negative MCD can be a manifestation of POEMS and hepatosplenomegaly is also common in this group of patients.

Morphology and Immunophenotyping

Histopathologically, CD is classified as hyaline vascular (HV) and plasma cell (PC) variants. PC variants can display HV features [52]. HV variants are characterized by altered nodal architecture by the increased number of follicles with regressed or atrophic germinal centers, hyalinized blood vessels penetrating in the follicles, and hypervascularization of the intrafollicular space, whereas in the PC variant there are hyperplastic germinal centers with infiltration of plasma cells in a sheet-like pattern [53].

Splenic involvement is rare and is often in HV morphology. Castleman disease in the liver is also very rare and reported only in nine cases thus far. Similar to the spleen, the involvement of the liver by CD often presents in UCD form as a single well-defined mass in the liver with hyaline-vascular type histomorphology [54–62]. The most common symptom is abdominal pain, though most of cases are asymptomatic. Common imaging finding is hypervascular lesion with or without calcification. Pathologic examination of the lesion is required as other benign and malignant entities are ought to be ruled out.

Diagnosis of CD is often based on clinical findings and histomorphologic features on routine hemotoxylin and eosin-stained sections. HHV8 IHC stain is necessary to determine the infection by the virus. The immunoglobulin light-chain expression by plasma cells is often polyclonal with a normal kappa:lambda ratio.

Differential Diagnosis

Histomorphologic features may mimic autoimmune diseases, HIV-associated lymphadenopathy, immunosuppression, and Hodgkin and non-Hodgkin lymphoma.

Prognosis

UCD often has an indolent course and surgery alone is considered curative. MCD patients may have more prominent clinical picture and complicated clinical course requiring intensive therapy. HHV8-positive MCD is often treated with rituximab and anti-HIV drugs when HIV-infected [63]. For HIV-negative patients, antiviral treatments for HHV8 are available [63]. Siltuximab, a monoclonal antibody binds to IL-6, is the only drug approved by the US Food and Drug Administration (FDA) for HHV8-negative MCD [64]. Also used are cytotoxic chemotherapies.

Kikuchi-Fujimoto Disease

Definition

Kikuchi-Fujimoto disease (KFD) is a benign disease characterized by histiocytic necrotizing lymphadenitis. It was first described in Japan by Japanese pathologists Kikuchi and Fujimoto.

Etiology

The etiology for KFD remains unknown. Several infectious agents including Epstein-Barr virus (EBV), cytomegalovirus (CMV), herpes simplex virus (HSV) type 1 and 2, varicella-zoster virus, human papillomavirus, parvovirus B19, hepatitis B virus, human herpesvirus [6–8], human T-lymphotropic virus 1, Brucella, Yersinia and Toxoplasma show no definitive evidence to link these agents to KFD [65]. The autoimmune hypothesis was also suggested by some authors.

Epidemiology

Kikuchi-Fujimoto disease affects both men and women near equally. Most patients are younger than 40 years of age, but can be seen at any age and most frequently seen in Asia [65].

Clinical Presentation

KFD clinically presents as cervical lymphadenopathy, fever, and leukopenia that tend to spontaneously resolve in a few months without treatment needed [66]. Cervical lymph nodes are most commonly involved followed by axillary and supraclavicular lymph nodes [65]. Additional symptoms including weight loss, nausea, vomiting, night sweats, and organomegaly can also be seen but not commonly.

Morphology and Immunophenotyping

The diagnosis can only be established by pathologic examination of the lymph node biopsy which shows areas of necrosis in cortex and paracortex, karyorrhectic nuclear debris mixed with rimming histiocytes and typically an absence of polymorphonuclear leukocytes [67]. In the majority of cases, KFD has a benign disease course with rare events of generalized lymphadenopathy and multisystemic involvement including hepatosplenomegaly leading to fatal outcomes [68–72]. KFD involvement in hepatic parenchyma can be associated with autoimmune diseases including autoimmune hepatitis [73] and often creates a diagnostic challenge as it

can mimic malignant process when presents with multiple liver lesions [74].

Histomorphologic evaluation on hemotoxylin and eosin-stained sections are often sufficient to render a diagnosis of KFD. CD68 and CD123 can be used to highlight numerous histiocytes and plasmacytoid dendritic cells, respectively, rimming the necrosis [75]. The CD68-positive histiocytes frequently express myeloperoxidase (MPO) [76].

Differential Diagnosis

Kikuchi-Fujimoto disease resembles several other benign and malignant diseases clinically and morphologically. In the spleen and liver, malignant neoplasms including Hodgkin and non-Hodgkin lymphoma should be ruled out. Also, other infectious diseases, i.e., EBV, HSV, and CMV infections, Cat-scratch disease, and mycobacterial and fungal infections should be excluded.

Prognosis

The disease is often self-limiting and prognosis is excellent.

IGG4-Related Disease

Definition

IgG4-related disease (IgG4-RD), formerly known as IgG4-related systemic disease, is a benign inflammatory entity that is characterized by increased serum IgG4 concentrations and tissue involvement by IgG4-secreting plasma cells and lymphocytes. IgG4 disease can involve a variety of organs, including the liver, pancreas, bile duct, lacrimal glands, salivary gland, thyroid, lung, and kidney and various inflammatory diseases including autoimmune pancreatitis, hypophysitis, Riedel thyroiditis, interstitial pneumonitis, interstitial nephritis, prostatitis, lymphadenitis, retroperitoneal fibrosis, inflammatory aortic aneurism, and inflammatory pseudotumor can be part of this entity [77].

Etiology

IgG4 overproduction causing elevated serum IgG4 levels and tissue infiltration by IgG4+ plasma cells are the main events in IgG4-RD [77]. Immune, autoimmune, and infectious etiologies have been studied as etiologic factors. Increased IgG4 production as a result of T_h2-regulated cytokine production has been reported [78]. Infectious agents including *Helicobacter pylori*, Gram-negative bacteria, and

Mycobacterium tuberculosis have been linked to IgG4-RD [77]. Additionally, antibodies such as carbonic anhydrase have been also reported in IgG4-RD [79].

Epidemiology

Due to heterogeneous clinical and histomorphologic features, the true prevalence of IgG4-RD is unknown. The estimated incidence in Japan is approximately 1/100,000 individuals with 336–1300 new patients per year [77]. The disease affects people in their middle to old age with a median age of 58 years [77]. IgG4-RD affects both men and women with a slight male predominance and more commonly seen in whites than other ethnicities [80].

Clinical Presentation

IgG4-RD often presents with multicentric masses in the involved system that can mimic malignant processes [81]. The most commonly involved organs include submandibular gland, lymph nodes, orbit, pancreas, retroperitoneum, lung, and parotid gland [82]. It is an incidental finding in approximately 30% of patients.

Morphology and Immunophenotyping

The diagnosis of IgG4-RD is rendered based on tissue biopsy and histomorphologic features, which include profound storiform fibrosis, obliterative phlebitis, and lymphoplasmacytic infiltrate in addition to elevated IgG4$^+$ cells and IgG4:IgG ratio greater than 40% supported by immunohistochemistry [83].

IgG4-RD commonly involves hepatobiliary system organs and the majority of the cases show bile duct lesions [82] and a portion of these patients has involvement of the intrahepatic bile ducts resulting in cholangitis [84, 85]. Histomorphologically, hepatic involvement is characterized by portal tract expansion by mixed inflammatory infiltrates containing lymphocytes, plasma cells, and eosinophils often without fibrosis [86]. A detailed morphologic and immunophenotypic evaluation is warranted as this entity can mimic several other benign autoimmune and cancerous lesions. Ghazale et al. described a diagnostic algorithm for IgG4-associated cholangitis [72] parallel to HISORt (histology, imaging, serology, other organ involvement and response to therapy) criteria [74] (Table 20.2). In this algorithm, >10 IgG4-positive plasma cells are often sufficient for diagnosis as in most cases bile duct biopsy samples are limited in size and do not provide adequate tissue for a definitive diagnosis [72].

Table 20.2 Diagnostic criteria for IgG4-associated cholangitis, HISORt criteria

Feature	Characteristic findings
Bile duct histology	Lymphoplasmacytic infiltrate with >10 IgG4 plasma cells within or around bile ducts Storiform fibrosis Obliterative phlebitis
Imaging	One or more strictures involving intrahepatic, proximal extrahepatic, or intrapancreatic bile ducts Fleeting/migrating biliary strictures
Serology	Increased serum IgG4 levels
Other organ involvement	Autoimmune pancreatitis Retroperitoneal fibrosis Renal lesions Salivary/lacrimal gland enlargement
Response to steroid therapy	Normalization of liver enzymes Resolution of structures

Modified from Refs. [72, 74]

Splenic involvement by IgG4-RD is extremely rare. A recent case report has described a splenic sclerosing angiomatoid nodular transformation with increased IgG4$^+$ cells [87].

CD38, CD138, and dimCD19-positive plasma cells expressing IgG4 are the hallmark of IgG4-RD. The presence of >50 IgG4$^+$ plasma cells per high-power field on immunostaining is highly specific for a diagnosis of IgG4-RD, whereas various organ-specific thresholds have been suggested. However, IgG4$^+$ plasma cell infiltration can be seen in profound inflammation. Therefore, a ratio of IgG4$^+$ plasma cells to IgG$^+$ plasma cells >40% has been determined as a cutoff value [83].

Differential Diagnosis

The clinical and morphological findings in IgG4-RD involving the liver are nonspecific and the differential diagnosis includes primary sclerosing cholangitis (PSC), Castleman disease, and infectious processes, i.e., hepatitis virus C. Also, vasculitic disease should be kept in mind when evaluating biopsy material.

Features that might be helpful to differentiate IgG4-RD from PSC include older age at onset (>50 years), increased serum IgG4 levels, pancreatic involvement, multiorgan involvement, absence of inflammatory bowel disease, and good response to steroid treatment [88].

Prognosis

Prognosis is often good in hepatic disease with response to steroid treatment.

References

1. Fremont RD, Rice TW. Splenosis: a review. South Med J. 2007;100:589–93.
2. Halpert B, Eaton WL. Lesions in accessory spleens. AMA Arch Pathol. 1954;57:501–4.
3. Kawamoto S, Johnson PT, Hall H, Cameron JL, Hruban RH, Fishman EK. Intrapancreatic accessory spleen: CT appearance and differential diagnosis. Abdom Imaging. 2012;37:812–27.
4. Abu Hilal M, Harb A, Zeidan B, Steadman B, Primrose JN, Pearce NW. Hepatic splenosis mimicking HCC in a patient with hepatitis C liver cirrhosis and mildly raised alpha feto protein; the important role of explorative laparoscopy. World J Surg Oncol. 2009; 7:1.
5. Madjar S, Weissberg D. Thoracic splenosis. Thorax. 1994;49: 1020–2.
6. Bajwa SA, Kasi A. Spleen, accessory. Treasure Island: StatPearls; 2018.
7. Tandon YK, Coppa CP, Purysko AS. Splenosis: a great mimicker of neoplastic disease. Abdom Radiol. 2018;43:3054.
8. Dodds WJ, Taylor AJ, Erickson SJ, Stewart ET, Lawson TL. Radiologic imaging of splenic anomalies. AJR Am J Roentgenol. 1990;155:805–10.
9. Gayer G, Zissin R, Apter S, Atar E, Portnoy O, Itzchak Y. CT findings in congenital anomalies of the spleen. Br J Radiol. 2001;74:767–72.
10. Imbriaco M, Camera L, Manciuria A, Salvatore M. A case of multiple intra-abdominal splenosis with computed tomography and magnetic resonance imaging correlative findings. World J Gastroenterol. 2008;14:1453–5.
11. Stanek A, Stefaniak T, Makarewicz W, Kaska L, Podgorczyk H, Hellman A, Lachinski A. Accessory spleens: preoperative diagnostics limitations and operational strategy in laparoscopic approach to splenectomy in idiopathic thrombocytopenic purpura patients. Langenbeck's Arch Surg. 2005;390:47–51.
12. Sohawon D, Lau KK, Lau T, Bowden DK. Extra-medullary haematopoiesis: a pictorial review of its typical and atypical locations. J Med Imaging Radiat Oncol. 2012;56:538–44.
13. Kim CH. Homeostatic and pathogenic extramedullary hematopoiesis. J Blood Med. 2010;1:13–9.
14. Macki M, Bydon M, Papademetriou K, Gokaslan Z, Bydon A. Presacral extramedullary hematopoiesis: an alternative hypothesis. J Clin Neurosci. 2013;20:1664–8.
15. Johns JL, Christopher MM. Extramedullary hematopoiesis: a new look at the underlying stem cell niche, theories of development, and occurrence in animals. Vet Pathol. 2012;49:508–23.
16. Miwa Y, Hayashi T, Suzuki S, Abe S, Onishi I, Kirimura S, Kitagawa M, Kurata M. Up-regulated expression of CXCL12 in human spleens with extramedullary haematopoiesis. Pathology. 2013;45:408–16.
17. O'Malley DP, Orazi A, Wang M, Cheng L. Analysis of loss of heterozygosity and X chromosome inactivation in spleens with myeloproliferative disorders and acute myeloid leukemia. Mod Pathol. 2005;18:1562–8.
18. Konoplev S, Hsieh PP, Chang CC, Medeiros LJ, Lin P. Janus kinase 2 V617F mutation is detectable in spleen of patients with chronic myeloproliferative diseases suggesting a malignant nature of splenic extramedullary hematopoiesis. Hum Pathol. 2007;38:1760–3.
19. Thambi R, Devi L, Balachandran K, Poothiode U. Extramedullary hematopoiesis as a 'clue' to diagnosis of hepatoblastoma on fine needle aspiration cytology: a report of two cases. J Cytol. 2013;30:198–200.
20. von Schweinitz D, Schmidt D, Fuchs J, Welte K, Pietsch T. Extramedullary hematopoiesis and intratumoral production of cytokines in childhood hepatoblastoma. Pediatr Res. 1995;38: 555–63.
21. Zhang HZ, Li Y, Liu X, Chen BR, Yao GH, Peng YN. Extramedullary hematopoiesis: a report of two cases. Exp Ther Med. 2016;12:3859–62.
22. Papavasiliou C. Clinical expressions of the expansion of the bone marrow in the chronic anemias: the role of radiotherapy. Int J Radiat Oncol Biol Phys. 1994;28:605–12.
23. Gupta P, Naran A, Auh YH, Chung JS. Focal intrahepatic extramedullary hematopoiesis presenting as fatty lesions. AJR Am J Roentgenol. 2004;182:1031–2.
24. Roberts JL, Fishman EK, Hartman DS, Sanders R, Goodman Z, Siegelman SS. Lipomatous tumors of the liver: evaluation with CT and US. Radiology. 1986;158:613–7.
25. Murakami T, Nakamura H, Hori S, Nakanishi K, Mitani T, Kozuka T, Kimura Y, Monden M, Wakasa K, Sakurai M. Angiomyolipoma of the liver. Ultrasound, CT, MR imaging and angiography. Acta Radiol. 1993;34:392–4.
26. Littrell LA, Carter JM, Broski SM, Wenger DE. Extra-adrenal myelolipoma and extramedullary hematopoiesis: imaging features of two similar benign fat-containing presacral masses that may mimic liposarcoma. Eur J Radiol. 2017;93:185–94.
27. Burke JS, Osborne BM. Localized reactive lymphoid hyperplasia of the spleen simulating malignant lymphoma. A report of seven cases. Am J Surg Pathol. 1983;7:373–80.
28. Straus SE, Cohen JI, Tosato G, Meier J. NIH conference. Epstein-Barr virus infections: biology, pathogenesis, and management. Ann Intern Med. 1993;118:45–58.
29. Siliezar MM, Munoz CC, Solano-Iturri JD, Ortega-Comunian L, Mollejo M, Montes-Moreno S, Piris MA. Spontaneously ruptured spleen samples in patients with infectious mononucleosis: analysis of histology and lymphoid subpopulations. Am J Clin Pathol. 2018;150:310–7.
30. Rieux-Laucat F, Magerus-Chatinet A, Neven B. The autoimmune lymphoproliferative syndrome with defective FAS or FAS-ligand functions. J Clin Immunol. 2018;38:558–68.
31. Price S, Shaw PA, Seitz A, Joshi G, Davis J, Niemela JE, Perkins K, Hornung RL, Folio L, Rosenberg PS, Puck JM, Hsu AP, Lo B, Pittaluga S, Jaffe ES, Fleisher TA, Rao VK, Lenardo MJ. Natural history of autoimmune lymphoproliferative syndrome associated with FAS gene mutations. Blood. 2014;123:1989–99.
32. Neven B, Magerus-Chatinet A, Florkin B, Gobert D, Lambotte O, De Somer L, Lanzarotti N, Stolzenberg MC, Bader-Meunier B, Aladjidi N, Chantrain C, Bertrand Y, Jeziorski E, Leverger G, Michel G, Suarez F, Oksenhendler E, Hermine O, Blanche S, Picard C, Fischer A, Rieux-Laucat F. A survey of 90 patients with autoimmune lymphoproliferative syndrome related to TNFRSF6 mutation. Blood. 2011;118:4798–807.
33. Lim MS, Straus SE, Dale JK, Fleisher TA, Stetler-Stevenson M, Strober W, Sneller MC, Puck JM, Lenardo MJ, Elenitoba-Johnson KS, et al. Pathological findings in human autoimmune lymphoproliferative syndrome. Am J Pathol. 1998;153:1541–50.
34. Neuhauser TS, Derringer GA, Thompson LD, Fanburg-Smith JC, Aguilera NS, Andriko J, Chu WS, Abbondanzo SL. Splenic inflammatory myofibroblastic tumor (inflammatory pseudotumor): a clinicopathologic and immunophenotypic study of 12 cases. Arch Pathol Lab Med. 2001;125:379–85.
35. Cheuk W, Chan JK, Shek TW, Chang JH, Tsou MH, Yuen NW, Ng WF, Chan AC, Prat J. Inflammatory pseudotumor-like follicular dendritic cell tumor: a distinctive low-grade malignant intra-abdominal neoplasm with consistent Epstein-Barr virus association. Am J Surg Pathol. 2001;25:721–31.
36. Horiguchi H, Matsui-Horiguchi M, Sakata H, Ichinose M, Yamamoto T, Fujiwara M, Ohse H. Inflammatory pseudotumor-like follicular dendritic cell tumor of the spleen. Pathol Int. 2004;54:124–31.
37. Li XQ, Cheuk W, Lam PW, Wang Z, Loong F, Yeong ML, Browett P, McCall J, Chan JK. Inflammatory pseudotumor-like

follicular dendritic cell tumor of liver and spleen: granulomatous and eosinophil-rich variants mimicking inflammatory or infective lesions. Am J Surg Pathol. 2014;38:646–53.

38. Chen Y, Shi H, Li H, Zhen T, Han A. Clinicopathological features of inflammatory pseudotumour-like follicular dendritic cell tumour of the abdomen. Histopathology. 2016;68:858–65.

39. Fajgenbaum DC, Shilling D. Castleman disease pathogenesis. Hematol Oncol Clin North Am. 2018;32:11–21.

40. Nagy A, Bhaduri A, Shahmarvand N, Shahryari J, Zehnder JL, Warnke RA, Mughal T, Ali S, Ohgami RS. Next-generation sequencing of idiopathic multicentric and unicentric Castleman disease and follicular dendritic cell sarcomas. Blood Adv. 2018;2:481–91.

41. Chang KC, Wang YC, Hung LY, Huang WT, Tsou JH, M Jones D, Song HL, Yeh YM, Kao LY, Medeiros LJ. Monoclonality and cytogenetic abnormalities in hyaline vascular Castleman disease. Mod Pathol. 2014;27:823–31.

42. Fajgenbaum DC, van Rhee F, Nabel CS. HHV-8-negative, idiopathic multicentric Castleman disease: novel insights into biology, pathogenesis, and therapy. Blood. 2014;123:2924–33.

43. Liu AY, Nabel CS, Finkelman BS, Ruth JR, Kurzrock R, van Rhee F, Krymskaya VP, Kelleher D, Rubenstein AH, Fajgenbaum DC. Idiopathic multicentric Castleman's disease: a systematic literature review. Lancet Haematol. 2016;3:e163–75.

44. Fajgenbaum DC, Uldrick TS, Bagg A, Frank D, Wu D, Srkalovic G, Simpson D, Liu AY, Menke D, Chandrakasan S, et al. International, evidence-based consensus diagnostic criteria for HHV-8-negative/idiopathic multicentric Castleman disease. Blood. 2017;129:1646–57.

45. Casper C. The aetiology and management of Castleman disease at 50 years: translating pathophysiology to patient care. Br J Haematol. 2005;129:3–17.

46. Kujat C, Muller-Leisse C, Lorbacher P, Seufert R, Falk S, Stutte HJ. A unifocal manifestation of Castleman's disease (angiofollicular lymphatic hyperplasia) in the spleen. Rofo. 1990;152:615–7.

47. Taura T, Takashima S, Shakudo M, Kaminou T, Yamada R, Isoda K. Castleman's disease of the spleen: CT, MR imaging and angiographic findings. Eur J Radiol. 2000;36:11–5.

48. Lee HJ, Jeon HJ, Park SG, Park CY. Castleman's disease of the spleen. World J Gastroenterol. 2015;21:1675–9.

49. Sbrana F, Zhou D, Zamfirova I, Leonardi N. Castleman's disease: a rare presentation in a retroperitoneal accessory spleen, treated with a minimally invasive robotic approach. J Surg Case Rep. 2017;2017:rjx195.

50. Mantas D, Damaskos C, Dailiani P, Samarkos M, Korkolopoulou P. Castleman's disease of the spleen. Acta Chir Belg. 2017;117:203–8.

51. Kawabata H, Takai K, Kojima M, Nakamura N, Aoki S, Nakamura S, Kinoshita T, Masaki Y. Castleman-Kojima disease (TAFRO syndrome): a novel systemic inflammatory disease characterized by a constellation of symptoms, namely, thrombocytopenia, ascites (anasarca), microcytic anemia, myelofibrosis, renal dysfunction, and organomegaly : a status report and summary of Fukushima (6 June, 2012) and Nagoya meetings (22 September, 2012). J Clin Exp Hematop. 2013;53:57–61.

52. Soumerai JD, Sohani AR, Abramson JS. Diagnosis and management of Castleman disease. Cancer Control. 2014;21:266–78.

53. Yu L, Tu M, Cortes J, Xu-Monette ZY, Miranda RN, Zhang J, Orlowski RZ, Neelapu S, Boddu PC, Akosile MA, et al. Clinical and pathological characteristics of HIV- and HHV-8-negative Castleman disease. Blood. 2017;129:1658–68.

54. Rahmouni A, Golli M, Mathieu D, Anglade MC, Charlotte F, Vasile N. Castleman disease mimicking liver tumor: CT and MR features. J Comput Assist Tomogr. 1992;16:699–703.

55. Cirillo RL Jr, Vitellas KM, Deyoung BR, Bennett WF. Castleman disease mimicking a hepatic neoplasm. Clin Imaging. 1998;22:124–9.

56. Uzunlar AK, Ozates M, Yaldiz M, Buyukbayram H, Ozaydin M. Castleman's disease in the porta hepatis. Eur Radiol. 2000;10:1913–5.

57. Karami H, Sahebpour AA, Ghasemi M, Karami H, Dabirian M, Vahidshahi K, Masiha F, Shahmohammadi S. Hyaline vascular-type Castleman's disease in the hilum of liver: a case report. Cases J. 2010;3:74.

58. Jang SY, Kim BH, Kim JH, Ha SH, Hwang JA, Yeon JW, Kim KH, Paik SY. A case of Castleman's disease mimicking a hepatocellular carcinoma: a case report and review of literature. Korean J Gastroenterol. 2012;59:53–7.

59. Miyoshi H, Mimura S, Nomura T, Tani J, Morishita A, Kobara H, Mori H, Yoneyama H, Deguchi A, Himoto T, et al. A rare case of hyaline-type Castleman disease in the liver. World J Hepatol. 2013;5:404–8.

60. Dong A, Dong H, Zuo C. Castleman disease of the porta hepatis mimicking exophytic hepatocellular carcinoma on CT, MRI, and FDG PET/CT. Clin Nucl Med. 2014;39:e69–72.

61. Maundura M, Hayward G, McKee C, Koea JB. Primary Castleman's disease of the liver. J Gastrointest Surg. 2017;21:417–9.

62. Lv K, Zhang CL, Xu MS. Primary Castleman's disease in the liver: a case report and literature review. Mol Clin Oncol. 2018;8:579–81.

63. Bower M. How I treat HIV-associated multicentric Castleman disease. Blood. 2010;116:4415–21.

64. Casper C, Munshi N, Ke X, Fosså A, Simpson D, Capra M, Liu T, Hsieh RK, Goh YT, Zhu J, et al. A multicenter, randomized, double-blind, placebo-controlled study of the efficacy and safety of siltuximab, an anti-interleukin-6 monoclonal antibody, in patients with multicentric Castleman's disease. Blood. 2013;122:505.

65. Masab M, Farooq H. Kikuchi disease. Treasure Island: StatPearls; 2018.

66. Quintas-Cardama A, Fraga M, Cozzi SN, Caparrini A, Maceiras F, Forteza J. Fatal Kikuchi-Fujimoto disease: the lupus connection. Ann Hematol. 2003;82:186–8.

67. Pileri S, Kikuchi M, Helbron D, Lennert K. Histiocytic necrotizing lymphadenitis without granulocytic infiltration. Virchows Arch A Pathol Anat Histol. 1982;395:257–71.

68. Turner RR, Martin J, Dorfman RF. Necrotizing lymphadenitis. A study of 30 cases. Am J Surg Pathol. 1983;7:115–23.

69. O'Neill D, O'Grady J, Variend S. Child fatality associated with pathological features of histiocytic necrotizing lymphadenitis (Kikuchi-Fujimoto disease). Pediatr Pathol Lab Med. 1998;18:79–88.

70. Chan JK, Wong KC, Ng CS. A fatal case of multicentric Kikuchi's histiocytic necrotizing lymphadenitis. Cancer. 1989;63:1856–62.

71. Tsai MK, Huang HF, Hu RH, Lee PH, Lee CJ, Chao SH, Hsu HC, Ko WJ, Chu SH. Fatal Kikuchi-Fujimoto disease in transplant recipients: a case report. Transplant Proc. 1998;30:3137–8.

72. Rudniki C, Kessler E, Zarfati M, Turani H, Bar-Ziv Y, Zahavi I. Kikuchi's necrotizing lymphadenitis: a cause of fever of unknown origin and splenomegaly. Acta Haematol. 1988;79:99–102.

73. Shusang V, Marelli L, Beynon H, Davies N, Patch D, Dhillon AP, Burroughs AK. Autoimmune hepatitis associated with Kikuchi-Fujimoto's disease. Eur J Gastroenterol Hepatol. 2008;20:79–82.

74. Toral Revuelta JR, Martinez Ruiz M, Llobell Segui G, Peralba Vano JI, Mellado del Rey F, Martos Pelegrin J. Pseudometastatic hepatic lesions and Kikuchi necrotizing lymphadenitis. An Med Interna. 1993;10:346–8.

75. Pepe F, Disma S, Teodoro C, Pepe P, Magro G. Kikuchi-Fujimoto disease: a clinicopathologic update. Pathologica. 2016;108:120–9.

76. Pileri SA, Facchetti F, Ascani S, Sabattini E, Poggi S, Piccioli M, Rondelli D, Vergoni F, Zinzani PL, Piccaluga PP, et al. Myeloperoxidase expression by histiocytes in Kikuchi's and Kikuchi-like lymphadenopathy. Am J Pathol. 2001;159:915–24.

77. Umehara H, Nakajima A, Nakamura T, Kawanami T, Tanaka M, Dong L, Kawano M. IgG4-related disease and its pathogenesis-

cross-talk between innate and acquired immunity. Int Immunol. 2014;26:585–95.

78. Zen Y, Fujii T, Harada K, Kawano M, Yamada K, Takahira M, Nakanuma Y. Th2 and regulatory immune reactions are increased in immunoglobin G4-related sclerosing pancreatitis and cholangitis. Hepatology. 2007;45:1538–46.

79. Aparisi L, Farre A, Gomez-Cambronero L, Martinez J, De Las Heras G, Corts J, Navarro S, Mora J, Lopez-Hoyos M, Sabater L, et al. Antibodies to carbonic anhydrase and IgG4 levels in idiopathic chronic pancreatitis: relevance for diagnosis of autoimmune pancreatitis. Gut. 2005;54:703–9.

80. Chen JH, Deshpande V. IgG4-related disease and the liver. Gastroenterol Clin North Am. 2017;46:195–216.

81. Stone JH, Zen Y, Deshpande V. IgG4-related disease. N Engl J Med. 2012;366:539–51.

82. Wallace ZS, Deshpande V, Mattoo H, Mahajan VS, Kulikova M, Pillai S, Stone JH. IgG4-related disease: clinical and laboratory features in one hundred twenty-five patients. Arthritis Rheumatol. 2015;67:2466–75.

83. Deshpande V, Zen Y, Chan JK, Yi EE, Sato Y, Yoshino T, Kloppel G, Heathcote JG, Khosroshahi A, Ferry JA, et al. Consensus statement on the pathology of IgG4-related disease. Mod Pathol. 2012;25:1181–92.

84. Hirota M, Satoh K, Kikuta K, Masamune A, Kume K, Hamada S, Satoh A, Kanno A, Unno J, Ito H, et al. Early detection of low enhanced pancreatic parenchyma by contrast-enhanced computed tomography predicts poor prognosis of patients with acute pancreatitis. Pancreas. 2012;41:1099–104.

85. Ghazale A, Chari ST, Zhang L, Smyrk TC, Takahashi N, Levy MJ, Topazian MD, Clain JE, Pearson RK, Petersen BT, et al. Immunoglobulin G4-associated cholangitis: clinical profile and response to therapy. Gastroenterology. 2008;134:706–15.

86. Deshpande V, Sainani NI, Chung RT, Pratt DS, Mentha G, Rubbia-Brandt L, Lauwers GY. IgG4-associated cholangitis: a comparative histological and immunophenotypic study with primary sclerosing cholangitis on liver biopsy material. Mod Pathol. 2009;22:1287–95.

87. Gaeta R, Donati F, Kauffmann EF, Campani D. A splenic IgG4+ Sclerosing Angiomatoid Nodular Transformation (SANT) treated by Hemisplenectomy: a radiologic, histochemical, and immunohistochemical study. Appl Immunohistochem Mol Morphol. 2017; https://doi.org/10.1097/PAI.0000000000000560.

88. Joshi D, Webster GJ. Biliary and hepatic involvement in IgG4-related disease. Aliment Pharmacol Ther. 2014;40:1251–61.

Raul S. Gonzalez and Andrew G. Evans

Introduction

Benign or malignant diseases confined to the liver can be associated with inflammation, including lymphoid or plasmacytic infiltrate, and can rarely mimic neoplastic hematopoietic disorders. These differential diagnoses have received limited attention in the literature. Understanding the patterns of liver histology caused by lymphoma and various non-neoplastic inflammatory pathologies is essential, as the differential diagnosis varies depending on whether an inflammatory infiltrate primarily involves portal tracts, primarily involves sinusoids, or forms a discrete mass lesion [1].

The differential diagnosis for pathologic enlargement of the spleen is broad. As a hematopoietic organ, the spleen is a site of primary lymphoma, but also manifests pathologic abnormalities in a variety of infectious diseases, hematologic disorders, and systemic inflammatory disorders that may mimic primary or secondary involvement by a hematopoietic malignancy. The pathologic differential for splenomegaly differs depending on whether it exhibits diffuse homogenous enlargement or radiographically discrete heterogenous masses. Careful gross examination and radiographic correlation are critical to determine areas for proper histologic sampling. Furthermore, ancillary studies are often needed, including flow cytometry and genetic analysis. In the chapter, we will focus on common systemic infections as well as non-infectious inflammatory disorders involving the liver and spleen. Pathologists should be familiar with the etiology and histologic changes in these diseases.

R. S. Gonzalez
Department of Pathology, Beth Israel Deaconess Medical Center, Boston, MA, USA

A. G. Evans (✉)
Department of Pathology and Laboratory Medicine, Strong Memorial Hospital, University of Rochester Medical Center, Rochester, NY, USA
e-mail: Andrew_Evans@URMC.rochester.edu

Systemic Infections

Epstein-Barr Virus

Epstein-Barr virus (EBV) belongs to the *Gammaherpesvirinae* subfamily of herpes viruses. Similar to other herpes viruses, it also exhibits the tendency of establishing latency in the host [2]. Acute viral infection gives rise to lifelong latent infection and affects nearly 90% of individuals depending on geographic location. The exact role of EBV infection in chronic liver disease may be either as a silent companion or as a causative agent [3]. In healthy individuals, primary EBV infection results in transient viremia and activation of cytotoxic T cells, while in an immune-compromised setting, the repeated activation of EBV infection or reactivation leads to B-cell immortality and eventually development of a clonal B-cell lymphoproliferative disorder or lymphoma [4, 5].

Mononucleosis is a systemic response to acute EBV infection (also refer to Chap. 20) and clinically can manifest with hepatosplenomegaly in addition to acute infectious signs and symptoms (fever, sore throat, swollen glands). Rupture of the spleen can occur with rapid increase in splenic size [6, 7]. When a patient develops B symptoms, weight loss, lymphadenopathy, and/or organomegaly, lymphoma may be clinically suspected until laboratory study demonstrates a positive Monospot (heterophile antibody) test. Positive serology for EBV infection [antiviral capsid antigen, anti-VCA IgM and IgG, anti-early antigen (EA) IgG, and anti-EBV nuclear antigen (anti-EBNA)] usually develops weeks or months after Monospot test [6, 8, 9]. Thus, the diagnosis of infectious mononucleosis is primarily based on clinical observation and immediate laboratory assessment, while a biopsy of spleen or liver is not indicated clinically.

Forms of chronic hepatic EBV infection include chronic active EBV infection (CAEBV), EBV-associated chronic hepatitis, EBV infection/reactivation post-transplant, and EBV-associated hepatocellular carcinoma. The former two entities are included in differential diagnoses of primary

© Springer Nature Switzerland AG 2020
L. Zhang et al. (eds.), *Diagnostic Pathology of Hematopoietic Disorders of Spleen and Liver*,
https://doi.org/10.1007/978-3-030-37708-3_21

EBV-positive hepatic lymphomas, while the latter two settings are not discussed in the chapters. CAEBV, though rare, is observed in patients with or without liver disease. It is diagnosed by abnormal EBV serology, histologic findings consistent with infection (e.g., hepatitis), and EBV genome integration into the affected tissue [3]. The clinical course resembles a chronic or recurrent infectious mononucleosis [10].

EBV infection could be the trigger for other forms of hepatitis, including infectious (e.g., hepatitis B and C) or autoimmune-mediated disease [3, 11, 12]. The mechanisms are underinvestigated. It is proposed that EBV-specific T cells play an important role by producing various cytokines, including interleukin (IL)-1, IL-2, IL-10, and interferon-gamma (INF-gamma) [13].

Microscopic Features

Liver An important mimic of hematopoietic neoplasia in the liver is involvement by Epstein-Barr virus (EBV), which can resemble hepatosplenic T-cell lymphoma (HSTCL) among other lymphomas. In EBV infection (mononucleosis), the sinusoids become engorged with numerous bland lymphocytes, which may also be present in portal tracts (Fig. 21.1) [14]. These lymphocytes are predominantly cytotoxic T cells (CD8-positive) [6]; scattered B cells are present in portal tracts and are infected with the virus, which can be demonstrated with EBV-encoded RNA (EBER) in situ hybridization [15].

A liver biopsy is usually not performed for chronic active EBV infection (CAEBV). However, EBV can be identified in EBV-associated chronic hepatitis via in situ hybridization

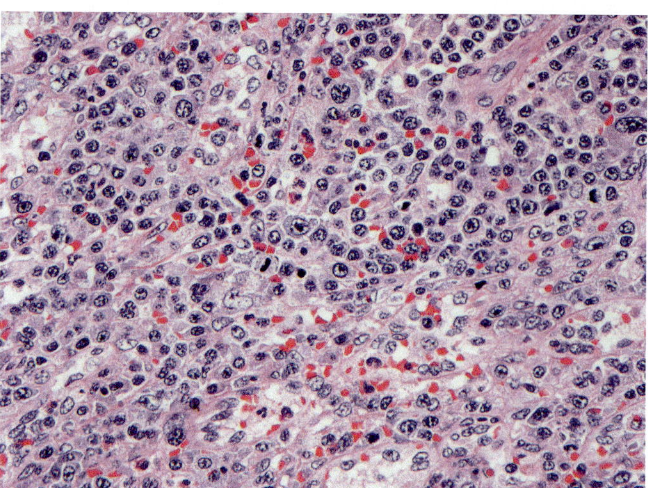

Fig. 21.2 Post-transplant lymphoproliferative disorder may have polymorphous morphology, with a wide spectrum of B-cell differentiation and even overt plasmacytoid appearance, as seen here. Individual large scattered immunoblasts are also present, not unlike the reactive atypical cells that can be seen in infectious mononucleosis

assay using EBER [12] in addition to histologic evidence of chronic hepatitis.

Spleen Acute EBV infection (i.e., infectious mononucleosis) is commonly associated with splenomegaly, and is an important differential to consider or exclude in the evaluation of lymphoma. Florid follicular hyperplasia may give way to a marked atypical lymphoid hyperplasia that includes large reactive immunoblasts, which mimic lymphoma cells. Based on morphology, it is sometimes difficult to differentiate between acute EBV infection and a B-cell lymphoma such as diffuse large B-cell lymphoma. EBV infection in patients with a history of prior organ transplant can result in a polymorphous post-transplant lymphoproliferative disorder (PTLD) (Fig. 21.2).

Differential Diagnosis

The differential between acute self-limited EBV infection and malignant lymphoproliferative disorder can be extremely challenging by morphology alone, and correlation with additional studies, including B cell clonality studies by flow cytometry, and genetic evaluation for chromosomal abnormalities by karyotyping, is advised.

In self-limited acute EBV infection, the large immunoblasts of concern typically provide a mottled appearance, alongside reactive histiocytes, plasma cells, and small lymphocytes, and should not extend into large sheets comparable to diffuse large B-cell lymphoma. Several aggressive T- or B-cell lymphomas must be excluded in accordance with clinicopathologic findings.

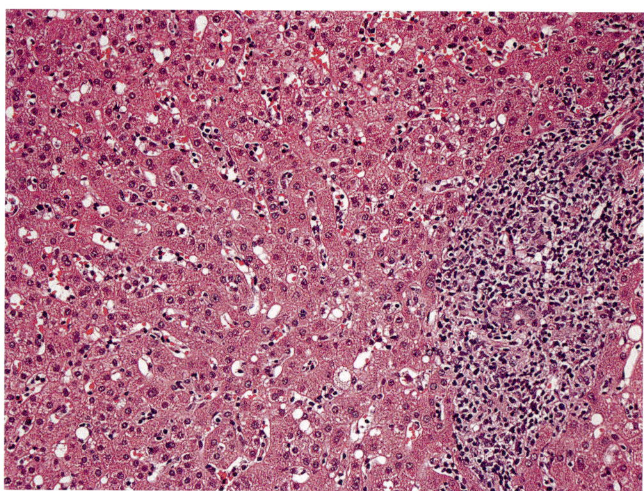

Fig. 21.1 Periportal infiltration by numerous small lymphocytes, which are also present in sinusoids. Lymphocytes are comprised of phenotypically normal T cells, and few interspersed EBV+ cells may be present

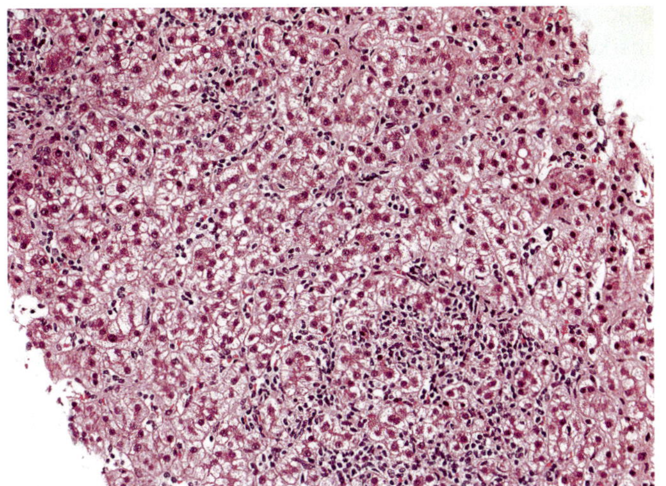

Fig. 21.3 HSTCL has a distinctive and almost exclusively sinusoidal infiltration pattern. Atypical lymphoid cells of small-to-medium size with clear cytoplasm and coarse chromatin may engorge sinusoids. Phenotypically, these are usually T-cell receptor (TCR) gamma/delta positive

Hepatosplenic T-Cell Lymphoma

In a similar fashion, hepatosplenic T-cell lymphoma (HSTCL) occupies the sinusoids of the liver (Fig. 21.3) [16, 17]. Three findings can help distinguish this T-cell neoplasm, frequently expressing gamma-delta TCR, from EBV infection. First, the lymphoma cells should not involve the portal tracts, unlike the lymphocytes in EBV infection. Second, damaged or dying hepatocytes can be seen in severe EBV infection but should not be seen in lymphoma. Third, the cells in EBV infection retain CD5 immunoreactivity, whereas CD5 is usually negative in HSTCL [17, 18]. Clinical symptoms may overlap somewhat, as both processes can cause fever and hepatomegaly.

Other T- or B-Cell Lymphomas/Leukemias

Burkitt lymphoma, classic Hodgkin lymphoma, and a subset of diffuse large B-cell lymphoma, not otherwise specified, are frequently associated with EBV [19]. Involvement by the aforementioned lymphoma in the liver and/or spleen can occur [16, 20, 21]. A previously diagnosed lymphoma and the corresponding immunophenotypic changes help to confirm hepatic involvement by the lymphoma. Identification of clonal B cells via flow cytometry, immunohistochemical staining, or PCR study aids a final diagnosis. Coexisting CAEBV infection/reactivation and EBV-associated chronic hepatitis should be carefully sought in the liver biopsy if there are laboratory data supporting EBV infection.

Of note, hairy cell leukemia can also involve the liver sinusoids, though the appearance is often sufficiently distinct [22, 23]. In the spleen, hairy cell leukemia exhibits a unique infiltrating pattern: red pulp expansion and a "blood lake" appearance [24]. The hepatic infiltrating pattern is similar to chronic EBV infection. However, the unique immunophenotype of hairy cell leukemia (CD20+, CD11c+, CD25+, CD103+, Annexin 1+, and TRAP+) and *BRAF* V600E mutation provide an important diagnostic distinction [25].

Hairy cell leukemia is usually not associated with EBV infection. However, EBV-positive cells can be detected in the liver biopsy as bystanders if a chronic EBV hepatitis is present.

Cytomegalovirus

Cytomegalovirus (CMV) is a member of the *Herpesviridae* family. Reactivation of CMV often occurs in immunocompromised individuals, while acute infection could be acquired before or after birth or even in the adult [26]. Clinically, the infection is usually asymptomatic but can manifest with infectious mononucleosis-like signs or symptoms (fever, pharyngitis, lymphadenopathy, hepatosplenomegaly) [26]. Several laboratory methods (viral culture, direct immunofluorescence, DNA in situ hybridization, immunohistochemical staining, PCR for CMV DNA, and antigen tests) are used for diagnosis of CMV infection, in addition to morphologic assessment [26–28]. PCR is the most reliable way for monitoring the viral infection [28].

CMV hepatitis presents with a long-lasting fever, mildly elevated transaminases, and a low ratio of alanine aminotransferase to LDH. There are only mild histopathological changes found on liver biopsy. Atypical lymphocytosis and splenomegaly are two common findings [29].

Liver While CMV infection may be associated with chronic inflammation, it is typically limited and involves a patchy periportal lymphocytic infiltrate and mild lobular hepatitis [29]. Apoptosis can be observed. However, there is no overt damage of hepatocytes, such as bridging necrosis, as can be found in hepatitis A, B, and, C [29]. In acute infection, or the mononucleosis-like syndrome, infiltrates within portal tracts and sinusoids may become more prominent. Micro abscesses may also be seen. The pathognomonic finding in CMV hepatitis is a classic cytomegalic cytopathic effect that may be seen in enlarged hepatocytes, endothelial cells, biliary epithelium, or sinusoidal macrophages (Kupffer cells) [29, 30]. There is massive nuclear and cytoplasmic enlargement with intranuclear inclusions (Cowdry type A) typical of herpesvirus infection (Fig. 21.4) [30]. Immunostaining for CMV antigen is often useful for highlighting virally infected cells.

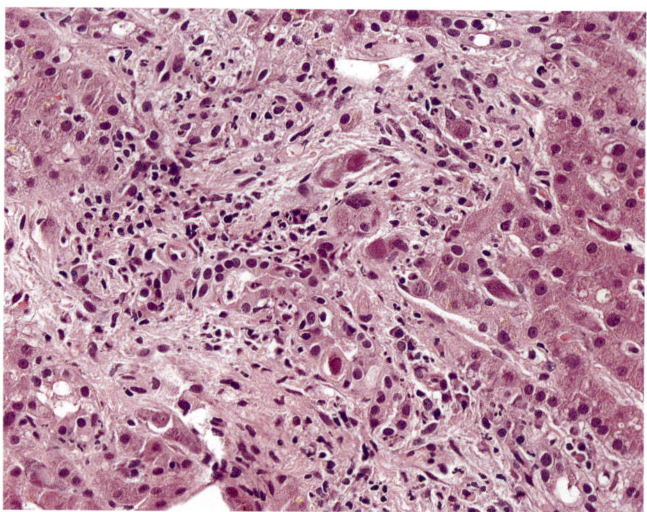

Fig. 21.4 Cytopathic effect of CMV hepatitis includes cell enlargement and eosinophilic nuclear inclusions in hepatocytes

Differential Diagnosis

Differential diagnoses should include, but not be limited to, EBV-driven infectious mononucleosis, other viral hepatitis, lymphoma, and graft-versus-host disease in patients status post solid organ transplantation. Morphologic evidence of cytomegalic cytopathic effect, Cowdry type A cells, and positive CMV immunohistochemical staining helps to confirm the presence of CMV infection [30].

Spleen Architectural changes within the spleen attributable to CMV are somewhat similar to the mononucleosis-like changes of EBV, albeit typically less pronounced. Follicular hyperplasia, marginal zone proliferation, and sinusoidal proliferations of immunoblasts or plasma cells may be seen. In some severe cases, vasculitis and lymphocyte depletion may be seen. As above, characteristic cell enlargement and viral inclusions can be expected, and immunostaining for CMV is particularly helpful.

Human Immunodeficiency Virus

Human immunodeficiency virus (HIV) is the virus causing acquired immunodeficiency syndrome (AIDS) and is spread via contacting with the blood, semen, fluids, or breast milk of an HIV-positive individual. HIV infection can be divided into 4 clinical stages from asymptomatic to advanced disease, according to the WHO clinical staging system for HIV/AIDS. Opportunistic infections are commonly accompanied in stage IV disease [31].

Liver A variety of histologic liver abnormalities are commonly seen in the setting of HIV, but virtually none are spe-

cific to this virus. Common findings include steatosis, marked iron deposition (related to transfusion history), granulomas associated with a variety of opportunistic infections, and high co-incidence of primary hepatotropic virus infection [32]. Importantly, when co-infection with HIV and hepatitis C virus (HCV) occurs, the severity of histologic damage from HCV may be worse, particularly with respect to more severe fibrosis and piecemeal necrosis [33, 34].

Spleen Likewise, the most notable pathologic changes of the spleen associated with HIV/AIDS are not directly attributable to the virus itself, but largely reflect the sequelae of disease such as secondary opportunistic infections (e.g., CMV and atypical *Mycobacterium*) and AIDS-related malignancies/lymphomas. In the era before highly active antiretroviral therapy (HAART), white pulp depletion was more commonly seen [35]. Other histologic patterns that are likely attributable to systemic HIV infection include follicular hyperplasia and intraparenchymal plasmacytosis [36].

Malaria (*Plasmodium* species)

Malaria is caused by protozoan parasites of the genus *Plasmodium* spread through the bites of infected female *Anopheles* mosquitoes. It can cause life-threatening disease, but it is preventable and curable [37]. The two most common species (5 in total) – *P. falciparum* and *P. vivax* – are the most causative [37].

Diagnostic evaluation for presence and speciation of *Plasmodium* species is effectively performed on a routine blood smear. That being said, studies of the liver and spleen histopathology in malaria have revealed some correlative findings. The laboratory methods used for diagnosing malaria have been well established, including microscopic examination of peripheral blood films (thick and thin preparation), QBC staining, anti-malaria antibody (rapid diagnostic tests), serological tests, and molecular tests [37].

The liver stage of the disease is an obligatory phase in which sporozoites develop into merozoites, prior to red blood cell infection. In severe malaria, most commonly caused by *P. falciparum*, worsening liver damage is associated with severe hyperbilirubinemia and more extensive periportal inflammation, fatty change, and Kupffer cell hyperplasia [38].

Splenomegaly is also routinely found, and can be so severe as to cause splenic rupture. The degree of splenomegaly is likely attributable to a combination of congestion related to clearance of hemolyzed red cells, parasite clearance and sequestration, and cytokine-mediated inflammatory changes.

In endemic areas, hyperreactive malarial splenomegaly syndrome (HMSS) secondary to chronic malaria antigen stimulation is frequently observed, accounting for 31–76% of splenomegaly in different African countries, and which has a high mortality rate (up to 36% within 3 years) [39]. PCR is the most sensitive diagnostic tool when compared with histologic examination for microorganism inclusions in peripheral blood specimen, which is usually negative in the setting [40, 41].

Differential Diagnosis

Since histologic findings in both liver and spleen could be non-specific, identification of intracellular *Plasmodium* in red blood cells on peripheral smear or PCR study for the presence of *Plasmodium* DNA is critical for the establishment of malarial infection [37, 41].

Hemophagocytic Lymphohistiocytosis, Secondary (or Infection-Related)

Hemophagocytic lymphohistiocytosis (HLH) is a systemic inflammatory disorder (a.k.a. macrophage activation syndrome), in which natural killer (NK) and T-cell function become dysregulated, leading to uncontrolled immune system activation. The primary form of this disease is familial (i.e., genetic) and most frequently known to occur among patients with mutations in elements of the perforin cytotoxic pathway. Secondary HLH most commonly occurs in response to viral infection (HIV, EBV, or others), may be related to an underlying malignancy (e.g., T-cell lymphoma), and still in some cases is ultimately idiopathic [42]. Organomegaly (i.e., hepatosplenomegaly) is among one of the multiple diagnostic criteria; therefore, liver and splenic manifestations of HLH are important to recognize, as the liver may be among the most common tissues biopsied (following bone marrow) to document hemophagocytosis, and splenomegaly may be evaluated prior to clinical consideration of HLH in the diagnostic differential (also refer to Chap. 17).

Liver HLH is another process that can lead to increased inflammatory cells within the sinusoids, potentially mimicking a hematopoietic disorder. Microscopic changes can vary widely but generally include hemophagocytosis by macrophages within the sinusoids, portal tract, and lobules (Fig. 21.5), along with increased lymphocytic inflammation in these areas. In some cases, the portal infiltrate is sufficiently heavy that HLH can also mimic a portal or intrasinusoidal malignant lymphoma [43].

Spleen Massive histiocytic infiltration of splenic red pulp occurs in HLH, accompanied by marked erythrophagocytosis. Histiocytes expand both sinuses and cords, with expanded but intact splenic architecture. Atrophy of the white pulp may be seen. Due to the normally high number of resident macro-

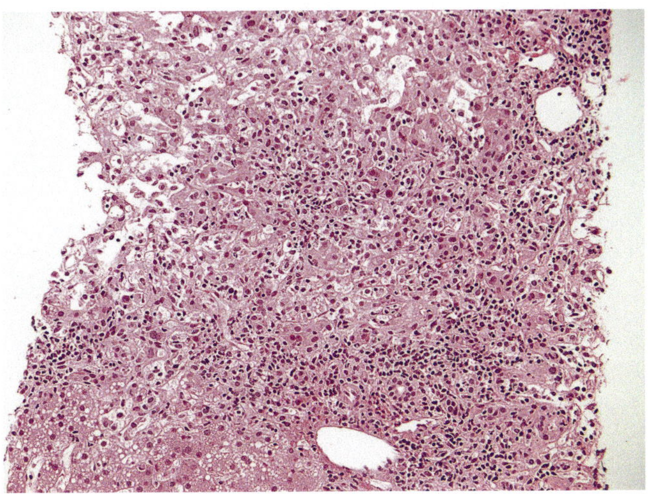

Fig. 21.5 Hemophagocytic lymphohistiocytosis can produce dense lymphocytic inflammation throughout the hepatic parenchyma and particularly within sinusoids. Careful histopathologic and clinical correlation is needed to exclude T-cell/histiocyte-rich large B-cell lymphoma, peripheral T-cell lymphoma, or hepatosplenic T-cell lymphoma

phages present in the splenic reticuloendothelial system, it may be difficult to surmise when HLH is present in less florid cases. As with other tissues, CD163 or CD68 immunostaining may help identify islands of erythrophagocytosis (i.e., nucleated red blood cells accumulated and enveloped within pockets of positively staining histiocytic cytoplasm).

Differential Diagnosis

The primary malignant differential for HLH in the liver is HSTCL or T-cell/histiocyte-rich large B-cell lymphoma (T/HRLBCL). Careful histologic evaluation and immunohistochemical staining for aberrant T cells and large atypical B cells is advised if lymphoma is suspected.

Granulomatous Infections

Necrotizing Granulomatous Inflammation Widespread or hematogenous dissemination of invasive fungus (e.g., histoplasmosis) or *Mycobacteria* species (e.g., *M. tuberculosis*) can give rise to the tumor-like formation of necrotizing granulomata in the liver or spleen [44–46].

In both liver and splenic parenchyma, infiltration by variably sized organized granuloma can occur, typically without regard to specific architectural elements. Well-formed palisading walls of histiocytes are rimmed by small lymphocytes (predominantly CD4-positive T cells) and typically abundant necrotic debris (Fig. 21.6). The presence of necrosis strongly favors an infectious etiology, but by comparison, the presence of abundant non-necrotizing granulomata (which may fre-

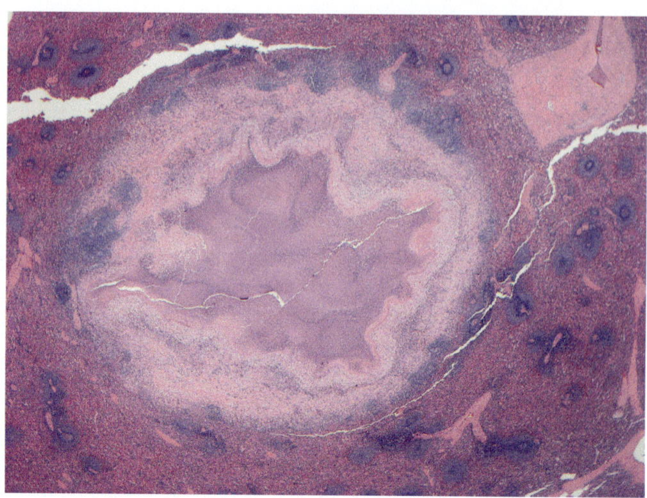

Fig. 21.6 Stellate necrotizing granuloma, with well-formed walls of palisading histiocytes surrounding central necrosis

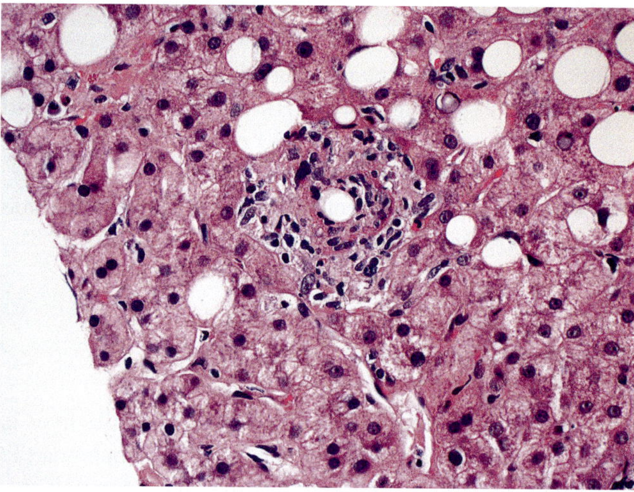

Fig. 21.7 Fibrin-ring granuloma in the liver of a patient with Q fever

quently be presumed to correlate with systemic sarcoidosis) is an important mimic of the granulomatous variant of classic Hodgkin lymphoma (see discussion below).

Fibrin-Ring Granulomas This peculiar type of granuloma is generally described in the liver. Small and rounded, they resemble epithelioid, non-caseating granulomas, though the center contains a damaged globule of fat surrounded by a fibrinous ring (hence the name) (Fig. 21.7). They are most strongly associated with Q fever, though they have been described in numerous other disease states, including EBV infection, cytomegalovirus hepatitis, and drug-induced liver injury (allopurinol, ipilimumab, and others) [47, 48]. They have also been described in patients with hepatic involvement by Hodgkin lymphoma, though most cases also show obvious evidence of involvement, with mixed inflammation and Reed-Sternberg cells involving portal tracts [16]. The presence of fibrin-ring granulomas in the liver should still at least raise the possibility of lymphoma, especially in patients with suggestive symptoms. Ultimately, however, a different diagnosis is more likely to be correct in any given case with this type of granuloma.

Parasitic Hydatid Cyst

Cystic parasitic lesions of the liver and spleen are rare, and due to their distinctive radiographic and gross appearance, they are not commonly included in the differential with hematopoietic disorders.

Hydatid cysts are caused by larval infection from the *Echinococcus* species of tapeworm, which is one step in a complicated developmental lifecycle that involves different stages in both intermediate and definitive hosts. Intermediate hosts develop the cystic form of the disease and are more severely affected due to disease dissemination of the onco-sphere, which hatches from an ingested egg to penetrate the intestinal wall and disseminates systemically before forming hydatid cysts. Symptoms are related to mass effects of the enlarging cysts, and potentially severe inflammatory reactions when cysts rupture. In the United States, the most common species is *E. granulosus*, which typically forms uniloculated cysts in the liver and spleen, among other organs. Other species include *E. multilocularis*, *E. oligarthus*, and *E. vogeli*, the latter of which forms multiloculated cysts [49]. The liver is the most commonly affected organ, while isolated splenic cysts are uncommon and typically result from abdominal dissemination of a ruptured hepatic cyst. Histologically, the cyst wall has a characteristic lamellated appearance, with an outer fibrous layer and inner germinative layers of the organism in which parasitic structures such as hooklets and scolices can be found. Surrounding the cyst is an inflammatory infiltrate comprised predominantly of chronic lymphocytic inflammation, macrophages, and eosinophils [49].

Differential Diagnosis

Comparatively non-parasitic cysts and pseudocysts are much more common in Western populations. Splenic pseudocysts, which are more common than true cysts, lack an epithelial lining, are comprised of well-formed fibrous tissue, and typically result from lack of resorption from post-traumatic hemorrhage or hematoma, post-splenic infarction, and local regional inflammation. True cysts may contain either epithelial, mesothelial, or epidermoid lining.

Miscellaneous

On a final note, with respect to systemic infections, there are a myriad of other infectious agents that cause splenomegaly but are not routinely considered in the differential with lymphoma. These include brucellosis, echinococcosis, histoplasmosis, leishmaniasis, schistosomiasis, syphilis, toxoplasmosis, trypanosomiasis, and typhoid fever. The details are not discussed in the chapter.

Inflammatory Liver Disease

Viral Hepatitis

Hepatitis C Virus

In chronic HCV, the portal tracts of the liver become filled with a moderately dense inflammatory infiltrate composed predominantly of lymphocytes (Fig. 21.8) [50]. Lobular inflammation may also be present, though less striking. The portal inflammation is generally contained to that region, creating round contours clearly delineating the portal areas from the lobules. Severely affected portal tracts may show evidence of germinal center formation (Fig. 21.9). However, the portal tracts are not equally affected, meaning inflammation may be sparse in some.

Differential Diagnosis

The main potential mimic of lymphoma in the liver is chronic viral hepatitis, particularly hepatitis C (HCV), which can resemble liver involvement by CLL/SLL. Hepatic involvement by CLL/SLL somewhat resembles chronic HCV at low

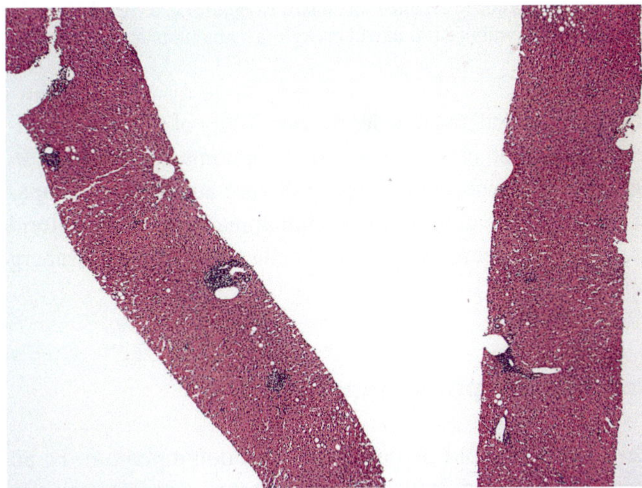

Fig. 21.8 Chronic HCV infection. Bland small lymphocytes forming dense infiltrates in periportal areas

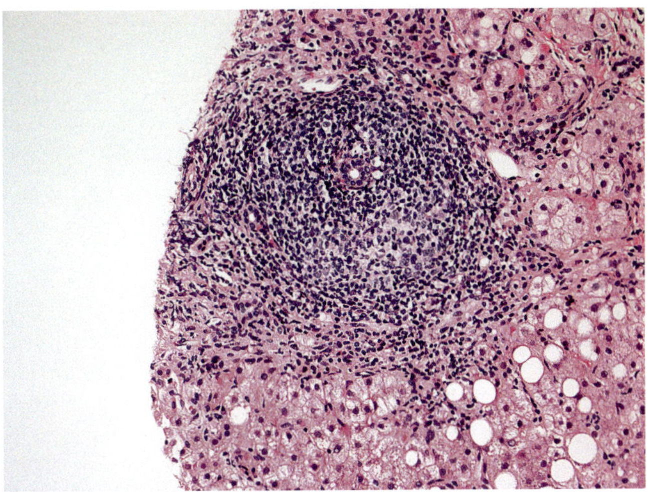

Fig. 21.9 Reactive germinal center formation in chronic HCV

power, with the portal tracts involved by a chronic inflammatory infiltrate [16]. On closer inspection, however, the lymphocytes are packed slightly more densely than in HCV, and they appear monomorphic (Fig. 21.10). All portal tracts are involved to a similar degree. Additionally, the inflammation often spills beyond the portal tracts, causing irregular contours around the inflammatory foci. CLL/SLL should not induce liver fibrosis, unlike chronic HCV, so the presence of liver fibrosis (portal, periportal, bridging, or cirrhotic) generally favors the latter diagnosis.

Immunostains for CD5, CD20, and CD23 should all be positive in the lesional cells of CLL/SLL, helping confirm the diagnosis. In contrast, the inflammation seen in chronic HCV is predominantly CD4- and CD8-positive T cells, meaning CD20 and CD23 should be negative; B cells may be seen, particularly in the center of lymphoid aggregates [51].

Clinical history is the best method of distinguishing HCV from hepatic CLL/SLL. Serologic testing can easily determine a patient's viral load. With the advent of new medication that can cure HCV (e.g., sofosbuvir), this once-common pathologic pattern of injury is becoming less frequently seen; loss of familiarity with this pattern may possibly increase the chance of misinterpretation.

Other Viral Hepatitides

In Western populations, other pathogens responsible for viral hepatitis include hepatitis A virus (HAV) and hepatitis B virus (HBV), as well as other less common primary hepatotropic viruses (hepatitis D, E, and F viruses), adenovirus, and less common human herpesviruses. In tropical regions and lesser developed nations, pathogens of concern include yellow fever virus and other rare flaviviruses, along with numerous tropical, zoonotic, and hemorrhagic

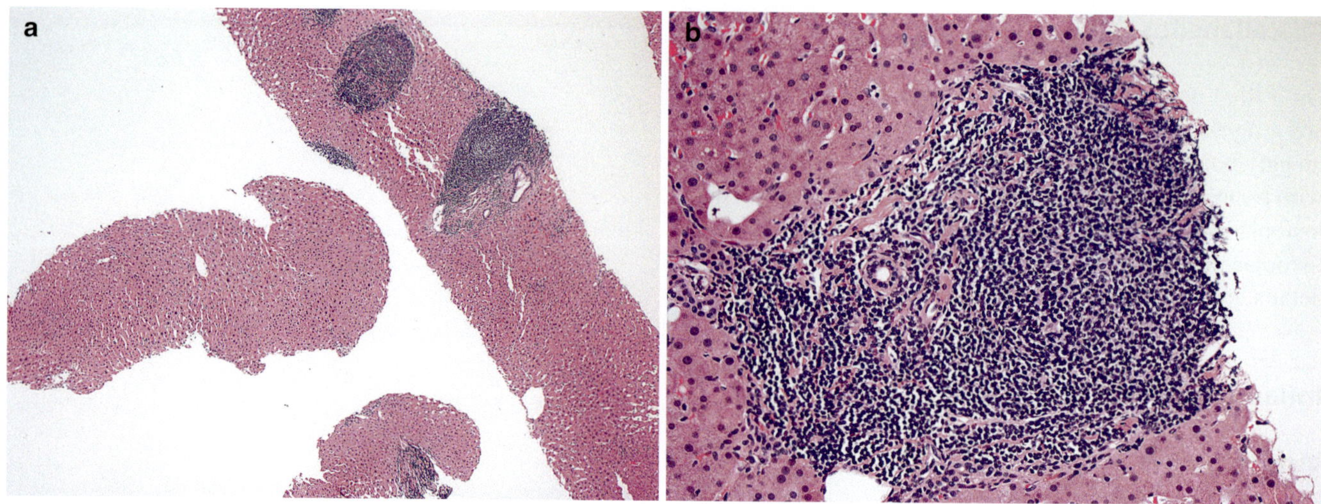

Fig. 21.10 (**a** and **b**) Involvement of the liver by chronic lymphocytic leukemia/small lymphocytic lymphoma (SLL/CLL) (**a**). Higher power shows monomorphic small atypical lymphoid morphology, which should stain for CD5, CD23, and a B-cell marker such as CD20 (perhaps weakly) or Pax5

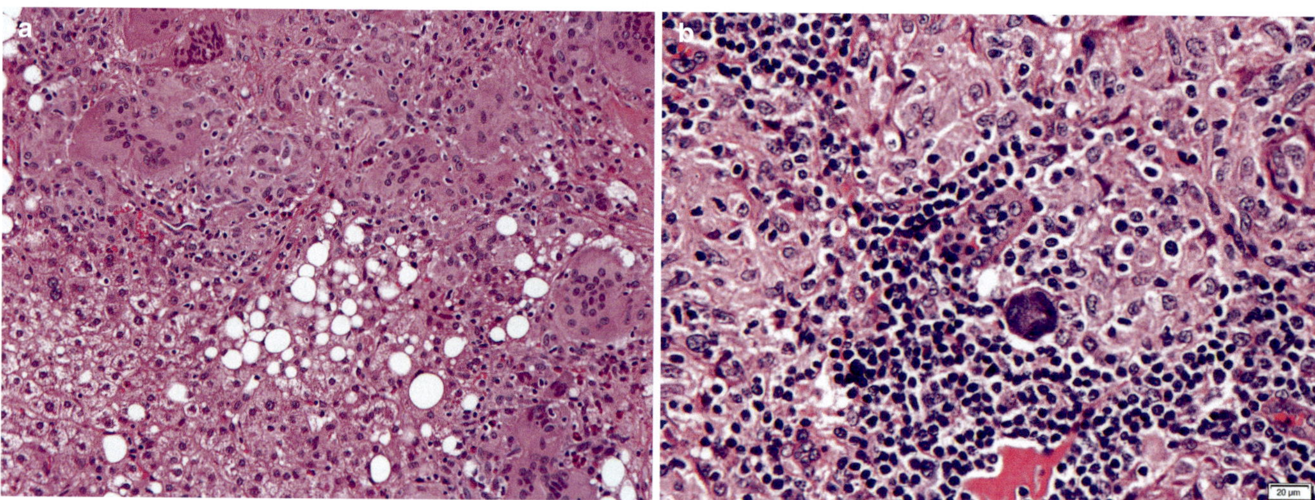

Fig. 21.11 (**a** and **b**) Abundant well-formed non-necrotizing granulomata and associated giant cells can be seen infiltrating throughout the liver parenchyma in sarcoidosis, among other inflammatory disorders (**a**). Care should be taken if there is any history or clinical suspicion of classic Hodgkin lymphoma to evaluate for elusive Hodgkin/Reed-Sternberg cells, which can hide within a prominent background granulomatous pattern (**b**)

viruses (*Filo-*, *Arena-*, *Bunya-*, *Corona-*, *Picorna-*, and *Reovirus* family members). Clinical and laboratory tests help diagnose other viral hepatitides.

Granulomatous Hepatitis, Non-infectious

Non-necrotizing granulomas of the liver have a broad differential, as they may be primary to the liver (e.g., primary biliary cholangitis, autoimmune hepatitis), or the result of systemic disease (e.g., sarcoidosis, Crohn's disease, systemic lupus erythematous). Approximately 80% of sarcoidosis have hepatosplenic involvement [52]. Given this broad differential, which will often not yet be narrowed at the time of pathologic evaluation, it is critical to consider the possibility of the granulomatous pattern of classic Hodgkin lymphoma (particularly in patients with suspected systemic disease and lymphadenopathy). Rarely, the granulomatous inflammation can be so florid as to nearly obscure the presence of diagnostic Reed-Sternberg cells (Fig. 21.11).

Reactive Lymphoid Hyperplasia

Reactive lymphoid hyperplasia (pseudolymphoma) is an unusual localized inflammatory process that may mimic hepatocellular carcinoma clinically or a lymphoma microscopically [53]. Histology shows a well-demarcated nodular region composed of mature lymphocytes (B cells) forming follicles with germinal centers. Adjacent portal tracts may show similar inflammation. The differential diagnosis includes any lymphoma that can present as an isolated liver mass (such as T-cell/histiocyte rich B-cell lymphoma). Molecular studies help confirm the benign, polyclonal nature of this rare process.

Splenomegaly, Non-infectious

Extramedullary Hematopoiesis (Also See Chap. 17)

Hematopoiesis occurs outside of the bone marrow (medullary) cavity in adults under a variety of malignant and benign conditions that impair or limit normal blood growth [54]. Examples include bone marrow irradiation, thalassemia, infectious and inflammatory syndromes, primary or secondary bone marrow fibrosis, and marrow infiltration by metastatic cancer [54]. Extramedullary hematopoiesis (EMH) in different organs or tissue is characterized by the appearance of trilineage hematopoietic precursors, including megakaryocytes, nucleated erythroid precursors, and early myeloid precursors (myelocytes, promyelocytes, and myeloblasts) (Fig. 21.12). The liver and spleen are the two most frequent sites of EMH secondary to myeloproliferative neoplasms (MPN) or EMH without MPN [54, 55]. Resultant splenomegaly easily triples or quadruples normal spleen size (e.g., easily exceeding 1000 grams in weight). Pathologic EMH must be conceptually distinguished from physiologic or primary EMH, which occurs as a normal part of embryologic development prior to 4–5 months' gestational age [56].

Fibrocongestive Splenomegaly

Longstanding portal hypertension, due to a variety of conditions including liver cirrhosis, congestive heart failure, portal vain stenosis, and thrombosis of portal veins, hepatic veins (i.e., Budd-Chiari syndrome) or splenic veins, may cause chronic red pulp congestion, sinusoidal dilatation, and fibrotic changes. Histologically dilated veins and sinuses can be seen (Fig. 21.13), along with hemosiderin-laden macrophages, fibrosis of red pulp, normal or attenuated white pulp, and Gamna-Gandy body formation (see below). Fibrocongestive splenomegaly is not an uncommon finding in patients with sickle cell disease (see separate chapter) [57].

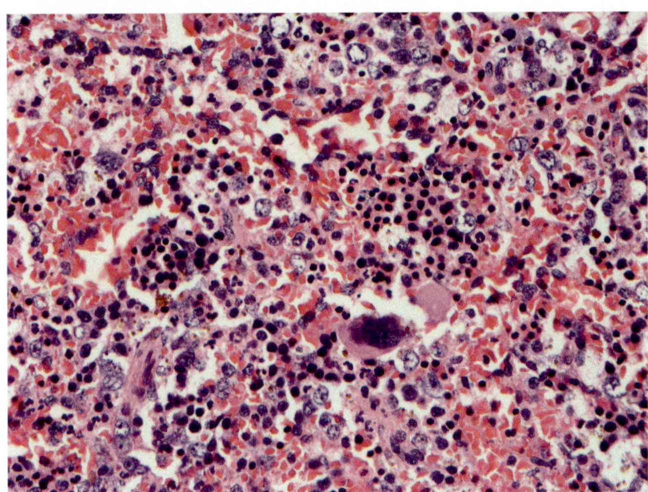

Fig. 21.12 Extramedullary hematopoiesis of the spleen is evident by the appearance of discrete islands of developing nucleated erythroid precursors, scattered immature myeloid cells, and most prominently large megakaryocytes with multilobulated nuclei

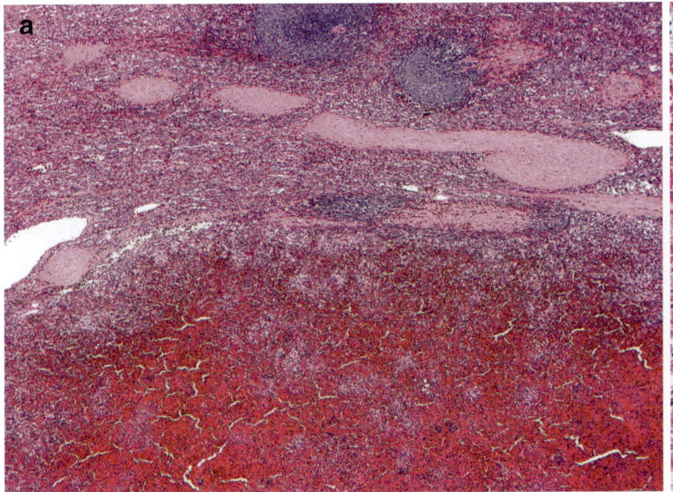

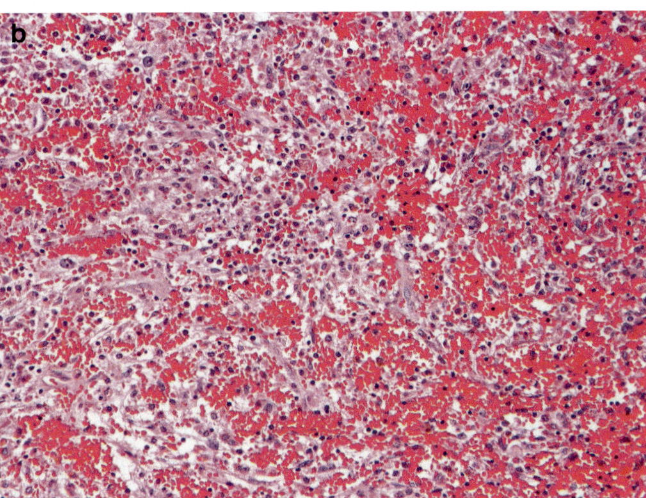

Fig. 21.13 (**a** and **b**) Fibrocongestive splenomegaly shows large areas of the spleen overtaken by congested sinusoids packed with red blood cells. Residual areas of normal splenic parenchyma may persist (**a**). At higher power, the most fibrocongestive areas are devoid of white pulp lymphocytes and contain fibroblastic and reticular cell proliferations (**b**)

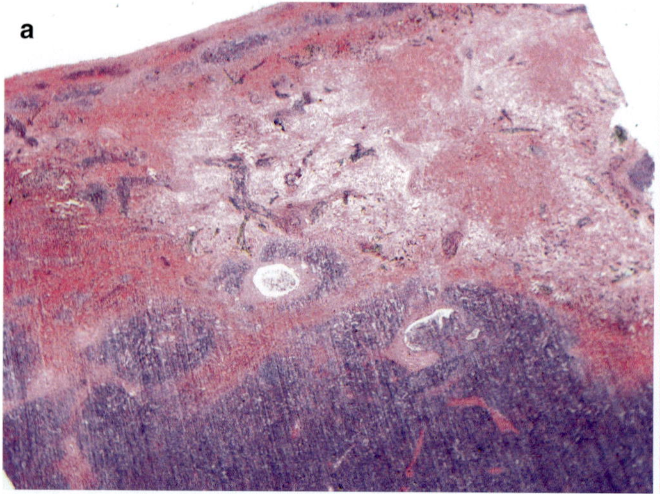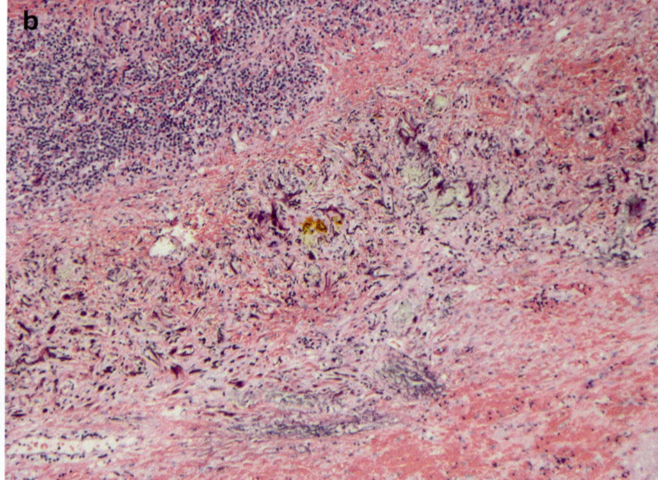

Fig. 21.14 (**a** and **b**) Gamna-Gandy bodies are discrete fibrotic nodules of the remotely infarcted spleen that exhibit prominent reticular fibers, hemosiderin, and iron deposition, often associated with intrapa-renchymal hemorrhage (**a**). At higher power, brightly powered pigment deposition can be seen (**b**)

Gamna-Gandy Bodies

Chronic hemolysis, infarction of the spleen, or fibrocongestive changes can result in excessive iron deposition and dystrophic calcification within dense fibrotic lesions of the spleen known as Gamna-Gandy bodies. This phenomenon most commonly occurs in sickle cell anemia, but other conditions where they may be seen include portal hypertension, acquired hemochromatosis, and patients with chronic blood transfusion [58]. These deposits are siderotic, pigment-laden lesions that show up on a variety of imaging techniques, including magnetic resonance imaging and ultrasound. They may be mistaken for tumor-forming masses within the spleen. On gross examination, these nodules more likely mimic desmoplastic reaction to metastatic tumor than the soft tissue appearance of lymphoma. Histologic sectioning reveals distinct pigment deposition that is rust-to-yellow-to-black in color (Fig. 21.14). They are pathologically insignificant, but in rare cases require clinical correlation with a preceding history of hemolysis or iron overload.

Diagnostic Caveats

1. Certain benign or malignant diseases confined to the liver can be associated with inflammation, including a lymphoid or plasmacytic infiltrate, that rarely mimics neoplastic hematopoietic disorders. Of note, dense lymphoid infiltrate in HCV hepatitis could mimic chronic lymphocytic leukemia/small lymphocytic lymphoma, and infectious mononucleosis may resemble hepatosplenic T-cell lymphoma. Acute or chronic EBV infection should be distinguished from EBV-associated lymphomas.
2. It is important to know the patterns of liver histology caused by lymphoma and various non-neoplastic inflammatory pathologies, since the differential diagnosis varies depending on whether an inflammatory infiltrate primarily involves portal tracts, primarily involves sinusoids, or forms a discrete mass lesion.
3. Whether a disease process causes diffuse homogenous enlargement or radiographically discrete heterogenous masses in the spleen provides diagnostic clues in patients with splenomegaly. Careful gross examination and radiographic correlation are critical to determine areas for proper histologic sampling.
4. It is important to correlate with clinical history as well as laboratory findings to identify infectious etiologies, and to distinguish autoimmune disease, secondary inflammatory conditions, or granulomatous processes from neoplastic hematopoietic disorders.
5. Furthermore, ancillary studies are often needed, including immunohistochemical study, flow cytometry, and genetic analysis, to exclude hematopoietic malignancy. In the situation, adequate tissue biopsy tissue is essential.

References

1. Baumhoer D, Tzankov A, Dirnhofer S, Tornillo L, Terracciano LM. Patterns of liver infiltration in lymphoproliferative disease. Histopathology. 2008;53(1):81–90.
2. Cohen JI. Epstein-Barr virus infection. N Engl J Med. 2000;343(7):481–92.

3. Petrova M, Kamburov V. Epstein-Barr virus: silent companion or causative agent of chronic liver disease? World J Gastroenterol. 2010;16(33):4130–4.

4. Maurmann S, Fricke L, Wagner HJ, et al. Molecular parameters for precise diagnosis of asymptomatic Epstein-Barr virus reactivation in healthy carriers. J Clin Microbiol. 2003;41(12):5419–28.

5. Richinson A, Kieff E. Epstein-Barr virus. In: Knipe D, Howley P, editors. Tields virology. Vol 1 and 2. Philadelphia: Lippincott Williams & Wilkins; 2001. p. 2575–627.

6. CDC. Epstein-barr virus and infectious mononucleosis: laboratory testing. https://www.cdc.gov/epstein-barr/laboratory-testing.html. Updated 2018.

7. Handin R. Blood: pricinples and practice of hematology. Philadelphia: Lippincott Williams & Wilkins; 2003.

8. Mononucleosis. https://www.mayoclinic.org/diseases-conditions/mononucleosis/diagnosis-treatment/drc-20350333. Accessed 6 Aug 2017.

9. Elgh F, Linderholm M. Evaluation of six commercially available kits using purified heterophile antigen for the rapid diagnosis of infectious mononucleosis compared with Epstein-Barr virus-specific serology. Clin Diagn Virol. 1996;7(1):17–21.

10. Straus SE. The chronic mononucleosis syndrome. J Infect Dis. 1988;157(3):405–12.

11. Vento S, Cainelli F. Is there a role for viruses in triggering autoimmune hepatitis? Autoimmun Rev. 2004;3(1):61–9.

12. Drebber U, Kasper HU, Krupacz J, et al. The role of Epstein-Barr virus in acute and chronic hepatitis. J Hepatol. 2006;44(5):879–85.

13. Jabs WJ, Wagner HJ, Schlenke P, Kirchner H. The primary and memory immune response to Epstein-Barr virus infection in vitro is characterized by a divergent production of IL-1beta/IL-6 and IL-10. Scand J Immunol. 2000;52(3):304–8.

14. Suh N, Liapis H, Misdraji J, Brunt EM, Wang HL. Epstein-Barr virus hepatitis: diagnostic value of in situ hybridization, polymerase chain reaction, and immunohistochemistry on liver biopsy from immunocompetent patients. Am J Surg Pathol. 2007;31(9):1403–9.

15. Niedobitek G, Agathanggelou A, Steven N, Young LS. Epstein-Barr virus (EBV) in infectious mononucleosis: detection of the virus in tonsillar B lymphocytes but not in desquamated oropharyngeal epithelial cells. Mol Pathol. 2000;53(1):37–42.

16. Loddenkemper C, Longerich T, Hummel M, et al. Frequency and diagnostic patterns of lymphomas in liver biopsies with respect to the WHO classification. Virchows Arch. 2007;450(5):493–502.

17. Shi Y, Wang E. Hepatosplenic T-cell lymphoma: a clinicopathologic review with an emphasis on diagnostic differentiation from other T-cell/natural killer-cell neoplasms. Arch Pathol Lab Med. 2015;139(9):1173–80.

18. Kaplan D, Smith D, Meyerson H, Pecora N, Lewandowska K. CD5 expression by B lymphocytes and its regulation upon Epstein-Barr virus transformation. Proc Natl Acad Sci U S A. 2001;98(24):13850–3.

19. Castillo JJ, Beltran BE, Miranda RN, Paydas S, Winer ES, Butera JN. Epstein-barr virus-positive diffuse large B-cell lymphoma of the elderly: what we know so far. Oncologist. 2011;16(1):87–96.

20. Fugl A, Andersen CL. Epstein-Barr virus and its association with disease – a review of relevance to general practice. BMC Fam Pract. 2019;20(1):62.

21. Biemer JJ. Hepatic manifestations of lymphomas. Ann Clin Lab Sci. 1984;14(4):252–60.

22. Yam LT, Janckila AJ, Chan CH, Li CY. Hepatic involvement in hairy cell leukemia. Cancer. 1983;51(8):1497–504.

23. Choi WT, Gill RM. Hepatic lymphoma diagnosis. Surg Pathol Clin. 2018;11(2):389–402.

24. Wotherspoon A, Attygalle A, Mendes LS. Bone marrow and splenic histology in hairy cell leukaemia. Best Pract Res Clin Haematol. 2015;28(4):200–7.

25. Kreitman RJ, Arons E. Update on hairy cell leukemia. Clin Adv Hematol Oncol. 2018;16(3):205–15.

26. Kaye K. Cytomegalovirus (CMV) infection. https://www.merckmanuals.com/home/infections/herpesvirus-infections/cytomegalovirus-cmv-infection. Accessed 27 May 2019.

27. Eguchi H, Horita N, Ushio R, et al. Diagnostic test accuracy of antigenaemia assay for PCR-proven cytomegalovirus infection-systematic review and meta-analysis. Clin Microbiol Infect. 2017;23(12):907–15.

28. Weinberg A, Hodges TN, Li S, Cai G, Zamora MR. Comparison of PCR, antigenemia assay, and rapid blood culture for detection and prevention of cytomegalovirus disease after lung transplantation. J Clin Microbiol. 2000;38(2):768–72.

29. Kunno A, Abe M, Yamada M, Murakami K. Clinical and histological features of cytomegalovirus hepatitis in previously healthy adults. Liver. 1997;17(3):129–32.

30. Colina F, Juca NT, Moreno E, et al. Histological diagnosis of cytomegalovirus hepatitis in liver allografts. J Clin Pathol. 1995;48(4):351–7.

31. Weinberg JL, Kovarik CL. The WHO clinical staging system for HIV/AIDS. Virtual Mentor. 2010;12(3):202–6.

32. Wilkins MJ, Lindley R, Dourakis SP, Goldin RD. Surgical pathology of the liver in HIV infection. Histopathology. 1991;18(5):459–64.

33. Garcia-Samaniego J, Soriano V, Castilla J, et al. Influence of hepatitis C virus genotypes and HIV infection on histological severity of chronic hepatitis C. The Hepatitis/HIV Spanish Study Group. Am J Gastroenterol. 1997;92(7):1130–4.

34. Mohsen AH, Easterbrook PJ, Taylor C, et al. Impact of human immunodeficiency virus (HIV) infection on the progression of liver fibrosis in hepatitis C virus infected patients. Gut. 2003;52(7):1035–40.

35. Diaz LK, Murphy RL, Phair JP, Variakojis D. The AIDS autopsy spleen: a comparison of the pre-anti-retroviral and highly active anti-retroviral therapy eras. Mod Pathol. 2002;15(4):406–12.

36. Falk S, Muller H, Stutte HJ. The spleen in acquired immunodeficiency syndrome (AIDS). Pathol Res Pract. 1988;183(4):425–33.

37. Tangpukdee N, Duangdee C, Wilairatana P, Krudsood S. Malaria diagnosis: a brief review. Korean J Parasitol. 2009;47(2):93–102.

38. Viriyavejakul P, Khachonsaksumet V, Punsawad C. Liver changes in severe Plasmodium falciparum malaria: histopathology, apoptosis and nuclear factor kappa B expression. Malar J. 2014;13:106.

39. Leoni S, Buonfrate D, Angheben A, Gobbi F, Bisoffi Z. The hyperreactive malarial splenomegaly: a systematic review of the literature. Malar J. 2015;14:185.

40. Mothe B, Lopez-Contreras J, Torres OH, Munoz C, Domingo P, Gurgui M. A case of hyper-reactive malarial splenomegaly. The role of rapid antigen-detecting and PCR-based tests. Infection. 2008;36(2):167–9.

41. SM AE, El-Rayah el A, Giha HA. Validation of PCR for detection and characterization of parasitaemia in massive splenomegaly attributed clinically to malaria infection. Diagn Microbiol Infect Dis. 2011;70(2):207–12.

42. George MR. Hemophagocytic lymphohistiocytosis: review of etiologies and management. J Blood Med. 2014;5:69–86.

43. Chen JH, Fleming MD, Pinkus GS, et al. Pathology of the liver in familial hemophagocytic lymphohistiocytosis. Am J Surg Pathol. 2010;34(6):852–67.

44. Kauffman CA. Histoplasmosis: a clinical and laboratory update. Clin Microbiol Rev. 2007;20(1):115–32.

45. Lee DG, Choi JH, Kim YJ, et al. Hepatosplenic tuberculosis mimicking disseminated candidiasis in patients with acute leukemia. Int J Hematol. 2001;73(1):119–21.

46. Gupta PP, Fotedar S, Agarwal D, Sansanwal P. Tuberculosis of spleen presenting with pyrexia of unknown origin in a non-immunocompromised woman. Lung India. 2008;25(1):22–4.

47. Everett J, Srivastava A, Misdraji J. Fibrin ring granulomas in checkpoint inhibitor-induced hepatitis. Am J Surg Pathol. 2017;41(1):134–7.

48. Marazuela M, Moreno A, Yebra M, Cerezo E, Gomez-Gesto C, Vargas JA. Hepatic fibrin-ring granulomas: a clinicopathologic study of 23 patients. Hum Pathol. 1991;22(6):607–13.

49. Pedrosa I, Saiz A, Arrazola J, Ferreiros J, Pedrosa CS. Hydatid disease: radiologic and pathologic features and complications. Radiographics. 2000;20(3):795–817.

50. Goodman ZD, Ishak KG. Histopathology of hepatitis C virus infection. Semin Liver Dis. 1995;15(1):70–81.

51. Tucci FA, Broering R, Lutterbeck M, Schlaak JF, Kuppers R. Intrahepatic B-cell follicles of chronically hepatitis C virus-infected individuals lack signs of an ectopic germinal center reaction. Eur J Immunol. 2014;44(6):1842–50.

52. Vardhanabhuti V, Venkatanarasimha N, Bhatnagar G, et al. Extra-pulmonary manifestations of sarcoidosis. Clin Radiol. 2012;67(3):263–76.

53. Lv A, Liu W, Qian HG, Leng JH, Hao CY. Reactive lymphoid hyperplasia of the liver mimicking hepatocellular carcinoma: incidental finding of two cases. Int J Clin Exp Pathol. 2015;8(5):5863–9.

54. Fan N, Lavu S, Hanson CA, Tefferi A. Extramedullary hematopoiesis in the absence of myeloproliferative neoplasm: Mayo Clinic case series of 309 patients. Blood Cancer J. 2018;8(12):119.

55. Tefferi A. Primary myelofibrosis: 2019 update on diagnosis, risk-stratification and management. Am J Hematol. 2018;93(12):1551–60.

56. Kim CH. Homeostatic and pathogenic extramedullary hematopoiesis. J Blood Med. 2010;1:13–9.

57. Chopra R, Al-Mulhim AR, Al-Baharani AT. Fibrocongestive splenomegaly in sickle cell disease: a distinct clinicopathological entity in the Eastern province of Saudi Arabia. Am J Hematol. 2005;79(3):180–6.

58. Selcuk D, Demirel K, Kantarci F, Mihmanli I, Ogut G. Gamna-Gandy bodies: a sign of portal hypertension. Turk J Gastroenterol. 2005;16(3):150–2.

Index

© Springer Nature Switzerland AG 2020

L. Zhang et al. (eds.), *Diagnostic Pathology of Hematopoietic Disorders of Spleen and Liver*,

https://doi.org/10.1007/978-3-030-37708-3

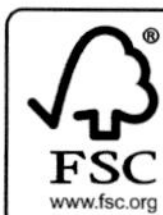

MIX
Papier aus verantwortungsvollen Quellen
Paper from responsible sources
FSC® C105338

If you have any concerns about our products,
you can contact us on
ProductSafety@springernature.com

In case Publisher is established outside the EU,
the EU authorized representative is:
Springer Nature Customer Service Center GmbH
Europaplatz 3, 69115 Heidelberg, Germany

Printed by Libri Plureos GmbH
in Hamburg, Germany